ADOLESCENT GYNECOLOGY AND ENDOCRINOLOGY: BASIC AND CLINICAL ASPECTS

ANNALS OF THE NEW YORK ACADEMY OF SCIENCES

Volume 816

ADOLESCENT GYNECOLOGY AND ENDOCRINOLOGY: BASIC AND CLINICAL ASPECTS

Edited by George Creatsas, George Mastorakos, and George P. Chrousos

The New York Academy of Sciences
New York, New York
1997

∞ *The paper used in this publication meets the minimum requirements of American National Standard for Information Sciences—Permanence of Paper for Printed Library Materials, ANSI Z39.48-1984.*

Cover art shows one of the six caryatids from the Erechtheum, a small temple on the Acropolis of Athens. The caryatids were draped figures of adolescent girls used instead of a column as an architectural support. The caryatids of the Erechtheum are the most famous example (450–415 B.C.). Caryatids are sometimes called "Canephorae" or "Korai" (maiden). Thus, a caryatid was chosen as an artistic representation of female adolescent beauty.

Library of Congress Cataloging-in-Publication Data

Adolescent gynecology and endocrinology : basic and clinical aspects / edited by George Creatsas, George Mastorakos, and George P. Chrousos.

p. cm. — (Annals of the New York Academy of Sciences : ISSN 0077-8923 v. 816)

Contains the proceedings of an international congress, held in Athens, Greece in the fall of 1995.

Includes bibliographical references and index.

ISBN 1-57331-038-7 (cloth : alk. paper). — ISBN 1-57331-039-5 (pbk. : alk. paper)

1. Adolescent gynecology—Congresses. 2. Pediatric endocrinology—Congresses. I. Creatsas, G. II. Mastorakos, George. III. Chrousos, George P. IV. Series.

[DNLM: 1. Genitalia, Female—physiology—congresses. 2. Endocrine Glands—physiology—congresses. 3. Endocrine Diseases—in adolescence—congresses. 4. Puberty—physiology—congresses. 5. Puberty—psychology—congresses. W1 AN626YL v.816 1997 / WS 360 A2394 1997]

[RJ478.A353 1997]

618'.083—dc21

DNLM/DLC

for Library of Congress 97-13702

CIP

&/PCP

Printed in the United States of America

ISBN 1-57331-038-7 (cloth)

ISBN 1-57331-039-5 (paper)

ISSN 0077-8923

ANNALS OF THE NEW YORK ACADEMY OF SCIENCES

Volume 816
June 17, 1997

ADOLESCENT GYNECOLOGY AND ENDOCRINOLOGY: BASIC AND CLINICAL ASPECTS[a]

Editors
GEORGE CREATSAS, GEORGE MASTORAKOS, AND GEORGE P. CHROUSOS

Conference Organizers
D. ARAVANTINOS, G. CREATSAS, E. DELIGEOROGLOU, N. GOUMALATSOS, E. HASSAN, G. KALLIPOLITIS, D. LOUTRADIS, A. MALAMITSI-PUCHNER, G. MASTORAKOS, AND N. SALAKOS

Advisory Board
M. BATRINOS, G. CHROUSOS, CH. COUTIFARIS, J. DEWHURST, A. R. GENAZZANI, G. MAROULIS, P. MCDONOUGH, S. MICHALAS, M. NEW, A. PSYCHOYOS, J. SANFILIPPO, AND G. TOLIS

CONTENTS

[a]This volume is the result of the Third International Congress, entitled **Update on Adolescent Gynecology–Endocrinology,** which was sponsored by the Hellenic Society of Pediatric and Adolescent Gynecology, Fédération Internationale de Gynécologie Infantile et Juvénile (International Federation of Pediatric and Adolescent Gynecology), and the National Institute of Child Health and Human Development and held on December 6 through 9, 1995, in Athens, Greece.

Part II. From Adolescence to Adulthood

Part III. Endometrium

Part IV. Menstrual Cycle

Part V. Disorders of the Ovarian Cycle

Part VI. Pubertal Endocrinological Disorders

Part VII. Endometriosis

Part VIII. Female Genital Tract Malignancies during Adolescence

Part IX. Gynecological Surgical Procedures during Adolescence

Part X. Genetic Disorders in Adolescence

Part XI. Adolescent Sexuality

Part XII. The Future in Contraception

Part XIII. The Reproductive Revolution

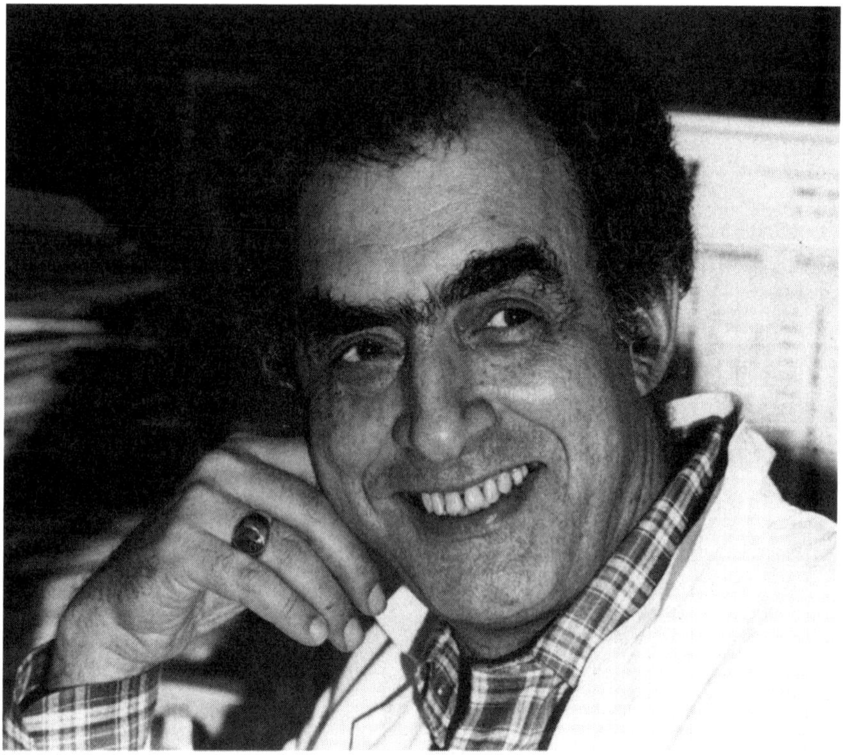

Alexander Psychoyos
May 15, 1927–October 18, 1995

A Tribute to the Work of Alexander Psychoyos

MARIE-CLAIRE LEBEAU

INSERM U 33, Bâtiment Gregory Pincus
80, rue du Général Leclerc
94276 Le Kremlin Bicêtre, France

Understanding the complex mechanism of egg implantation was the essential preoccupation of Aleko Psychoyos' professional life. He started to work on this subject in the late 50s, when, after completing his medical studies in Athens in 1954, he entered the Department of Experimental Morphology and Endocrinology at the Collège de France in Paris, which was directed by Professor Robert Courrier, a pioneer in the field of experimental endocrinology.

Aleko Psychoyos first developed a very useful biological test to determine the initiation of the implantation process: Evans blue, injected i.v. into rats, produced blue spots in the uterus at the nidation sites. He was then able to determine the hormonal control of uterine receptivity, with the definition of an optimal period (receptive phase) and a refractory period (nonreceptive phase) for egg implantation. This biphasic phenomenon is determined by a basic hormonal sequence, namely a minimum three-day period of uterine priming with progesterone, and a minute amount of estrogen superimposed at the end of this period. Although the data were first obtained in rats, later studies showed that this hormonal sequence is also valid for primates, and recent clinical studies have demonstrated the importance of this hormonal regimen for successful *in vitro* fertilization.

Since the 1960s, Aleko Psychoyos had studied ultrastructural changes of the rat luminal uterine epithelium under transmission electron microscopy (TEM) and had observed some bulbous cytoplasmic projections at the expected time of implantation. Pursuing these observations when scanning electron microscopy (SEM) became available, he was astonished to see that the walls of the uterine lumen were covered with a thick carpet of microvilli, like a sea floor, with here and there some sea-anemone-like formations, which appeared to correspond to the projections observed under TEM. He suggested that these peculiar protrusions, which were termed pinopodes (from the Greek πίνω = drink and πόδες = feet), were involved in the uptake of material released by the blastocyst. In fact, they were shown to mediate epithelial uptake of fluid (pinocytosis) and macromolecules (endocytosis). In rodents during the nidation window, there is a closure of the uterine lumen that could be attributed to the withdrawal of uterine fluid by the pinopodes, which are present precisely at that time. Having determined the progesterone dependence of pinopode formation, Aleko Psychoyos and his colleagues extended their observations to the human uterus and investigated the timing of the appearance of pinopodes on the luminal surface epithelium. They were able to define an implantation window, using pinopodes as markers of uterine receptivity. The results of these studies have been tested in clinical practice and have significantly improved the success rates in *in vitro* fertilization. In some cases, RU 486 could be used to displace the window, so that the uterus is at the optimal phase at the time of egg transfer (reviews in Refs. 1 and 2).

Intrigued by the alternation of receptive and nonreceptive phases of the uterus, Aleko Psyĉhoyos searched for the inhibitory, blastotoxic factor(s) that could be repsonsible for the nonreceptive phase, that is, the period when the uterine environment becomes hostile and when the survival of transferred embryos in the uterus becomes impossible. He and his colleagues isolated from rat or human flushings a small molecule that reached a maximum concentration at that period. This molecule, which has strong spermicidal and anti-viral properties, was later identified as cholic acid. Given its *in vitro* properties, cholic acid should be an efficient agent for use in barrier contraception and control of sexually transmitted diseases (STDs).[3] Aleko Psychoyos truly hoped that some day this discovery would give birth to a simple, safe, and inexpensive contraceptive device, which could be used in the control of world population and to curtail STDs, including AIDS.

Among his other interests were the phenomenon of delayed implantation, the localization of estrogen and progesterone receptors at the time of implantation in the rat and during the menstrual cycle in the baboon, as well as the role of prostaglandins in blastocyst implantation.

Aleko Psychoyos died suddenly on October 18, 1995. His friends and colleagues will keep the memory of his creative and original intelligence, his warm and generous personality, his love of life, and his unforgettable smile. He was always speaking about writing a book on implantation, but never managed to take the time to do it. It is now up to young researchers to continue to explore the complex mechanism of blastocyst implantation, which fascinated Aleko Psychoyos so much that he devoted his professional life to its study.

REFERENCES

1. PSYCHOYOS, A. 1973. Endocrine control of egg implanation. *In* Handbook of Physiology. Section 7, Endocrinology. Vol. II, Part 2. R. O. Greep & E. B. Astwood, Eds. 187–215. Williams and Wilkins. Baltimore.
2. PSYCHOYOS, A. 1995. Nidation window: From basic to clinic. *In* Molecular and Cellular Aspects of Periimplantation Processes. S. K. Dey, Ed. 1–14. Springer-Verlag. New York.
3. PSYCHOYOS, A., G. CREATSAS, E. HASSAN, V. GEORGOULAS & A. GRAVANIS 1993. Spermicidal and antiviral properties of cholic acid: Contraceptive efficacy of a new vaginal sponge (Protectaid®) containing sodium cholate. Hum. Reprod. **8:** 866–869.

Preface

During this century, marked social, cultural, ethical, and technological changes have taken place. The impact of these changes on the growth, development, health, and social status of women has been major. In addition, women's causes have gained a great deal of momentum and received international recognition. Childhood, puberty, and adolescence determine a great deal of an individual's adult behavior and health. Thus, understanding the physiological and psychological changes that take place during this period is crucial for intervening to prevent ills that afflict the adult society, all the way from health problems to dysfunctional family units to dysfunctional, valueless societies. The study of childhood and puberty/adolescence is multidisciplinary, and the fields of pediatric and adolescent gynecology and endocrinology serve primary roles.

This volume comprises the edited proceedings of an international congress, entitled Update on Adolescent Gynecology and Endocrinology, held in Athens, Greece, in the fall of 1995, under the auspices of the Hellenic Society for Pediatric and Adolescent Gynecology in collaboration with the Fédéracion Internationale de Gynécologie Infantile et Juvénile (International Federation of Infantile and Juvenile Gynecology), the National Institute of Child Health and Human Development, and the European Society of Contraception. Both basic and clinical information is presented, without neglecting the psychological and social behavior of teenaged girls. The first part covers gynecological and endocrinological physiology from childhood to adulthood, including novel information on the endometrium and the menstrual cycle. The second part deals with surgical procedures. The third and last part approaches the subjects of adolescent sexuality and reproduction in relation to recent trends in contraception. We hope that the biomedical community will increasingly focus its interest on this particularly vulnerable and important period in a woman's life.

George Creatsas
George Mastorakos
George P. Chrousos

The Future of Pediatric and Adolescent Gynecology

ALVIN F. GOLDFARB[a]

Professor of Obstetrics and Gynecology
Jefferson Medical College of Thomas Jefferson University
Philadelphia, Pennsylvania

INTRODUCTION

On May 10, 1967, volume 142 of the *Annals of the New York Academy of Sciences* was devoted to pediatric and adolescent gynecology. My good friend Warren R. Lang was consulting editor. In his preface he pointed out, "This volume represents the first major attempt to review attitudes, research, and progress in the field of pediatric and adolescent gynecology." In his opening remarks, the Director of Professional Affairs of Ortho Pharmaceutical Corporation, R. V. Chapple, M.D., wrote, "We are all aware of the folklore taboos that militate against adequate vaginal examination of little girls with unresponsive vaginal infections. And yet we realize, as scientifically trained persons, that these so-called simple infections may lead to future problems of infertility. In fact, their origin may be a congenital anomaly that demands investigation."

At the present moment in the United States, we do not do pelvic examinations or look at the genitalia of pediatric or adolescent patients unless they have a problem. As a matter of fact, it is state of the art, as of the date I am writing this, (July 15, 1996) that to examine an adolescent before her having had a sexual experience or without a gynecologic complaint is not acceptable before age 18. We are attempting to change that by having all young women by the age of 14 be seen for an educational and informational experience called a "well girl examination." Also, we are trying to make sure all pediatricians examine the external genitalia of their female patients at all ages. Have we made any progress? Anecdotally, it would appear not. In the 30 years since the first *Annals* on pediatric and adolescent gynecology was written, there have been tremendous changes in pediatric and adolescent gynecology. These changes are not only informational and scientific, but also therapeutic. What can we discuss with reference to the future of pediatric and adolescent gynecology?

In the period of time before the end of this millennium, I think that we have to talk about the patient, the environment, sexuality, nutrition, and problems of pain. This is where the future of pediatric and gynecology lies. Not in the surgical approach to the management of this patient, but to the behavioral and endocrinological approach to the management of this patient. In this volume, the major subsets are endocrinology and gynecology. My remarks will relate only to gynecologic problems. The first problem we have is our understanding of the patient. The informational age that we live in and the environmental changes have made today's patient different than her

[a]Address for correspondence: Alvin F. Goldfarb, M.D., North American Society for Pediatric and Adolescent Gynecology, 1015 Chestnut St., Ste. 1225, Philadelphia, PA 19107-4302.

counterpart in 1967. Today, most adolescents are influenced by media, violence, and sociologic factors all of which have an impact on their health.

With a change in attitude regarding sexuality, there has been an increase in teenage pregnancies and of sexually transmitted diseases in the adolescent. These have become major health care problems for the adolescent. These problems, along with contraceptive choices, represent a large portion of adolescent gynecologic care. It is interesting that in the United States the problems of adolescent premarital sexual activity have mainly been approached from an ethical and moral point of view, whereas in Europe, and the Nordic countries in particular, they have primarily been concerned about the health consequences of early sexual activity. Therefore, the approach to this problem has been different in the United States and Europe. As of today the Europeans have much better data regarding a reduction in teenage pregnancies than the United States.

Along with the increase in sexual activity, not only was there an increase in unintended pregnancies, there was also an increase in the number of persons who developed sexually transmitted diseases. The appearance of AIDS in the 1980s changed the focus of health promotion strategies. The problem of teenage pregnancies had been replaced by a truly complicated dilemma—HIV and other sexually transmitted diseases. We now had problems that allowed us to begin to think in terms of adolescent sexuality not only as a medical problem, but also as a problem involving mental and social health with long-term effects on the life of the adolescents and their newborns. I first used the concept of ambulatory reproductive health care in a paper that appeared in 1980 and was published in a text by Wallace and Gold in which we talked about ambulatory reproductive health services.

The second major problem that will affect the future of adolescent gynecology is the problem of nutrition. In the last two decades, eating disorders have become a worldwide problem. Many decades ago we talked about malnutrition: It was second to poverty. Now we talk about malnutrition that is self-induced. I refer to the anorectic and to the bulimic adolescent. In addition, as more and more pediatric and adolescent-aged women become involved in athletics and they begin to trim their weight and loose adipose tissue, we begin to see its effects on menstrual function, estrogen production, and an increased risk for the development of osteoporosis. The adolescent who feels that she is obese, even if she is not, develops psychosocial problems that lead to anorexia. These problems are usually found in persons who have low self-esteem and poor self-images. Each year many more young women develop anorexia to the point where their health is threatened, and many die as a result of this.

Another problem that impinges on the future of adolescent gynecologic health is violence. Violence, substance abuse, and unprotected sexual activity have a negative impact on the health of adolescent women. Teenagers today experience and witness a great deal of violence in their families and communities which puts them at risk for a number of health problems. These problems are not only emotional and psychological but also physical. There may be trauma to the genitalia that can influence the transmission of sexually transmitted diseases as well as future reproduction.

The last item that will influence the future of adolescent gynecology is the recognition and management of chronic pelvic pain. In evaluating an adolescent with chronic pelvic pain, it is important to recognize the varying somatic, physiological, and social factors that either alone or in combination may play a role in the pain syndrome. We have always been rather organic in our structuring of the evaluation and diagnosis of pelvic pain, but today we must understand that there is a biopsychosocial model of pain that must be understood and used in managing this problem. The causes of pelvic pain are not only gynecological, but may well be urologic, gastrointestinal, musculoskeletal, or psychosocial. The use of laparoscopic surgical instruments and newer diagnostic radiologic procedures improves our ability to diagnose and manage pelvic pain. Therefore, we as clinicians must be comfortable evaluating pelvic pain in a holistic manner.

If I can become Janus and look backwards to the 1960s, our interest in pediatric and adolescent gynecology was then based on our understanding of puberty and the reproductive endocrine changes during adolescence. Genetics was just becoming an area of interest, gynecologic cancer was a major concern, and we were more interested in the scientific aspects of the vagina, with reference to its biology and to its cytology. Today we talk about examining the patient, empowering the patient to participate in the decision-making process and evaluating in a more thorough fashion the biopsychosocial aspects of adolescent sexuality.

What about the future? In the information presented in this volume, we can foresee in the future the development of a philosophy for earlier examinations of the adolescent female, empowering the patient, and allowing her a greater role in the decision-making process concerning her health. During this examination, we would offer the patient improved informational services regarding her general health as well as her reproductive health. As physicians, we must improve our ability to listen and become more nonjudgmental in managing the general health and the gynecologic care of these patients.

The Future of Pediatric and Adolescent Endocrinology

GEORGE P. CHROUSOS

Pediatric Endocrinology Section
Developmental Endocrinology Branch
National Institute of Child Health and Human Development
National Institutes of Health
Bethesda, Maryland 20892

Traditionally, pediatric and adolescent endocrinology has encompassed the study of growth and development, including psychosexual differentiation and maturation, and of diseases of the endocrine system that occur during the "dynamic" periods of childhood and adolescence. The latter period, which was indistinguishable from that of puberty in earlier societies, is clearly distinct from it in the modern world. This is reflected in the use of the word "hebe" as synonymous to both "puberty" and "adolescence" in classic Greek.

Literally speaking, the latin roots of "puberty" and "adolescence" are, respectively, the words "*pubis-esce,*" meaning development of pubic hair and, hence, sexual maturation, and "*adult-esce*" or becoming a grown-up and, hence, a self-sustaining, financially and psychologically independent member of the adult society, who can raise and support his or her own family.[1] Whereas the duration of puberty, that is, the process of complete sexual maturation, is 4 or 5 years, the duration of adolescence in today's developed societies has been extended by an additional 5 to 10 years. Thus, the periods of puberty and adolescence, which include endocrine, somatic, psychological, and socioeconomic changes and are under the purview of pediatric endocrinology, are now characterized by a major disengagement, which is bound to interfere with the psychological and physical health of our youth.

The last 50 years have seen profound progress in pediatric and adolescent endocrinology. We have dramatically enhanced our understanding of the physiology and pathophysiology of the developing endocrine system; we have markedly improved our diagnostic capacity; and, we have immensely increased our therapeutic efficacy.[2] Also, during the past two decades, we have seen an enlargement of the scope of our field. This has been aided by the realization that there are "critical" periods within childhood and puberty/adolescence, during which psychological and physical vulnerabilities develop; several classic hormones appear to participate in this phenomenon. Also, the same period is characterized by the onset of life-long medical/psychological problems, which have a strong genetic predisposition; these include obesity, addictive behaviors, depression, eating disorders, insulin-dependent diabetes mellitus type I, and the severe forms of schizophrenia, referred to as hebephrenia from the above mentioned root *hebe.*[1] Finally, the vicious cycle of teenage pregnancy–poverty and unhappiness/development of vulnerabilities, which plagues a significant proportion of some modern societies, takes place in the population of patients that pediatricians and pediatric endocrinologists serve.

Recently, it has become apparent that a large number of common pathological conditions occur in parallel and in conjunction with each other and in varying combinations and degrees.[3–5] These states have a genetic vulnerability background, which is not simple Mendelian but polygenic and which allows expression of the clinical phenotype in the presence of triggers from the environment. These states include anxiety disorders, depression, alcohol and substance abuse, eating disorders, juvenile delinquency, personality and conduct disorders and several "psychosomatic" diseases, such as the various generalized or organ-specific chronic pain and/or fatigue syndromes. There is no question that there is a very complex genetic background continuum in the population of human beings, from extreme resilience to extreme vulnerability to the above "co-morbidity" states and that environmental triggers (stressors) of diminishing size would be required to cause expression of these conditions in an individual (FIG. 1**A**).

What appears to be of crucial importance is that the above environmental triggers or stressors have not a transient but a permanent effect on the organism, quite reminiscent of the "critical" effects of several hormones exerted on certain target tissues and lasting well after the exposure to the hormone has ceased. The prenatal and early life periods are particularly sensitive to these permanent effects of stressors and are, hence, critical periods, although sufficiently strong stressors may have permanent effects on the organism throughout the lifespan, as the existence of adult posttraumatic stress disorder suggests.[3] Nevertheless, it seems that the vulnerability of the subpopulation of human beings to developing one or more of the co-morbid states can be altered by exogenous triggers, with adverse stimuli shifting the entire bell-shaped curve of that subpopulation to the right, and with a propitious, supportive environment shifting the same curve to the left (FIG. 1**B**).

The above phenomenon appears to be mediated to some extent by two key hormones of the stress system and the hypothalamic–pituitary adrenal axis, corticotropin-releasing hormone (CRH) and the glucocorticoids.[3,6] Thus, presence of stressors in the prenatal or early postnatal life is associated with concurrent elevations of these and other hormones and alterations in the responsiveness of the stress system, which are permanent and, hence, present for the remaining life of the individual. Proper responsiveness of the stress system to stressors is a crucial prerequisite for sense of well-being, adequate performance of tasks, and positive social interactions. Improper responsiveness has been associated with inadequacies in the above functions and increased vulnerability to one or more of the co-morbid states. Thus, depending on the genetic background of the individual exposed to adverse stimuli in early life, one might develop any of the co-morbid states in any combination and degree of severity.

The above concepts of genetic vulnerability and permanent alterations of this vulnerability by exogenous stimuli at critical periods of life aided by hormones of the stress system have been amply demonstrated in convincing rodent and nonhuman primate studies.[3,7–9] Human data appear to agree with the experimental animal studies. An excellent example comes from the study of sexually abused preadolescent girls, who, when studied at least 2 years after the last episode of abuse took place, had changes of their hypothalamic–pituitary–adrenal axis similar to previously characterized changes observed in adult patients with melancholic depression.[10] Interestingly, all young patients studied had mood disorders ranging from dysthymia to de-

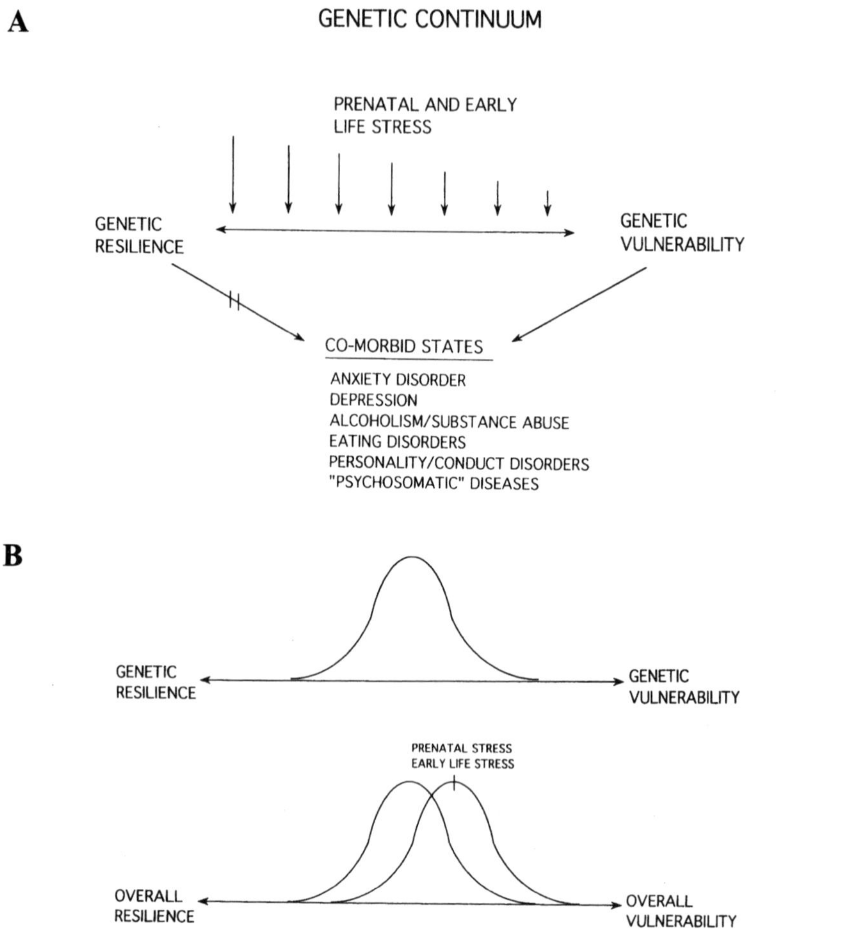

FIGURE 1. (**A**) The genetic continuum defining background resiliency–vulnerability to develop one or more common states of major epidemiologic and societal impact. The vertical arrows indicate the size of environmental stressors necessary to produce a morbid state. (**B**) Shift in vulnerability of a subpopulation affected by an environmental stressor.

pression at the time of the study. In concordance with these data, there has recently been an epidemiologic association of history of sexual abuse in patients with a psychosomatic disorder and of history of "stressful life events" in patients with melancholic depression.[11,12] The adverse environmental stimuli in both conditions took place most frequently during the periods of childhood and puberty/adolescence.

The importance of this information in understanding some of the evils plaguing human societies are obvious. Poverty and lack of education lead to prenatal and early life stress with many adverse consequences, including the production of physically,

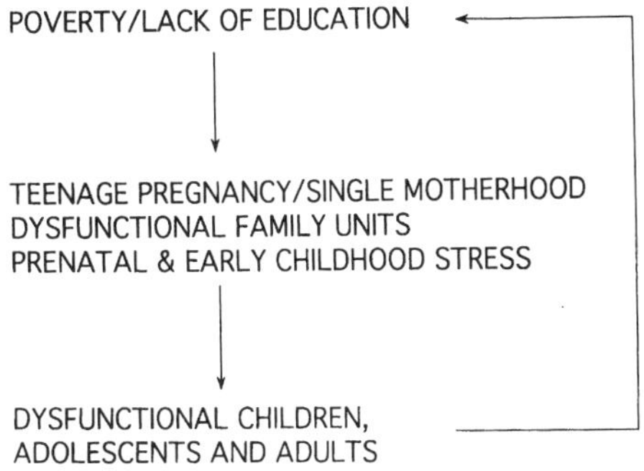

FIGURE 2. The vicious cycle plaguing a significant subpopulation of human societies.

psychologically, and socially dysfunctional individuals, who are bound to serve as links of a perpetual vicious cycle through continuing poverty, lack of education, teenage pregnancy, and fetal and child abuse and neglect (FIG. 2).

The next 50 years are expected to be a period of rapid growth and conquest for pediatric and adolescent endocrinology. The monogenic disorders will be fully understood at a molecular level, new sensitive and accurate diagnosis methods will be developed, and novel preventive and fully curative pharmacotherapies and, hopefully, gene therapies will be developed for these disorders. The polygenic disorders will also be unraveled, the principal responsible genes, and I expect a finite number of such genes, will be defined, and we will be able to estimate the vulnerability risks of individuals, which will allow us to take the necessary preventive or therapeutic measures to prevent or cure. These disorders include not only the co-morbid states, but also insulin-dependent diabetes mellitus and endocrine malignancies, some of which are devastating and incurable at the present time. Finally, a major challenge would be to extricate our young patients from the vicious cycle of poverty, lack of education, early life stress, and dysfunctional teenage and adult behaviors. The intervention will hopefully be at many levels of this cycle, and our role will be to study these phenomena, educate the patients and the state, and act preventively and therapeutically whenever we can. Although the task of breaking this vicious cycle appears daunting at the present time, there is no doubt that knowledgeable, multifaceted, and coordinated activity can result in its elimination. The input of medicine and its allied fields for accomplishing this worthy goal is pivotal.

REFERENCES

1. DORN, L. D. & G. P. CHROUSOS. 1993. The endocrinology of stress and stress system disorders in adolescence. *In* Adolescent Endocrinology. R. Rosenfield, Ed. Endocrinol. Metab. Clinics N. Am. **22:** 685–700.
2. CHROUSOS, G. P. 1996. Organization and integration of the endocrine system. *In* Pediatric Endocrinology. M. Sperling, Ed.: pp. 1–14. W.B. Saunders. Philadelphia, PA.
3. CHROUSOS, G. P. & P. W. GOLD. 1992. The concepts of stress and stress system disorders: Overview of physical and behavioral homeostasis. JAMA **267:** 1244–1252.

4. Kendler, K. S., E. E. Walters, M. C. Neals, R. C. Kessler, A. C. Heath & L. J. Eaves. 1995. The structure of the genetic and environmental risk factors for six major psychiatric disorders in women. Arch. Gen. Psychiatry **52:** 374–383.
5. Kendler, K. S., L. J. Eaves, E. E. Walters, M. C. Neals, A. C. Heath & R. C. Kessler. 1996. The identification and validation of distinct depressive syndromes in a population-based sample of female twins. Arch. Gen. Psychiatry **53:** 391–399.
6. Piazza, P. V., V. Deroche, J. Deminière, S. Maccari, M. Le Moal & H. Simon. 1993. Corticosterone in the range of stress-induced levels possesses reinforcing properties: Implications for sensation-seeking behaviors. Proc. Natl. Acad. Sci. USA **90:** 11738–11742.
7. Johnson, E. O., T. C. Kamilaris, A. E. Calogero, P. W. Gold & G. P. Chrousos. 1996. Effects of early parenting on growth and development in a small primate. Ped. Res. **39:** 999–1005.
8. Johnson, E. O., T. C. Kamilaris, C. S. Carter, A. E. Calogero, P. W. Gold & G. P. Chrousos. 1996. The biobehavioral consequences of psychogenic stress in a small, social primate (*Callithrix jacchus jacchus*). Biol. Psychiatry **40:** 317–337.
9. Coplan, J. D., M. W. Andrews, L. A. Rosenblum, M. J. Owens, S. Friedman, J. M. Gorman & C. B. Nemeroff. 1996. Persistent elevations of cerebrospinal fluid concentrations of corticotropin-releasing factor in adult nonhuman primates exposed to early-life stressors: Implications for the pathophysiology of mood and anxiety disorders. Proc. Natl. Acad. Sci. USA **93:** 1619–1623.
10. DeBellis, M., G. P. Chrousos, L. Dorn, L. Burke, K. Helmers, M. A. Kling, P. K. Trickett & F. W. Putnam. 1994. Hypothalamic–pituitary–adrenal axis dysregulation in sexually abused girls. J. Clin. Endocrinol. Metab. **78:** 249–255.
11. Scarinci, I. C., J. MacDonald-Haile, L. A. Bradley & J. E. Richter. 1994. Altered pain perception and psychosocial features among women with gastrointestinal disorders and history of abuse: A preliminary model. Am. J. Med. **97:** 108–118.
12. Kendler, K. S., R. C. Kessler, E. E. Walters, C. J. MacLean, P. C. Sham, M. C. Neale, A. C. Heath & L. J. Eaves. 1995. Stressful life events, genetic liability and onset of an episode of depression in women. Am. J. Psychiatry **152:** 833–842.

Development of the Hypothalamic–Pituitary–Ovarian Axis

DAN APTER[a]

Department of Obstetrics & Gynecology
Helsinki University
00290 Helsinki, Finland

INTRODUCTION

The basic clock mechanism that turns on the process of puberty is still largely unknown, although it seems to be a centrally driven process affecting the gonadotropin releasing hormone (GnRH) pulse generator.[1] Based on lesions including various parts of the central nervous system (CNS), both removal of inhibition and activatory pathways can be involved in the pubertal activation of the GnRH pulse generator.[2] The GnRH neuronal network has by itself an intrinsic pulsatile activity.[3] Advances in the basic understanding of neuronal regulation of puberty have recently been summarized.[4,5] This review will focus on data obtained by sensitive new techniques on hormonal events in females concerning hypothalamic–pituitary–ovarian interaction during infancy, childhood, and puberty.

INFANCY

The hypothalamic–pituitary axis becomes functionally active with gonadotropin secretion under GnRH control during the second trimester of pregnancy.[1] The negative feedback of steroids is operative towards term, causing a decrease of gonadotropin secretion. With removal of placental steroids, gonadotropin secretion is again activated, with serum LH concentrations in girls up to 1 IU/l but in boys even up to 10 IU/l during the first 4 months.[6] Serum FSH is much higher in girls than in boys, with concentrations even exceeding adult values at this age. The high gonadotropin concentrations cause gonadal activation with increased steroid secretion especially in boys[7] but also in girls.[7,8] The biological significance of this early hypothalamic–pituitary–gonadal activation is not known. After 4 to 6 months of age, gonadotropin and steroid concentrations decrease to very low levels by 1 to 2 years of age.[1,6,7]

CHILDHOOD

New, very sensitive immunofluorometric (IFMA; Delfia®, Wallac, Turku, Finland)[9–12] and immunochemiluminometric[6,13] assays have for the first time permitted

[a]Address for correspondence; Dan Apter, Finnish Student Health Service, 00260 Helsinki, Finland. Fax + 350-9-4050 500; Telephone +358-9-4050 740.

accurate measurements of gonadotropin concentrations during the midchildhood nadir lasting from about 1 to 9 years of age in girls. The sensitivity of these assays is about 50- to100-fold that of traditional radioimmunoassay. Random daytime LH concentrations seem to be below 0.15 IU/l with mean concentrations of 0.04 IU/l in girls at this age.[6,9] Compared to LH, prepubertal girls have relatively high FSH concentrations with a range of 0.3 to 2.0 IU/l and a mean about 1 IU/l.[9]

In the same way that a 100-fold increase in sensitivity of LH measurements is changing our conception of gonadotropin secretion, a similar improvement in estradiol measurements by a recombinant cell bioassay changes the perception of prepubertal estradiol secretion. With this unique assay, mean serum estradiol concentration was found to be 2.2 pmol/l in prepubertal girls, which is lower than reported earlier, but much higher than the level of 0.3 pmol/l found in prepubertal boys.[14] This finding implies that the ovaries of midchildhood girls significantly secrete estradiol.

During childhood, continous follicular growth and atresia occur in the ovaries. The first observations were based on autopsy materials,[15,16] and recently ultrasonography has confirmed the findings.[17–20] The very early follicular development to the stage of antrum formation (approximately 0.25-mm diameter) is regarded to be independent of gonadotrophic stimulation.[21] Antrum formation and further growth to the stage at which follicles become potentially able to begin preovulatory development (2–5 mm diameter) is considered to require stimulation by FSH. In midchildhood, follicles up to 5 mm in diameter are seen. From 7 to 10 years of age, the number of follicles exceeding 5 mm in diameter increases significantly.[20] The size of the largest visible follicle expressed in millimeters corresponds to the age in years; for example, 9-year-old girls may display 9-mm follicles. Before the onset of puberty, blood concentrations of FSH do not rise sufficiently to sustain development beyond this stage; therefore, all antral follicles become atresic. However, even in the 7- to 9-year-old prepubertal girls, ovarian volume correlates significantly with FSH concentrations.[20] It remains to be examined with the new sensitive estradiol assay, whether the follicular growth seen at this age is indeed reflected in changes in serum estradiol levels.

The hypothalamic–pituitary unit is under peripheral feedback regulation. Gonadally produced sex steroids and peptide hormones cause a diminution of hypothalamic GnRH release and a decrease of pituitary gonadotropin secretion. This feedback system is operative and very sensitive in prepubertal children,[1] although the main constraint is of central CNS origin. Clinically important is the observation that girls with precocious puberty due to autonomous ovarian function in the McCune–Albright syndrome may have FSH concentrations clearly below the prepubertal normal range.[22] The fact that lacking normal negative feedback effect of prepubertal gonads results in increased secretion of especially FSH is evident in studies of hypogonadal children.[23] In all six hypogonadal boys studied,[24] the mean FSH level was above the range of the normal prepubertal boys, whereas the LH level was elevated in only one boy. All boys had LH and FSH pulses.[24] As the normal range of gonadotropins in prepubertal girls has been better defined, patients with Turner syndrome seem to have increased pulsatile FSH levels (Apter and Dunkel, manuscript in preparation). Some of the prepubertal girls with Turner syndrome have high FSH, others only marginally elevated, as presumably also the degree of ovarian insufficiency varies.

LH and FSH are secreted in discrete bursts separated by intervals without secretory activity. During childhood, normal gonadotropin secretion involved episodic fluctuations in a sleep-entrained diurnal rhythm as revealed by studies using sensitive enough assays. It is not a period of complete quiescence, as earlier radioimmunoassay (RIA)-based results mainly indicated.

In one study observing LH and FSH pulses in mid-childhood, blood samples were withdrawn at 20-min intervals from 2000 to 0800 in 16 boys and 6 girls 4 to 8 years of age.[12] Comparisons of immunoradiometric assays and IFMA results were made. Pulses were detectable only with IFMA at very low concentrations, but a good correlation was seen at higher levels. As measured by IFMA, a mean of 2 pulses per 12 hr in both sexes for both hormones were seen with a close temporal association between sleep onset and the appearance of nocturnal pulsatile gonadotropin secretion. The mean LH concentration of 0.19 in girls was not different from that of 0.10 IU/l in boys, whereas girls had much higher FSH concentrations than boys (1.95 versus 0.46). No maturational changes in gonadotropin patterns with chronological age or bone age were seen. Thus the occurrence of nocturnal low amplitude, low frequency pulsatile gonadotropin secretion does not indicate that puberty is imminent, but is typical of midchildhood.

We have conducted studies to further define the prepubertal restraint and neuroendocrine activation of pulsatile LH and FSH secretion. Blood samples were collected for 24 hours with 10-minute intervals in 10 prepubertal, 7 early pubertal, and 23 postmenarcheal, healthy, normal girls 7 to 18 years ot age. GnRH pulse generator activity was evaluated by the use of a GnRH-antagonist, and pituitary sensitivity was assessed by responses to GnRH stimulation.[25] Measurements were performed with the Delfia system. A pulsatile pattern of LH and FSH secretion was observed in girls of all ages. Prepubertal girls had irregular LH pulses with very low amplitude during day-time, but LH and FSH pulses with increased amplitude were evident within one hour after onset of sleep (FIG. 1**A**). Older prepubertal girls (FIG. 1**B**) had more regular and higher amplitude pulses throughout sleep than younger prepubertal girls. The sleep-related LH and FSH pulses in the prepubertal girls were abolished with Nal-Glu GnRH antagonist treatment (FIG. 1 **A B**, *right panels*), indicating that these pulses are GnRH dependent.

An increase in LH and especially FSH concentrations anticipated the onset of puberty, as prepubertal girls within about half a year of the beginning of breast developmcnt had higher gonadotropin concentrations during both sleep and wake periods than those who had a longer time before the appearance of breast stage II.[25] No differences were seen in steroid, growth hormone, and IGF-I concentrations. Thus FSH concentrations in prepubertal subjects may give information about how close the onset of physical puberty is. Reference values and timing of blood sampling must be time-specific in prepubertal patients, as FSH concentrations decrease continuously during the day only to be interrupted by the sleep-related rise (FIG. 1**A** and **B**, *left panels*).

PUBERTY

Puberty involves the reactivation of the GnRH pulse generator, the removal of CNS restraint. It is initiated independent of gonadal activity, as it occurs in patients

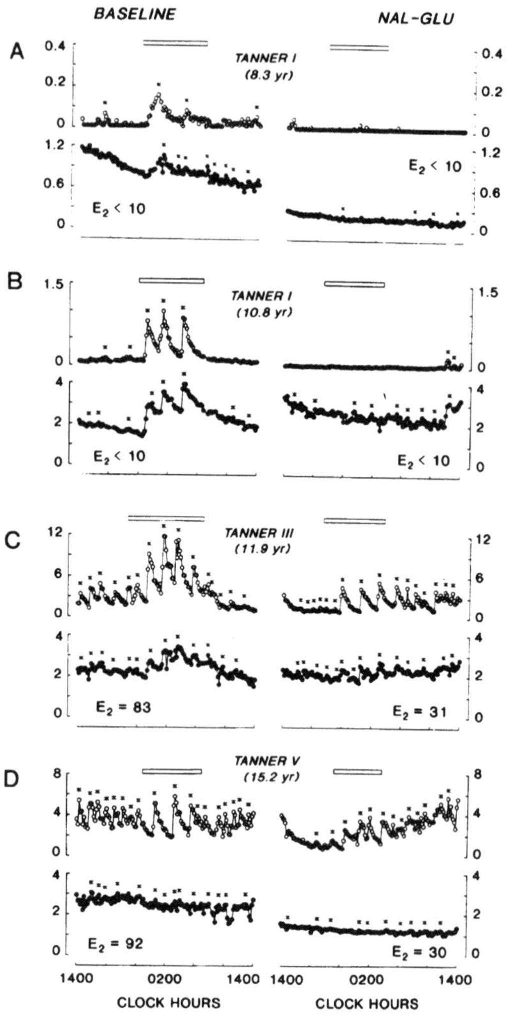

FIGURE 1. Representative plots of serum LH (*open circles, upper panels*) and FSH (*closed circles, lower panels*) concentrations during 24-hr baseline studies and during Nal-Glu GnRH antagonist treatment in four girls of different development. Note the change of scales. Significant pulses are marked with *. E_2 concentrations are in pmol/l. Sleep is marked with a bar. (From Apter *et al.*[25]; used with permission.)

with gonadal dysgenesis,[26,27] and puberty can be activated by exogenous pulses of GnRH in infantile monkeys[28] and in girls with delayed puberty.[29] Further, prepubertal monkeys can be stimulated to release GnRH and gonadotropins, when stimulated with an excitatory amino acid, *N*-methyl-D-aspartate.[30,31] This confirms the potential for adult levels of GnRH production during prepubertal years, identifying the hypothalamus, pituitary, and gonads as components of the system that are capable of operating at any time.[1]

With the onset of puberty, a very steep increase occurs, especially in daytime LH concentrations.[25] Mean wake-time LH increased 60-fold from prepubertal to early pubertal girls (TABLE 1). Pulses were seen at regular frequence throughout daytime (FIG. 1**C**). Even using single samples, serum LH concentrations exceeded 0.2 IU/l in all subjects in breast stage at least II,[6,9] with no or very minimal overlapping with stage I subjects. Further, a 10-fold difference was found in mean LH concentrations between breast stage I and II subjects within the same chronological age.[9]

The emergence of regular daytime LH pulses was closely related to increases in serum androstenedione, testosterone, and estradiol concentrations (FIG. 2). Daytime LH levels exceeding approximately 0.5 IU/l seem to be associated with a measurable increase in ovarian steroid production.[25] Similar conclusions about a threshold of LH concentrations needed for sustained ovarian androgen and estrogen production have been derived based on ovulation induction with human recombinant FSH in patients with hypogonadotropic hypogonadism or GnRH agonist suppression.[32,33]

The ovaries have a typical multifollicular appearance by ultrasonography in early puberty.[18–20,34] They are full of 5- to 12-mm follicles, but have scanty stroma, which distinguish this pattern from polycystic ovaries. The increasing steroid concentrations in turn induce the appearance of secondary sexual characteristics.

In early puberty, the sleep-entrained amplification of LH pulses is very marked

TABLE 1. Wake and Sleep LH and FSH Pulse Characteristics in Three Stages of Peripubertal Girls

		Group (No.)					
		Prepuberty (10)		Early Puberty (7)		After Menarche (23)	
		Wake	Sleep	Wake	Sleep	Wake	Sleep
LH							
Amplitude (IU/l)	Mean	0.06*	0.36	1.89**c***	4.08**c**	1.94***	3.69
	SE	0.01	0.08	0.53	0.87	0.18	0.34
Pulse Number/8 hr	Mean	0.68***	2.28	3.91**c**	4.30**b**	5.75**c*****	3.84
	SE	0.26	0.32	0.60	0.45	0.23	0.30
Transverse Mean (IU/l)	Mean	0.04**	0.20	2.51**c***	4.69**c**	3.61	3.5
	SE	0.01	0.05	0.71	1.21	0.23	0.25
	Range	0.0–0.1	0.0–0.4	0.4–5.1	0.5–8.9	2.3–5.9	1.2–5.6
FSH							
Transverse Mean (IU/l)	Mean	1.04*	1.66	3.20**c**	3.42**c**	3.97**a**	3.93
	SE	0.15	0.32	0.43	0.38	0.15	0.17
	Range	0.5–2.0	0.5–3.1	2.0–5.0	1.8–4.7	2.2–5.3	2.0–5.4

NOTE: **a** = $p < 0.05$, **b** = $p < 0.01$, and **c** = $p < 0.001$, compared to the preceding group of same wake or sleep state (Fisher post-hoc testing). Wake–sleep comparisons within the groups are marked with *, **, and ***, denoting $p < 0.05$, $p < 0.01$, and $p < 0.001$, respectively. Sleep includes the time from sleep onset to sleep offset of about 7–9 hr, wake time the rest of the 24-hr period. Modified from Apter *et al.*[25]

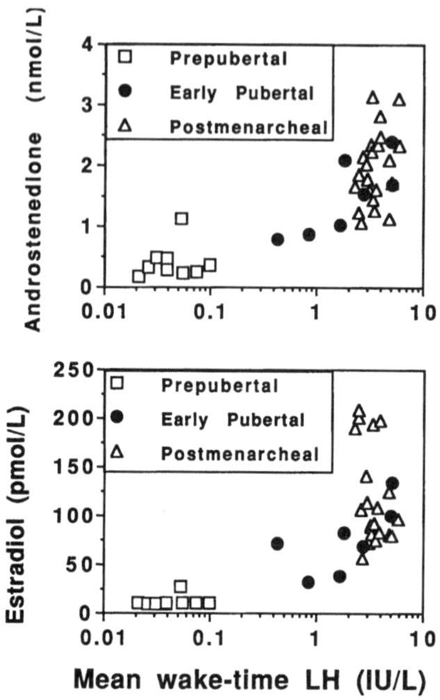

FIGURE 2. Androstenedione and estradiol concentrations in relation to mean wake–time LH levels in individual subjects (r = 0.81 and 0.62, respectively, $p < 0.0001$). The difference between prepubertal and early pubertal girls is evident, with no overlap in LH. (From Apter *et al.*[25]; used with permission.)

(FIG. 1**C**), although the greatest ratio between sleep and wake time concentrations are found in prepubertal subjects (TABLE 1). The sleep amplification is gradually reduced with age. Based on regression analysis of mean sleep/wake LH concentrations on age in our 7- to 18-year-old group, it was estimated that after 15.7 years of age LH concentrations during sleep are lower than during wake time, as seen in adult females in the early follicular phase.[35] An example of this adult pattern is seen in FIG. 1**D**, with the typical sleep-related slowing of pulse frequence.

The ontogeny of LH rise during pubertal development was mainly related to an increase of the pulse amplitude (ninefold), and to a lesser extent due to an increase in the number of pulses (fourfold),[25] a finding confirming the reports of Wennink *et al.*[36] and Dunkel *et al.*[37] The physiological effects of the changes in amplitude and frequence are difficult to differentiate. Mean 24-hr LH increased 40-fold from the prepubertal to the postmenarcheal group, and this incremental change occurred primarily during wake-time with an 80-fold increase as compared to 20-fold during sleep. The difference between the highest individual mean wake-time LH in the prepubertal group and the lowest in the early pubertal group (TABLE 1) was greater than the corresponding difference during sleep-time. Thus, daytime LH measurements seem to be more reflective of pubertal stage than sleep-time values.

Urinary LH and FSH measurements with immunofluorometric assays reveal a very similar pattern with age as serum measurements, and might be clinically more practical.[38]

The time course of LH and FSH release in response to an i.v. bolus of 10-μg GnRH was not different in the prepubertal, early pubertal, and postmenarcheal groups.[25] Maximal LH concentrations occurred at 20 to 30 minutes and maximal FSH concentrations at 30 to 40 minutes. In the prepubertal group, the FSH response was much greater than the LH response, whereas in the pubertal and postmenarcheal groups, the LH response was greater than that of FSH.[25] The magnitude of LH response to GnRH in this study is quite different from earlier results obtained by RIA. Of the three groups studied, the prepubertal group displayed the largest relative LH increase, more than 100-fold (FIG. 3**B**, *left lower panel*). The early pubertal group had the largest absolute LH increase (FIG. 3**A**, *left upper panel*). The prepubertal group also had the greatest FSH response both in relative and in absolute increase (FIG. 3, *right panels*), as previously observed with RIA.[39] A 7.9-year-old girl with the

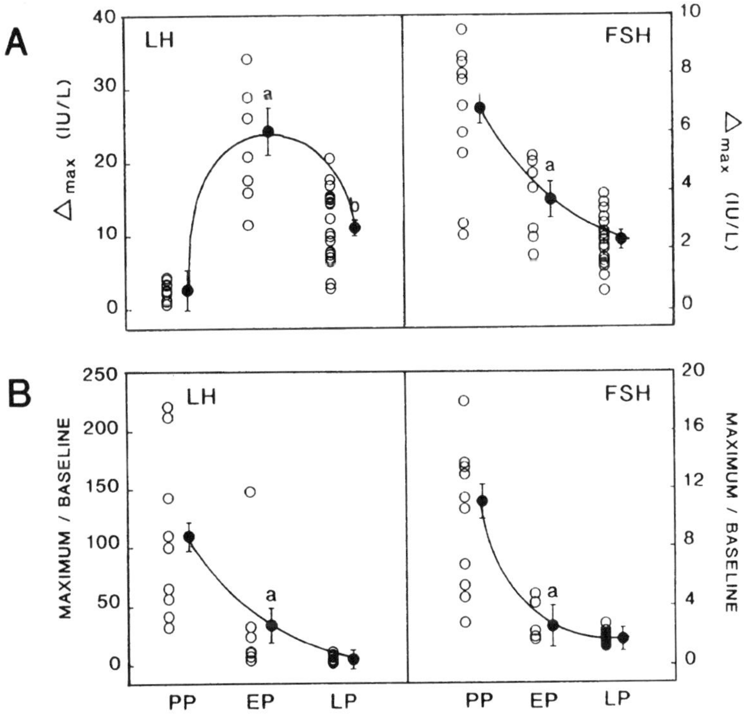

FIGURE 3. LH and FSH maximal absolute increase from baseline (*upper panels*) and maximal relative increase (*lower panels*) in response to 10 μg GnRH in three groups of girls. PP denotes prepubertal, EP early pubertal, and LP postmenarcheal subjects. The *open circles* represent individual values: the *closed circles* mean ± SE for each group; **a** denotes $p < 0.05$ and **b** $p < 0.01$ compared to the preceding group. (From Apter *et al.*[25]; used with permission.)

lowest mean LH and FSH concentrations clearly had the highest FSH response of all subjects. Thus, the prepubertal pituitary is highly sensitive to GnRH stimulation. This remarkably high pituitary sensitivity to GnRH stimulation in the face of relatively low levels of gonadotropin secretion may reflect infrequency and smaller amplitude of GnRH secretion, which provides priming action without inducing functional release.[25]

The disparity between patterns of LH and FSH secretion in different age groups is evident. The most striking difference was found in the prepubertal group, where FSH mean levels were 10- to 20-fold those of LH.[25] FSH/LH ratio decreased to about one in postmenarcheal subjects. A likely explanation for the differential regulation of FSH and LH is the gonadal feedback effect.[40] Before ovarian activation, FSH secretion appears to be more highly GnRH dependent than after pubertal onset when estradiol and inhibin may exert their modulatory influence.[40] This is indicated by a greater FSH response to GnRH stimulation and to Nal-Glu GnRH antagonist suppression (73% versus 30%) in the prepubertal than in the other two groups.[25] The suppression of LH with Nal-Glu GnRH antagonist (70%), on the other hand, was similar in all three groups. These responses are remarkably different from those found in adults for FSH but similar to adult women for LH.[41] Thus, profound changes in the hypothalamic–pituitary–ovarian interaction occur.

An interesting new finding by Aittomäki *et al.*[42] suggests that FSH may have a more fundamental role in ovarian development than was earlier thought. Hypergonadotropic ovarian dysgenesis with normal karyotype is relatively common in Finland with an estimated incidence of 1 in 8300 females. Patients with primary amenorrhea frequently have streak ovaries or hypoplastic ovaries. In several of these patients, hereditary XX pure gonadal dysgenesis was demonstrated to be caused by a mutation of the FSH receptor gene in the extracellular ligand-binding domain.[42] Thus, FSH seems to have a pivotal role in the development of the ovary into a mature, cycling, and hormonally active organ.

MENSTRUAL CYCLICITY

Estrogen and androgen concentrations oscillate with increasing magnitude as puberty progresses.[43,44] Under the stimulation of gonadotropins, increasing follicular maturation takes place. Androgens are produced by the first-maturing follicles and thecal tissue. At a certain critical androgen/estrogen concentration, the development of the follicles is arrested,[45] they undergo atresia, and steroid production decreases.[46] By midpuberty, there is sufficient estrogen priming of the endometrium, followed by withdrawal, to result in the first menstrual bleeding. The first menstrual cycles are usually anovulatory. Under the influence of increasing GnRH and estrogens, the pituitary develops the ability to respond with a surge of LH after estrogen stimulation. The development of this positive feedback loop requires that the sensitivity of the negative feedback system has decreased enough to allow GnRH and gonadotropin levels to increase rather than fall as estradiol concentrations are rising. Eventually, a follicle under FSH stimulation escapes the critical microenvironmental leading to atresia and produces sufficient estradiol to elicit the preovulatory gonadotropin surge.

The establishment of regular ovulatory menstrual cycle takes a surprisingly long time. The length of the menstrual cycle is rather long and variable during the first years after menarche.[47,48] Based on basal body temperature measurements, Döring[49] estimated that the percentage of complete menstrual cycles was 16% in 15- to 17-year-old girls, and a maximal proportion of normal cycles was not observed before the age of 26 to 30 years. With repeated serum progesterone measurements, we found 15% of the cycles to be ovulatory during the first year after menarche, 41% during the third, and 74% during the sixth year (TABLE 2[50–52]). Similar results have also been obtained with urinary pregnanediol[53] and salivary progesterone[54,55] measurements.

Even when ovulation takes place, the first luteal phases are frequently deficient. They are of short duration, and the progesterone concentration is low.[56] When 15- to-16-year-old adolescents were compared to 25- to 35-year-old adult women with frequent sampling during one ovulatory menstrual cycle,[57] it was found that the early follicular FSH increase occurred significantly later in the adolescent group. Adults had peak FSH concentrations by cycle day 4, whereas the "early follicular phase" peak occurred on day 10 in adolescents. This was followed by a slower increase both in serum estradiol concentration and in follicular growth (TABLE 3), with ovulation occurring later and from a smaller follicle in the adolescent group, followed by lower progesterone concentrations in the luteal phase.

The lability of the hypothalamic–pituitary–ovarian axis in adolescence is reflected in the frequent occurrence of menstrual cycle disturbances. These are described in other papers. Even a minor form of stress such as a journey or examination period may cause temporary amenorrhea. This is especially seen in lean subjects. Obese girls frequently have hyperandrogenic oligomenorrhea. Metabolic factors affect the hypothalamic–pituitary–ovarian axis at all levels. We need more information about who will later have a normal development, and what signs might indicate future reproductive dysfunction.

TABLE 2. Development of Ovulatory Cycles in Relation to Time since Menarche

Years since Menarche	Number of Cycles	% Ovulatory Cycles[a]
0.0–0.9	34	15
1.0–1.9	41	34
2.0–2.9	41	41
3.0–3.9	33	58
4.0–4.9	37	70
5.0–5.9	20	74
8.0–12	33	85
12–18	28	96

[a]Ovulatory cycle = serum progesterone > 6.4 nmol/l (>2.0 ng/ml, 10 × follicular mean) in specimens drawn on days 20–23 and/or later in the cycle. Data combined from longitudinal follow-up.[50,51,52]

TABLE 3. Characteristics of Ovulatory Menstrual Cycles in 15- to 16-Year-Old Adolescents ($n = 8$) and 25- to 35-Year-Old Adult Women ($n = 12$).

	Cycle Day			
Estradiol (nmol/l)	10	14	Immediate Preovulatory	Maximal Luteal Progesterone
Adolescents	0.15 ± 0.02*	0.51 ± 0.14*	0.94 ± 0.09*	29 ± 4.3*
Adults	0.37 ± 0.05	1.18 ± 0.18	1.37 ± 0.16	44 ± 4.1
Diameter of Largest Follicle (mm)				Day of Ovulation
Adolescents	7.5 ± 0.6**	12.3 ± 1.1***	17.5 ± 0.8*	19.0 ± 0.7***
Adults	12.0 ± 07	19.6 ± 0.8	20.2 ± 0.7	14.0 ± 0.4

NOTE: Significance of difference between adolescents and adults is marked with *, **, and ***, denoting $p < 0.05$, $p < 0.01$, and $p < 0.001$, respectively. (From Apter *et al.*[57]; used with permission.)

SUMMARY

The onset of puberty is a centrally driven process, the detailed mechanisms of which are not known. It is translated into an increased activity of the hypothalamic GnRH pulse generator. This in turn is seen as increased pituitary pulsatile secretion of LH and FSH. LH pulses are observed even in midchildhood, particularly after the onset of sleep. Onset of puberty is associated with a greater increase in LH pulse amplitude than frequency and a much greater increase in LH and FSH. A progressive increase in daytime pulsatility occurs, with a gradual reduction of sleep-entrained amplification. Prepubertal FSH concentrations are relatively high in girls, and continous ovarian follicular growth and atresia take place, with estradiol concentrations being higher than in boys. Only after the steep early pubertal increase in LH, ovarian steroidogenesis is activated, with increases in androgen and estrogen secretion. Under further FSH stimulation, follicular growth and maturation proceed. The first menstrual cycles are mostly anovulatory for 1 to 2 years. Luteal phase insufficiency is common the first five years after menarche.

REFERENCES

1. GRUMBACH, M. M. & D. M. STYNE. 1992. Puberty: Ontogeny, neuroendocrinology, physiology and disorders. *In* Williams' Textbook of Endocrinology. J. D. Wilson & D. W. Foster, Eds.: 1139–1221. 8th edit. WB Saunders. Philadelphia.
2. SIEGEL-WITCHEL, S. 1995. CNS lesions, neurological disorders, and puberty in man. *In* The Neurobiology of Puberty. T. M. Plant & P. A. Lee, Eds.: 229–239. Journal of Endocrinology Ltd. Bristol.
3. GOLDSMITH, P. C. & K. K. THIND. 1995. Morphological basis for neuronal control of GnRH secretion in the monkey. *In* The Neurobiology of Puberty. T. M. Plant & P. A. Lee, Eds.: 73–85. Journal of Endocrinology Ltd. Bristol.
4. BOURGUIGNON, J. P., A. GERARD, M. L. ALVAREZ GONZALEZ, G. PURNELLE & P. FRANCHI-

MONT. 1995. The role of excitatory amino acids in triggering the onset of puberty. *In* The Neurobiology of Puberty. T. M. Plant & P. A. Lee, Eds.: 129–138. Journal of Endocrinology Ltd. Bristol.
5. PLANT, T. M. 1995. Fourth international conference on the control of the onset of puberty. *In* The Neurobiology of Puberty. T. M. Plant & P. A. Lee, Eds.: 337–342. Journal of Endocrinology Ltd. Bristol.
6. NEELY, E. K., R. L. HINTZ, D. M. WILSON, P. L. LEE, T. GAUTIER, *et al.* 1995. Normal ranges for immunochemiluminometric gonadotropin assays. J. Pediatr. **127:** 40–46.
7. WINTER, J. S., I. A. HUGHES, F. I. REYES & C. FAIMAN. 1976. Pituitary-gonadal relations in infancy: 2. Patterns of serum gonadal steroid concentrations in man from birth to two years of age. J. Clin. Endocrinol. Metab. **42:** 679–686.
8. BIDLINGMAIER, F., M. WAGNER-BARNACK, O. BUTENANDT & D. KNORR.1973. Plasma estrogens in childhood and puberty under physiologic and pathologic conditions. Pediatr. Res. **7:** 901–907.
9. APTER, D., B. CACCIATORE, H. ALFTHAN & U.-H. STENMAN. 1989. Serum luteinizing hormone concentrations increase 100-fold in females from 7 years of age to adulthood, as measured by time-resolved immunofluorometric assay. J. Clin. Endocrinol. Metab. **68:** 53–57.
10. DUNKEL, L., H. ALFTHAN, U.-H. STENMAN, P. TAPANAINEN & J. PERHEENTUPA. 1990. Pulsatile secretion of LH and FSH in prepubertal and early pubertal boys revealed by ultrasensitive time-resolved immunofluorometric assays. Pediatr. Res. **27:** 215–219.
11. GOJI, K. & S. TANIKAZE. 1992. Comparison between spontaneous gonadotropin concentration profiles and gonadotropin response to low-dose gonadotropin-releasing hormone in prepubertal and early pubertal boys and patients with hypogonadotropic hypogonadism: Assessment by using ultrasensitive, time-resolved immunofluorometric assay. Pediatr. Res. **31:** 535–539.
12. WU, F. C. W., G. E. BUTLER, C. J. H. KELNAR, H. F. STIRLING & I. HUHTANIEMI. 1991. Patterns of pulsatile luteinizing hormone and follicle stimulating hormone secretion in prepubertal (midchildhood) boys and girls and patients with idiopathic hypogonadotropic hypogonadism (Kallmann's syndrome): A study using an ultrasensitive time-resolved immunofluorometric assay. J. Clin. Endocrinol. Metab. **72:** 1229–1237.
13. PANDIAN, M. R., W. D. ODELL, E. CARLTON & D. A. FISHER. 1993. Development of third-generation immunochemiluminometric assays for follitropin and lutropin and clinical applicationin determining pediatric reference ranges. Clin. Chem. **39:** 1815–1819.
14. KLEIN, K. O., BARON, M. J. COLLI, D. P. MCDONNELL & G. B. CUTLER, JR. 1994. Estrogen levels in childhood determined by an ultrasensitive recombinant cell bioassay. J. Clin. Invest. **94:** 2475–2480.
15. SAURAMO, H. 1954. Histology and function of the ovary from the embryonic period to the fertile age. Acta Obstet. Gynecol. Scand. **33:** 3–25.
16. PETERS, H., R. HIMELSTEIN-BRAW & M. FABER 1976. The normal development of the ovary in childhood. Acta Endocrinol. **82:** 617–630.
17. STANHOPE, R., J. ADAMS, H. S. JACOBS & C. G. D. BROOK. 1985. Ovarian ultrasound assessment in normal children, idiopathic precocious puberty and during low dose pulsatile gonadotropin releasing hormone treatment of hypogonadotropic hypogonadism. Arch. Dis. Child. **60:** 116–119.
18. GIORLANDINO, C., N. GLEICHER, C. TARAMANNI, A. VIZZONE, P. GENTILI *et al.* 1989. Ovarian development of the female child and adolescent. I. Morphology. Int. J. Gynecol. Obstet. **29:** 57–63.
19. WINER-MURAM, H., D. EMERSON, D. MURAM & T. BOULDEN. 1989. The sonographic features of the peripubertal ovaries. Adolesc. Pediatr. Gynecol. **2:** 160–163.
20. CACCIATORE, B., D. APTER, H. ALFTHAN & U.-H. STENMAN. 1991. Ultrasonic characteristics of the uterus and ovaries in relation to pubertal development and serum LH, FSH and estradiol concentrations Adolesc. Pediatr. Gynecol. **4:** 15–20.

21. Hillier, S. G. 1994. Current concepts of the roles of follicle stimulating hormone and luteinizing hormone in folliculogenesis. Hum. Reprod. **9:** 188–191.
22. Apter, D. 1993. Ultrasensitive new immunoassays for gonadotropins in the evaluation of puberty. Curr. Opin. Pediatr. **5:** 481–487.
23. Winter, J. S. D. & C. Faiman. 1972. Serum gonadotropin levels in agonadal children and adults. J. Clin. Endocrinol. Metab. **35:** 561–564.
24. Dunkel, L., H. Alfthan, U. H. Stenman & J. Perheentupa. 1990. Gonadal control of pulsatile secretion of luteinizing hormone and follicle-stimulating hormone in prepubertal boys evaluated by ultrasensitive time-resolved immunofluorometric assays. J. Clin. Endocrinol. Metab. **70:** 107–114.
25. Apter, D., T. L. Bützow, G. A. Laughlin & S. S. C. Yen. 1993. GnRH pulse generator activity during pubertal transition in girls: Pulsatile and diurnal patterns of circulating gonadotropins. J. Clin. Endocrinol. Metab. **76:** 940–949.
26. Conte, F. A., M. M. Grumbach & S. L. Kaplan. 1975. A diphasic pattern of gonadotropin secretion in patients with the syndrome of gonadal dysgenesis. J. Clin. Endocrinol. Metab. **40:** 670–674.
27. Ross, J. L., D. L. Loriux & G. B. Cutler. 1983. Developmental changes in neuroendocrine regulation of gonadotropin secretion in gonadal dysgenesis. J. Clin. Endocrinol. Metab. **57:** 288–293.
28. Wildt, L., G. R. Marshall & E. Knobil. 1980. Experimental induction of puberty in the female rhesus monkey. Science **207:** 1373–1375.
29. Stanhope, R., C. G. D. Brook, P. P. J., J. Adams & H. S. Jacobs. 1987. Induction of puberty by pulsatile gonadotropin releasing hormone. Lancet **2:** 552–555.
30. Medhamurthy, R., H. L. Dichek, T. M. Plant, I. Bernardini & G. B. Cutler, Jr. 1990. Stimulation of gonadotropin secretion in prepubertal monkeys after hypothalamic excitation with aspartate and glutamate. J. Clin. Endocrinol. Metab. **71:** 1390–1392.
31. Brann, D. W. & V. B. Mahesh. 1994. Excitatory amino acids: Function and significance in reproduction and neuroendocrine regulation. Front. Neuroendocrinol. **15:** 3–49.
32. Devroey, P., B. Mannaerts, J. Smitz, B. H. Coelingh & S. A. Van. 1994. Clinical outcome of a pilot efficacy study on recombinant human follicle-stimulating hormone (Org 32489) combined with various gonadotrophin-releasing hormone agonist regimens. Hum. Reprod. **9:** 1064–1069.
33. Schoot, B. C. 1995. Exogenous Follicle-Stimulating Hormone and Development of Ovarian Follicles. The Parthenon Publishing Group. Pearl River, N.Y.
34. Holm, K., E. Mosfeldt Laursen, V. Brocks & J. Müller. 1995. Pubertal maturation of the internal genitalia: An ultrasound evaluation of 166 healthy girls. Ultrasound Obstet. Gynecol. **6:** 175–181.
35. Kapen, S., R. Boyar, L. Hellman & E. D. Weitzman. 1976. The relationship of luteinizing hormone secretion to sleep in women during the early follicular phase: Effects of sleep reversal and a prolonged three-hour sleep–wake schedule. J. Clin. Endocrinol. Metab. **42:** 1031–1040.
36. Wennink, J. M., H. A. Delemarre-van de Waal, R. Schoemaker, H. Schoemaker & J. Schoemaker. 1990. Luteinizing hormone and follicle stimulating hormone secretion patterns in girls throughout puberty measured using highly sensitive immunoradiometric assays. Clin. Endocrinol. Oxf. **33:** 333–344.
37. Dunkel, L., H. Alfthan, U.-H. Stenman, G. Selstam, S. Rosberg & K. Albertsson-Wikland. 1992. Developmental changes in 24-hour profiles of luteinizing hormone and follicle-stimulating hormone from prepuberty to midstages of puberty in boys. J. Clin. Endocrinol. Metab. **74:** 890–897.
38. Demir, A., L. Dunkel, U. H. Stenman & R. Voutilainen. 1995. Age-related course of urinary gonadotropins in children. J. Clin. Endocrinol. Metab. **80:** 1457–1460.

39. DICKERMAN, Z., R. PRAGER-LEWIN & Z. LARON. 1976. Response of plasma LH and FSH to synthetic LH-RH in children at various pubertal stages. Am. J. Dis. Child. **130:** 634–638.
40. YEN, S. S. C. 1991. The human menstrual cycle: Neuroendocrine regulation. *In* Reproductive Endocrinology. S. S. C. Yen & R. B. Jaffe, Eds.: 273–308. Third edit. W. B. Saunders. Philadelphia.
41. MORTOLA, J. F., M. SATHANANDAN, S. PAVLOOU, K. D. DAHL, A. J. W. HSUEH, *et al.* 1995. Suppression of bioactive and immunoreactive follicle-stimulating hormone and luteinizing hormone levels by a potent gonadotropin-releasing hormone antagonist: Pharmacodynamic studies. Fertil. Steril. **51:** 957–963.
42. AITTOMÄKI, K., J. L. D. LUCENA, P. PAKARINEN, P. SISTONEN, J. TAPANAINEN *et al.* 1995. Mutation in the follicle-stimulating hormone receptor gene causes hereditary hypergonadotropic ovarian failure. Cell **82:** 959–968.
43. WINTER, J. S. D. & C. FAIMAN. 1973. The development of cyclic pituitary–gonadal function in adolescent females. J. Clin. Endocrinol. Metab. **37:** 714–718.
44. PENNY, R., A. F. PARLOW, N. O. OLAMBIWONNU & S. D. FRASIER. 1977. Evolution of the menstrual pattern of gonadotropin and sex steroid concentrations in serum. Acta Endocrinol. **84:** 729–737.
45. MCNATTY, K. P., D. M. SMITH, A. MAKRIS, R. OSATHANONDH & K. J. RYAN. 1979. The microenvironment of the human antral follicle: Interrelationships among the steroid levels in antral fluid, the population of granulosa cells, and the status of the oocyte in vivo and in vitro. J. Clin. Endocrinol. Metab. **49:** 851–860.
46. VIHKO, R. & D. APTER. 1980. The role of androgens in adolescent cycles. J. Steroid Biochem. **12:** 369–373.
47. TRELOAR, A. E., R. E. BOYNTON, B. G. BEHN & B. W. BROWN.1967. Variation of the human menstrual cycle through reproductive life. Int. J. Fertil. **12:** 77–126.
48. WIDHOLM, O. & R.-L. KANTERO. 1971. Menstrual patterns of adolescent girls according to chronological and gynelogical ages. Acta Obstet. Gynaecol. Scand. **14(Suppl.):** 19–29.
49. DÖRING, G. K. 1969. The incidence of anovular cycles in women. J. Reprod. Fertil. Suppl. **6:** 77–81.
50. APTER, D. 1980. Serum steroids and pituitary hormones in female pubert: A partly longitudinal study. Clin. Endocrinol. **12:** 107–120.
51. APTER, D. & R. VIHKO. 1985. Hormonal patterns of the first menstrual cycles. *In* Adolescence in Females. S. Venturoli, C. Flamigni & J. R. Givens, Eds.: 215–238. Year Book Medical Publishers. Inc. Chicago.
52. APTER, D. & R. VIHKO. 1990. Endocrine determinants of fertility: Serum androgen concentrations during follow-up of adolescents into the third decade of life. J. Clin. Endocrinol. Metab. **71:** 970–974.
53. METCALF, M. G., D. S. SKIDMORE, G. F. LOWRY & J. A. MACKENZIE. 1983. Incidence of ovulation in the years after the menarche. J. Endocrinol. **97:** 213–219.
54. READ, G., D. WILSON, I. HUGHES & K. GRIFFITHS. 1984. The use of salivary progesterone assays in the assessment of ovarian function in postmenarcheal girls. J. Endocrinol. **102:** 265–268.
55. VUORENTO, T. & I. HUHTANIEMI. 1992. Daily levels of salivary progesterone during menstrual cycle in adolescent girls. Fertil. Steril. **58:** 685–690.
56. APTER, D., L. VIINIKKA & R. VIHKO. 1978. Hormonal pattern of adolescent menstrual cycles. J. Clin. Endocrinol. Metab. **47:** 944–954.
57. APTER, D., I. RÄISÄNEN, P. YLÖSTALO & R. VIHKO. 1987. Follicular growth in relation to serum hormonal patterns in adolescent compared to adult menstrual cycles. Fertil. Steril. **47:** 82–88.

Ovarian Aging

GEORGE B. MAROULIS

Division of Reproductive Endocrinology & Fertility
Department of Obstetrics and Gynecology
University of South Florida College of Medicine
4 Columbia Drive, #529
Tampa, Florida 33606

Aging is a process occurring with advancing age, and it influences all biological systems. The human ovary and, as a consequence, the woman's reproductive potential starts showing aging-related changes from the age of 30 years.[1] The ovary has two main functions: (1) The production and release of oocytes and (2) the secretion of steroid hormones, that is, estrogens, progestins, and androgens. The ovarian hormones' role in reproduction is primarily through their effect on the endometrium and implantation, although they also significantly influence the skeletal, cardiovascular, and nervous systems. After menopause the ovary primarily produces androgens.

Premenopausal ovarian aging is characterized by (1) Changes in the quality and quantity of oocytes released and (2) changes in the hormonal production of the preovulatory follicle as reflected by estradiol levels and the post-ovulatory corpus luteum as reflected by the lenght of the luteal phase and the serum levels of progesterone.

The decline of ovarian function and its reserve with age is progressive and subtle. More specifically, these age-related changes pertain to the oocyte reservoir, the quality of oocytes, and the ovarian responsiveness to gonadotropin stimulation.

Oocyte depletion is an ongoing process from birth until a few years after menopause. During fetal life, as many as seven million oocytes are present in a female's ovaries; by birth this number has been reduced to two million, and at menarche 300,000 remain. It is estimated that no more than about 400 oocytes are actually released throughout a womans reproductive life.[2,3] It is hypothesized that human ovarian follicles are composed of two populations: nongrowing follicles and the early growing follicles. In younger women depletion of the nongrowing follicles enter the pool in an accelerated fashion. The mechanisms that accelerate the entrance of the nongrowing follicles into a growth stage may depend on the increasing level of FSH levels observed with increasing age.[4]

Oocyte depletion, as far as is currently known, cannot be arrested or delayed. However, data from women taking oral contraceptives suggest that menopause in these women may be slightly delayed.[5] Factors that may accelerate oocyte depletion are familiar predisposition, radiation therapy, chemotherapeutic agents, infection, galactosemia, smoking and the presence of mumps, oophoritis, and autoimmune diseases.

Existing data also suggest that oocyte aging may affect the nucleus possibly leading to defective nuclear development or chromosomal aberrations.[6,7] In fact, a number of studies suggest that advanced maternal age increases the rate of aneuploidy in oocytes.[8,9] The change in the quality of the oocytes with advancing age may be the reason for the observed increase of fetal chromosomal anomalies with increasing age.

However, these chromosomal anomalies, including Down's syndrome, may be a consequence of the decreased number of oocytes in the pool rather than the effect of age perse.[10] The possible relation of fetal anomalies to the dwindling oocyte number is suggested by animal data, which show that unilateral ovariectomy in mice led to an increase of fetal aneuploidy with maternal age.[11] This increase of congenital defects due to oocyte disturbances may be even more significant considering that a relationship between Down's syndrome and Alzheimer's disease has been recently described.[7] This relationship has only been reported in children who have this chromosomal defect.[12]

In older women, oocytes are fertilized, but the resulting conceptuses have a decreased implantation rate. The reason for this decreased implantation rate is not clear, but may be related to decreased embryo quality and not to the quality of the uterine environment.

The probability that oocyte aging is the key to the decreased implantation rate in older women is demonstrated by the increase of the implantation rates when embryos developing from oocytes obtained from younger women are implanted in older women.[13] Another possible reason for the decreased implantation rate has been proposed by Cohen, who has postulated it is due to an impairment of hatching of embryos of older women.[14]

These age-related changes of ovarian function may affect hormonal levels and menstrual cyclicity, particularly after the age of 40. The menstrual cycles usually become shorter and irregular as early as nine and as late as one to two years before the onset of menopause. This shortening of the follicular phase is associated with a decrease in the serum estradiol level and a shortening of the menstrual cycle length. The serum FSH level slightly increases with age while the LH remains unchanged. Following the LH surge the serum progesterone level and the length of the luteal phase usually also remain unchanged.[15] However, in one study aging was associated with an increased incidence of a short luteal phase, while in another study the progesterone levels were decreased in most of the women, suggestive of inadequate corpus luteum function.[16,17]

The observed age-related decrease of ovarian function is associated with a decrease in ovarian responsiveness and decreased fertility potential. Although ovarian reserve generally decreases with age, a wide variation is observed among women. There are two markers for this decline of ovarian responsiveness and fecundability potential: a rise of the early follicular phase (day 2 to 3) serum FSH level and a decrease of inhibin, a polypeptide hormone secreted by the granulosa cells.[18,19] FSH stimulates follicular production of estradiol and inhibin. With increasing age, there is a decrease in follicular inhibin production that precedes the decrease of follicular estradiol and is therefore the earliest sign of ovarian aging and the most probable cause for the rise of serum FSH.[20]

The rise of the follicular phase serum FSH with advancing age is correlated with decreased reproductive potential, a decrease in the number and the quality of oocytes, and a decreased implantation rate. Indeed when cycle day 3 serum FSH exceeds the level of 15 mIU/ml, implantation and fertility rates decrease.[21] A level of serum FSH between 15 and 25 mIU/ml is associated with a further reduction in fertility, whereas a level over 25 mIU/ml is usually associated with zero pregnancy rate. It should be pointed out, however, that the decreased oocyte quality that is observed with increasing age can be seen even if the FSH levels are normal.[21] For this reason, two tests have been proposed to further identify individuals with poor ovarian reserve; the clomiphene citrate challenge test (CCCT) and the GnRH analog stimulation test.[22,23]

The CCCT is based on the premise that, although in response to the clomiphene the serum FSH level is supposed to rise, women with normal ovarian reserve produce enough estrogen and inhibin to keep serum FSH levels within the normal range. After an intake of 100 milligrams of clomiphene citrate from day 5 to day 9 serum FSH level is measured on day 10. With aging, less inhibin is secreted per follicle, thus leading to less suppression of serum FSH which then rises above 20 mIU/ml (Leeco). This decrease in the production of inhibin reflects a decreasing ovarian reserve, which accellerates with age so that 3% of patients had such a response below the age of 30, 7% at 30–34, 10% at 35–39, and 26% at age 40 and above.[22] The GnRH agonist stimulation test is designed to stimulate ovarian function. According to this test, on cycle day 2, leuprolide acetate (1.0 mg/ml) is given, and the estradiol measurement is obtained 24 hours later. An increase in the estradiol production following GnRHa is associated with increasing pregnancy rates so that a change of E_2 of less than 10 picograms per ml is associated with a pregnancy rate of less than 5%, while a change of more than 100 picograms per ml is associated with a pregnancy rate of 35%.[23] These two tests seem to enhance the predictability of ovarian response, but it should again be mentioned that age, even in the presence of a normal test, is a determining factor, so that these tests of ovarian responsiveness should be evaluated within the framework of each age group.

All these changes in ovarian function due to age are not clearly understood. It is not clear whether it is the decreasing number of follicles or the follicular milieu or the age that are responsible for the change of the menstrual cycle pattern and the ovarian function. Possible changes of the vascularity of the ovaries may play a role in ovarian aging. In a study by Gonzalez, ovaries from postmenopausal women were compared with those of women during their earlier reproductive years, and it was found that in postmenopausal ovaries the arteries, the veins, and the arterioles have a lumen diminution up to 88.5% and 94.2% had a thickened wall, which may support the hypothesis that vascular aging including thickening of the blood vessels and diminished lumen may lead to a decreased blood supply and change in the function of the ovaries.[24] Further studies of ovarian blood supply are needed to confirm these findings. A recent study using Doppler ultrasound found that the impendance (resistance index) of the ovarian artery progressively increased from 5 to 10 years after menopause, suggesting a progressive decrease of blood flow with age.[25]

The change of the quality of oocytes with age as well as the associated changes in the embryos may be the most significant cause for the increase of spontaneous abortions observed with increasing age.[27] This further decreases the overall potential for fertility in older women. Studies from normal populations have shown that the incidence of spontaneous abortions in women over the age of 40 is approximately 30%, but it is likely that this is underestimating the actual incidence rate since many early abortions are not recognized. Indeed, in longitudinal studies as many as 60% of conceptions detected by the rising β-hCG abort within the first 12 weeks of pregnancy.[1] Results from the pregnancies of normal fertile women as well as those who became pregnant following IVF, GIFT, or AID show that compared with an abortion rate of 7–15% in women between the ages of 20 and 29, women 40 years of age or older have an abortion rate that exceeds that of 40%.[1] The increase in abortion rate observed with age is observed in both chromosomally normal and abnormal conceptuses. The increase in abortions of chromosomally normal conceptuses suggests that factors other than gross chromosomal abnormalities influence embryo survival or that possibly the endometrial environment may be influenced by age. The increase in chromosomal abnormalities is primarily due to trisomies, which suggests a loss of oocyte integrity with advancing age.[8] Cytogenetic studies of abortuses show that more than 50% of the abortuses are chromosomally abnormal.[26] Most are aneuploid, 17% are triploid, and some are structural rearrangements, mosaics, sex chromosome trisomies, and autosomal monosomies. A recent study by a group at Cornell who did pre-implantation biopsies showed an increase in chromosomal abnormalities of embryos of women over the age of 40.[27]

POSTMENOPAUSAL OVARIES

The postmenopausal ovary is active but only functions as a hormone-producing and not an oocyte-releasing organ. Following menopause there is obviously a lack of follicular development, and consequently estrogen and progesterone production are nonexistent. The primary source, therefore, of hormonal production in postmenopausal ovaries is the stroma and their cells, which still produce a significant amount of testosterone and androstenedione. The conversion of this androgen precursor contributes to the small amount of estrogen circulating in the blood of postmenopausal women.[28]

REFERENCES

1. MAROULIS, G. B. 1991. Effect of aging on fertility and pregnancy. Sem. Reprod. Endocrinol. **9:**165.
2. BLOCK, E. 1952. Quantitative morphological investigations of follicular system in women. Variations at different ages. Acta. Anat. **14:** 1088–1123.
3. BAKER, T. G. 1963. A quantitative and cytological study of germ cells of human ovaries. Proc. R. Soc. London. (Biol.) **158:** 417–433.
4. GOUGON, A., R. ECHOLARD & C. PHALABARD. 1994. Age related changes of the population of human ovarian follicles; Increase in the disappearance rate of non-growing and early growing follicles in aging women. Biol. Reprod. **50:** 653–663.
5. VANKEEP, P. A., P. C. BRAND & P. HEHERT. 1979. Factors affecting the age at menopause. J. Biosoc. Sci. (Suppl.) **6:** 37–55.
6. KEEFE, D. L., T. NIVEN-FAIRCHILD, S. POWER & S. BURADAGUNTA. 1995. Mitochondrial deoxyribonucleic acid deletions in oocytes and reproductive aging in women. Fertil. Steril. **64:** 577.
7. FINCH, C. E. 1994. The evolution of ovarian oocyte decline with aging and possible relationships to Down Syndrome and Alzheimer's disease. Exp. Gerontol. **29:** 299.
8. MACAS, E., E. FLOERSHEIM, E. HOTZ, *et al.* 1990. Abnormal chromosomal arrangements in human oocytes. Hum Reprod. **5:** 703.
9. PLANCHOT, M. J. DEGROUCHY, A. M. JUNCA, *et al.* 1988. Chromosomal analysis of human oocytes and embryos in an in-vitro fertilization program. Am. N. T. Acad. Scien. **541:** 384–397.

10. KLINE, J. & B. LEVIN. 1992. Trisomy and age at menopause predicted association given a link with rate of oocyte atresia. Pediatr. Perinat. Epidemiol. **6:** 225–239.
11. BROOK, J., G. GROSDEN & A. C. CHANDLEY. 1984. Maternal aging and aneuploid embryos: Evidence for the mouse that biological and not chronological age is the important influence. Hum. Genet. **66:** 41–45.
12. FARRER, L. A., LA. CUPLES, L. CONNER & P. A. WOLF, *et al.* 1993. ASSOCIATION OF DECREASED PATERNAL AGE AND LATE ONSET OF ALZHEIMER'S DISEASE: AN EXAMPLE OF GENETIC IMPRINTING. ARCH. NEUROL. **48:** 599–604.
13. SAUER, M. V., R. J. PAULSON, B. A. ARY & A. LOBO. 1994. Three hundred cycles of oocyte donation at the University of Southern California assessing the effect of age and infertility diagnosis on pregnancy and implantation rates. J. Asst. Reprod. Genet. **11:** 92–96.
14. COHEN, J., M. ALIKANI, J. TROWBRIDGE & Z. ROSENWAKS. 1992. Implantation enhancement by selective assisted hatching using zona drilling of human embryos with poor prognosis. Hum. Reprod. **7:** 685–691.
15. SHERMAN, B. M. & S. G. KOREMAN. 1975. Hormonal characteristics of the human menstrual cycle throughout reproductive life. J. Clin Investig. **55:** 699-706.
16. LENTON, E. A. & B. M. LANDGREN. 1985. The normal menstrual cycle. *In* clinical Reproductive Endocrinology. Spearman, Churchill Livingston. R. P. Ed.: 92–93. London.
17. REYES, F., J. WINTER & L. FAIMAN. 1977. Pituitary–ovarian relationships preceding the menopause. Am. J. Obstet. Gynecol. **129:** 557.
18. LENTON, E. A., L. SEXTON, S. LEE & I. D. COOKE. 1988. Progressive changes in LH/FSH ration in women throughout reproductive life. Maturitas **10:** 35–43.
19. PELLICER, A., M. MARI & M. DELOSSANTOS, *et al.* 1994. Effect of aging of the human ovary: The secretion of immunoreactive l-inhibin and progesterone. Fertil. Steril. **61:** 663.
20. BUCKLER, H. M., C. A. EVANS & H. MAMTORA, *et al.* 1991. Gonadotropin steroid and inhibin levels in women with incipient ovarian failure during anovulatory and ovulatory rebound cycles. J. Clin. Endocrinol. Metab. **72:** 116–124.
21. SCOTT, R. D., J. P. TONER & S. I. MUASHER. 1989. Follicle-stimulating hormone levels on cycle day 3 are predictive of in-vitro fertilization outcome. Fertil. Steril. **51:** 651.
22. SCOTT, R. T., M. R. LEONARDI & G. E. HOFFMAN, *et al.* 1993. A prospective evaluation of clomiphene citrate challenge test screening to the general infertility population. Obstet. Gynecol.**82:** 539–544.
23. WINSLOW, K. L., J. P. TONER, R. G. BRESKI, A. C. OEHNINGER, A. A. ACOSTA & S. J. MUASHER. 1991. The gonadotropin-releasing hormone agonist stimulation test: A sensitive predictor of performance in the flare-up in-vitro fertilization cycle. Fertil. Steril. **56:** 711–717.
24. GONZALEZ, O. V., N. L. MARTINEZ, G. RODRIQUEZ & J. ANCER. 1992. Pattern of vascular aging of the post-menopausal ovary. Ginecol. Obstet. Mexico. **60:** 1–3.
25. KURJAK, A. & S. KUPESIC. 1995. Ovarian senescence and its significance on uterine and ovarian perfusion. Fertil. Steril. **64:** 352.
26. EIBEN, B., S. BORGMANN, I. SCHUBBE & I. HANSMANN. 1987. Cytogenetic study directly from chorionic villi of 140 spontaneous abortions. Hum. Genet. **77:** 137–141.
27. MICHAELI, G., M. FELJGI, Y. GHETLER, I. BENNUM, Y. BEYTH & A. AMIEL. 1990. Chromosomal analysis of unfertilized oocytes and morphologically abnormal pre-implantation embryos from an in-vitro fertilization program. JIVF ET **7:** 341.
28. ADASHI, E. T. 1991. The climacteric ovary: A viable endocrine organ. Sem. Reprod. Endocrinol. **9:** 200.

Autocrine–Paracrine Role of Ovarian Corticotropin-Releasing Hormone

GEORGE MASTORAKOS,[a,b,c] LUCIA GHIZZONI,[d]
ELIZABETH L. WEBSTER,[c] AND GEORGE P. CHROUSOS[c]

[b]*Endocrine Unit*
Evgenidion Hospital
Athens University
11528, Athens, Greece

[c]*DEB/National Institute of Child Health and Human Development*
National Institutes of Health
Bethesda, Maryland 20892

[d]*Department of Pediatrics*
University of Parma
43100 Parma, Italy

Corticotropin-releasing hormone (CRH), the principal neuropeptide regulator of pituitary ACTH secretion, is also produced at several peripheral locations, such as inflammatory sites and the Leydig cell of the testis. We demonstrated immunoreactive (Ir) CRH in the cytoplasm of thecal and luteinized stromal cells and in cells within the corpora lutea in the ovaries of adult Sprague-Dawley rats, at all phases of the estrous cycle; and we identified, characterized, and localized CRH receptors in rat ovarian theca and stroma. We detected no CRH binding sites in the ovaries of prepubertal rats. We found immunoreactive CRH in normal human ovaries with a distribution similar to that of rat ovarian IrCRH, with no IrCRH present in oocytes of primordial follicles. Human ovaries from women with polycystic ovary syndrome (PCOS) also had IrCRH in their theca; however, IrCRH was less prominent in the stroma or the sparsely present corpora lutea, whereas it was detected in oocytes of primordial follicles. Low but detectable levels of IrCRH were measured in human follicular fluid samples collected from women undergoing *in vitro* fertilization. The mobility of rat and human ovarian IrCRH was similar to that of rat/human CRH-(1-41) by reversed-phase HPLC. To examine the potential role of ovarian CRH on granulosa–lutein cell steroidogenesis, we obtained follicular aspirates of seven patients undergoing *in vitro* fertilization and incubated these cells with increasing concentrations of CRH (10^{-9}–10^{-6} M). Estradiol and progesterone production by these cells was inhibited by CRH. We conclude that ovarian CRH may play a regulatory role in one or more of the various functions of the ovary, and this includes inhibition of female sex steroid production by this organ. There are differences in the location and levels of CRH in ovaries from women with PCOS when compared to ovaries from normal women.

[a]Address for correspondence: Dr. George Mastorakos, Evgenidion Hospital, Endocrine Unit, Athens University, Papadiamantopoulou 20, 11528 Athens, Greece.

INTRODUCTION

CRH, a 41-amino-acid neuropeptide secreted by the paraventricular nucleus of the hypothalamus, is a principal regulator of ACTH secretion. It was named for its property of stimulating anterior pituitary secretion of adrenocorticotropin hormone (ACTH).[1–3] Later, CRH and its receptors were found in many extrahypothalamic sites of the central nervous system (CNS),[4–7] and it became clear that this peptide was a major coordinator of the stress response, including activation of arousal and sympathetic system and central suppression of the immune/inflammatory reaction via glucocorticoid and catecholamine elevations.[8–10] On the other hand, CRH immunoreactivity and mRNA have also been detected outside the CNS, in resting subpopulations of human white blood cells and in rat and human active inflammatory sites.[11–13] More specifically, immunoreactive (Ir) CRH is found in the cytoplasm of accessory cells of the immune system, such as macrophages, tissue fibroblasts, and endothelial cells,[11,14–16] and we recently found IrCRH in the eyes of rodents suffering from experimentally induced uveitis.[17] In contrast to its systemic indirect immunosuppressive effects, in inflammatory sites CRH acts as an autocrine or paracrine proinflammatory peptide.[11,14,15] In addition, CRH and its receptors were also identified in Leydig cells of the rat testis, where CRH was shown to exert autocrine inhibitory actions on testosterone biosynthesis.[18–21]

Ovulation, luteolysis, and, perhaps, follicular atresia have characteristics of an aseptic immune/inflammatory reaction.[22] Resident macrophages constitute a major cellular component of the interstitial ovarian compartment[23–25] and macrophage-generated cytokines, such as interleukin (IL)-1, IL-6, and tumor necrosis factor α (TNFα) have been proposed as auto/paracrine regulators of ovulation, luteinization, and steroidogenesis.[26,27] Furthermore, the theca cell has been suggested to be the embryological and functional equivalent of the Leydig cell.[28] On the basis of the above, we examined rat and human ovaries for presence of CRH and/or its receptors and studied the potential effect of this neuropeptide on ovarian sex steroid biosynthesis.

PRESENCE OF IMMUNOREACTIVE CRH AND CRH-BINDING SITES IN THE RAT OVARY[29,30]

We examined ovaries from adult, normally cycling Sprague-Dawley rats (2–3 months old), in which normal cycling was verified by daily vaginal smears. The intracellular localization of CRH was done immunohistochemically, employing a rabbit polyclonal, highly specific anti-r/hCRH antiserum, affinity-purified by adsorption to synthetic r/hCRH.[29] To localize the peptide, we performed immunohistochemistry using a Biotin-Avidin/horseradish peroxidase system. Sections were incubated with the affinity-purified rabbit antibody to r/hCRH, and control sections were incubated either with the affinity-negative IgG fraction or nonimmune normal rabbit IgG. Specific staining for CRH was localized mainly in the cytoplasm of theca and stromal cells (FIG. 1**A**), regardless of size or maturity of ovarian follicles, as well as in the cytoplasm of the oocyte of graafian follicles (FIG. 1**B**). The granulosa cells had no CRH immunostaining. Immunoreactive CRH was also detected in the cytoplasm of a subpopulation of cells within the corpora lutea (FIG. 1**C**). These cells were found

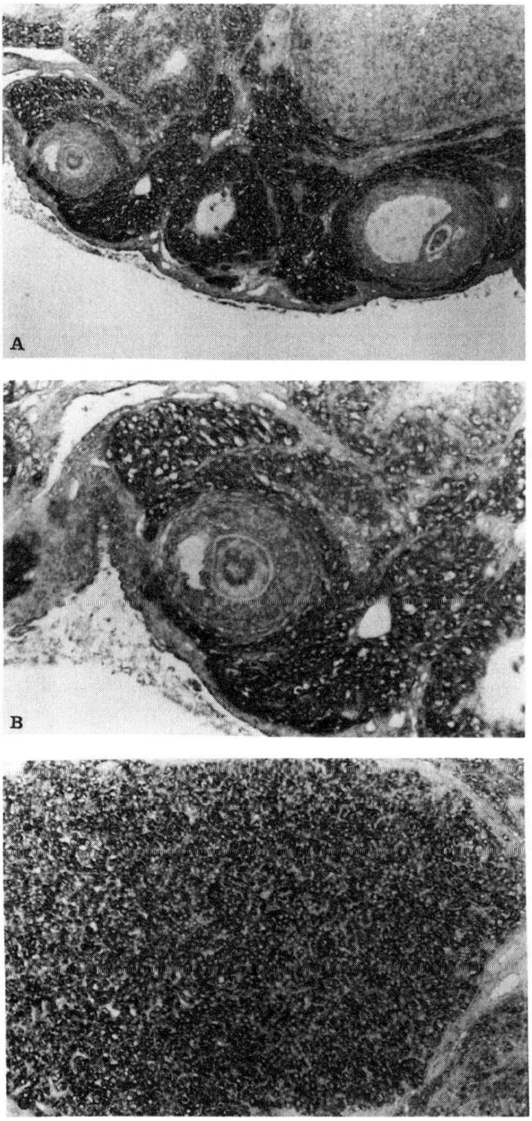

FIGURE 1. Immunohistochemical localization of IrCRH in the rat ovary. Positive staining is revealed as black-dark spots. (**A**) Positively stained theca and stromal cells around follicles (×50; here reduced by 40%). (**B**) Positively stained theca and stromal cells around a follicle on a higher magnification (×100; here reduced by 40%). Interestingly, IrCRH is detected within the cytoplasm of the intrafollicular oocyte. (**C**) Positively stained cells of a corpus luteum (×100; here reduced by 40%).

throughout all stages of corpus luteum maturation and at all phases of the estrous cycle. Since the ≈14 day half-life of a rat corpus luteum is longer than the duration of the 4- to 5-day rat estrous cycle, corpora lutea of different maturation stages were found in the rat ovaries at all stages of the estrous cycle. Most of the CRH-positive cells were large, luteinized cells, although one could not exclude the possibility that some of them were ovarian-resident macrophages.

The chromatographic mobility of ovarian CRH examined by reversed-phase, high-pressure liquid chromatography (HPLC) was similar to that of synthetic r/hCRH 1–41, the form produced by the rat and human hypothalamus and the human placenta. There were also immunoreactive bands with higher mobility than r/hCRH 1–41, indicating the presence of CRH-degradation products and/or aggregates/precursors with different hydrophobicity. Quantification of CRH ovarian content was performed with a specific and sensitive radioimmunoassay after acid extraction of the ovaries.[31] CRH content in ovaries from all phases of the ovarian estrous cycle varied from 0.042 to 0.126 pmol per gram wet tissue.

To investigate the presence of specific, high-affinity, saturable binding sites for CRH in the ovary, we measured binding of ^{125}I-labeled Tyr-ovine(o)CRH in homogenates of rat ovaries using assay conditions identical to those described for membrane preparations from mouse pituitaries and spleens.[6,7,32] Specific binding of radiolabeled Tyr-oCRH was linear with increasing tissue concentrations. Competitive displacement curves of ^{125}I-labeled Tyr-oCRH binding in ovarian homogenates incubated with increasing concentrations of r/hCRH demonstrated that the specific binding was saturable. Scatchard analyses employing the nonlinear curve-fitting program LIGAND, revealed a single, high-affinity binding site. The apparent dissociation constant (K_d) of oCRH-binding sites was 6.34 ± 2.3 nM (mean ± SEM), and the concentration of the receptor was 61.17 ± 15.6 fmoles/mg protein. The regional distribution of ^{125}I-labeled Tyr-oCRH receptors within the rat ovary was examined with *in vitro* autoradiographic techniques (FIG. 2). CRH receptors were diffusely distributed in ovarian stroma and theca areas surrounding follicles as well, as on the cumulus oophorus (FIG. 2**B**). There was a notable absence of specific binding in the granulosa areas, while specific ^{125}I-labeled Tyr-oCRH binding sites in the corpora lutea were sparse. In contrast to the clearcut presence of ^{125}I-labeled Tyr-oCRH binding sites in the ovaries of adult animals, we were not able to conclusively demonstrate the presence of such sites in the ovaries of prepubertal rats (23 days old).[33]

PRESENCE OF CRH IN NORMAL AND POLYCYSTIC HUMAN OVARIES[34]

To determine whether CRH is also present in human ovaries, we examined 26 normal ovaries or portions thereof, removed from women in the course of gynecological operations for nonovarian malignancies, and in follicular fluids collected from 10 women after ovarian hyperstimulation with the GnRH analogue buserelin (Suprefact) and hCG (Pregnyl) for assisted reproduction. To investigate whether ovarian CRH might participate in the pathophysiology of PCOS, we also examined nine ovaries or portions thereof, removed from women with PCOS.

In normal human ovaries, IrCRH had a distribution similar to that of rat ovarian

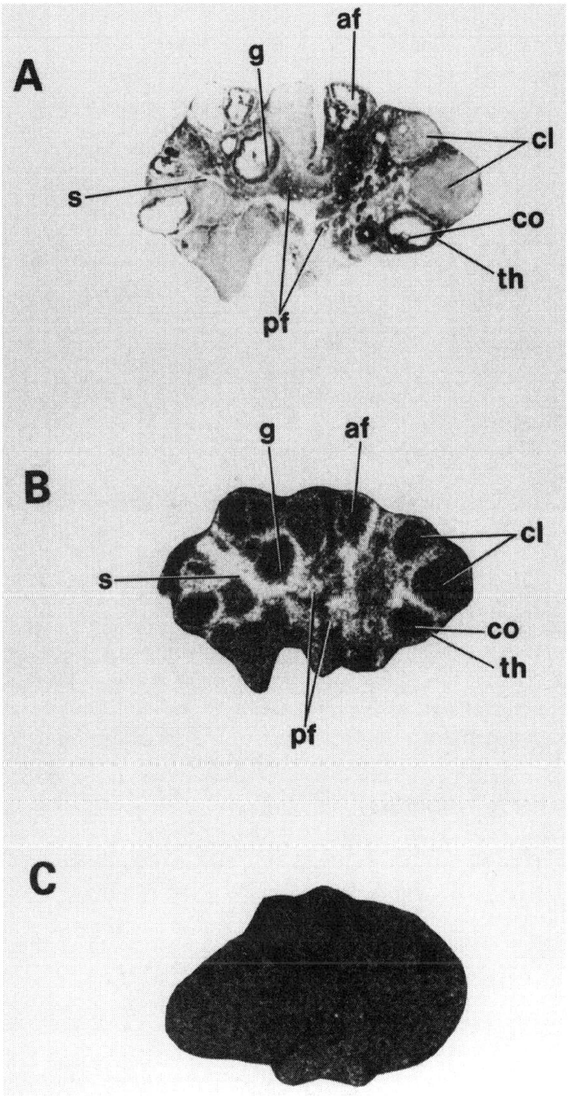

FIGURE 2. Autoradiographic localization of CRH receptors in the rat ovary. **(A)** Bright-field photomicrograph showing the histology of the section of rat ovary used to generate the autoradiogram shown in **B. (B)** Direct print of the autoradiogram generated on tritium-sensitive Ultrofilm, which shows the distribution of autoradiographic grains (*white spots*) in the section of ovary shown in **A. (C)** Nonspecific binding determined in the presence of 1 mM r/hCRH was uniform. Proestrous ovary sections are shown here. *s*: stroma; *g*: granulosa; *af*: atretic follicle; *cl*: corpus luteum; *co*: cumulus oophorus; *th*: theca; *pf*: primordial follicles.

IrCRH, as determined by immunohistochemistry. Thus, immunoreactivity was intense in the cytoplasm of thecal cells surrounding the ovarian follicles, in luteinized cells of the stroma, and in a subpopulation of cells within developing corpora lutea (FIG. 3). The latter were both small theca-derived and large granulosa-derived, luteinized cells. The staining pattern in the corpora lutea was heterogeneous, with the strongest CRH immunoreactivity in cells localized at the periphery, and the weakest

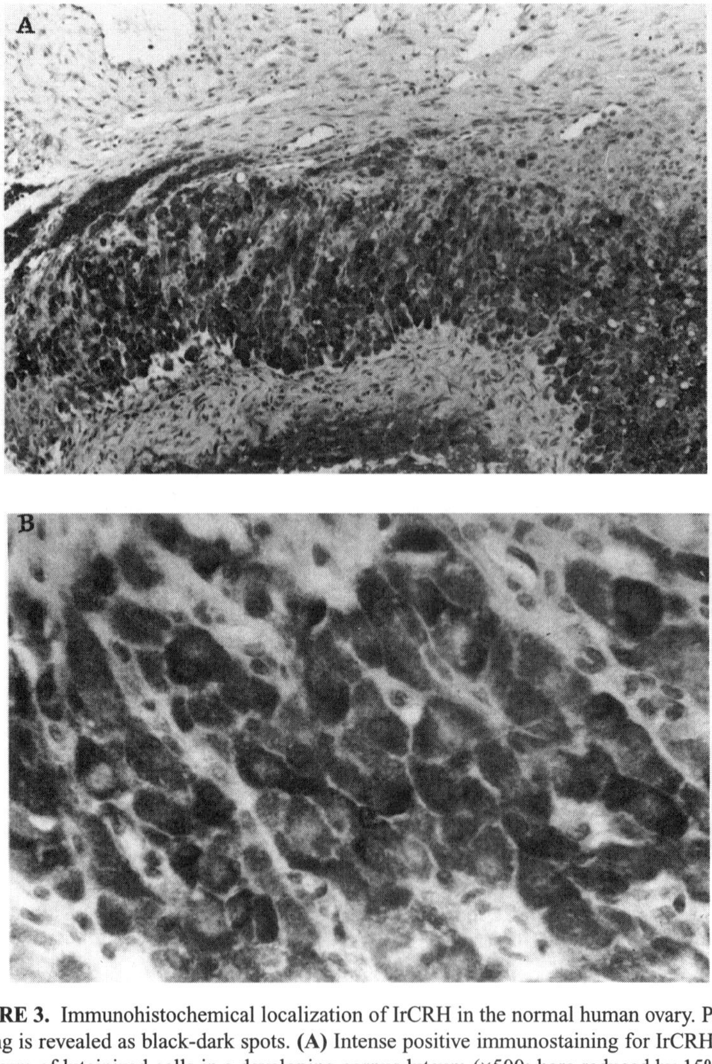

FIGURE 3. Immunohistochemical localization of IrCRH in the normal human ovary. Positive staining is revealed as black-dark spots. **(A)** Intense positive immunostaining for IrCRH in the cytoplasm of luteinized cells in a developing corpus luteum (×500; here reduced by 15%). **(B)** Positively stained luteinized cells of a developing corpus luteum on a higher magnification (×2000; here reduced by 15%).

in cells localized at the center of the structure. On the other hand, IrCRH staining was less prominent or totally absent in regressing corpora lutea, characterized by small-sized granulosa-lutein cells with pycnotic nuclei and abundant cytoplasmic lipids, indicating near completion or completion of functional luteolysis. Histologically characterized macrophages in these structures were weakly stained for IrCRH. Immunoreactive CRH was absent from the primary oocytes of primordial follicles of normal ovaries. Immunoreactive CRH of normal human ovaries had similar chromatographic mobility to r/hCRH-(1–41) (FIG. 4**A**). Total ovarian IrCRH content, measured in extracts of normal human ovaries at all phases of the menstrual cycle, varied between 0.047 and 0.105 pmol/g wet tissue (mean ± SD, 0.075 ± 0.02 pmol/g).

Immunoreactive CRH was also detected by specific RIA[31] in extracts of follicular fluids from hormonally stimulated human ovaries. The amount varied between 3.2 and 6.7 pmol/l (mean ± SD, 4.975 ± 1.179 pmol/l). Its chromatographic mobility was similar to that of r/hCRH-(1–41) (FIG. 4**B**).

Immunoreactive CRH was also localized in theca cells of polycystic ovaries; however, it was less prominent in the sparse corpora lutea in the latter. CRH immunostaining was absent in the stroma of polycystic ovaries, in which no luteinized cells were observed. Interestingly, unlike the findings in normal ovaries, IrCRH was detected within the primary oocytes of primordial follicles in all of the polycystic ovaries studied. Immunoreactive CRH of polycystic ovaries had the same chromatographic mobility to r/hCRH-(1–41) (FIG. 4**C**). A peak of IrCRH corresponding to the retention time (18 min) of the sulfoxide form of CRH, $Met(O)^{21,38}$-CRH, was eluted before the retention time (25 min) of r/hCRH-(1–41). Total ovarian IrCRH content, measured in extracts of polycystic ovaries varied between 0.025 and 0.052 pmol/g wet tissue (mean ± SD, 0.038 ± 0.09 pmol/g).

ROLE OF AGING AND STRESS ON OVARIAN CRH[35]

To examine the effects of aging and stress on ovarian CRH, we studied the ovaries of groups of healthy young (3–4 mo) and old (24 mo) female Fischer 344/N rats, before and after a 120-min immobilization stress. Young females were all in proestrous, and old females were in constant anestrous. Pre-immobilization corticosterone (CORT) levels were similar in both age groups, whereas immobilization produced a dramatic increase in CORT in both groups. Immunoreactive CRH was detected in the ovaries of all rats, and its distribution and intensity were quantified in the theca, granulosa, stroma, and corpora lutea. At baseline, IrCRH was 50% lower in old than in young rats in the theca and stroma by both distribution and intensity (FIG. 5**A** and **C**). Stress was associated with a decrease of IrCRH levels in the theca in both age groups (FIG. 5**B** and **D**), albeit to a significantly lesser extent in old rats (old 35% versus young 70%).

CRH INHIBITS STEROIDOGENESIS BY GRANULOSA-LUTEIN CELLS[36]

To investigate the role of CRH on ovarian steroid biosynthesis granulosa-lutein cells were obtained from follicular aspirates of nine patients with spontaneous ovula-

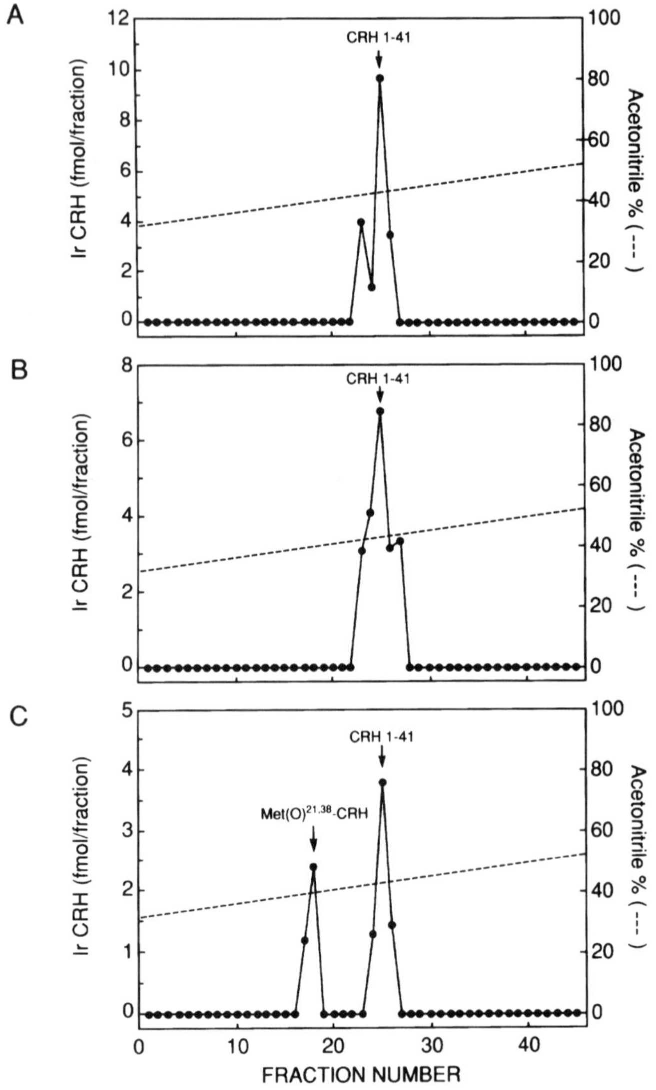

FIGURE 4. Reverse HPLC characterization of IrCRH extracted from a normal human ovary (**A**), human follicular fluid (**B**), and human PCO ovary (**C**). The amount of IrCRH in individual fractions was determined by RIA. Synthetic r/hCRH-(1–41) and Met(O)^{21,38}-CRH were eluted from this column in fractions 25 and 18, respectively, as indicated.

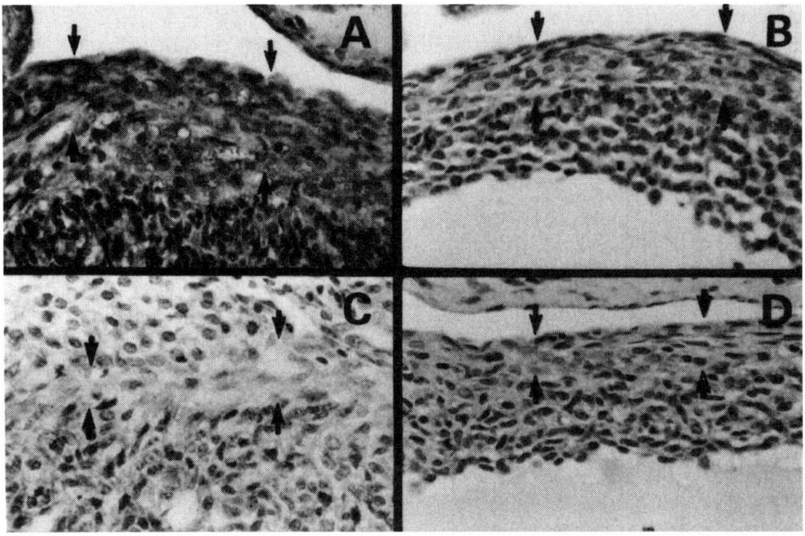

FIGURE 5. Immunohistochemical distribution of IrCRH in the rat ovary. In the left side of this four-panel figure, representative of our data, the distribution of CRH in the theca of nonstressed young (**A**) and nonstressed old (**C**) rats is shown. In the right side of this figure, the immunohistochemical distribution of IrCRH obtained from young (**B**) and old (**D**) rats immobilized for 2 hours is shown. It should be noticed (*arrows*) that the intense positive staining (*black-dark spots*) for IrCRH in the theca of young nonstressed rats in **A** is in contrast to its diminution in old unstressed and both young and old stressed rats.

tory cycles undergoing IVF for infertility due to uni- or bilateral tubal impatency or male factor. All patients received a GnRH analogue (Decapeptyl; Ipsen, Paris, France; 3.75 mg i.m.), one month before FSH therapy was started. Subsequently, superovulation for *in vitro* fertilization/embryo transfer was induced with purified urinary FSH (Metrodin, Serono, Rome, Italy; 75 IU FSH/ampule): two ampules/day from day 1–3 and individualized thereafter, depending on daily plasma estradiol (E_2) levels and measurements of follicular growth by transvaginal ultrasound. When at least one follicle reached 16 mm in diameter and plasma E_2 levels were greater than 200 pg/ml, hCG (Profasi, Serono, Rome, Italy; 10,000 IU) was administered. Follicular aspiration for oocyte retrieval was performed by laparoscopy under general anesthesia 34 to 38 hours after hCG administration. After oocyte recovery, granulosa cells were obtained from follicular fluid by centrifugation at 800 rpm for 15 min; cells were resuspended with a 1:1 mixture of medium 199 and Hank's salt solution, and pools were prepared from each individual patient. The suspension (10 ml) was layered in 10 ml of lymphocyte separation medium (Ficoll) and centrifuged at 1800 rpm at room temperature for 30 min. Granulosa cells were recovered from the Ficoll interface, washed three times with Hank's and resuspended with 3 ml medium 199. Aliquots of the cell suspension were counted with a hemocytometer to determine the number of cells, and plated (5×10^5 cell/well) for 24 hr in multiwell dishes in 1 ml medium 199 with Earle's salt supplemented with 2% L-glutamine, 1% nonessential amino acids, 1% penicillin-streptomycin, 1% tylosin, 10% fetal bovine serum. Cultures were maintained in humidified 95% air–5% CO_2 at 37°C. After 24 hr, culture media were replaced with 1 ml serum-free media containing 10^{-7} mol/l of androstenedione as substrate for E_2 production. The *in vitro* effect of CRH was tested by adding increasing doses of oCRH (10^{-11}–10^{-6} mol/l) to the culture media. Culture media were removed after 24 hr, and stored at –20°C until tested for E_2 or progesterone content by specific RIA. We tested for E_2 or progesterone content by specific RIA. We found that the levels of both E_2 (FIG. 6) and progesterone in the culture media were inhibited by CRH. This effect of CRH was abolished by α-helical CRH 9-41, a CRH antagonist, suggesting that it was a CRH receptor-mediated effect.

DISCUSSION

CRH is present in theca cells of ovarian follicles, in luteinized stromal cells, and in luteinized cells and macrophages in the corpora lutea in rat and normal human ovaries.[29,34] The chromatographic mobility of ovarian CRH immunoreactive peptide is similar to that of r/hCRH-(1–41). CRH mRNA was recently reported in the mouse and human ovary by a highly sensitive reverse transcription–polymerase chain reaction, suggesting that some or all of CRH is locally produced.[37,38] Ovarian CRH may

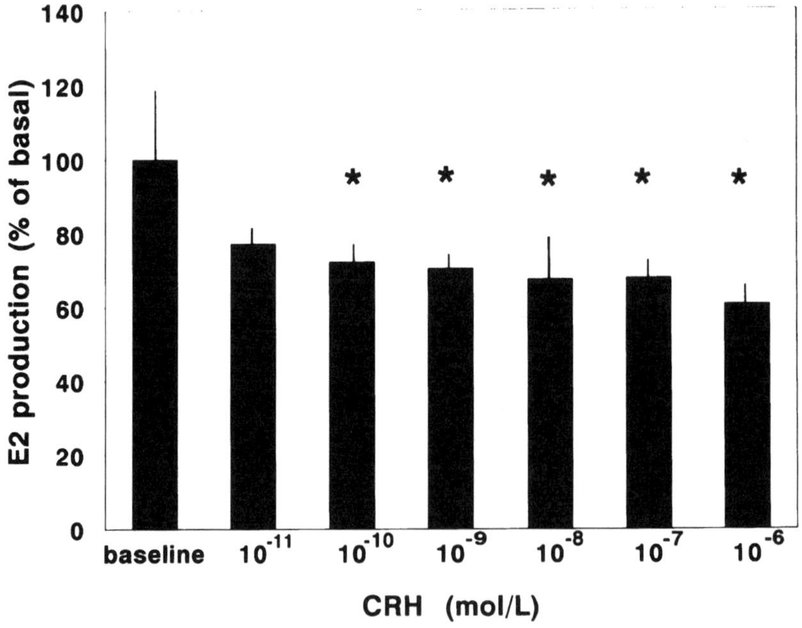

FIGURE 6. Effect of increasing concentrations of oCRH on E_2 production by cultured granulosa-lutein cells. *: $p < 0.05$ versus baseline.

be derived from various cell types. It may be produced by immune accessory cells normally residing in the ovary, such as *in situ* macrophages, tissue fibroblasts, and/or endothelial cells.[23–25] CRH mRNA and peptide have been shown in peripheral blood mononuclear cells[39] and in spleen and inflammatory synovia from arthritic Lewis rats.[12] Ovarian macrophages constitute a major cellular component of the interstitial ovarian compartment and are mostly concentrated near perifollicular capillaries.[23–25] On the other hand, ovarian CRH could be transported to the ovary through postganglionic sympathetic and/or unmyelinated sensory neurons type C and Aδ. The theca is richly innervated, and CRH may be produced by either of these fibers. The sympathetic ganglia and the dorsal root ganglia, where the cell bodies of these neurons reside, are replete with CRH.[40,41] Finally, we must consider that the theca and stroma cells, luteinized cells of the corpora lutea, and oocytes, all of which contain IrCRH, may also themselves produce this peptide.

Follicular fluid CRH could be derived from the CRH-immunopositive cells described above, after diffusion into the follicular antrum, through the granulosa layer and/or it could be produced by the mature oocyte itself, which shows intense cytoplasmic IrCRH staining.[29]

The specific high-affinity CRH receptors identified in homogenates of rat ovaries were similar to the high-affinity receptor previously identified in rat pituitary, hypothalamus, brain,[6,7] Leydig cells,[21] and arthritic synovial tissues.[12] Recently, evidence by *in situ* hybridization studies was provided that the ovarian CRH receptor is of subtype 1.[38,42] The presence of CRH receptors on the cumulus oophorus, taken together with the localization of IrCRH in the ovum, as well as in follicular fluid, might indicate that CRH might participate within a local intrafollicular cross-talk.

Compared with normal ovaries, CRH was absent from the ovarian stroma of PCOS patients, probably because of the absence of luteinized stromal cells in the latter group.[34] Also, immunostaining for CRH was less prominent in the sparse corpora lutea of polycystic ovaries than in those of normal ovaries, probably because the former were in an advanced stage of regression. This is compatible with the overall decreased IrCRH content of PCOS ovaries compared to normal ovaries. If CRH is a suppressor of androgen biosynthesis by the theca, in analogy to its effect in the Leydig cell, the decreased presence of IrCRH in the PCOS ovary might facilitate hyperandrogenism.[20,21] On the other hand, the detection of IrCRH in primary oocytes of primordial follicles in ovaries from patients with PCOS, in contrast to its absence in those of primordial follicles of normal ovaries, might suggest that CRH is relevant to the known oocyte dysfunction of patients with PCOS.[43]

Immunoreactive CRH was significantly lower in the stroma and theca of old than young rats both before and after immobilization.[35] Acute immobilization stress decreased IrCRH in the ovarian theca of young, and to a lesser extent, old rats. By contrast, no age- or stress-associated effects in IrCRH were observed in the granulosa or corpus luteum compartments. In old rats, stress was less effective in decreasing ovarian IrCRH, probably because of a "floor" effect. The decrease observed in ovarian IrCRH as a consequence of stress, together with the parallel increase of their plasma corticosterone levels, suggest that ovarian CRH may be acutely downregulated by glucocorticoids. This is compatible with previous studies showing that, like hypothalamic CRH, peripheral CRH is also inhibited by glucocorticoids.[12] Recently, the human CRH gene was shown to possess estrogen-responsive elements and to be activated by E_2.[44] Because ovarian CRH and plasma estrogen levels are both high during young age, it is possible that ovarian estrogens upregulate CRH expression in the ovary of the young rat, as they do with hypothalamic CRH during the estrous cycle or after being administered to ovariectomized rats.[45] Conversely, age-related reductions in the amount or action of estrogens may contribute to the basal and stress-related decreases in ovarian CRH observed with aging.

Ovarian CRH appears to participate in the regulation of ovarian E_2 and progesterone biosynthesis. Specifically, CRH seems to exert an inhibitory effect on aromatase activity and on nonaromatase-dependent steroidogenesis by cultured granulosa-lutein cells. This effect of CRH might be mediated by secretion of cytokines by macrophages, contaminating the cultures. Many of the effects of this neuropeptide on peripheral blood mononuclear cells are mediated by IL-1.[46] Granulosa cells respond to IL-1 with reductions in steroidosynthesis.[47] Therefore, CRH might exert an inhibitory action on ovarian estrogen and progesterone production either directly or through an immune-mediated mechanism. Further studies are needed to define the relevance of CRH to ovarian physiology.

CONCLUSIONS

The ovary is another extrahypothalamic ("peripheral") site of CRH and CRH-receptor localization. The decrease of ovarian CRH as a consequence of stress suggests that ovarian CRH may be acutely downregulated by circulating glucocorticoids. Ovarian CRH and plasma estrogen levels are high during young age, suggesting that estrogens may upregulate ovarian CRH, possibly through the estrogen-responsive elements present in the regulatory region of the CRH gene. Ovarian CRH may play a role in the ovary through auto/paracrine inhibitions of steroid biosynthesis; it also may participate in the aseptic inflammatory phenomena of the ovary (ovulation/luteolysis/follicular atresia) through its proinflammatory properties. The presence of Ir-CRH in primary oocytes and its overall reduction in PCOS ovaries might be related to the oocyte dysfunction and excessive ovarian androgen production observed in this condition.

REFERENCES

1. Saffran, M., A. V. Schally & B. G. Bentey. 1955. Stimulation of the release of corticotropin from the adenohypophysis by a neurohypophysial factor. Endocrinology **57:** 439–444.
2. Guillemin, R. & B. Rosenberg. 1955. Humoral hypothalamic control of anterior pituitary: A study with combined tissue cultures. Endocrinology **57:** 599–607.
3. Vale, W., J. Spiess, C. Rivier & J. Rivier. 1981. Characterization of a 41-residue ovine hypothalamic peptide that stimulates secretion of corticotropin and β-endorphin. Science (Washington, DC) **213:** 1394–1397.
4. Fischman, A. J. & R. L. Moldow. 1982. Extrahypothalamic distribution of CRF-like immunocreativity in the rat brain. Peptides (Elmsford) **1:** 149–153.
5. Swanson, L. W., P. E. Sawchenko, J. Rivier & W. Vale. 1983. Organization of ovine corti-

cotropin-releasing factor immunocreactive cells and fibers in the rat brain: An immunohistochemical study. Neuroendocrinology **36:** 165–186.
6. Wynn, P. C., R. L. Hauger, M. C. Holmes, M. A. Millan, K. J. Catt & G. Aguilera. 1984. Brain and pituitary receptors for corticotropin-releasing factor: Localization and differential regulation after adrenalectomy. Peptides (Elmsford) **5:** 1077–1084.
7. De Souza, E. B. 1987. Corticotropin-releasing factor receptors in the rat central nervous system: Characterization and regional distribution. J. Neurosci. **7:** 88–100.
8. Chrousos, G. P. & P. W. Gold. 1992. The concepts of stress and stress system disorders. J. Am. Med. Assoc. **267:** 1244–1252.
9. Brown, M. R., L. A. Fisher, J. Spiess, C. Rivier, J. Rivier & W. Vale. 1982. Corticotropin-releasing factor: Actions on the sympathetic nervous system and metabolism. Endocrinology **111:** 928–931.
10. Brown, M. R. 1991. Neuropeptide-mediated regulation of the neuroendocrine and autonomic responses to stress. *In* Stress, Neuropeptides and Systemic Disease. J. McCubbin, P. Kaufman & C. Nemeroff, Eds.: 73–93. Academic Press. New York.
11. Karalis, K., H. Sano, J. Redwine, S. Listwak, R. L. Wilder & G. P. Chrousos. 1991. Autocrine or paracrine inflammatory actions of corticotropin-releasing hormone *in vivo.* Science **254:** 421–423.
12. Crofford, L. J., H. Sano, K. Karalis, E. L. Webster, E. A. Goldmuntz, G. P. Chrousos & R. L. Wilder. 1992. Local secretion of corticotropin-releasing hormone in the joints of Lewis rats with inflammatory arthritis. J. Clin. Invest. **90:** 2555–2564.
13. Crofford, L. J., H. Sano, K. Karalis, T. C. Friedman, H. R. Epps, E. F. Remmers, P. Mathern, G. P. Chrousos & R. L. Wilder. 1993. Corticotropin-releasing hormone in synovial fluids and tissues of patients with rheumatoid arthritis and osteoarthritis. J. Immunol. **151:** 1–10.
14. Karalis, K., G. Mastorakos, H. Sano, R. L. Wilder & G. P. Chrousos. 1995. Somatostatin may participate in the antiinflammatory actions of glucocorticoids. Endocrinology **136:** 4133–4138.
15. Karalis, K., G. Mastorakos, G. P. Chrousos & G. Tolis. 1994. Somatostatin analogues suppress the inflammatory reaction *in vivo.* J. Clin. Invest. **93:** 2000–2006.
16. Scopa, C. D., G. Mastorakos, T. C. Friedman, M. Melachrinou, M. J. Merino & G. P. Chrousos. 1994. Presence of immunoreactive corticotropin-releasing hormone in thyroid lesions. Am. J. Pathol. **145:** 1159–1167.
17. Mastorakos, G., E. A. Bouzas, P. B. Silver, G. Sartani, T. C. Friedman, C. C. Chan, R. R. Caspi & G. P. Chrousos. 1995. Immune corticotropin-releasing hormone is present in the eyes of and promotes experimental autoimmune uveoretinitis in rodents. Endocrinology **136:** 4650–4658.
18. Yoon, D. J., C. Sklar & R. David. 1988. Presence of immunoreactive corticotropin-releasing factor in rat testis. Endocrinology **122:** 759–761.
19. Audhya, T., C. S. Hollander, D. H. Schlesinger & B. Hutchinson. 1989. Structural characterization and localization of corticotropin-releasing factor in the testis. Biochem. Biophys. Acta **995:** 10–16.
20. Fabbri, A., J. C. Tinajero & M. L. Dufau. 1990. Corticotropin-releasing factor is produced by rat Leydig cells and has a major local antireproductive role in the testis. Endocrinology **127:** 1541–1543.
21. Ulisse, S., A. Fabbri & M. L. Dufau. 1989. Corticotropin-releasing factor receptors and actions in rat Leydig cells. J. Biol. Chem. **264:** 2156–2163.
22. Espey, L. L. 1980. Ovulation as an inflammatory reaction: A hypothesis. Biol. Reprod. **22:** 73–106.
23. Bulmer, D. 1964. The histochemistry of ovarian macrophages in the rat. J. Anat. **98:** 313–319.

24. HUME, D. A., D. HALPIN, H. CHARLTON & S. GORDON. 1984. The mononuclear phagocyte system of the mouse defined by immunohistochemical localization of antigen F4/80: Macrophages of endocrine organs. Proc. Natl. Acad. Sci. USA **81:** 4174–4177.
25. KATABUCHI, H., Y. FUKUMATSU & H. OKAMURA. 1989. Immunohistochemical and morphological observations of macrophages in the human ovary. *In* Growth Factors and the Ovary. A. N. Hirshfield, Ed.: 409–413. Plenum. New York.
26. ADASHI, E. Y. 1989. Cytokine-mediated regulation of ovarian function: Encounters of a third kind. (Editorial.) Endocrinology **124:** 2043–2045.
27. ADASHI, E. Y. 1990. The potential relevance of cytokines to ovarian physiology: The emerging role of resident ovarian cells of the white blood cell series. Endocrinol. Rev. **11:** 454–464.
28. ERICKSON, G. F., D. A. MAGOFFIN, C. A. DYER & C. HOFEDITZ. 1985. The ovarian androgen producing cells: A review of structure/function relationships. Endocrinol. Rev. **6:** 371–399.
29. MASTORAKOS, G., E. L. WEBSTER, T. C. FRIEDMAN & G. P. CHROUSOS. 1993. Immunoreactive corticotropin-releasing hormone and its binding sites in the rat ovary. J. Clin. Invest. **92:** 961–968.
30. MASTORAKOS, G., E. L. WEBSTER & G. P. CHROUSOS. 1993. Corticotropin-releasing hormone and its receptors in the ovary: Physiological implications. *In* Intraovarian Regulators and Polycystic Ovarian Syndrome: Recent Progress on Clinical and Therapeutic Aspects. G. Tolis, J. Bringer & G. P. Chrousos, Eds. Ann. N. Y. Acad. Sci. **687:** 20–28.
31. CALOGERO, A. E., R. BERNARDINI, A. N. MARGIORIS, G. BAGDY, W. T. GALLUCCI, P. J. MUNSON, L. TAMARKIN, T. P. TOMAI, L. BRADY, P. W. GOLD & G. P. CHROUSOS. 1989. Effects of serotonergic agonists and antagonists on corticotropin-releasing hormone secretion by explanted rat hypothalami. Peptides (Elmsford) **10:** 189–200.
32. WEBSTER, E. L. & E. B. DE SOUZA. 1988. Corticotropin-releasing factor receptors in mouse spleen: Identification, autoradiographic localization, and regulation by divalent cations and guanine nucleotides. Endocrinology **122:** 609–610.
33. WEBSTER, E. L., G. MASTORAKOS & G. P. CHROUSOS. 1992. Identification and characterization of corticotropin-releasing hormone receptors in rat ovary. IX Ovarian workshop "Ovarian cell interactions: Genes to Physiology." Serono Symposia, Chapel Hill, North Carolina.
34. MASTORAKOS, G., C. D. SCOPA, A. VRYONIDOU, T. C. FRIEDMAN, D. KATTIS, C. PHENEKOS, M. J. MERINO & G. P. CHROUSOS. 1994. Presence of immunoreactive corticotropin-releasing hormone in normal and polycystic human ovaries. J. Clin. Endocrinol. Metab. **79:** 1191–1197.
35. MASTORAKOS, G., G. CIZZA, R. KVETNANSKY, E. BERGAMINI, M. R. BLACKMAN, P. W. GOLD & G. P. CHROUSOS. 1995. Aging and acute stress decrease corticotropin-releasing hormone in the ovary of the Fischer 344/N rat. Life Sci. **56:** 1065–1071.
36. GHIZZONI, L., G. MASTORAKOS, A. VOTTERO, A. BARRECA, M. FURLINI, A. CESARONE, B. FERRARI, G. P. CHROUSOS & S. BERNASCONI. Corticotropin-releasing hormone-induced inhibition of steroid biosynthesis by cultured granulosa-lutein cells is mediated by interleukin-1 receptors. J. Clin. Endocrinol. Metab. Submitted.
37. MUGLIA, L. J., N. A. JENKINS, D. J. GILBERT, N. G. COPELAND & J. A. MAJZOUB. 1994. Expression of the mouse corticotropin-releasing hormone gene *in vivo* and targeted inactivation in embryonic stem cells. J. Clin. Invest. **93:** 2066–2072.
38. ASAKURA, H., I. ZWAIN & S. S. C. YEN. 1996. Gene expression and cellular localization of corticotropin-releasing factor (CRF), CRF-binding protein (CRF-BP) and type-1 CRF receptors (CRF-R) in the human ovary. 10th International Congress of Endocrinology, San Francisco, CA.

39. STEPHANOU, A., D. S. JESSOP, R. A. KNIGHT & S. L. LIGHTMAN. 1990. Corticotropin-releasing factor-like immunoreactivity and mRNA in human leukocytes. Brain Behav. Immun. **4:** 67–73.
40. MERCHENTHALER, I., M. A. HYNES, S. VIGH, A. V. SCHALLY & P. PETRUSZ. 1983. Immunocytochemical localization of corticotropin-releasing factor (CRF) in the rat spinal cord. Brain Res. **275:** 373–377.
41. UDELSMAN, R., J. P. HARWOOD, M. A. MILLAN, G. P. CHROUSOS, D. S. GOLDSTEIN, R. ZIMLICHMAN, K. J. CATT & G. AGUILERA. 1986. Functional corticotropin-releasing factor receptors in the primate peripheral sympathetic nervous system. Nature (London) **319:** 147–150.
42. NAPPI, R. E. & S. RIVEST. 1996. Stress-induced genetic expression of a selective corticotropin-releasing factor-receptor subtype within the rat ovaries: An effect dependent on the ovulatory cycle. Biol. Reprod. **53:** 1417–1428.
43. CHROUSOS, G. P., J. BRINGER & G. TOLIS. 1993. Introduction. *In* Intraovarian Regulators and Polycystic Ovarian Syndrome: Recent Progress on Clinical and Therapeutic Aspects. G. Tolis, J. Bringer, G. P. Chrousos, Eds. Ann. N. Y. Acad. Sci. **687:** xiii–xv.
44. VAMVAKOPOULOS, N. C. & G. P. CHROUSOS. 1993. Evidence of direct estrogen regulation of human corticotropin-releasing hormone gene expression: Potential implications for the sexual dimorphism of the stress response and immune/inflammatory reaction. J. Clin. Invest. **92:** 1896–1902.
45. BURGESS, L. H. & R. J. HANDA. 1992. Chronic estrogen-induced alterations in adrenocorticotropin and corticosterone secretion and glucocorticoid receptor-mediated functions in female rats. Endocrinology **131:** 1261–1269.
46. KAVELAARS, A., R. E. BALLIEUX & C. J. HEIJNEN. 1989. The role of IL-1 in the corticotropin-releasing factor and arginine-vasopressin-induced secretion of immunoreactive β-endorphin by human peripheral blood mononuclear cells. J. Immunol. **142:** 2338–2342.
47. HURWITZ, A., D. W. PAYNE, J. N. PACKMAN, C. L. ANDREANI, C. E. RESNICK, E. R. HERNANDEZ & E. Y. ADASHI. 1991. Cytokine-mediated regulation of ovarian function: Interleukin-1 inhibits ganodotropin-induced androgen biosynthesis. Endocrinology **129:** 1250–1256.

The Hypothalamic-Pituitary-Adrenal Axis and the Female Reproductive System

M. A. MAGIAKOU,[a,b] G. MASTORAKOS,[c] E. WEBSTER,[d]
AND G. P. CHROUSOS[d]

[b]*Second Department of Pediatrics*
"P & A Kyriakou" Children's Hospital and

[c]*Endocrine Unit*
"Evgenidion" Hospital
University of Athens
115 27 Athens, Greece

[d]*Pediatric Endocrinology Section*
Developmental Endocrinology Branch
National Institute of Child Health and Human Development
National Institutes of Health
Bethesda, Maryland 20892

AN OVERVIEW OF THE STRESS AND REPRODUCTIVE SYSTEMS

Definition of Stress and the Stress Syndrome

Living organisms survive by maintaining an immensely complex dynamic and harmonious equilibrium, homeostasis, that is constantly challenged or outright threatened by intrinsic or extrinsic disturbing forces or stressors.[1] The steady state required for successful adaptation is maintained by counteracting/reestablishing forces, or adaptive responses. Stress, thus, is a state of dysharmony or threatened homeostasis.

Both physical and emotional stressors set into motion central and peripheral responses designed to preserve homeostasis.[1–4] Centrally, there is a facilitation of neural pathways mediating, among other functions, arousal, alertness, vigilance, cognition, and focused attention, as well as appropriate aggression, with concurrent inhibition of pathways that subserve vegetative functions, such as feeding and reproduction. Peripheral changes occur principally to promote an adaptive redirection of energy, that is, oxygen and nutrients directed to the central nervous system (CNS) and stressed body site(s), mediated by increases in cardiovascular tone, blood pressure, heart rate and respiratory rate, stimulation of gluconeogenesis and lipolysis, inhibition of growth and reproductive function, and containment of the inflammatory/immune response.

[a]Address for correspondence: Maria Alexandra Magiakou, M.D., Clinical Associate, 2nd Department of Pediatrics, University of Athens, "P & A Kyriakou" Children's Hospital, 11527 Athens, Greece.

Stress System

Because the general stress response is both essential for survival and remarkably consistent in its presentation, it has been suggested that a discrete, dedicated stress system has evolved specifically for its coordination.[1–4] The two principal components of this system are the corticotropin-releasing hormone (CRH) and the locus ceruleus-norepinephrine (LC-NE)/autonomic (sympathetic) nervous systems.[1–4] The

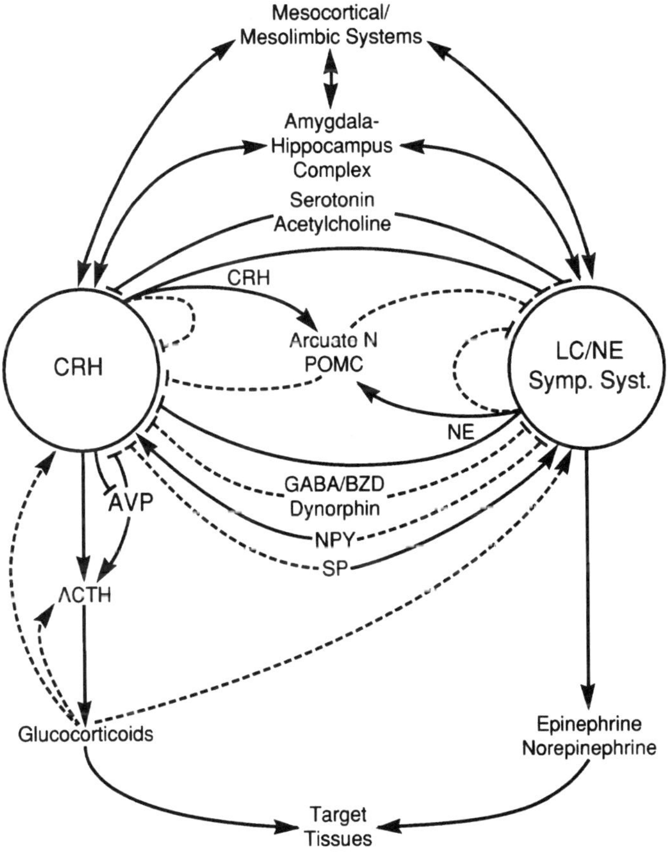

FIGURE 1. A simplified, heuristic representation of the central and peripheral components of the stress system, their functional interrelations, and their relationships to other central nervous system systems involved in the stress response. The hypothalamic corticotropin-releasing-hormone (CRH) neuron in the paraventricular nucleus and the centers of the arousal and autonomic systems in the brain stem represent major centers of this system connected anatomically and functionally to each other. POMC indicates proopiomelanocortin; LC/NE Symp Syst, locus ceruleus-norepinephrine/sympathetic system; AVP, arginine vasopressin; GABA, γ-aminobutyric acid; BZD, benzodiazepine; and ACTH, corticotropin. (Taken from Chrousos and Gold[2]; used with permission from the *Journal of the American Medical Association.*)

former is widespread throughout the brain, but has been best characterized in the paraventricular nucleus of the hypothalamus,[5–9] whereas the latter are located in the brainstem.[10] The reciprocal interaction of CRH with the LC/NE-sympathetic system, the parallel regulation of both components of the stress system by various agonists and antagonists, and the interactions of the stress system with the mesocorticolimbic system and the amygdala/hippocampus are schematically demonstrated in FIGURE 1 and extensively discussed in an earlier report.[2]

The Hypothalamic–Pituitary–Adrenal (HPA) Axis

The adrenal cortex consists of three anatomic zones: the outer zona glomerulosa, the intermediate zona fasciculata, and the inner zona reticularis. The zona glomerulosa is responsible for the production of aldosterone, the zona fasciculata for the production of cortisol, and the zona reticularis for the production of adrenal androgens. ACTH, synthesized and secreted by the corticotropes of the anterior pituitary, is the primary regulator of cortisol and adrenal androgen secretion. ACTH is part of a larger 245-amino-acid precursor molecule, propiomelanocortin (POMC). Adrenal androgens are also synthesized under the influence of other as yet unidentified putative pituitary factor(s), which act synergistically with ACTH and have been called adrenal androgen-stimulating factor(s).[11,12]

Hypothalamic control of ACTH secretion is exerted primarily by CRH, a 41-amino-acid peptide, produced by parvocellular neurons of the paraventricular nucleus (PVN) and secreted into the hypophyseal–portal system. Another hypothalamic hormone involved in a major fashion in the regulation of ACTH is arginine-vasopressin (AVP). This hormone is also produced by parvocellular neurons of the PVN and secreted into the hypophyseal-portal system, as well as by magnocellular neurons of the same nucleus secreted via the posterior pituitary into the systemic circulation. CRH is permissive for the secretion of ACTH, whereas AVP is a major synergistic factor in the production of this hormone.[13]

The basal activity of the HPA axis is under the influence of one or more circadian pacemakers. During stress, the HPA axis is activated in response to a variety of stressors, and CRH appears to mediate the metabolic, circulatory, and behavioral adaptations that take place in such demanding situations. There are also several regulatory negative feedback loops that function to constrain the activity of HPA axis. Prominent negative feedback loops are those exerted by glucocorticoids on CRH and ACTH secretion. The adrenal cortisol secretion rate under basal conditions is 12–15 mg/m^2 per day. In normal individuals, the highest plasma cortisol levels are between 6:00 and 8:00 A.M. and the lowest at about midnight. Cortisol secretion increases by two- to fourfold in stress. Plasma cortisol concentrations are elevated during physical and/or emotional stress, including illness, trauma, surgery, and starvation.[14]

The Female Reproductive Cycle

The hypothalamic–pituitary–ovarian (HPO) axis, through the circulating levels of gonadotropins, estradiol, and progesterone, regulates structural and functional changes in its target organs, including the fallopian tubes, uterus, and vagina. The menstrual cycle is divided into a follicular, ovulatory, and luteal phase.

The first half of the follicular phase begins in the late luteal phase of the preceding cycle, with initiation of follicular growth and a rise of serum levels of FSH. LH levels also rise one or two days later than those of FSH, while ovarian secretion of estradiol ensues. *The second half of the follicular phase* begins 7–8 days before the preovulatory LH surge and is characterized by a marked increase in ovarian secretion of estradiol. The latter reaches a maximum on the day before the LH peak. The rise in plasma estradiol is accompanied by a decrease in FSH, and an increase in LH levels. Briefly before the onset of the midcycle LH surge, there is a small rise in plasma progesterone, which is followed by the ovulatory LH surge. At this time, there is a rapid rise in the plasma LH level, which leads to the final maturation of the graafian follicle and its rupture 16–24 hours after the LH peak. There is a simultaneous increase in FSH. The preovulatory peak of estradiol and the first appearance of progesterone are related to the rapid follicular maturation and reflect the increased functional activity of the theca and granulosa cells of the ripening follicle, destined to ovulate. During *the luteal phase* the follicular cells are luteinized, and the postovulatory follicle becomes increasingly vascularized. The life span and function of spontaneously luteinized follicular cells are limited. LH is required for normal survival and function of the corpus luteum during the menstrual cycle. The most important feature of this period is the marked increase in progesterone secretion by the corpus luteum, which reaches a maximum about 8 days after the midcycle LH peak. There is a parallel but smaller increase in estradiol. As progesterone increases, plasma LH and FSH decline throughout most of the luteal phase; however, FSH begins to rise at the end of the luteal phase to initiate follicular growth for the next cycle.[15]

INTERACTIONS OF THE HPA AXIS WITH THE REPRODUCTIVE, GROWTH, AND THYROID AXES AND THE IMMUNE SYSTEM

Reproductive Axis

The reproductive axis is inhibited at all levels by various components of the HPA axis (FIG. 2).[16–18] Thus, either directly or via arcuate POMC neuron β-endorphin, CRH suppresses the gonadotropin hormone-releasing hormone (GnRH) neuron of the arcuate nucleus of the hypothalamus. Glucocorticoids, on the other hand, exert inhibitory effects at the level of the GnRH neuron, the pituitary gonadotroph, and the gonads themselves and render target tissues of sex steroids resistant to these hormones.[17] These effects of the HPA axis participate in the "hypothalamic" amenorrhea of stress and depressive, anxiety, and eating disorders, and the hypogonadism of Cushing's syndrome. The interaction between CRH and the gonadal axis appears to be bidirectional. We recently showed direct regulation of the human CRH gene expression by estrogens[19] (see below).

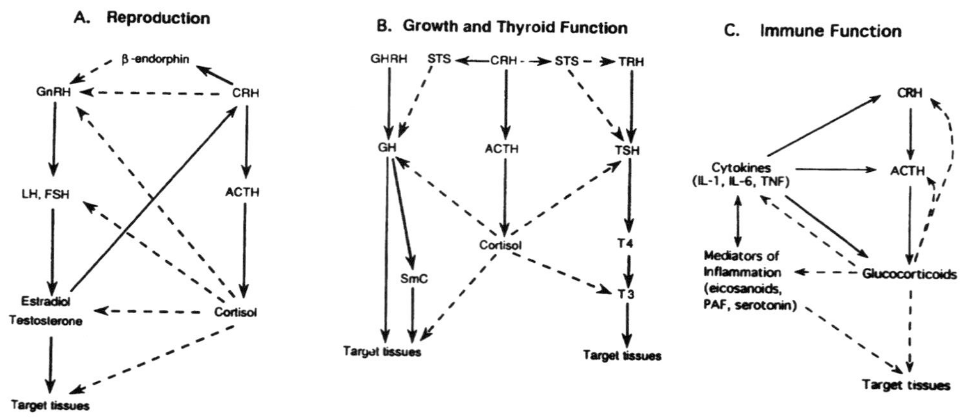

FIGURE 2. A simplified, heuristic representation of the interactions between the hypothalamic–pituitary–adrenal axis and other neuroendocrine systems, including the reproductive axis (**A**), the growth and thyroid axis (**B**), and the immune system (**C**). LHRH indicates luteinizing hormone-releasing hormone; CRH, corticotropin-releasing hormone; LH, luteinizing hormone; FSH, follicle-stimulating hormone; ACTH, corticotropin; GHRH, growth hormone-releasing hormone; STS, somatostatin; TRH, thyrotropin-releasing hormone; GH, growth hormone; TSH, thyroid-stimulating hormone; T_4, thyroxine; SmC, somatomedin C; T_3, triiodothyronine; IL-1, interleukin 1; IL-6, interleukin 6; TNF, tumor necrosis factor; and PAF, platelet-activating factor. (Taken from Chrousos and Gold[2]; used with permission from the *Journal of the American Medical Association.*)

Growth and Thyroid Axes

Activation of the HPA axis also leads to suppression of the growth axis (FIG. 2).[20–21] CRH-induced secretion of somatostatin, which inhibits GH secretion, glucocorticoid-mediated suppression of GH secretion, a decrease in effective circulating levels of free insulin-like growth factor 1 (IGF-1), and glucocorticoid-induced target tissue insensitivity to IGF-1 and other growth factors, are the pathophysiological mechanisms implicated.[22–24] A parallel phenomenon is the suppression of thyroid axis function. Glucocorticoid-induced suppressed secretion of TSH and decreased conversion of the relatively inactive thyroxine (T4) to the potent triiodothyronine (T3) in peripheral tissues occur during stress.[25,26] In addition, endogenous TRH and TSH secretion may be suppressed by CRH-induced somatostatin.

Immune System

Activation of the HPA axis also leads to suppression of the immune system, primarily via glucocorticoid-induced changes in the traffic and function of immune system cells (FIG. 2). Production of several proinflammatory cytokines and mediators of inflammation is decreased, and their action on several target cells diminished. The immune system in turn activates the stress system, primarily by an inflammation-mediated stimulation of the CRH neuron perhaps via the inflammatory cytokines (TNFα, IL-1, IL-6).[27–32] Hence, a full negative feedback cycle exists between the HPA axis and the immune/inflammatory reaction.

Gender Differences in Stress Response and Immune Regulation—Regulation of CRH Gene by Estrogens

Sex differences in the regulation of the stress response in general, and the HPA axis in particular, as well as sexual dimorphism of the immune/inflammatory reaction including susceptibility to autoimmune disease, have been described in various species, including the mouse, rat, and human.[3,4,33–36] These studies have suggested that gonadal steroids interact in a regulatory manner with CNS and peripheral substrates of the stress response, including the HPA axis, and the immune/inflammatory reaction. Estrogens and androgens have been implicated in these differences; however, whether their effects are direct or via estrogen- or androgen-dependent mediators is unclear. The exact site(s) of this interaction and its mechanism(s) are not well understood, but the central role that CRH plays in these functions suggests that this hormone may be a common key point of such regulation.

We recently demonstrated the presence of estrogen-responsive elements in the promoter area of the CRH gene and direct stimulatory estrogen effects on CRH gene expression.[19] This might explain the slight hypercortisolism of females and the preponderance of depressive, anxiety, and eating disorders; Cushing's disease; and autoimmune phenomena in women.

PERIPHERAL CRH AND THE FEMALE REPRODUCTIVE SYSTEM

Ovarian CRH

CRH is also produced at peripheral inflammatory sites, where it acts as a proinflammatory cytokine, and by the Leydig cells of the testis, where it exerts autocrine inhibition of testosterone biosynthesis.[37–42] Because key ovarian functions, such as ovulation and luteolysis, represent aseptic inflammatory responses, and because the theca cell of the ovary is the functional equivalent of the Leydig cell, we explored the CRH presence in the ovary by specific CRH immunohistochemistry of adult cycling female Sprague-Dawley rat ovaries and demonstrated cytoplasmic ir-CRH in theca and stromal cells and in cells within the corpora lutea, at all phases of the estrous cycle. The mobility of the ovarian ir-CRH molecule was similar to that of rat/human CRH by reversed-phase HPLC. Furthermore, we demonstrated the presence of CRH-binding sites in the rat ovary by autoradiography, which revealed CRH receptors primarily in ovarian theca and stroma.[43] By specific binding assay, binding was linear with increasing tissue concentrations, saturable, and of high affinity.

Subsequently to the rat studies, we found that ir-CRH was present also in normal human ovaries. By immunohistochemistry it had a similar distribution to that of rat ovarian ir-CRH.[44] Polycystic ovaries also had ir-CRH in thecal cells; however, CRH was less prominent or completely absent from the stroma or the sparse corpora lutea. Human follicular fluid samples also contained low, but detectable levels of ir-CRH.

The presence of ir-CRH and CRH receptors in rat ovaries, and the presence of ir-CRH in normal human ovaries suggests that this neuropeptide may play a regulatory role in one or more of the various functions of this gonad, such as ovulation and/or luteolysis, perhaps through its proinflammatory properties and/or by participating in the auto/paracrine regulation of steroid biosynthesis.[43,44] Interestingly, ir-CRH was localized in primary oocytes of polycystic but normal ovaries, and this might be related to the increased androgen biosynthesis by the theca and stroma and/or to the oocyte dysfunction of women with this syndrome.[44]

Endometrial CRH

Recently, CRH was localized *in vitro* in both cultured human endometrial epithelial and decidualized stromal cells.[45,46] These findings suggested that CRH should be present *in vivo* in the human endometrium. In a recent study we identified, quantitated, and localized CRH in human endometrial tissue biopsies, which were performed by linear endometrial curettage for diagnostic purposes at all stages of the menstrual cycle. Intense ir-CRH staining was localized in the cytoplasm of cells of the endometrial glands, in endometrial stromal cells exhibiting decidual reaction, and in local immune accessory cells. The presence of CRH in the endometrium, and more specifically in the glandular epithelium, during the proliferative and secretory phases of the menstrual cycle, together with its known proinflammatory properties, suggest that it may participate in the inflammatory-like phenomena of endometrial physiology, such as menstrual shedding, surface epithelium repair, and/or implantation of the blastocyst.[47] The presence of CRH in decidualized stromal cells is in accordance with its previously reported production from *in vitro* decidualized cultured endometrial stromal cells, as well as from the placental decidua.[45,46]

Placental CRH and the HPA Axis in Human Pregnancy

During pregnancy, the plasma concentrations of total and free cortisol steadily increase, reaching their zenith at the third trimester.[48,49] The degree of hypercortisolism in pregnancy is similar to that observed in severe depression and anorexia nervosa or in strenuously exercising athletes. Plasma ACTH concentrations rise in parallel with those of total and free cortisol, but remain within the normal range of nonpregnant women,[50] whereas substantially elevated levels of plasma CRH are observed.[51] This CRH, identical to hypothalamic CRH in structure, immunoreactivity and bioactivity, is synthesized in the placenta, decidua, and fetal membranes.[45,52] CRH-ir rises exponentially as pregnancy advances, peaking during labor, and rapidly falling to low or undetectable levels after parturition.[53–55] Although it appears that to a large extent circulating CRH in pregnancy is bound with a high affinity to the CRH binding protein (CRHbp), which circulates in human plasma and is thought to reduce the bioactivity of placental CRH,[56,57] circulating "free" CRH may be responsible for the hypercortisolism observed in pregnancy. CRHbp concentrations are similar to those of nonpregnant women until late gestation (36 weeks), when they fall to about 1/3 of those of earlier stages of pregnancy and of the nonpregnant state.[58]

The physiological importance of the activation of the hypothalamic-pituitary-adrenal (HPA) axis during pregnancy in humans and other primates is not clearly understood as yet. It has been suggested that placental CRH may be a modulator of both maternal and fetal pituitary-adrenal function during part of pregnancy, and/or that it may participate in fetal maturation and adaptation to intrauterine stress and in the physiological mechanisms of parturition.[59] Recently, Clifton *et al.* found that CRH is a potent vasodilator of the uterine arteries and suggest that it may participate in the regulation of placental blood flow.[60]

In a recent study we investigated the detailed pattern of circulating ir-CRH, ACTH, cortisol, estradiol, and progesterone during the third trimester of pregnancy over 24 hr, in plasma samples drawn serially every 30 min from 22 healthy pregnant women between the 34th and 36th week of gestation.[61] All five hormones were secreted in a pulsatile fashion. There was no apparent circadian rhythm of CRH or estradiol secretion, whereas there was a clear circadian rhythm in plasma ACTH, cortisol, and progesterone secretion, with the latter in reverse phase. These data, taken together with other observations,[62,63] suggest that even though the overall increased activity of the HPA axis in the last trimester of pregnancy is generated by placental CRH, the circadian and pulsatile secretion of ACTH and cortisol is driven, presumably, by another major ACTH-secretagogue, most likely AVP of parvocellular paraventricular nucleus origin.[61]

The HPA Axis in the Postpartum Period

As mentioned above, the increased activity of the HPA axis during the third trimester of human pregnancy might be driven by progressively increasing circulating levels of placental CRH, and gradually decreasing levels of CRH-binding protein. The resetting of the HPA axis and, especially, the recovery of the CRH neuron has not yet been studied in detail during the postpartum period. This period is characterized by an increased vulnerability to psychiatric (postpartum blues, depression, and psychosis) and autoimmune (Hashimoto thyroiditis, rheumatoid arthritis) manifestations, both phenomena compatible with suppressed hypothalamic CRH secretion.[64–66] The development of "postpartum blues" might represent a transient "steroid withdrawal" syndrome based on the fact that, although postpartum cortisol levels may not be lower than normal nonpregnant values, they are lower than values observed in the third trimester of pregnancy.

To investigate the hypothesis that the postpartum period is associated with hypothalamic CRH suppression, we studied prospectively 17 healthy women starting on the 20th week of gestation.[67] In them we performed serial psychometric testing monthly during pregnancy and in the postpartum period, and serial oCRH tests in the postpartum at 3, 6 and 12 weeks. Upon entering the study and, while pregnant, all 17 women were euthymic, whereas in the postpartum period seven women developed the "blues" and one developed depression. The ACTH response to oCRH was markedly blunted at 3 and 6 weeks, but normal at 12 weeks postpartum, whereas the cortisol response was at the upper limit of normal at all three time-points. The relatively high cortisol response at all three time points suggests that postpartum women have hypertrophic adrenal cortices that respond well to the blunted exogenous CRH-induced elevations of plasma ACTH.

These findings are compatible with a suppressed hypothalamic CRH neuron, which gradually recovers, in parallel to a progressive "relative" downsizing of the adrenal cortices. This transient suppression of the CRH neuron was more severe in the women who developed the "blues" or depression than in euthymic women, and is compatible to what is observed in patients with atypical depression or seasonal affective disorder[68] (FIG. 3). This significant central suppression of hypothalamic CRH secretion in the postpartum period might explain the increased vulnerability to psychiatric diseases observed during this period.[64] It might also explain the vulnerability to autoimmune diseases observed in postpartum.[65] One could further test this hypothesis by showing hyporesponsiveness of hypothalamic CRH to inflammatory stimuli, such as interleukin-6 during this period.[27,69] In FIGURE 4 we include a heuristic model of the adaptation of the HPA axis in the non-pregnant, pregnant, and postpartum states.

SUMMARY

The hypothalamic-pituitary-adrenal (HPA) axis and the female reproductive system are intertwined and exhibit a complex relationship. Thus, the HPA axis exerts profound, mostly inhibitory effects, on the reproductive axis, with corticotropin-releasing hormone (CRH) and CRH-induced propiomelanocortin peptides inhibiting hypothalamic GnRH secretion, and with glucocorticoids inhibiting pituitary LH and ovarian estrogen and progesterone secretion and rendering estrogen-target tissues, such as the endometrium, resistant to the gonadal steroid. These effects of the HPA axis are responsible for the "hypothalamic" amenorrhea of stress, depression and eating disorders, and the hypogonadism of Cushing's syndrome. Conversely, estrogen

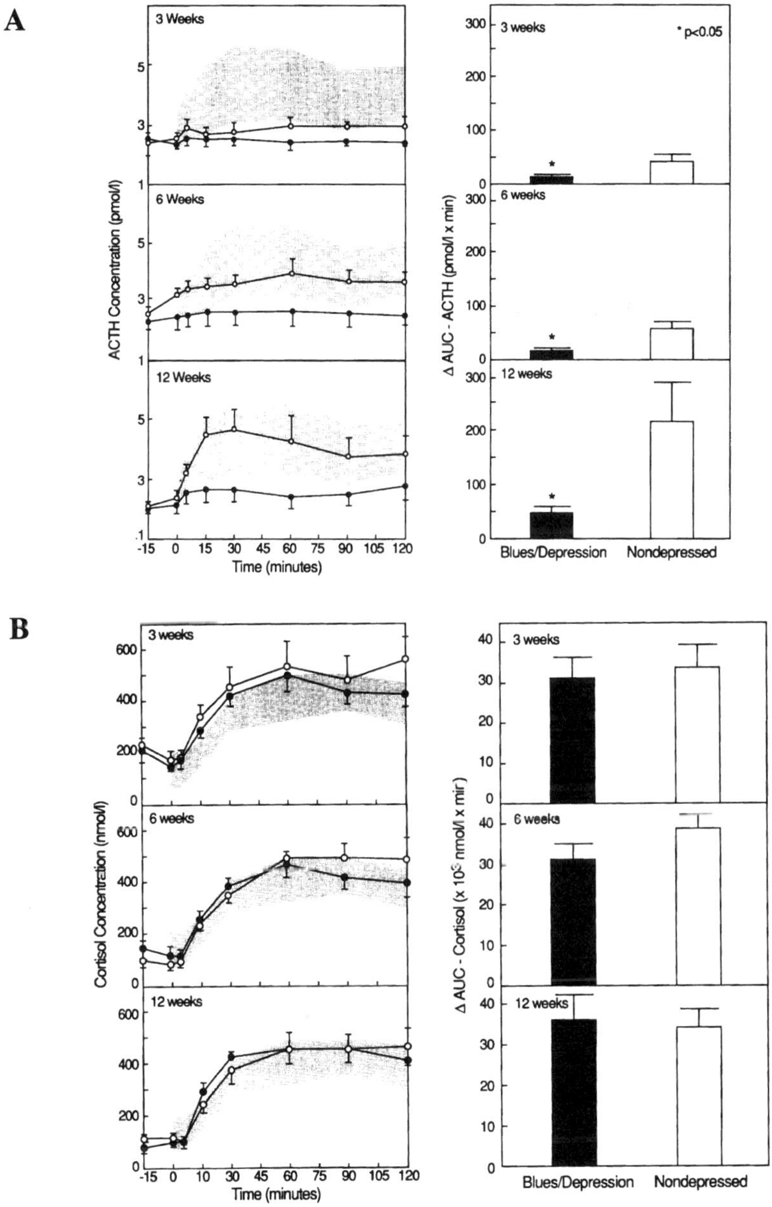

FIGURE 3. *Left panels*: Mean ± SE plasma ACTH and cortisol response to oCRH in postpartum euthymic women (*open circles*) and women with blues/depression (*solid circles*) 3, 6, and 12 weeks after delivery. The grey area includes the mean ± 2 SE values from nonpregnant control women. *Right panels*: Mean ± SE net area under the curve values of plasma ACTH and cortisol in postpartum euthymic women (*white bars*) and women with blues/depression (*black bars*) 3, 6, and 12 weeks after delivery. (Taken from Magiakou *et al.*[67]; used with permission from the *Journal of Clinical Endocrinology and Metabolism.*)

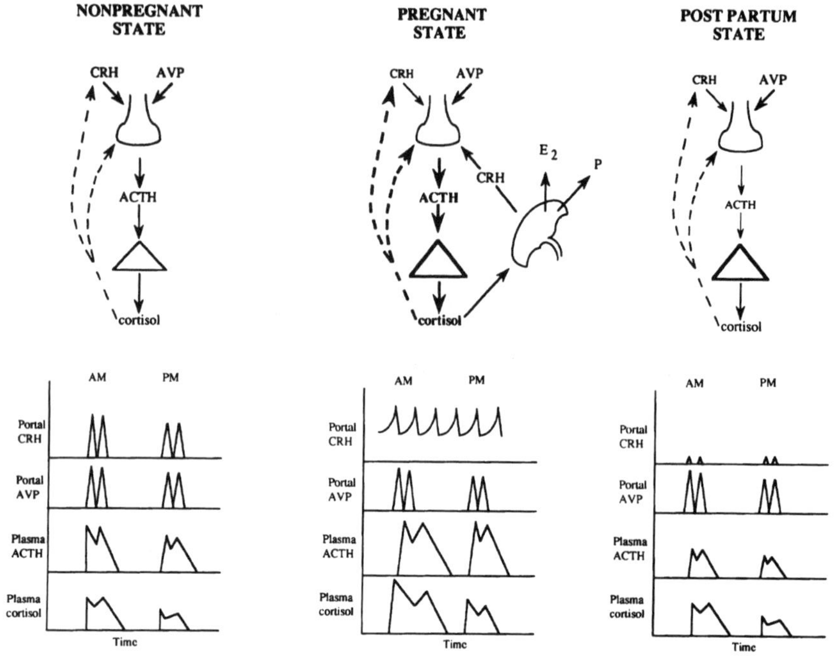

FIGURE 4. Heuristic model of the hypothalamic–pituitary–adrenal axis in the nonpregnant, pregnant, and postpartum state. CRH indicates corticotropin-releasing hormone; AVP, arginine vasopressin; ACTH, corticotropin; E_2, estradiol; P, progesterone.

directly stimulates the CRH gene, which may explain the slight hypercortisolism of females and the preponderance of depressive, anxiety, and eating disorders, as well as Cushing's disease in women. Interestingly, several components of the HPA axis and their receptors are present in reproductive tissues, as autocoid regulators of their various functions. These include ovarian and endometrial CRH, which may participate in the inflammatory processes of the ovary, that is, ovulation and luteolysis, and of the endometrium, that is, implantation and menstruation. Finally, the hypercortisolism of the latter half of pregnancy can be explained by high levels of placenta CRH in plasma. This hypercortisolism causes a transient adrenal suppression in the postpartum period, which may explain the postpartum blues/depression and autoimmune phenomena of this period.

REFERENCES

1. Chrousos, G. P., D. L. Loriaux & P. W. Gold, Eds. 1988. Mechanisms of Physical and Emotional Stress. Advances in Experimental Medicine and Biology. Vol. 245. Plenum Press. New York.

2. CHROUSOS, G. P. & P. W. GOLD. 1992. The concepts of stress and stress system disorders: Overview of physical and behavioral homeostasis. JAMA **267**(9): 1244–1252.
3. GOLD, P. W., F. GOODWIN & G. P. CHROUSOS. 1988. Clinical and biochemical manifestations of depression: Relationship to the neurobiology of stress, part 1. N. Engl. J. Med. **319:** 348–353.
4. GOLD, P. W., F. GOODWIN & G. P. CHROUSOS. 1988. Clinical and biochemical manifestations of depression: Relationship to the neurobiology of stress, part 2. N. Engl. J. Med. **319:** 413–420.
5. CUMMINGS, S., R. ELDER, J. ELLIS & A. LINDALL. 1983. Corticotropin-releasing factor immunoreactivity is widely distributed within the central nervous system of the rat: An immunohistochemical study. J. Neurosci. **3:** 1355–1368.
6. SWANSON, L. W., P. E. SAWCHENKO, J. RIVIER & W. W. VALE. 1983. Organization of ovine corticotropin-releasing factor immunoreactive cells and fibers in the rat brain: An immunohistochemical study. Neuroendocrinology **36:** 165–186.
7. SWANSON, L. W. & P. E. SAWCHENKO. 1983. Hypothalamic integration: Organization of the paraventricular and supraoptic nuclei. Ann. Rev. Neurosci. **6:** 269–324.
8. DESOUZA, E. B., T. R. INSEL, M. H. PERRIN, J. RIVIER, W. W. VALE & M. KUHAR. 1985. Corticotropin-releasing factor receptors are widely distributed within the rat central nervous system: An autoradiographic study. J. Neurosci. **5:** 3189–3203.
9. DUNN, A. J. & C. W. BERRIDGE. 1990. Physiological and behavioral responses to corticotropin-releasing factor administration: Is CRF a mediator of anxiety or stress responses? Brain Res. Rev. **15:** 17–100.
10. NAUTA, W. J. H. & M. FEIRTAG. 1986. Fundamental Neuroanatomy. Freeman. New York.
11. MASTORAKOS, G. & G. P. CHROUSOS. 1996. Adrenal androgens. *In* Reproductive Endocrinology, Surgery, and Technology. E. Y. Adashi, J. A. Rock & Z. Rosenwaks, Eds.: 1539–1553. Raven Press. New York.
12. PARKER, L. N., E. T. LIFRAK & W. D. ODELL. 1983. A 60,000 molecular weight human pituitary glycopeptide stimulates adrenal androgen secretion. Endocrinology **113:** 2092–2096.
13. KAMILARIS, T. & G. P. CHROUSOS. 1989. Adrenal Diseases. *In* Diagnostic Endocrinology, W. T. Moore & R. Eastman, Eds.: 79–109. B. C. Decker, Inc. Toronto, CA.
14. UDELSMAN, R., W. T. GALLUCCI, J. RAMP, *et al.* 1986. Adaptation during surgical stress: A reevaluation of the role of glucocorticoids. J. Clin. Invest. **77:** 1377–1381.
15. YEN, S. S. C. 1978. The human menstrual cycle. *In* Reproductive Endocrinology. S. S. C. Yen & R. B. Jaffe, Eds.: 126. Saunders. Philadelphia, PA.
16. MACADAMS, M. R., R. H. WHITE & B. E. CHIPPS. 1986. Reduction in serum testosterone levels during chronic glucocorticoid therapy. Ann. Intern. Med. **140:** 648–651.
17. RABIN, D., P. W. GOLD, A. MARGIORIS, *et al.* 1988. Stress and reproduction: Interactions between the stress and reproductive axis. *In* Mechanisms of Physical and Emotional Stress. G. P. Chrousos, D. L. Loriaux & P. W. Gold, Eds.: 377–387. Plenum Press. New York.
18. RIVIER, C., J. RIVIER & W. W. VALE. 1986. Stress-induced inhibition of reproductive function: Role of endogenous corticotropin releasing factor. Science **231:** 607–609.
19. VAMVAKOPOULOS, N. C. & G. P. CHROUSOS. 1993. Evidence of direct estrogen regulation of human corticotropin releasing hormone gene expression: Potential implications for the sexual dimorphism of the stress response and immune/inflammatory reaction. J. Clin. Invest. **92:** 1896–1902.
20. DIEGUEZ, C., M. D. PAGE & M. F. SCANLON. 1988. Growth hormone neuroregulation and its alterations in disease states. Clin. Endocrinol. (Oxford) **28:** 109–143.
21. RIVIER, C. & W. W. VALE. 1985. Involvement of corticotropin releasing factor and somatostatin in stress-induced inhibition of growth hormone secretion in the rat. Endocrinology **117:** 2478–2482.

22. BURGUERA, B., C. MURUAIS, A. PENALVA, *et al.* 1990. Dual and selective action of glucocorticoids upon basal and stimulated growth hormone release in man. Neuroendocrinology **51:** 51–58.
23. UNTERMAN, T. G. & L. S. PHILLIPS. 1985. Glucocorticoids effects on somatomedins and somatomedin inhibitors. J. Clin. Endocrinol. Metab. **61:** 618–626.
24. MAGIAKOU, M. A., G. MASTORAKOS, M. T. GOMEZ, S. R. ROSE & G. P. CHROUSOS. 1994. Suppressed spontaneous and stimulated growth hormone secretion in patients with Cushing's disease before and after surgical cure. J. Clin. Endocrinol. Metab. **78:** 131–137.
25. BENKER, G., M. RAIDA, T. OLBRICHT, *et al.* 1990. TSH secretion in Cushing's syndrome: Relation to glucocorticoid excess, diabetes, goiter, and the "sick euthyroid syndrome." Clin. Endocrinol. **33:** 777–786.
26. DUICK, D. S. & H. W. WAHNER. 1979. Thyroid axis in patients with Cushing's syndrome. Arch. Intern. Med. **139:** 767–772.
27. MASTORAKOS, G., G. P. CHROUSOS & J. S. WEBER. 1993. Recombinant interleukin 6 activates the hypothalamic–pituitary–adrenal axis in humans. J. Clin. Endocrinol. Metab. **77:** 1690–1694.
28. BERNARDINI, R., T. C. KAMILARIS, A. E. CALOGERO, *et al.* 1990. Interactions between tumor necrosis factor-alpha, hypothalamic corticotropin-releasing hormone, and adrenocorticotropin secretion in the rat. Endocrinology **126:** 2876–2881.
29. BESEDOVSKY, H. O. & A. DEL REY. 1992. Immune-neuroendocrine circuits: Intergrative role of cytokines. Front. Neuroendocrinol. **13:** 61–94.
30. BUSBRIDGE, N. J. & A. B. GROSSMAN. 1991. Stress and the single cytokine: Interleukin modulation of the pituitary-adrenal axis. Mol. Cell. Endocrinol. **82:** C209.
31. NAITOH, Y., J. FUKATA, T. TOMINAGA, *et al.* 1988. Interleukin-6 stimulates the secretion of adrenocorticotropin hormone in conscious freely moving rats. Biochem. Biophys. Res. Commun. **155:** 1459–1063.
32. SAPOLSKY, R., C. RIVIER, G. YAMAMOTO, *et al.* 1987. Interleukin-1 stimulates the secretion of hypothalamic corticotropin releasing factor. Science **238:** 522–524.
33. HALEEM, D. J., G. KENNETT & G. CURZON. 1990. Hippocampal 5-hydroxytryptamine synthesis is greater in female rats than in males and more decreased by the 5-HT1A agonist 8-OH-DPAT. J. Neural. Transm. Gen. Sect. **79:** 93–101.
34. DEVRIES, G. J., J. P. C. DEBRUIN, H. B. M. UYLINGS & M. A. CORNER, Eds. 1984. Progress in Brain Research. Vol. **61:** 3–508. Elsevier. Amsterdam.
35. DEVRIES, G. J. 1990. Sex differences in neurotransmitter systems. J. Neuroendocrinol. **2:** 1–13.
36. AHIMA, R. S., A. N. L. LAWSON, S. Y. S. OSEI & R. E. HARLAN. 1992. Sexual dimorphism in regulation of type II corticosteroid receptor immunoreactivity in the rat hippocampus. Endocrinology **131:** 1409–1416.
37. KARALIS, K., H. SANO, J. REDWINE, S. LISTWAK, R. L. WILDER & G. P. CHROUSOS. 1991. Autocrine or paracrine inflammatory actions of corticotropin releasing hormone in vitro. Science **254:** 421–423.
38. CROFFORD, L. J., H. SANO, K. KARALIS, *et al.* 1993. Corticotropin releasing hormone in synovial fluids and tissues of patients with rheumatoid arthritis and osteoarthritis. J. Immunol. **151:** 1–10.
39. YOON, D. J., C. SKLAR & R. DAVID. 1988. Presence of immunoreactive corticotropin releasing factor in rat testis. Endocrinology **122:** 759–761.
40. AUDHYA, T., C. S. HOLLANDER, D. H. SCHLESINGER & B. HUTCHINSON. 1989. Structural characterization and localization of corticotropin releasing factor in the testis. Biochem. Biophys. Acta **995:** 10–16.
41. FABRI, A., J. C. TINAJERO & M. L. DUFAU. 1990. Corticotropin releasing factor is produced

by rat Leydig cells and has a major local antireproductive role in the testis. Endocrinology **127:** 1541–1543.

42. ULISSE, S., A. FABBRI & M. L. DUFAU. 1989. Corticotropin releasing factor receptors and actions in rat Leydig cells. J. Biol. Chem. **264:** 2156–2163.
43. MASTORAKOS, G., E. L. WEBSTER, T. C. FRIEDMAN & G. P. CHROUSOS. 1993. Immunoreactive corticotropin releasing hormone and its binding sites in the rat ovary. J. Clin. Invest. **92:** 961–968.
44. MASTORAKOS, G., C. D. SCOPA, A. VRYONIDOU, *et al.* 1994. Presence of immunoreactive corticotropin releasing hormone in normal and polycystic human ovaries. J. Clin. Endocrinol. Metab. **79:** 1191–1197.
45. PETRAGLIA, F., S. TABANELLI, M. C. GALASSI, G. C. GARUTI, A. C. MANCINI, A. R. GENAZZANI & E. GURPIDE. 1992. Human decidua and in vitro decidualized endometrial stromal cells at term contain immunoreactive corticotropin-releasing factor (CRF) and CRF messenger ribonucleic acid. J. Clin. Endocrinol. Metab. **74:** 1427–1431.
46. MAKRIGIANNAKIS, A., E. ZOUMAKIS, A. N. MARGIORIS, P. THEODOROPOULOS, C. STOURNARAS & A. GRAVANIS. 1995. The corticotropin releasing hormone in normal and tumoral epithelial cells of human endometrium. J. Clin. Endocrinol. Metab. **80:** 185–189.
47. MASTORAKOS, G., C. D. SCOPA, L. C. KAO, *et al.* 1996. Presence of immunoreactive corticotropin releasing hormone in human endometrium. J. Clin. Endocrinol. Metab. **81:** 1046–1050.
48. ROSENTHAL, H. E., W. R. SLAUNWHITE, JR. & A. A. SANDBERG. 1969. Transcortin: A corticosteroid-binding protein of plasma. X. Cortisol and progesterone interplay and unbound levels of these steroids in pregnancy. J. Clin. Endocrinol. Metab. **29:** 352–367.
49. ABOU-SAMRA, A. B., M. PUGEAT, H. DECHAUD, *et al.* 1984. Increased plasma concentrations of *N*-terminal β-lipotropin and unbound cortisol during pregnancy. Clin. Endocrinol. (Oxford) **20:** 221–228.
50. LAATIKAINEN, T., T. VIRTANEN, I. RAISANEN & K. SALMINEN. 1987. Immunoreactive corticotropin releasing factor and corticotropin in plasma during pregnancy, labor and puerperium. Neuropeptides **10:** 343–353.
51. GOLAND, R. S., S. L. WARDLAW, R. I. STARK, L. S. BROWN & A. G. FRANTZ. 1986. High levels of corticotropin-releasing hormone immunoreactivity in maternal and fetal plasma during pregnancy. J. Clin. Endocrinol. Metab. **63:** 1199–1203.
52. GRINO, M., G. P. CHROUSOS & A. N. MARGIORIS. 1987. The corticotropin releasing hormone gene is expressed in human placenta. Biochem. Biophys. Res. Commun. **148:** 1208–1214.
53. SASAKI, A., S. OSAMU, A. N. MARGIORIS, *et al.* 1987. Immunoreactive corticotropin releasing hormone in human plasma during pregnancy labour and delivery. J. Clin. Endocrinol. Metab. **64:** 224–229.
54. CAMPBELL, E. A., E. A. LINTON, C. D. A. WOLFE, P. R. SCRAGGS, M. T. JONES & P. J. LOWRY. 1987. Plasma corticotropin releasing hormone concentrations during pregnancy and parturition. J. Clin. Endocrinol. Metab. **64:** 1054–1059.
55. SMITH, R., J. CUBIS, M. BRINSMEAD, *et al.* 1990. Mood changes, obstetric experience and alterations in plasma cortisol, beta-endorphin and corticotrophin releasing hormone during pregnancy and the puerperium. J. Psychosomat. Res. **34:** 53–69.
56. ORTH, D. N. & C. D. MOUNT. 1987. Specific high-affinity binding protein for human corticotrophin-releasing hormone in normal human plasma. Biochem. Biophys. Res. Commun. **143:** 411–417.
57. POTTER, E., D. P. BEHAN, W. H. FISCHER, E. A. LINTON, P. J. LOWRY & W. W. VALE. 1991. Cloning and characterization of the cDNAs for human and rat corticotropin-releasing factor-binding proteins. Nature **349:** 423–426.

58. LINTON, E. A., A. V. PERKINS, R. J. WOODS, F. EBEN, C. D. A. WOLFE, D. P. BEHAN, E. POTTER, W. W. VALE & P. J. LOWRY. 1993. Corticotropin-releasing hormone-binding protein (CRH-BP): Plasma levels decrease during the third trimester of normal human pregnancy. J. Clin. Endocrinol. Metab. **76:** 260–262.
59. GOLAND, R. S., I. M. CONWELL, W. B. WARREN & S. L. WARDLAW. 1992. Placental corticotropin-releasing hormone and pituitary–adrenal function during pregnancy. Neuroendocrinology **56:** 742–749.
60. CLIFTON, V. L., M. A. READ, I. M. LEITCH, *et al.* 1994. Corticotropin-releasing-hormone-induced vasodilation in the human fetal placental circulation. J. Clin. Endocrinol. Metab. **79:** 666–669.
61. MAGIAKOU, M. A., G. MASTORAKOS, D. RABIN, *et al.* 1996. Placental CRH secretion and the maternal hypothalamic–pituitary–adrenal axis in human pregnancy. Clin. Endocrinol. (Oxford) **44:** 419–428.
62. SCHULTE, H. M., D. WEISNER & B. ALLOLIO. 1990. The corticotrophin releasing hormone test in late pregnancy: Lack of adrenocorticotrophin and cortisol response. Clin. Endocrinol. (Oxford) **33:** 99–106.
63. GOLAND, R. S., S. JOZAK & I. CONWELL. 1994. Placental corticotropin-releasing hormone and the hypercortisolism of pregnancy. Am. J. Obstet. Gynecol. **171:** 1287–1291.
64. DAVIDSON, J. & E. ROBERTSON. 1985. A follow-up study of postpartum illness, 1946–1978. Acta Psychiatr. **71:** 451–457.
65. LIVOLSI, V. A. 1993. Postpartum thyroiditis—the pathology slowly unravels (editorial). Am. J. Clin. Pathol. **100:** 193–195.
66. CHROUSOS, G. P. 1995. The hypothalamic–pituitary–adrenal axis and immune-mediated inflammation. N. Engl. J. Med. **332:** 1351–1360.
67. MAGIAKOU, M. A., G. MASTORAKOS, D. RABIN, B. BUBBERT, P. W. GOLD & G. P. CHROUSOS. 1996. Hypothalamic CRH suppression during the postpartum period: Implications for the increase of psychiatric manifestations in this period. J. Clin. Endocrinol. Metab. **81:** 1912–1917.
68. GOLD, P. W., D. L. LORIAUX, A. ROY, *et al.* 1986. Responses to corticotropin-releasing-hormone in the hypercortisolism of depression and Cushing's disease: Pathophysiologic and diagnostic implications. N. Engl. J. Med. **314:** 1329–1335.
69. MASTORAKOS, G., J. S. WEBER, M. A. MAGIAKOU, H. GUNN & G. P. CHROUSOS. 1994. Hypothalamic–pituitary–adrenal axis activation and stimulation of systemic vasopressin secretion by recombinant interleukin-6 in humans: Potential implications for the syndrome of inappropriate vasopressin secretion. J. Clin. Endocrinol. Metab. **79:** 934–939.

Adrenarche

JOHN PAPADIMAS[a]

Department of Endocrinology
University of Thessaloniki
Thessaloniki, Greece

INTRODUCTION

Adrenarche occurs at the beginning of secretion by the adrenal glands of increased amounts of androgens in normal girls and boys between 6 and 8 years of age. This hormonal phenomenon definitely occurs before puberty and in the absence of increased ACTH or cortisol secretion. It is accompanied clinically by the appearance of pubic and axillary hair and by a transient and slight acceleration of bone maturation and growth.

MECHANISM AND ETIOLOGY OF ADRENARCHE

The conversion of 21-carbon steroids to 19-carbon androgens in the adrenals, and particularly by the zona reticularis, the step characteristic of adrenarche, is mediated by the enzyme C_{17-20} desmolase (FIG. 1). The main androgen of the zona reticularis is DHEA, with a secretion rate of approximately 25 mg/day. Most of the DHEA circulates as sulfate. Another important adrenal androgen is androstenedione (Δ_4), whereas testosterone (T) is synthesized by the adrenal cortex in very small amounts. Reversible reduction of the 17-keto group of Δ_4 to T is catalyzed by the non-P_{450} enzyme 17β-hydroxysteroid oxidoreductase, the congenital absence of which results in lack of external genital masculinization at birth. In conclusion, adrenal androgens include mainly DHEA and DHEA-S, Δ_4, 11β-OHΔ_4, and T in small amounts (FIG. 1).

Several investigators[1,2] have found that these adrenal androgens increase between the ages of 6 and 8 years in both sexes, before the increase in FSH and LH concentrations and while ACTH and cortisol values remain stable[3] (FIGS. 2 and 3). Dexamethasone-suppressible plasma values of Δ_4 have also been found to increase during adrenarche.[1]

The possibility of altered sensitivity to ACTH of adrenal cells has been investigated as a potential factor in the adrenarche. In fact, an increased DHEA response to an acute synthetic ACTH stimulation with an unchanged cortisol response has been reported in normal adrenarchal and pubertal children.[5] Epidermal growth factor (EGF) was also reported to stimulate DHEA-S secretion by human fetal adrenal cells *in vitro*. However, an investigation of normal children showed a decrease in urinary excretion of EGF after the age of two years.[6]

Intrinsic adrenal factors have also been suggested to be responsible for adrenarche

[a]Address for correspondence: Dr. John Papadimas, 76 Mitropoleos St., 54622 Thessaloniki, Greece.

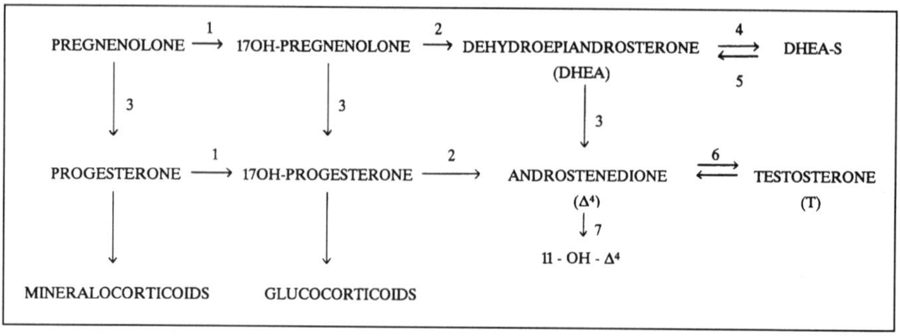

FIGURE 1. Human adrenocortical metabolic pathways. Enzymes: (1) 17α-hydroxylase, (2) C_{17-20} desmolase, (3) 3β-hydroxysteroid dehydrogenase-isomerase, (4) steroid sulfotransferase, (5) steroid sulfatase, (6) 17β-hydroxysteroid oxidoreductase, (7) 11-hydroxylase.

and are related to histologic observations of the zona reticularis. This zona is known to be the major source of adrenal androgens. Increased amounts of these androgens and cortisol have been shown in the zona reticularis compared to the zona fasciculata.[7] The zona reticularis has also been found to be the major site of DHEA sulfation in the human adrenals.[8] Based on these findings, it has been postulated that a high concentration of cortisol in the adrenal portal blood supply, which flows from the cortex toward the medulla, may stimulate zona reticularis cells to synthesize androgens and cause the adrenarche to occur.[9]

In castrated and hypophysectomized chimpanzees, it was shown that ACTH replacement therapy was adequate for maintenance of normal cortisol but not sufficient for normal DHEA or DHEA-S production. This finding is consistent with the existence of a non-ACTH pituitary substance, as a regulator of adrenal androgen production.[10] In fact, a non-ACTH human fetal pituitary factor was shown to stimulate the DHEA-S secretion by human fetal adrenal glands.[11] Similar findings have also been reported as a factor for human adult pituitary, that is, causing the production of adrenal androgens. This was called cortical androgen-stimulating hormone (CASH) and was suggested to be identical with a portion of the joining peptide of pituitary POMC.[12]

THE BIOLOGIC ROLE OF ADRENARCHE

Adrenarche in normal conditions occurs before puberty and may play a role in the activation of GnRH-gonadotrophin axis and the acceleration of the pubertal process. It has been suggested that adrenal androgen secretion causes the decrease in the serum concentrations of sex hormone-binding globulin (SHBG) seen in normal boys and, therefore, accelerates the pubertal process by causing an increase in free-testosterone levels.[13] This increase of the biologically active free testosterone causes in boys and girls a small but significant growth spurt between 6 and 8 years of age. This growth spurt is due to a transient increase in long-bone growth, which thereafter resumes a preadrenarchal rate until the beginning of puberty.[14]

In conclusion, adrenarche may cause a transient acceleration of bone growth and maturation and the appearance of axillary and pubic hair and may also serve as a permissive factor in puberty but does not seem to be necessary for the initiation of normal puberty.

REFERENCES

1. Forest, M. 1989. Physiological changes in circulating androgens. *In* Androgens in Childhood. M. Forest, Ed.: 104. Karger. Basel.
2. Zemel, B. & S. Katz. 1986. The contribution of adrenal and gonadal androgens to the growth in height of adolescent males. Am. J. Phys. Anthropol. **71:** 479.
3. Apter, D., A. Pakkerinenen, G. Hammond, *et al.* 1979. Adrenocortical function in puberty. Acta Paediatr. Scand. **68:** 599.
4. Ranke, M. & W. Gupta. 1982. Responsiveness of cortisol and DHEA to ACTH in children. Horm. Res. **16:** 32.
5. Sklar, C., S. Kaplan & M. Grumbach. 1981. Lack of effect of estrogens on adrenal androgen secretion in children and adolescents. Clin. Endocrinol. **14:** 311.
6. Herman, B., A. Arthur-Smith, M. A. Hammock, *et al.* 1988. Ontogeny of β-endorphin and cortisol in the plasma of children and adolescents. J. Clin. Endocrinol. Metab. **67:** 186.
7. Maroulis, G. & G. Abraham. 1980. Concentration of androgens and cortisol in the zones of the adrenal cortex. *In* Adrenal Androgens. A. Genazzani, Ed.: 49. Raven. New York.
8. Kennerson, A., D. McDonald & J. Adams. 1983. DHA sulfotransferase localization in human adrenal glands: A light and electron microscopic study. J. Clin. Endocrinol. Metab. **86:** 786.
9. Anderson, D. 1980. The adrenal androgen-stimulating hormone does not exist. Lancet **2:** 454.
10. Albertson, B., W. Hobson, B. Burnett, *et al.* 1984. Dissociation of cortisol and adrenal androgen secretion in the hypophysectomized ACTH-replaced chimpanzee. J. Clin. Endocrinol. Metab. **59:** 13.
11. Brubaker, P., *et al.* 1982. Corticotropic peptides in the human fetal pituitary. Endocrinology **111:** 1150.
12. Parker, L., *et al.* 1989. Human adrenal gland cortical androgen-stimulating hormone (CASH) is identical with a portion of the joining peptide of pituitary POMC (Abstract 299). *In* Program and Abstracts of the 71st Annual Meeting of the Endocrine Society (Seattle, WA) p. 97.
13. Maruyama, Y., N. Aoki, Y. Suzuki, *et al.* 1987. SHBG, testosterone, estradiol and DHA in prepuberty and puberty. Acta Endocrinol. (Copenhagen) **114:** 60.
14. Molinari, L., R. Largo & A. Prader. 1980. Analysis of the growth spurt at age seven. Helv. Paediatr. Acta **35:** 325.

Modifications of Growth Hormone Secretion during Female Puberty

J. E. TOUBLANC

Hôpital St. Vincent de Paul
82 avenue Denfert-Rochereau
75014 Paris France

INTRODUCTION

The acquisition of secondary sexual characteristics, through which we recognize the onset of puberty, leads to reproductive maturity. These phenomena are largely dependent on sex steroids.

Growth hormone (GH) is mainly responsible for the pubertal growth spurt, which is also a secondary sexual characteristic because it shows sexual dimorphism. The secretion of GH and insulin-like growth factor-1 (IGF-1) is modified during puberty under the influence of sex steroids.

Here, we review these physiological events and also provide information on some pathologic conditions.

PHYSIOLOGIC BACKGROUND

GH is synthesized by the somatotroph cells of the pituitary gland as a pre-growth hormone, a 217-amino-acid molecule. Subsequent cleavage leads to the classical form of GH of 191 amino acids (21.5K daltons). A smaller form with a deletion of 15 amino acids is due to alternative splicing of GH pre-messenger RNA (mRNA).[1]

GH circulates in both free and bound forms, the main binding protein being identical to the extracellular domain of the GH receptor.[2,3] A second site on the receptor permits homodimerization and signal transduction through the membrane.[4]

The binding protein activity increases just before puberty and continues to increase throughout puberty until a maximal level is reached in young adulthood.[5,6]

REGULATION OF GH SECRETION

The secretion of GH is possible through the balanced equilibrium in the secretion of two hormones: One is stimulatory, growth hormone releasing hormone (GHRH), and other is inhibitory, somatotropin release inhibiting hormone (SRIH) or growth hormone inhibiting hormone (GHIH) or somatostatin (SS) (see FIG. 1).[7]

GHRH is synthesized in the hypothalamic arcuate and ventromedial nuclei. Only

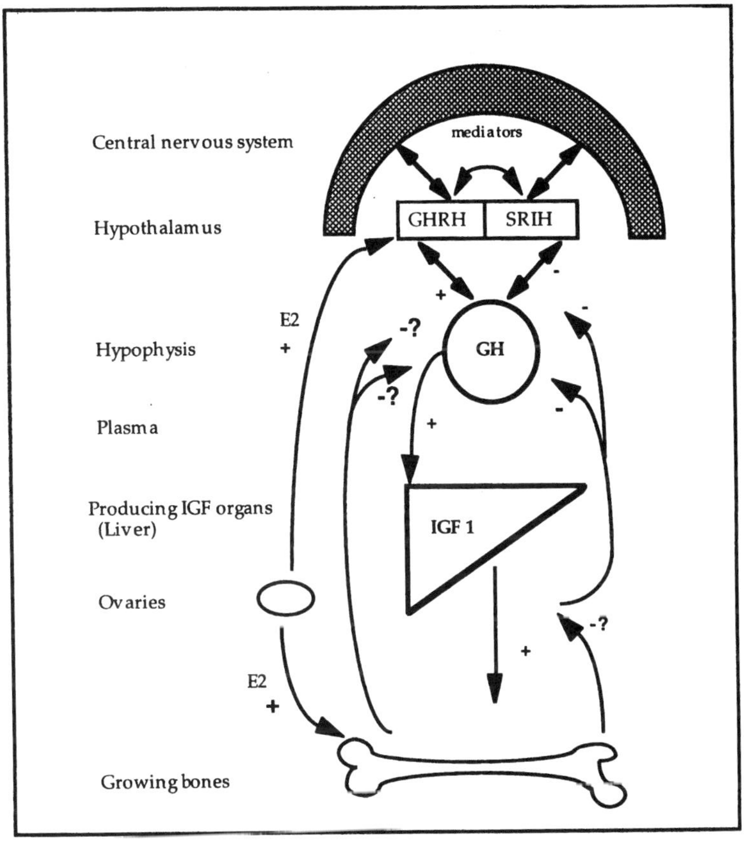

FIGURE 1. Regulatory system for GH secretion (based on the work of M. B. Ranke and P. Haber[7]).

a few scattered cells can be detected in the lateral basal hypothalamus and paraventricular dorso- and ventromedial nuclei.[8] Additional sites of GHRH production are the placenta, small intestine, and pancreas; rarely, paraneoplastic secretions have been reported. SRIH is produced in the periventricular and amygdaloid nuclei of the medial basal hypothalamus. SRIH-immunoreactive axons are found in the ventrolateral part of the nucleus area containing GHRH-synthesizing cells.[9] There is morphological evidence of connections between SRIH-positive axon varicosities and GHRH-producing neurons in this part of the hypothalamus. Some peripheral organs could also produce SRIH and these include components of the gastrointestinal or urinary tracts.[8]

Axons from GHRH- and SRIH-containing neurons terminate in the median eminence. This site is close to the fenestrated capillaries of the primary plexus of the hypophyseal portal system.[8] In this way, both hormones can reach the somatrophic cells of the pituitary gland. The pulsatile pattern of GH secretion is due to episodic, coordinated secretion of GHRH and SRIH. In the rat, both hormones have a secretory frequency of and pulse every 3–4 hours and are virtually 180° out of phase with each other.[10,11] The amount of GHRH determines the amplitude of GH secretory episodes, while the pattern of SRIH secretions determine the duration of the peaks.[12,13] GHRH and SRIH influence each other's secretions through bidirectional synapses between the neurons that produce them.[14] GHRH stimulates SRIH secretion,[15] while SRIH inhibits GHRH secretion.[16] Combination of both hormones could maximize the response of GH by somatotrophic cells.[17] The oscillatory control of these rhythmic GHRH and SRIH patterns may be at the hypothalamic level or may be influenced by higher neural mechanisms[18] and by GH itself.[19]

At least in the rat, there are sexual differences in the GH surges: In males the peaks are less numerous but of greater amplitude and the GH baseline is low, while in females there are more peaks of a lower amplitude combined with a high GH baseline. Both GHRH and SRIH are regulated by androgens, and the mRNAs of these neuropeptides are higher in males than in females mainly at the first stages of development, although these differences decrease afterwards.[20] However, testosterone is required to achieve and maintain the male pattern of GH secretion post pubertally.[21] Conversely, estradiol has a negative influence on SRIH, but does not increase the concentrations of GHRH and SRIH mRNAs.[22] *In vitro,* gender differences appear to exist[23,24] between testosterone, which enhances the production of GH by pituitary cells,[25,26] and estradiol, which increases the number of these cells[27] and the production of GH mRNA.[28] All of these actions put together induce in the pubertal period a gender-specific circulating GH profile.[8]

OTHER CONTROLS OF GH SECRETION

The amino acids that are used in stimulatory tests of GH secretion (arginine, ornithine) increase GH levels through direct actions on GHRH secretion.[29] Different types of short or long loops exist between IGF-1 and GH or GHRH–SRIH secretions (FIG. 1). One loop is at the hypothalamic level: inhibition of GHRH by IGF-1[16] and, conversely, stimulation of SRIH.[30] Another one is at the pituitary level with IGF-1 inhibiting GH cells in culture.[31] IGF-1 may come from the circulation or be produced locally in the pituitary.[32]

GH is capable of inhibiting its own production[18] through direct action on both hypothalamic regulatory hormones (GHRH-SRIH) and also via intermediate metabolic pathways.[33]

GH PHYSIOLOGY IN THE PUBERTAL PERIOD

The relationship between the modifications of GH and puberty has been facilitated by advances in various fields: miniaturization of samples, the possibility of harmless repeated sampling,[34] and utilization of sophisticated methods of analysis of several samples in order to describe GH spontaneous secretion variations.[35,36]

Two categories of these methods have been used. The first evaluate the pulsatile pattern of GH secretion: among them, CLUSTER, DETECT, PULSAR, ULTRA, and CYCLE DETECTOR (reviewed in Ref. 37). The ability of detecting the pulses is directly related to the frequency of the samples; decreasing the intervals between samples also decreases the accuracy of these methods. The second category is known as deconvolution analysis or convolution modeling.[38] This method appreciates and analyzes different parameters of GH secretion: the bursts of GH secretion by the frequency of occurrence, the mass of hormone released, the rate of hormone secretion and the duration of the secretory processes. Half-life and estimates of GH production can be calculated from the resultant data. Accuracy of these methods has been demonstrated by comparison with direct measures of these parameters.[8]

PUBERTAL GROWTH SPURT

As soon as elevated concentrations of estradiol (E_2) appear in girls, a change in growth velocity is observed between 11 and 12 years, which is different than boys, in whom the pubertal growth spurt occurs two years later between 13 and 14 years.[34] The size of the pubertal growth spurt is not much different in boys than in girls; at the very most, 2 cm less is observed in girls. Girls grow less after their pubertal growth spurt than boys. At least the main difference for the final height is due to the two more years of prepubertal growth observed in boys after the onset of puberty, which added to the 2-cm difference of the growth spurt represents the difference in mean final height between the sexes. When related to pubertal stages, the growth spurt occurs in girls between stages P3 and P4, and when menarche appears at least 95% of the final height has been attained.

TABLE 1. GH Plasma Concentration (Day vs. Night) in Healthy Girls of Normal Height[a]

Group of Children				GH Values			
				Mean (μg/l)			
Age (years)	(*n*)	Height	Stage of Puberty	Day	Night	Mean Peak Amplitude	Number of Peaks
7.2–7.9	2	Normal	1	0.90	4.18	56.8	6.0
10.8–12.7	4		2	0.76	3.22	26.1	6.0
12.6–12.8	3		3	4.66	8.13	120.4	6.0
13.3–14.6	4		4 – m	5.50	9.11	123.8	9.5
12.6–14.5	10		4 + m	3.95	7.53	98.6	8.5
12.9–14.8	10		5	2.68	4.36	62.6	8.0

NOTE: Mode of sampling was discrete sampling at 10-min intervals. The sampling took place over 6 hours (1200–1800 hours)[45] or 9 hours (2100–0600 hours).[46] Mode of analysis, pulsar: G: 3.8, 2.7, 7.9, 1.5, 1.2.

[a]Authors: Delamarre-Van de Waal *et al.*[45] (1991) and Wennink *et al.*[46] (1991).

TABLE 2. GH Plasma Concentrations (5–12 hr) in Healthy Girls of Normal or Short Stature

Author	Mode of Sampling (Interval)	Time (hr)	Mode of Analysis	Group of Children: Age (years)	Group of Children: (*n*)	Group of Children: Height	Group of Children: Stage of Puberty	GH Values: Mean (μg/l)	GH Values: Sum of Peak Amplitude	
Edge *et al.* (1990)	Continuous integrated (15 min)	12 (night)	Pulsar G: 3.2, 2.6, 1.9, 1.5, 1.2	(9–21)	34					
								4.0	32 ± 4	
				4	17	1	9.1 ± 2.9	91 ± 23		
				3		2; 3	5.5	51 ± 8		
				8		4; 5				
								Mean (ng/ml)	Mean Peak Amplitude	Number of Peaks
Miller *et al.*[41] (1982)	Discrete sampling (20 min)	6 (09–15)[a]	GH peak GH value, ≥ 5 ng/ml		12		1	3.27 ± 0.34	12.3 ± 1.7	1.9 ± 0.27
					1		2	1.9	10.6	2.0
					7		3; 5	3.5 ± 0.32	12.7 ± 1.7	2.1 ± 0.38
					3		Adult	2.3 ± 0.99	10.3 ± 2.6	1.3 ± 0.33
								Mean	AUC	
Garnier *et al.*[43] (1988)	Discrete sampling (20 min)	7; 9 (9/10–18)[b]	AUC[a] mean				1	8 ± 2.8	1786 ± 788	
					19				2263 ± 990	
								9.7 ± 2.95	(653 ± 4048)	
					16		2; 3		(589 ± 5562)	

								GH Values		
								Mean (μg/l)	Mean Peak Amplitude	Number of Peaks
Rose *et al.*[44] (1991)	Discrete sampling (20 min)	12	Trapezoid x, 36 values pulse: 20% increase of preceding nadir	5; 18	122	Normal	1 early	2.8 ± 1.3	7.0 ± 3.7	4.5 ± 1.5
							1 late	4.2 ± 1.8	10.7 ± 4.3	3.9 ± 1.0
							2	4.2 ± 3.3	11.0 ± 4.3	4.3 ± 1.2
							3	6.8 ± 3.5	15.0 ± 6.3	4.1 ± 1.2
							4	6.9 ± 3.1	12.4 ± 4.8	4.3 ± 1.3
							5	3.0 ± 1.9	9.8 ± 4.4	3.7 ± 1.3
						Short	1 early	3.6 ± 1.1	7.7 ± 1.9	4.4 ± 1.0
							1 late	4.0 ± 2.0	11.2 ± 5.6	3.9 ± 1.1
							2	4.4 ± 1.9	12.6 ± 5.0	3.5 ± 0.8
							3	6.2 ± 3.8	14.9 ± 11.1	4.3 ± 0.8
							4	3.9 ± 2.1	10.2 ± 2.9	3.8 ± 0.4
							5	1.5	7.2	3.0

[a]Represents time of day during which sampling took place, e.g. 0900–1500 hours.
[b]Area under the curve.

GROWTH HORMONE MODIFICATIONS IN FEMALE PUBERTY

Before puberty, the plasma concentration of GH is related to the quality of growth.[39] Nevertheless growth hormone is not the only factor responsible for prepubertal growth; factors such as nutrition, genetics, socioeconomic status of the family, and emotional and psychological climate play an important part.[8]

GH has been extensively studied in male, but less in female, puberty.[40–47] The progressive increment of GH is related to pubertal stage (see TABLES 1–4). Several studies, many of them cross-sectional, have demonstrated a clear rise in GH secretion, and this has been supported by studies using methods of continuous sampling.[34,40]

The peak amplitude of GH secretory episodes increases at puberty, while the frequency of peaks remains constant. Another characteristic of GH secretion in the pubertal period is the appearance of significant daytime peaks, while in prepubertal children most GH pulses occur during the night.[41] This is similar to the secretory profile of LH, FSH, and prolactin.[48] The peak amplitude starts decreasing at stage P4, and at stage P5 it is similar to that in the prepubertal stage.[40] In adulthood GH levels fall, but not in the same proportion for all parameters: Thus, GH concentrations are tenfold lower than in puberty, whereas, in comparison, the peak amplitudes are only fourfold lower, indicating that the hypothalamic regulatory hormones of GH secretion are not altered in the same way.[34] Urinary measures of GH excretion show differences between prepubertal and pubertal children[49–53] and a decrease at the end of puberty with small differences between girls and boys.[53] The evolution of urinary secretion is parallel to that of plasma related to pubertal stages[53,54] (see TABLE 5). Using the hormone-to-creatinine concentration ratio, the difference does not appear at the beginning of puberty[51,52]; it occurs later (TABLE 5).

As for prepubertal children, the concentration of GH is related to the quality

TABLE 3. GH Secretion Rate as Estimated by Deconvolution Technique in Healthy Girls of Normal Height[a]

Group of Children			Stage of Puberty	GH Secretion Rate (mU/kg × 24 hr)
Age (years)	(*n*)	Height		
	99	Normal		
9.8 ± 0.5	9		1	20.8 ± 2.7
11.0 ± 0.3	10		2	32.5 ± 2.0
12.7 ± 0.4	8		3	59.0 ± 4.4
13.9 ± 0.3	11		4	60.7 ± 11.1
14.6 ± 0.8	8		5	24.0 ± 4.4

NOTE: Mode of sampling: integrated continuous withdrawal; interval: 20 min. Sampling took place over 24 hours. Mode of analysis was deconvolution.

[a]Authors: Albertsson-Wikland and Rosberg, 1992.[40]

TABLE 4. GH Plasma Concentrations over 24 Hours in Healthy Girls with Normal Height

Author	Mode of Sampling Interval (min)	Time (hr)	Mode of Analysis	Group of Children: Age (years)	(*n*)	Height	Stage of Puberty	GH Values: Mean (μg/l)		
Zadik *et al.*[47] (1985)	30 Integrated	24			4	Normal	1	5.5 ± 1.6		
					7	Normal	2; 4	6.2 ± 1.0		
					10	Normal	5	8.1 ± 2.4		
								Mean (ng/ml)	AUC[a] Korr	Number of Peaks
Albertsson-Wikland and Rosberg[40] (1992)	20 Integrated continuous withdrawal	24	Pulsar G: 4.0; 2.4; 1.7; 1.2; 0.9		144	Normal				
				11.0 ± 0.3	18		1	4.8 ± 0.6	87 ± 10	8.4 ± 0.9
				11.9 ± 0.4	12		2	7.4 ± 0.9	148 ± 18	6.9 ± 0.4
				12.7 ± 0.4	12		3	13.4 ± 2.0	241 ± 28	8.8 ± 0.7
				13.9 ± 0.3	19		4	14.1 ± 2.6	264 ± 48	7.6 ± 0.2
				14.6 ± 0.8	8		5	5.5 ± 1.0	112 ± 19	9.3 ± 0.9

[a]AUC, area under curve.

TABLE 5. Values of Urinary Growth Hormone in Female Puberty

Authors	Pubertal Stages	ng/night	Creatinine (ng/g)
K. M. Main *et al.*[53] (1994)	1	1.8 (0.5–5.5)	10.2 (3.2–32.5)
	2	2.4 (0.7–8.4)	10.9 (4.6–25.7)
	3	3.6 (1.3–10.0)	12.5 (6.7–23.3)
	4	3.4 (1.3–9.0)	10.8 (4.0–29.6)
	5	3.0 (1.1–8.2)	8.4 (3.2–22.4)
	Adults	2.3 (0.7–7.2)	6.8 (2.2–20.7)
Authors	**Pubertal Stages**	**ng/24 hr**	**Creatinine (pmol/mmol)**
D. Porquet *et al.*[52] (1993)	1	2.9 ± 2.0	0.031 ± 0.021
	2	4.1 ± 1.6	0.028 ± 0.010
	3	11.5 ± 6.2	0.061 ± 0.021
	4	10.5 ± 4.0	0.050 ± 0.025
	5	6.9 ± 3.6	0.030 ± 0.015

of growth in pubertal subjects.[39] Sex steroids, however, also play a major role at this time. These hormones act in synergy with GH to induce the pubertal growth spurt, and one may calculate that each hormone is responsible for approximately half of the height gain during this period.[34] This is clear in patients with isolated growth hormone deficiency, where in the absence of GH treatment, the pubertal growth spurt is lowered by 50 to 60%.[54–56] On the other hand, in castrated patients with androgen insensitivity, estradiol treatment permits a normal pubertal growth spurt.[57]

In early puberty, changes in IGF1 concentrations are roughly parallel to those of GH, but the correlation with growth velocity is not as clear as for GH, since IGF1 is still increasing after the growth spurt, reaching a peak, one year after peak growth velocity is achieved. IGF1 levels remain elevated for four years after this, despite the fact that growth rate is decreasing at this time.[58] The evaluation of IGF1 concentrations is complicated by the fact that IGF1 is intimately related to its binding proteins (IGF BPs), mainly IGF BP 1 and IGF BP 3, which can be modified by factors other than IGF1 during puberty.[34,58] In addition, one must take into account the great discrepancies in the methods used for measuring IGF-1.[34]

MODIFICATIONS OF GH SECRETION IN PUBERTAL PATHOLOGY

Various pathologic conditions might influence pubertal GH secretion either spontaneously or because of a specific therapy. Thus, longitudinal studies of GH secretion were possible through induction of puberty with pulsatile GnRH injections in gonadotropin-deficient patients.[59] These approaches gave a better insight into the biology of GH modifications due to endogenous sex steroid rises induced by GnRH injections. On the other hand, in patients with precocious puberty, GH secretion mimics the changes observed in normal puberty, but resumes a prepubertal pattern as soon as the GnRH analogue treatment is applied.[60,61] In rare cases of precocious puberty associated with GH deficiency, no such elevation of GH secretion occurs.[62] In addition, one can observe the modifications of GH secretion occurring under exogenous estrogen treatments mimicking puberty. A classic example of this is Turner syndrome: In this pathologic condition one can observe a progressive decrease of GH concentrations in puberty due to lack of estrogen.[63] Conversely, treatment with ethinyl-estradiol (EE_2) (doses of 100 ng/kg per day) reproduces the physiologic pubertal elevation of GH in these patients.[69]

One can also demonstrate this by augmentation of the GH response to pharmacological stimuli after a short-term period of treatment with EE_2 in prepubertal children with short stature.[65] The usual dose of EE_2 is 50–100 μg given 3 days before the test.[7]

SPECIFIC ACTIONS OF GH ON ADULT BONE MINERAL DENSITY

During and immediately after puberty the skeleton acquires its adult bone mineral density (BMD). GH has two main actions on bone growth: one direct, through the division of chondrocytes of the growth plate, and indirect, through stimulation of osteoblast formation and activity, all phenomena in which local production of IGF-1 by bone itself plays a major role.[66]

During puberty, the bone mineral density increases between four- and sixfold over a 3-year period in girls and a 4-year period in boys. Mineralization of the femoral neck in girls is already well established in stage III and increases slowly afterwards to adult level. The mineral bone density of the lumbar spine is quite high at stage IV and completed through stage V. Boys acquire their adult BMD later at the end of puberty.[67]

During puberty, GH concentrations are correlated with osteocalcin, which is an indicator of bone turnover, as well as with IGF-1.[68] Bone mineral deposition is the highest during mid-puberty at the very period where GH attains its highest level and decreases afterwards as GH does. The actions of GH on bone mineral content is not only on the bone itself, but also through modification of kidney reabsorption of phosphorus.

Sex steroids also exert their effects on bone turnover directly and through local stimulation of IGF-1 production. Androgens and to a greater extent E_2 also stimulate the maturation of chondrocytes, leading to epiphyseal fusion.

GH plays a role in the acquisition of BMD that is difficult to demonstrate in normal conditions, but quite evident in pathologic conditions. The relation of GH and BMD can be demonstrated by GHD patients in whom the onset of GHD occurred during puberty[69] or at a prepubertal age.[70] Such patients cannot achieve a normal adult BMD without GH treatment.[71] Sometimes, GH treatment should be given to patients who have reached their adult height for the benefit of a normal bone density.[72]

In adolescents with Turner syndrome who have received no estrogen therapy, GH treatment stimulates BMD.[73] In contrast, in patients who have received neither estrogen nor GH, osteopenia is a common finding on skeletal X-rays.

SUMMARY

Growth hormone levels rise steadily through normal puberty, in parallel with the pubertal stages but decline rapidly at the end of puberty (stage V). The general evolution of the secretory profile of GH is parallel to the growth velocity curve.

The frequency of GH pulses remains unchanged; however, their amplitude, mean integrated concentrations, area under the curve, and urinary growth hormone are elevated at midpuberty. The main action of GH is to ensure, together with sex steroids, the pubertal growth spurt.

However, the role of pubertal GH is not confined to inducing the pubertal growth spurt. It also participates, together with sex steroids, in the acquisition of adult bone mineral density.

REFERENCES

1. Lewis, U. J., R. N. P. Singh, G. F. Tutweller, M. B. Sigel, E. F. Van der Laan & W. P. Van der Laan. 1980. Human growth hormone: A complex of proteins. Recent Prog. Horm. Res. **36:** 477–408.
2. Baumann, G., M. W. Stolar, K. Ambrum, C. P. Baesano & B. C. De Vries. 1986. A specific growth hormone binding protein in human plasma: Initial characterization. J. Clin. Endocrinol. Metab. **62(1):** 134–141.
3. Leung, D. W., S. A. Spencer, G. Chiacanes, R. G. Hammonds, C. Clollins, W. J. Henzel, R. Barnard, M. J. Waters & W. I. Wood. 1987. Growth hormone receptor and serum binding protein: Purification, cloning and expression. Nature **330(6148):** 537–543.
4. Cunniggham, B. C., M. Ultsch, A. M. de Vos, M. G. Mulkerrin, K. R. Clauser & J. A. Wells. 1991. Dimerization of the extracellular domain of the human growth hormone receptor by a single hormone molecule. Science **254(5033):** 821–825.
5. Silbergeld, A., L. Lazar, B. Ester, R. Keret, R. Tepper & Z. Laron. 1989. Serum growth hormone binding protein activity in healthy neonates, children and young adults: Correlations with age, height and weight. Clin. Endocrinol. (Oxford) **31(3):** 295–303.
6. Tar, A., J. F. Hocquette, J. C. Soubervielle, J. P. Clot, R. Brauner & C. Postel-Vinay. 1990. Evaluation of the growth hormone-binding proteins in human plasma using HPLC gel filtration. J. Clin. Endocrinol. Metab. **71(5):** 1202–1207.
7. Ranke, M. B. & P. Haber. 1992. Growth hormone stimulation tests. *In* Functional Endocrinologic Diagnostics in Children and Adolescents. M. B. Ranke, Ed.: 61–75. J & J Verlag. Mannheim.

8. KERRIGAN, J. R. & A. D. ROGOL. 1992. The impact of gonadal steroid hormone action on growth hormone secretion during childhood and adolescence. Endocrinol. Rev. **13(2):** 281–298.
9. LIPOSITS, Z. S., D. MERCHANTELER, C. PHELIX & W. K. PARELL. 1988. Synaptic communication between somatostatinergic axons and growth hormone releasing factor synthesizing neurons in the arcuate nucleus of the rat. Histochemistry **89(2):** 247–252.
10. TANNENBAUM, G. S. & N. LING. 1984. The interrelationship of growth hormone (GH)-releasing factor and somatostatin in generation of the ultradian rhythm of GH secretion. Endocrinology **115(5):** 1952–1957.
11. PLOSTSKY, P. M. & W. VALE. 1985. Patterns of growth hormone releasing factor and somatostatin. Science **230(4626):** 461–463.
12. KRAICIER, J., J. S. COWAN, M. S. SHEPPARD, B. LUSSIER & B. C. MOOR. 1986. Effect of somatostin withdrawal and growth hormone (GH)-releasing factor on GH release in vitro: Amount available for release after desinhibition. Endocrinology **119(4):** 2047–2051.
13. KRAICIER, J., M. S. SHEPPARD, J. LUKE, B. LUSSIER & B. C. MOOR. 1988. Effect of somatostin and growth hormone (GH)-releasing factor on GH release in vitro. Endocrinology **122(5):** 1810–1815.
14. HORVATH, S., M. PALKOVITS, T. GORCS & A. AMIRA. 1989. Electron microscopic immunocytochemical evidence for the existence of bidirectional synaptic connections between growth hormone releasing hormone and somatostatin containing neurons in the hypothalamus of the rat. Brain Res. **481(1):** 8–15.
15. KATAKAMI, H., A. ARIMURA & L. A. FROHMAN. 1986. Growth hormone (GH)-releasing factor stimulates somatostatin: An inhibitory feedback effect on GH secretion. Endocrinology **118(5):** 1872–1877.
16. KATAKAMI, H., T. R. DOWNS & L. A. FROHMAN. 1988. Inhibitory effect of hypothalamic medial preoptic area somatostatin on growth hormone-releasing factor in rat. Endocrinology **123(2):** 1103–1109.
17. TANNENBAUM, G. S., J. C. PAINSON, A. LENGUYEL & P. BRAZEAU. 1989. Paradoxical enhancement of pituitary growth hormone (GH) responsiveness to GH releasing hormone in the face of high somatostatin tone. Endocrinology **124(3):** 1380–1388.
18. MÜLLER, E. E. 1987. Neural control of somatropic function. Physiol. Rev. **67(4):** 963–1053.
19. BURTON, K. A., D. K. CLIFTON & R. A. STEINER. 1992. The role of growth hormone (GH) itself in the generation of pulsatile GH secretion. *In* Human Growth: Basic and Clinical Aspects. M. Hernández & J. Argente, Eds.: 307–313. Excerpta Medica. Amsterdam.
20. ARGENTE, J., J. A. CHOWEN, P. ZEITLER, D. K. CLIFTON & R. A. STEINER. 1992. Sex steroid and developmental regulation of somatostatin and growth hormone-releasing hormone gene expression. *In* Human Growth: Basic and Clinical Aspects. M. Hernández & J. Argente, Eds.: 295–306. Excerpta Medica. Amsterdam.
21. ZEITLER, P., J. ARGENTE, J. CHOWEN-BREED, D. K. CLIFTON & R. A. STEINER. 1990. Growth hormone-releasing hormone messenger ribonucleic acid in hypothalamus of the adult male rat is increased by testosterone. Endocrinology **127(3):** 1362–1368.
22. ARGENTE, J., J. A. CHOWEN-BREED, R. A. STEINER & D. K. CLIFTON. 1990. Somatostatin messenger RNA in hypothalamic neurons is increased by testosterone through activation of androgen receptors and not by aromatization to estradiol. Neuroendocrinology **52(2):** 342–349.
23. HO, K. Y., D. A. LEONG, Y. N. SINHA, M. L. JONHSON, W. S. EVANS & M. O. THORNER. 1986. Sex-related differences in GH secretion in rat using reverse hemolytic plaque assay. Am. J. Physiol. **250(2):** E650–E654.
24. HOEFFLER, J. P. & L. S. FRAWLEY. 1986. Capacity of individual somatotropes to release

growth hormone varies according to sex: Analysis by reverse hemolytic plaque assay. Endocrinology **119(3):** 1037–1041.

25. HERTZ, P., M. SILBERMAN, L. EVEN & Z. HOCHBERG. 1989. Effects of sex steroid on the response of cultured rat pituitary cells to growth hormone-releasing hormone and somatostatin. Endocrinology **125(2):** 581–585.
26. EVANS, W. S., R. J. KRIEG, E. R. LIMBER, D. L. KAISER & M. O. THORNER. 1985. Effects of *in vivo* gonadal hormone environment on *in vitro* hGRF-40-stimulated GH release. Am. J. Physiol. **249(2):** E276–E280.
27. JIN, L., J. SONG & R. V. LLOYD. 1989. Estrogen stimulates both prolactin and growth hormone mRNAs expression in the mt/F4 transplantable pituitary tumor. Proc. Soc. Exp. Biol. Med. **192:** 225–229.
28. SIMARD, J., J. F. HUBERT, T. HOSSEINZADEH & F. LABRIE. 1986. Stimulation of growth hormone release and synthesis by estrogens in rat anterior pituitary cells in culture. Endocrinology **119(5):** 2004–2011.
29. ALBA-ROTH, J., O. A. MULLER, J. SCHOPOL & K. VON WERDER. 1988. Arginine stimulates growth hormone secretion by suppressing endogenous somatostatin secretion. J. Clin. Endocrinol. Metab. **67(6):** 1186–1189.
30. BERELOWITZ, M., M. SZABO, L. A. FROHMAN, S. FIRESTONE, L. CHU & R. L. HINTZ. 1981. Somatomedin mediates growth hormone negative feedback by effects on both hypothalamus and pituitary. Science **212(4510):** 1279–1281.
31. CEDA, G. P., G. P. DAVIS, R. G. ROSENFELD & A. R. HOFFMAN. 1987. The growth hormone (GH)-releasing hormone (GHRH)–GH–somatomedin axis: Evidence for rapid inhibition of GHRH elicited GH release by insulin-like growth factors I and II. Endocrinology **120(4):** 1658–1662.
32. NAMBA, H., S. MORITA & S. MELMED. 1989. Insuline factor-I action on growth hormone secretion and messenger ribonucleic acid levels; interaction with somatostatin. Endocrinology **124(4):** 1794–1799.
33. CASANUEVA, F. F., L. VILLANUEVA, C. DIEGUEZ, Y. DIAZ, J. A. CABRANES, B. SZOKE, M. F. SCALON, A. V. SCHALLY & A. FERNANDEZ-CRUZ. 1987. Free fatty acids block growth hormone (GH) releasing hormone stimulated GH secretion in man directly at the pituitary. J. Clin. Endocrinol. Metab. **65(4):** 634–642.
34. BROOK, C. G. D. & P. C. HINDMARSH. 1992. The somatrotropic axis in puberty. Endocrinol. Metab. Clinics N. Am. **21(4):** 767–782.
35. VELDHUIS, J. D. & M. L. JOHNSON. 1992. Computer-assisted algorithms to analyze growth hormone release. *In* Human Growth: Basic and Clinical Aspects. M. Hernández and J. Argente, Eds.: 43–57. Excerpta Medica. Amsterdam.
36. MERRIAM, G. R. & K. W. WACHTER. 1982. Algorithms for the study of episodic hormone secretion. Am. J. Physiol. **243(3):** E310–E318.
37. URBAN, R. J., W. S. EVANS, A. D. ROGOL, D. L. KAISER, M. L. JOHNSON & J. D. VELDHUIS. 1988. Contemporary aspects of discrete peak-detection algorithms. The paradigm of the luteinizing hormone pulse signal in men. Endocrinol. Rev. **9(1):** 3–37.
38. MARTHA, P. M., JR., K. M. GORMAN, R. M. BLIZZARD, A. D. ROGOL & J. D. VELDHUIS. 1992. Endogenous growth hormone secretion and clearance rate in normal boys as determined by deconvolution analysis: Relation to age, pubertal status and body mass. J. Clin. Endocrinol. Metab. **74(2):** 336–344.
39. ALBERTSSON-WIKLAND, K. & S. ROSBERG. 1994. Physiological growth hormone secretion: Changes with age, stature and puberty. *In* Frontiers in Paediatric Neuroendocrinology. M. O. Savage, J.-P. Bourguignon & A. B. Grossman, Eds.: 131–137. Blackwell Scientific Publications. Oxford.
40. ALBERTSSON-WIKLAND, K. & S. ROSBERG. 1992. Methods of evaluating spontaneous

growth hormone secretion. *In* Functional Endocrinologic Diagnostics in Children and Adolescents. M. B. Ranke, Ed.: 61–75. J & J Verlag. Mannheim.

41. Miller, J. D., G. S. Tannenbaum, E. Colle & H. J. Guyda. 1982. Daytime pulsatile growth hormone secretion increases during childhood and adolescence. J. Clin. Endocrinol. Metab. **55(5):** 989–994.
42. Edge, J. A., D. B. Dunger, D. R. Matthews, J. P. Gilbert & C. P. Smith. 1990. Increased overnight growth hormone concentrations in diabetics compared to normal adolescents. J. Clin. Endocrinol. Metab. **71(5):** 1356–1362.
43. Garnier, P., F. Raynaud & J. C. Job. 1988. Growth hormone during sleep. I. Comparison with GH responses to conventional pharmacologic stimuli in pubertal and early pubertal short subjects. Effects of treatment with human growth hormone in patients with discrepant measurements of GH secretion. Horm. Res. **29(4):** 133–139.
44. Rose, S. R., G. Municchi, K. M. Barnes, G. A. Kamp, M. M. Uridate, J. L. Ross, F. Cassorla & G. B. Cutler. 1991. Spontaneous growth hormone secretion increases during puberty in normal girls and boys. J. Clin. Endocrinol. Metab. **73(2):** 428–435.
45. Delamarre-van-de-Waal, H. A., J. M. B. Wennink & R. J. H. Odink. 1991. Gonadotrophin and growth hormone secretion throughout puberty. Acta Paediatr. Scand. **80**(Suppl. 372): 26–31.
46. Wennink, J. M. B., H. A. Delamarre-van-de-Waal, R. Schoemaker, G. Blaauw, C. van-den-Braken & J. Schoemaker. 1991. Growth hormone secretion patterns in relation to LH and estradiol secretion throughout normal female puberty. Acta Endocrinol. **124(1):** 129–135.
47. Zadik, Z., A. C. Stuart, Z. Guila & A. A. Kowarski. 1985. The influence of age on the 24-hr integrated concentrations of growth hormone. J. Clin. Endocrinol. Metab. **60(3):** 513–516.
48. Dunger, D. B., D. R. Matthews & J. A. Edge. 1990. Evidence for temporal coupling of GH, PRL, LH and FSH pulsatility during normal puberty. Horm. Res. **38**(Suppl.39): 1 (Abstr. 1).
49. Price, D. A., G. M. Addison & E. D. Hebert. 1991. Increase in urinary growth hormone excretion in puberty. Arch. Dis. Child. **65(5):** 1203–1204.
50. Marum, R. H., V. B. Daruis & W. Nicolau. 1992. Growth hormone in urine on three consecutive days. Acta. Pædiatr. **81**(Suppl. 383): 83 (Abstr. 2).
51. Georges, P., J. Liefooghe, G. Forzy, D. Ponchaux, L. Di Nicola & J. L. Chaussain. 1995. Urinary hGh: Pubertal related changes in normal subjects and in growth retardation. Horm. Res. **41(2–4):** 84 (Abstr. 110).
52. Porquet, D., J. Léger, C. Reverchon, S. Louis & J. Passagot. 1993. Dosages de l'hormone de croissance dans les urines. Établissement de valeurs usuelles chez l'enfant à l'aide d'une trousse commerciale. Immunanal. Biol. Spec. **8(1):** 51–56.
53. Main, K. M., M. Jarden, L. Angelo, B. Dinsen, N. T. Hertel, A. Juul, J. Müller & N. E. Skakkebæk. 1994. The impact of gender and puberty on reference values for urinary growth hormone excretion: A study of three morning samples in 517 children and adults. J. Clin. Endocrinol. Metab. **79(3):** 865–871.
54. Tanner, J. M., R. H. Whitehouse, P. C. R. Hughes & B. S. Carter. 1976. Relative importance of growth hormone and sex steroids for growth at puberty for trunk length, limb length and muscle width in growth hormone deficient children. J. Pediatr. **89(6):** 1000–1010.
55. Aynsley-Green, A., M. Zachmann & A. Prader. 1976. Interrelations of growth hormone and testosterone on growth in hypopituitarism. J. Pediatr. **89(6):** 992–999.
56. Zachman, M. 1992. Interrelations between growth hormone and sex hormones: Physiologic and therapeutic consequences. Horm. Res. **38**(Suppl. 1): 1–8.

57. Zachmann, M., A. Prader, E. M. Sobol, J. F. Crigler, Jr., E. M. Ritzen, M. Atarés & A. Fernandex. 1986. Pubertal growth in patients with androgen insensitivity: Indirect evidence for the importance of the estrogens in pubertal growth in girls. J. Pediatr. **108(5):** 694–697.
58. Blum, W. F. 1992. Insulin-like growth factors and their binding proteins. *In* Functional Endocrinologic Diagnostics in Children and Adolescents. M. B. Ranke, Ed.: 102–117. J & J Verlag. Mannheim.
59. Stanhope, R., P. J. Pringle & C. G. D. Brook. 1988. The mechanism of the adolescent growth spurt induced by low dose pulsatile GnRH treatment. Clin. Endocrinol. (Oxford) **28(1):** 83–91.
60. Mansfield, M. J., C. R. Rudlin, J. F. Crigler, Jr., K. A. Karol, J. D. Crawford, P. A. Boepple & W. F. Crowley, Jr. 1988. Changes in growth and serum growth hormone and plasma somatomedin-C levels during suppression of gonadal sex steroid secretion in girls with central precocious puberty. J. Clin. Endocrinol. Metab. **66(1):** 3–9.
61. Chaussain, J. L., S. de Oliveira, C. Swænepœl, K. Boudjema & M. Roger. 1992. Effects of a long-term therapy with a depot-preparation of DTRP6-LHRH (Decapeptyl®) on growth and bone maturation in children with precocious puberty. *In* Human Growth: Basic and Clinical Aspects. M. Hernández & J. Argente, Eds.: 316–321. Excerpta Medica. Amsterdam.
62. Attie, K. M., N. R. Ramirez, F. A. Conte, S. L. Kaplan & M. M. Grumbach. 1990. The pubertal growth spurt in eight patients with true precocious puberty and growth hormone deficiency: Evidence for a direct role of sex steroids. J. Clin. Endocrinol. Metab. **71(4):** 975–983.
63. Mauras, N., A. D. Rogol & J. D. Veldhuis. 1989. Specific, time-dependent actions of low dose ethinyl estradiol administration on the episodic growth hormone, follicle-stimulating hormone and luteinizing hormone in prepubertal girls with Turner's syndrome. J. Clin. Endocrinol. Metab. **69(5):** 1053–1058.
64. Mauras, N., A. D. Rogol & J. D. Veldhuis. 1990. Increased hGH production rate after low dose estrogen therapy in pre-pubertal girls with Turner's syndrome. Pediatr. Res. **28(6):** 626–630.
65. Moll, G., R. L. Rosefeld & V. S. Fang. 1986. Administration of low dose estrogen rapidly and directly stimulates growth hormone production. Am. J. Dis. Child. **140(2):** 124–127.
66. Wüster, C. 1993. Growth hormone and bone metabolism. Acta Endocrinol. (Copenhagen) **128**(Suppl. 1)**:** 14–18.
67. Ruiz, J. C., C. Mandel & M. Garabedian. 1995. Influence of spontaneous calcium intake and physical exercise on the vertebral and femoral bone mineral density of children and adolescents. J. Bone Min. Res. **10(5):** 675–682.
68. Blumsohn, A. 1994. Biochemical markers of bone turnover in girls during puberty. Clin. Endocrinol. (Oxford) **40(6):** 663–670.
69. Hyer, S. L., D. A. Rodin, J. H. Tobias, A. Leiper & S. S. Nussey. 1992. Growth hormone-deficiency during puberty reduces bone mineral density. Arch. Dis. Childh. **67(6):** 1472–1474.
70. Kaufman, J.-M., P. Taelman, A. Vermeulen & M. Vandeweghe. 1992. Bone mineral status in growth hormone-deficient males with isolated and multiple pituitary deficiencies of childhood onset. J. Clin. Endocrinol. Metab. **74(1):** 118–123.
71. O'Halloran, D. J., A. Tsatsoulis, R. W. Whitehouse, S. J. Homes, J. E. Adams & S. M. Shalet. 1993. Increased bone density after recombinant human growth hormone (GH) therapy in with isolated GH deficiency. J. Clin. Endocrinol. Metab. **76(5):** 1344–1348.

72. RANKE, M. B. 1995. Growth hormone therapy in children: When to stop? Horm. Res. **43(4):** 122–125.
73. NEELY, E. K., R. MARCUS, R. G. ROSENFELD & L. A. BACHRACH. 1993. Turner syndrome adolescents receiving growth hormone are not osteopenic. J. Clin. Endocrinol. Metab. **76(4):** 861–866.

Neuromodulatory Role of Opioidergic System on Hypothalamus–Pituitary–Gonadal Axis during Puberty

ALESSANDRO D. GENAZZANI,[a,b] OMBRETTA GAMBA,[a] LAURA SGARBI,[a] ANDREA GANDOLFI,[a] FABRIZIO CORAZZA,[a] NICOLA SURICO,[c] AND FELICE PETRAGLIA[a]

[a]*Physiopathology of Human Reproduction*
University of Modena
41100 Modena, Italy

[c]*Department of Obstetrics and Gynecology*
University of Novara
Novara, Italy

INTRODUCTION

The hypothalamus–pituitary–gonadal (HPG) axis changes its activity throughout life, and a number of years is required after birth to activate physiological functional regulation of the gonadal axis, which leads to optimal reproductive function in both sexes. Pubertal maturation occurs as a period of transition between childhood and adulthood during which deep biological, morphological, and psychological changes take place, leading to full sexual maturation. These physiological events are controlled by the interaction of several factors, and the maturation of the hypothalamic neuroendocrine mechanisms controlling pituitary gonadotropin secretion is fundamental for the onset of puberty. Many other factors, however, such as genetics, nutritional status, psychological state, and climate, may influence the onset of pubertal maturation.

Endogenous opioid peptides (EOPs) seem to have a prominent role in the maturation and control of the reproductive system.[1] In the brain EOPs represent an integrative pathway modulating GnRH secretion under endocrine or neuroendocrine influences, and they affect the reproductive functions at different levels. The involvement of EOPs in the control of pituitary gonadotropin secretion has been proposed and demonstrated by several reports.[2–4] Exogenous opiates also affect the reproductive capacity, as evidenced by the amenorrheic and/or hypogonadic status of heroin-addicted subjects.

ENDOGENOUS OPIOID PEPTIDES FAMILY

Opioid peptides derive from three common precursor molecules,[5] and their enzymatic degradation yields different fragments with and without opiatergic activity.

[b]Address for correspondence: Dr. Alessandro D. Genazzani, Physiopathology of Human Reproduction, University of Modena, Via del Pozzo 71, 41100 Modena, Italy. Fax: ++39 59 424394; E-mail: algen@unimo.it.

Three major EOPs have been identified in humans. β-Endorphin (βEP), a 31-amino-acid sequence, derives from the proopiomelanocortin (POMC) precursor, and it is considered the most important EOP in the neuroendocrine regulation of human reproduction. Met- and leu-enkephalins, both pentapeptides deriving from proenkephalin A, and the 17-amino-acid peptide dynorphin cleaved from prodynorphin are the other two components of the EOP family. βEP is produced in medial-basal hypothalamus and is widely distributed in the brain[6]; however, it is also synthesized and co-released with ACTH from the pituitary.[7]

Three major opioid receptor subtypes have been described: μ, δ, and κ receptors.[8] βEP binds to μ receptors, which also bind morphine with very high affinity.[8] The majority of μ receptors have been localized in the limbic system and in the hypothalamus.

EOPs are involved in the regulation and/or the modulation of many functions, such as pain and temperature perception, hunger and thirst control,[2,5] and reproduction.[2]

OPIOID MODULATION OF HYPOTHALAMUS–PITUITARY FUNCTIONS

In vitro experiments demonstrated that opioids and opiates inhibit GnRH release from the mediobasal hypothalamus,[4,8] thus confirming that EOP, mainly βEP, exert an inhibitory tone on the hypothalamic pulse generator.[10] In fact, acute morphine administration *in vivo* decreases circulating LH plasma levels in several species.[11] A possible action on anterior pituitary has been suggested but seems to have a lesser physiological relevance.[12]

The inhibitory role of EOPs on GnRH and LH release is considered dependent on the steroid milieau,[13] because in ovariectomized rats[14] or in postmenopausal women,[15] the administration of naloxone, a receptor opioid antagonist, fails to increase LH plasma levels. On this basis, the high LH pulse frequency and amplitude observed in postmenopausal women probably depend on a lack of opioidergic inhibition on GnRH-pulse generator.[16] When the hormonal replacement therapy is administered, the LH response to naloxone is restored.[15] Thus, the opioid negative tone on the GnRH pulse generator and LH release is modulated by steroid plasma levels, and several physiological and pathological conditions support this concept.

OPIOID PEPTIDES AND PUBERTAL MATURATION

The maturation of the HPG axis begins during the fetal period. GnRH is secreted in fetal hypothalamus beginning at the sixth week of gestation, and its presence stimulates the secretion of FSH and of LH by fetal pituitary by the 10th to 12th week of gestation, with a rapid increase of gonadotropin plasma levels until the 10th week. This determines the increase of plasma gonadal steroids levels in fetal circulation inhibiting the release of GnRH and then of FSH and LH. As a result, gonadotropin levels in the umbilical venous blood decrease significantly.

At birth, the fall of circulating gonadal steroid levels causes a rise of the secretion

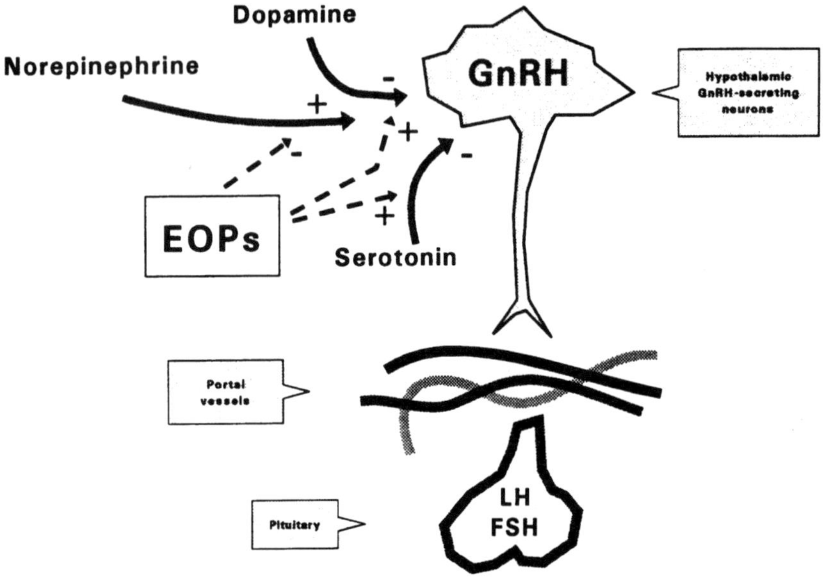

FIGURE 1. Schematic representation of the action of endogenous opioid peptides (EOPs) on the modulation exerted by various neuromediators on GnRH-secreting neurons. The integration of such signals affects the episodic GnRH discharge and drives the pulsatile release of LH and FSH at the pituitary level.

of LH and FSH, as a result of reduced inhibition of the hypothalamic release of GnRH. However, the sensibility of the hypothalamic–pituitary system to the negative feedback exerted by sex hormones gradually increases in the first months of life. After the second to fourth month, plasma LH and FSH begin to decrease, and circulating sex steroids reach the prepubertal levels at about the sixth month.

The pulsatile gonadotropin secretion is clearly present in neonates and in the first months of life.[17] More active FSH secretion can be observed in females, whereas LH secretion prevails in males. Thereafter, gonadotropin levels decline, and LH peaks are almost undetectable during the prepubertal period. Plasma FSH levels are higher than those of LH, and circulating sex steroids levels are low. By using a newly developed immunofluorimetric assay (IFMA) system, it has been shown that FSH secretion is pulsatile throughout pubertal development, and it is synchronized with LH as soon as LH is detectable in plasma.[18]

When puberty starts, important changes of gonadotropin secretory patterns take place. They reflect the maturation of the HPG axis, the predominant change being the progressive increase of plasma LH levels and the pulsatile nature of its secretion, selectively activated during sleep. Later on, pulsatile LH secretion extends into the daytime hours, and it is synchronized with FSH. Within a short time, the stimulation on the ovaries determines the occurrence of the first menstrual cycles. It is now generally accepted that pubertal changes affecting hypothalamus–pituitary axis are the result of reduced sensitivity to circulating sex steroids of the hypothalamic center (gonadostat), which is extremely sensitive to the negative feedback exerted even by small quantities of estradiol.

Inhibition of the activity of the hypothalamic GnRH-producing neurons by opioids has been proposed to represent the neurochemical substrate of the hypothalamic gonadostat[1]; however, the release of GnRH is modulated by LH (short-loop feedback), GnRH (ultrashort-loop feedback), and many other peptides and neurotransmitters such as dopamine, cholecystokinin (CCK), vasoactive intestinal peptide (VIP), neurotensin, substance P, and α-melanocyte-stimulating hormone (α-MSH). Hypothalamic βEP contents change during pubertal maturation, unmasking an age-related opioid modulation of LH secretion in rats[1] as well as in prepubertal children.[19] Moreover, the lack of circadian changes of hypothalamic βEP before puberty in rats has been reported, thus supporting the specific modulatory role of gonadal steroids on opioidergic pathway development and activity.[20]

Naloxone, an opiate receptor antagonist, has been widely used to clarify the mechanism underlying the inhibition of gonadotropin secretion by opioid peptides. In adult subjects, the acute infusion of naloxone increases plasma LH levels, acting on the frequency and the amplitude of the GnRH pulse.[21] In prepubertal and early pubertal children of both sexes the administration of naloxone does not change plasma LH levels.[22] On the contrary, naloxone only induces an LH response in children at the most advanced stages of pubertal maturation (Tanner PH 4-5).[19] This demonstrates a close relationship between the activity of the opioid system and gonadal maturation occurring during pubertal development. It is difficult to specify whether the primary change is central or peripheral, since the inability of the opioid antagonist to raise LH plasma levels in prepuberty might depend on the absence of any activity of the central opioid pathways on gonadotropin secretion during this period of life. Moreover, the evidence that naloxone injection is ineffective in children with gonadal dysgenesis or with idiopathic delayed puberty suggests that the increase in gonadal steroid production is the triggering event for the inhibition of gonadotropin secretion by opioids at puberty.[19] In fact, patients with Turner's or Klinefelter's syndrome do not show any change in plasma LH after naloxone administration, even following chronic replacement therapies.[23,24] Therefore, it may be suggested that the activity of the opioid system reflects the maturation of the HPG axis, and it is not simply related to the gonadal steroids: Girls with Turner's syndrome with spontaneous menarche are responsive to naloxone infusion. Age is not a critical factor in modulating the opioid control of LH because children with idiopathic delayed puberty or with precocious puberty do not show a significant increase in plasma LH after naloxone.[19] Moreover, Mauras *et al.*[25] demonstrated that naltrexone administration to prepubertal boys determined a reduction of LH plasma levels, suggesting that this paradoxical inhibitory response represented an agonist-like effect of chronic naltrexone administration. This implies that opiate pathways are not highly sensitive to opiate substances, and it may be proposed that physiological pubertal progression may be accompanied by the decreased sensitivity of the hypothalamic gonadostat to the inhibitory effects of opioids.[25]

The importance of the opioidergic control of gonadotropin secretion assumes a particular relevance when dealing with some cases of secondary amenorrhea not related to any other objective endocrine causal factor. Recent data support the specific

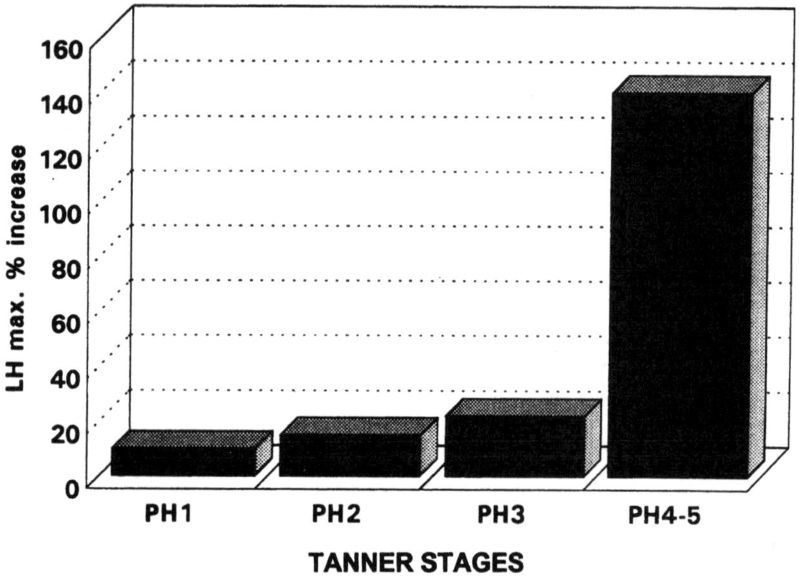

FIGURE 2. The opioidergic pathway seems to be activated only in the last stages of pubertal development. In fact, the LH response to naloxone acute infusion appears only at Tanner stages 4–5. The fact that children with central true precocious puberty show a response to naloxone, whereas children with delayed puberty or gonadal dysgenesis do not show any change in LH plasma levels demonstrated that the maturation of the opioidergic pathway is not related to age.

role of an impairment of the HGP axis due to an exaggerated inhibitory effect of opioids on GnRH secretion, especially in those cases of stress-induced menstrual disturbances. Indeed, the opioid activity increases following environmental changes as an adaptative response. When naltrexone was administered at a dosage of 50 mg/day for at least 3 to 4 months, the restoration of a regular menstrual cyclicity occurred in a high percentage of lean, amenorrheic patients.[26,27] In these patients with hypothalamic amenorrhea, a greater nocturnal melatonin increase has been described,[28] and it might be related to the increased opiatergic inhibitory tone on GnRH secretion. Moreover, melatonin administration has been reported to prevent the progressive loss of LH response to naloxone in aging rats,[29] thus suggesting that a specific complex modulation of GnRH release is exerted by melatonin via the opiatergic pathway. The lack of LH response to naloxone administration both in prepubertal children and in postmenopausal women might be related not only to a hypogonadal state, but also to age-dependent, not-yet-activated, or already-disactivated melatonin modulation of the opiatergic pathway.

In conclusion, EOPs play a fundamental role in determining the onset of the activity of the HPG axis. The EOPs, inhibitory action is strictly dependent on the steroid hormone melieu, as shown by the different responses to naloxone administration during the different phases of the menstrual cycle. EOP inhibition represents one of the key factors modulating the activity of gonadal steroids on the HPG axis throughout the different phases of human reproduction.

REFERENCES

1. BHANOT, R. & M. WILKINSON. 1983. Opiatergic control of gonadotropin secretion during puberty in the rat: A neurochemical basis for the hypothalamic "gonadostat"? Endocrinology **113:** 596–603.
2. GENAZZANI, A. R. & F. PETRAGLIA. 1989. Opioid control of luteinizing hormone secretion in humans. J. Steroid Biochem. **33:** 751–755.
3. KALRA, S. P. & P. S. KALRA. 1984. Neural regulation of luteinizing hormone secretion in the rat. Endocrinol. Rev. **4:** 311–351.
4. WILKES, M. M. & S. S. C. YEN. 1981. Augmentation by naloxone of efflux of LRF from superinfused medial basal hypothalamus. Life Sci. **24:** 1325–1331.
5. GUILLEMIN, R. 1980. Beta-lipotropin and endorphins: Implications of current knowledge. *In* Neuroendocrinology. D. T. Krieger & J. C. Haughes, Eds.: 67–74. Sinauer. Sunderland, MA.
6. WARDLAW, S. L., W. B. WEHRENBERG, M. FERIN, P. W. CARMEL & A. G. FRANTZ. 1980. High levels of β-endorphin in hypophyseal portal blood. Endocrinology **106:** 1323–1329.
7. CHAN, J. S. D., C. L. LU, N. G. SEIDAH & M. CHRETIEN. 1982. Corticotropin releasing factor (CRF): Effects on the release of pro-opiomelanocortin (POMC)-related peptides by human anterior pituitary cells in vitro. Endocrinology **111:** 1388–1394.
8. YEN, S. S. C. 1991. The human menstrual cycle: Neuroendocrine regulation. In Reproductive Endocrinology. S. S. C. Yen & R. B. Jaffe, Eds.: 273–308. Saunders. Philadelphia, PA.
9. SHOUPE, D., J. F. MONTZ & A. R. LOBO. 1985. The effects of estrogens and progestins on endogenous opioid activity in oophorectomized women. J. Clin. Endocrinol. Metab. **60:** 178–181.
10. VELDHUIS, J. D., A. D. ROGOL, M. L. JOHNSON & M. L. DUFAU. 1983. Endogenous opiates modulate the pulsatile secretion of biologically active LH in man. J. Clin. Invest. **72:** 2031 2036.
11. DELITALA, G., M. MANNELLI, M. GIUSTI, M. MAGGI, M. L. DE FEO, G. GIORDANO, G. GIUSTI & M. SERIO. 1984. Relation of opiates to hormonal secretion in man. *In* Opioid Modulation of Endocrine Function. G. Delitala, M. Motta & M. Serio, Eds.: 65–88. Raven Press. New York.
12. CACICEDO, L. & F. SANCHEZ-FRANCO. 1986. Direct action of opioid peptides and naloxone on gonadotropin secretion by cultured rat pituitary cell. Life Sci. **38:** 617–625.
13. GABRIEL, S. M., J. W. SIMPKINS & S. P. KALRA. 1983. Modulation of endogenous opioid influence on luteinizing hormone secretion of progesterone and estrogen. Endocrinology **113:** 1806–1811.
14. PETRAGLIA, F., A. PENALVA, V. LOCATELLI, D. COCCHI, A. E. PANERAI, A. R. GENAZZANI & E. E. MULLER. 1982. Effect of gonadectomy and gonadal steroid replacement on pituitary and plasma β-endorphin levels in rat. Endocrinology **111:** 1224–1229.
15. REID, R. L., M. E. QUIGLEY & S. S. C. YEN. 1983. The disappearance of opioidergic regulation of gonadotropin secretion in postmenopausal women. J. Clin. Endocrinol. Metab. **57:** 1107–1110.
16. PETRAGLIA, F., G. COMITINI, G. D'AMBROGIO, A. VOLPE, F. FACCHINETTI, G. ALESSANDRINI & A. R. GENAZZANI. 1985. Short-term effects of ovariectomy: The opioid control of LH secretion in fertile, climateric and postmenopausal women. J. Endocrinol. Metab. **8:** 325–329.

17. FILICORI, M. & C. FLAMIGNI. 1988. Physiology and pathophysiology of pulsatile gonadotropin secretion. Gynecol. Endocrinol. **2:** 73–85.

18. GENAZZANI, A. D., F. PETRAGLIA, C. VOLPOGNI, O. GAMBA, F. MASSOLO & A. R. GENAZZANI. 1994. Evidence suggesting an additional mechanism regulating LH and FSH episodic secretion in prepubertal and in postmenopausal women. Hum. Reprod. **9:** 1807–1812.

19. PETRAGLIA, F., S. BERNASCONI, L. IUGHETTI, S. LOCHE, F. ROMANINI, F. FACCHINETTI, C. MARCELLINI & A. R. GENAZZANI. 1986. Naloxone-induced LH secretion in normal, precocious and delayed puberty. J. Clin. Endocrinol. Metab. **63:** 1112–1116.

20. GENAZZANI, A. R., G. P. TRENTINI, F. PETRAGLIA, C. F. DE GAETANI, M. CRISCUOLO, G. FICARRA, B. M. DE RAMUNDO & M. CLEVA. 1990. Estrogens modulate the circadian rhythm of hypothalamic β-endorphin contents in female rats. Neuroendocrinology **52:** 221–224.

21. ELLINGBOE, J., J. D. VELDHUIS, J. H. MENDELSON, J. C. KUEHNLE & N. K. MELLO. 1982. Effect of endogenous opioid blockade on the amplitude and frequency of pulsatile luteinizing hormone secretion in normal men. J. Clin. Endocrinol. Metab. **54:** 854–857.

22. FRAIOLI, F., M. CAPPA, A. FABBRI, L. GNESSI, C. MORETTI, P. BORELLI & A. ISIDORI. 1984. Lack of endogenous opioid inhibitory tone on LH secretion in early puberty. Clin. Endocrinol. **20:** 299–303.

23. FORTI, G., M. L. DE FEO, M. MAGGI, A. D. GENAZZANI, V. FAZZI & G. DELITALA. 1987. Naloxone administration does not affect gonadotropin secretion in patients with Klinefelter's syndrome. Acta Endocrinol. **115:** 320–325.

24. PETRAGLIA, F., D. LARIZZA, M. MAGHNIE, F. FACCHINETTI, A. VOLPE, S. BERNASCONI, A. R. GENAZZANI & F. SEVERI. 1988. Impairment of the opioideric control of LH secretion in Turner's syndrome: Lack of effect of the gonadal steroid therapy. J. Clin. Endocrinol. Metab. **66:** 1024–1028.

25. MAURAS, N., J. D. VELDHUIS & A. D. ROGOL. 1986. Role of endogenous opioid in pubertal maturation: Opposing actions of naltrexone in prepubertal and late pubertal boys. J. Clin. Endocrinol. Metab. **62:** 1256–1263.

26. GENAZZANI, A. D., F. PETRAGLIA, M. GASTALDI, C. VOLPOGNI, O. GAMBA & A. R. GENAZZANI. 1995. Naltrexone treatment restores menstrual cycles in patients with weight loss-related amenorrhea. Fertil. Steril. **64:** 954–956.

27. GENAZZANI, A. D., M. GASTALDI., F. PETRAGLIA, C. BATTAGLIA, N. SURICO, A. VOLPE & A. R. GENAZZANI. 1995. Naltrexone administration modulates neuroendocrine control of LH secretion in hypotalamic amenorrhea. Hum. Reprod. **10:** 101–104.

28. YEN, S. S. C., S. L. BERGA & B. Y. SUH. 1988. Functional hypothalamic amenorrhea: Multiple neuroendocrine aberrations. *In* The Brain and Female Reproductive Function. A. R. Genazzani, U. Montemagno, C. Nappi & F. Petraglia, Eds.: 381–393. Parthenon. Casterton Hall, U.K.

29. TRENTINI, G. P., A. R. GENAZZANI, M. CRISCUOLO, F. PETRAGLIA, C. F. DE GAETANI, G. FICARRA, B. BIDZINSKA, M. MIGALDI & A. D. GENAZZANI. 1992. Melatonin treatment delays reproductive aging of female rat via the opiatergic system. Neuroendocrinology **56:** 364–370.

The Relationship between the Immune and Endocrine Systems

ATHANASSIOS CHRYSSIKOPOULOS[a]

Second Department of Obstetrics and Gynecology
University of Athens
"Areteion" Hospital
Athens, Greece

Our rapidly increasing understanding of the regulatory mechanisms of the immune system has revealed indications that this system is subject to neuroendocrine regulation. At the same time, substances produced by the immune system may cause responsive actions in both the nervous and the endocrinological systems.

Recent investigations have demonstrated that peptide receptors, which are characterized for their neuroendocrinological activity in cellular aggregates of the immune system, were isolated while, at the same time, it was shown that factors secreted by the immune cells exercise endocrine functions and are responsible for the communication between the endocrine and immune systems.[1] This review summarizes what is currently known about the interactions of derivatives of the immune system and the endocrine system, especially their effects on reproduction.

CYTOKINES (LYMPHOKINES, MONOKINES, INTERLEUKINS)

After the first demonstration of a lymphocyte activator in 1972,[2] a great number of similar mediating factors, which induce multiplication, differentiation, and maturation of the hemopoietic cells, were also discovered.

These factors, named cytokines, are peptides or glycoproteins and are secreted by activated mesenchymal cells or cells of the immune system. They are distinguished as lymphokines or monokines, according to their origin from lymphocytes or monocytes/macrophages, respectively. The interleukins have been characterized as substances mediating the communication of lymphocytes. The cytokines transport intracellular messages among the different cells of the immune system. The majority of immunological differentiations are of local character, as are the paracrine and autocrine activities of the cytokines. Recent investigations have concluded that the cytokines are able to exercise teleactivity as well, especially on the endocrine system.

A cytokine may act on fairly different cells of various series,[3] thus mediating a variety of activities of proliferation and differentiation. Moreover, the cytokines manifest a significant overlap in their biological activities in different target cells. Despite this overlap, the cytokine activities are not identical, and each cytokine induces the multiplication of a different subcategory of T-lymphocytes. At the same time, one

[a]Address for correspondence: Athanassios Chryssikopoulos, 2nd Dept. of Obstetrics and Gynecology, University of Athens, "Areteion" Hospital, 76 Vas. Sophias Ave., GR-115 28 Athens, Greece.

cell may respond and/or produce one group of cytokines, whereas another cell may induce or inhibit the synthesis of other cytokines. The large number and diversiform activity of cytokines suggest actions at some yet-to-be defined level of the immune system.[4,5]

THE INFLUENCE OF THE IMMUNE SYSTEM ON THE ENDOCRINE SYSTEM

Interleukin-1 (IL-1) constitutes a significant mediator between the immune and endocrine systems. Notably, IL-1 increases the secretion of the adrenocorticotropic hormone (ACTH) and, consequently, the secretion of the corticosteroids in the adrenals. This activity of IL-1 is absolutely specialized, because it does not concomitantly affect the secretion of prolactin (PRL),[6] growth hormone, vasopressin,[7] and oxytocin.[8] The last two hormones can substitute the needs of the T-lymphocytes to interleukin-2 (IL-2) for the production of interferon-γ (INF-γ) in cultures of rat spleen.[9]

Recent studies have shown that IL-1 does not exercise its activity at the pituitary level but at the level of the hypothalamus, increasing secretion of corticotropin-releasing factor (CRF)[7,8,10] (FIG. 1). The CRF increase is achieved either by greater synthesis of prostaglandin E (PGE) at the anterior and posterior section of the hypothalamus[11] (current understanding is that PGE acts by stimulating ACTH at the median eminence[12,13]) or by the fact that IL-1 increases the sensibility of the CRF neurons in the catecholamines.[14]

A megalomolecular peptide, IL-1 does not pass the blood–brain barrier.[15] Despite

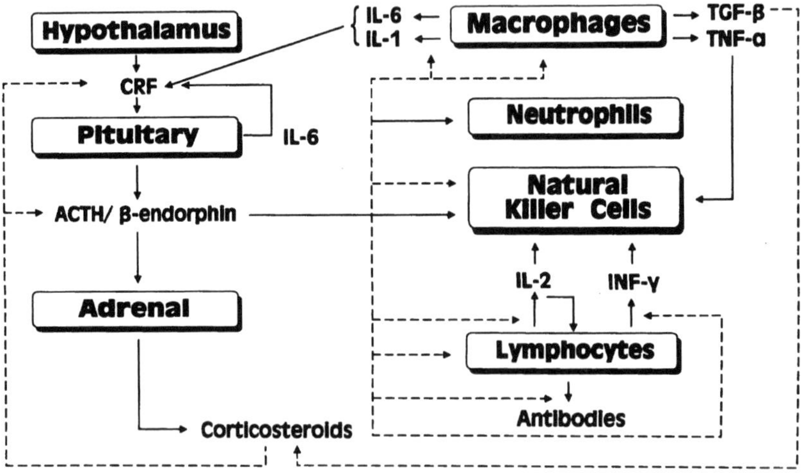

FIGURE 1. Interactions between the immunological and endocrinological system. CRF, corticotropin releasing factor; ACTH, adrenocorticotropic hormone; IL-1, IL-2, IL-6, interleukin-1, -2, -6; TNF-α, tumor necrosis factor-α, INF-γ, interferon-γ; TGF-β, transforming growth factor-β; (—) stimulation; (- - -) inhibition.

the fact that indications exist that IL-1 is synthesized at different sites of the brain[16] and that peripheral macrophages migrate within the brain,[17] most investigators believe that peripheral IL-1 enters the brain by teleactive means through areas in which the blood–brain barrier is absent, for example, the median eminence or the organum vasculosum of the laminae terminales.[18,19] Corticotropin-releasing factor and cytokines such as interleukin-6 (IL-6), tumor necrosis factor-α (TNF-α), and IL-2 also contribute to the increase of ACTH secretion through a different mechanism. TNF-α[13] and IL-2[20] stimulate the production and secretion of ACTH at the level of the pituitary, while IL-6[21] as well as IL-1 at the level of the hypothalamus, via CRF (FIG. 1).

Differentiations of the immunological system may cause increased secretion of IL-1 and consequently, via the CRF, increased production and secretion of ACTH, in turn resulting in the secretion of corticosteroids. The high level of corticosteroids inhibits further production and secretion of IL-1 in the macrophages, but at the same time inhibits the production and secretion of CRF[22] (FIG. 1). This feedback mechanism, in which substances from both the endocrine and the immune systems participate, constitutes a significant conquest of knowledge in the relationship between the two systems.

In addition to the cytokine activity in the hypothalamic–pituitary–adrenal (HPA) axis, its effect on the hypothalamic–pituitary–ovary axis (HPO) is also known. IL-1 inhibits gonadotropin-releasing hormone secretion (Gn-RH) as well as the preovulatory LH peak,[23] whereas TNF-α produces a rapid increase of LH, PRL, and ACTH secretion.[24] It is notable that, at least in experimental animals, IL-6 is produced in pituitary cells.[25] IL-1 and IL-6 both enhance gonadotropin secretion enough to compare with secretion produced by Gn-RH[26] (FIG. 2).

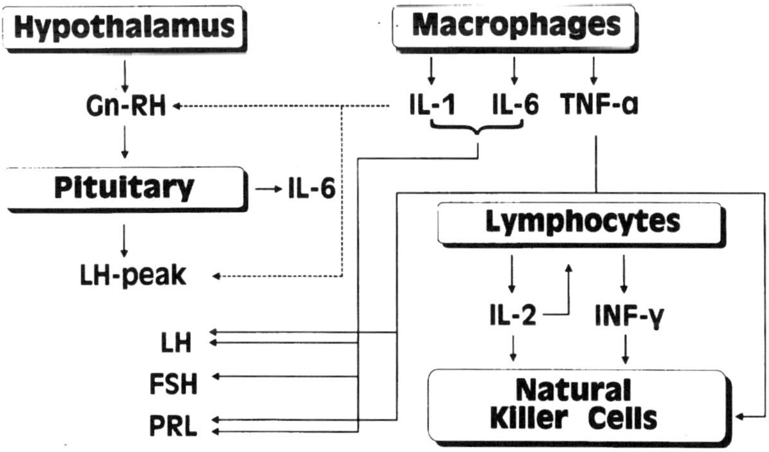

FIGURE 2. Interactions between the immunological and endocrinological system. Gn-RH, gonadotropin-releasing hormone; IL-1, IL-2, IL-6, interleukin-1, -2, -6; TNF-α, tumor necrosis factor-α; INF-γ, interferon-γ; FSH, follicle-stimulating hormone; LH, luteinizing hormone; PRL, prolactin; (—) stimulation; (---) inhibition.

The hypophyseal peptides, ACTH, α-, β-, γ-endorphin, and β-lipoprotein are derived from the same precursor protein, proopiomelanocortin (POMC).[27] Besides the hypophysis, there is a series of extra-hypophyseal organs, such as the brain,[28] the gastrointestinal system,[29] the placenta, and the gonads,[30] that are able to synthesize POMC products. It has now been generally accepted that the cellular units of the immune system synthesize and secrete POMC products.[31] The leukocytes can produce, other opioids in addition to β-endorphin,[32,33] whereas the production of mRNA preproenkephalin has been recorded in both activated T-lymphocyte-helpers[34] and macrophages.[35] These cells, in association with other extra-hypophyseal organs,[29,30] constitute a neuroendocrine complex of as-yet undetermined significance and extent. We do know that POMC product level, irrespective of source, is regulated by specific reactions of the immune system to various agents such as microbes, endotoxins, and viremias.

Up until this point, we have referred to cellular products of the immune system that act as stimulants on the HPA and HPO axes. Macrophage products exist, however, that exercise inhibitory activity. Transforming growth factor-β (TGF-β) is one such substance. The TGF-β belongs to the group that includes inhibin and the muellerian inhibiting substance.[36] Experimental evidence indicates that TGF-β inhibits both basic and ACTH-induced steroidogenesis in the adrenals, probably decreasing the enzymatic activity of 17a-hydroxylase/20,17-lyase[37–39] (FIG. 1).

Despite the fact that the normal role of inhibitory substances remains unclear, we should not overlook the observation that the adrenal cortex is, to a high degree, infiltrated by macrophages,[40] a fact that raises suspicion for a possible paracrinic association between the immune and endocrine systems. A similar paracrinic relationship exists among the products of the macrophages and the granulosa and luteal cells of the ovary. We thus observe the unusual phenomenon of some macrophages that synthesize polypeptides (IL-1) that stimulate the HPA and, at the same time, others (TGF-β) that inhibit it. The oddity of this phenomenon is significantly mitigated by the observation that the stimulating cytokines mainly have a central activity (IL-1), whereas the inhibition is exercised peripherically and occurs in the adrenals (FIG. 1).

THE EFFECT OF THE ENDOCRINE SYSTEM ON THE IMMUNE SYSTEM

The relationship between the two systems is not limited to positive or negative effects of the immune cell products on the functional activity of the HPA and HPO axes, but it is also extended to the retrograde effect of the hormonal products on both axes of the immune system. It is known that human phagocytes[41] and lymphocytes[42] have opioid receptors, but this opioid activity is not inhibited by naloxone. The activity of the natural killer (NK) cells is differentiated by β-endorphin and the enkephalines.[43–45] Moreover, β-endorphin increases the production of INF-γ in the mononuclear cells,[43] whereas ACTH inhibits the production of INF-γ in the spleen cells of the rat.[9]

Apart from these discrete observations is the whole complex of activities of corticosteroids. The negative feedback exercised by the corticosteroids in the production and secretion of IL-1, thus regulating its total production, has already been stated.

The effect of the corticosteroids to the immune system is multiple. They produce lymphocytopenia,[46] while at the same time they increase the neutrophil population.[47] They inhibit the production of IL-2,[48] which constitutes a significant growth factor of the T-lymphocytes, while cortisol inhibits the production of INF-γ,[49] which favors increased activity of NK-cells. The corticosteroids generally inhibit the activity of NK-cells[49,50] (FIG. 1).

EFFECT OF THE CYTOKINES ON THE OVARY

Apart from the teleactions between the two systems mentioned above, a dynamic correlation, paracrine or autocrine, seems to exist in the ovary. Low levels of gonadal steroids stimulate IL-1 production, although at higher levels they inhibit the production of both IL-1 and TNF-α.[51,52] On the other hand, cytokines seem to be significant regulators of ovarian function. The presence of macrophages in the corpus luteum of various experimental animals[53] suggests that their products come into dynamic play in paracrine and autocrine control of ovarian steroid production. Studies in rats corpora lutea (CL) have indicated that macrophages secrete substances that stimulate luteal cell progesterone (P) production and act as intragonadal luteotropic agents.[54] In another study, macrophages were demonstrated to be the dominant cell population in the rabbit CL during regression, whereas only a few were observed in young CL.[53] It has also been reported that the young CL produces significantly smaller quantities of TNF-α than the regressing CL,[53,55] while at the same time it affects the P production by the luteinizing granulosa cells.[56] Therefore, the macrophages probably play some kind of role in the commencement of CL regression with the production of the cytotoxic peptide TNF-α.[56]

Various studies report on the significant role of cytokines in folliculogenesis. Besides the macrophages, TNF-α is also produced by the granulosa cells,[57] and it is augmented by FSH. Cytokine concentration is higher in the preovulatory follicle, and its activity is biphasic.[56,57] FSH induced TNF-α production in the granulosa cells inhibits prostaglandin F_{2a} (PGF_{2a}) production which, in turn, suppresses the production of cytokine in the phagocytes.[3] Before ovulation, TNF-α increases short-term PGF_{2a} production,[58] and thus probably contributes to ovulation. In rats, TNF-α was shown to inhibit the induction of the FSH-induced aromatase activity[59] and the subsequent increase in P synthesis (FIG. 3). TNF-α also inhibits the hCG-induced increase of androsterone,[60] probably by inhibiting the activity of the enzymatic system of 17a-hydroxylase/17,20-lyase, although it does not affect the basic secretion of the hormone. Finally, TNF-α increases the production of 17-hydroxyprogesterone and androstendione in pre-ovulatory rat theca cells.[61] These observations reinforce the probability and possibility that this cytokine exercises different activities during the various phases of the follicle and the corpus luteum.

The other cytokine, IL-1, decreases FSH-induced LH receptor production in the granulosa cells and, consequently the P production.[62,63] At the same time TGF-β, produced in the lymphocytes, increases the production of the aromatase enzymes at low FSH levels,[64] whereas at high levels it decreases the LH receptor population (FIG. 4). IL-1 is also traced in the macrophages-free follicular fluid, indicating that the granulosa cells contribute to the production of cytokine. IL-1 inhibits the hCG-in-

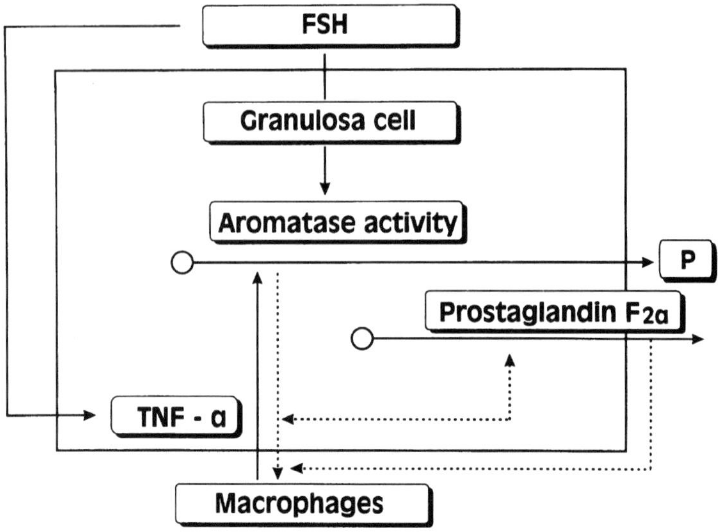

FIGURE 3. Paracrinic and autocrinic activity of tumor necrosis factor-α (TNF-α) in granulosa cells; P, progesterone; FSH, follicle-stimulating hormone.

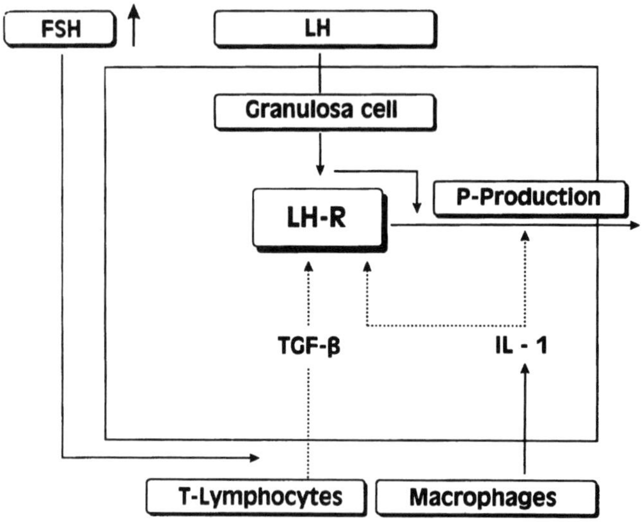

FIGURE 4. Paracrinic activity of interleukin-1 (IL-1) and transforming growth factor-β (TGF-β) in granulosa cells. LH-R, receptors of LH; P, progesterone; FSH, follicle-stimulating hormone; LH, luteinizing hormone; (—) stimulation; (--) inhibition.

duced androgen production (androstendione) in the young rat.[65] The evolution of steroidogenesis in cultured cells of the theca, in the presence of IL-1, suggests, precisely as in the case of TNF-α, the inhibition of the enzymic system of 17a-hydroxylase/17,20-lyase with contemporary stimulation of the enzyme of 20-hydroxysteroid dehydrogenase.[65] Recent studies indicate that IL-1 induces de-differentiation and growth of cells in the process of proliferating or differentiating but has no effect on the functions of fully differentiated cells.[66]

In conclusion, a significant complex of indications may prove that a well-controlled circuit exists between the immune and endocrine systems, functioning at several levels. Immunological differentiations stimulate the hormonal HPA axis via cytokines, and the corticosteroids produced control the production of cytokines. On the other hand, in the HPO axis, cytokines in collaboration with growth factors play a significant role in the development and differentiation of the human reproductive system.

Our current knowledge allows us to anticipate that eventually our understanding of the delicate mechanisms of interaction between the immune and endocrine systems will allow us to develop therapies for the improved reproductive efficiency.

SUMMARY

Increasing evidence links the immune and endocrine systems. Cytokines produced by activated immune and immune accessory cells can affect, positively or negatively, the secretion of hormones from the hypothalamic–pituitary–adrenal or hypothalamic–pituitary–ovarian axes. On the other hand, adrenal and ovarian hormones affect the secretion of cytokines by cells of the immune system. The interaction also occurs at a local level in paracrine or autocrine fashion. Cytokines produced by resident ovarian macrophages or ovarian cells can affect the follicle and the corpus luteum and, consequently, ovarian steroidogenesis at both phases of the menstrual cycle. Conversely, the ovarian steroids influence, positively or negatively, the secretion of cytokines from both the resident macrophages and local endocrine cells.

REFERENCES

1. Wegmann, T.E. 1990. The cytokine basis for cross-talk between the maternal immune and reproductive systems. Curr. Opin. Immunol. **2:** 765–769.
2. Gery, I., R. K. Gershow & B. H. Waksman. 1972. Potentiation of the T-lymphocyte response to mitogens. I. The responding cells. J. Exp. Med. **136:** 128–142.
3. Dinarello, C. A. 1989. Interleukin-1 and its related cytokines. Adv. Immunol. **44:** 205–211.
4. Trotta, P. P. 1991. Cytokines: An overview. Am. J. Reprod. Immunol. **25:** 137–141.
5. Garcia-Lioret, M. I. & J. Ignasio Santos. 1990. Cytokines and their role as health and disease mediators, new approaches to old problems. Bull. Med. Hosp. Infant Mex. **17:** 797–808.
6. Uehara, A., P. E. Gottschall, R. R. Dahl & A. Arimura. 1987. Interleukin-1 stimulates ACTH release by an indirect action which requires endogenous corticotropin releasing factor. Endocrinology **121:** 1580–1588.

7. Berkenbosch, F., J. Van Oers, A. Del Rey, F. Tiders & H. Besedovsky. 1987. Corticotropin releasing factor producing neurons in the rat activated by interleukin-1. Science **238:** 524–530.
8. Sapolsky, R., C. Rivier, G. Yamamoto, P. Plotsky & W. Yale. 1987. Interleukin-1 stimulates the secretion of hypothalamic corticotropin releasing factor. Science **238:** 522–524.
9. Johnson, H. M., B. A. Torres, E. M. Smith, L. D. Dion & J. E. Blalock. 1984. Regulation of lymphokine (γ-interferon) production by corticotropin. J. Immunol. **132:** 246–250.
10. Bateman, A., A. Singh, T. Kral & S. Solomon. 1989. The immune–pituitary–adrenal axis. Endocrinol. Rev. **10:** 92–112.
11. Dinarello, C. A. & H. A. Bernheim. Ability of human leukocyte pyrogen to stimulate brain prostaglandin synthesis in vitro. J. Neurochem. **37:** 702–710.
12. Hedge, G. A. & S. D. Hanson. 1972. The effects of prostaglandin on ACTH secretion. Endocrinology **91:** 925–932.
13. Sharp, B. M., S. G. Matta, P. K. Peterson, R. Newton, C. Chao & K. Meallen. 1989. Tumor necrosis factor is a potent ACTH secretagogue: Comparison to interleukin-1β. Endocrinology **124:** 3131–3138.
14. Dunn, A. J. 1988. Systematic interleukin-1 administration stimulates hypothalamic norepinephrine metabolism paralleling the increased plasma corticosterone. Life Sci. **43:** 429–438.
15. Coceani, F., J. Lees & C. A. Dinarello. 1988. Occurrence of interleukin-1 in cerebrospinal fluid of the conscious rat. Brain Res. **446:** 245–255.
16. Giulan, D., T. J. Baker, L.-C. N. Shih & L. B. Lachman. 1986. Interleukin-1 of the central nervous system is produced by ameboid microglia. J. Exp. Med. **164:** 594–601.
17. Schackert, G., R. D. Simmons, T. M. Buzbee, D. A. Hume & I. J. Fidler. 1988. Macrophage infiltration into experimental brain metastases occurrence through an intact blood barrier. J. Natl. Cancer Inst. **80:** 1027–1033.
18. Stitt, J. T. 1985. Evidence for the involvement of the organum vasculosum laminae terminalis in the febrile response of rabbits and rats. J. Physiol. (London) **368:** 501–510.
19. Morimoto, A., N. Murakami, T. Nakamori & T. Watanabe. 1988. Multiple control of fever production in the central nervous system of rabbits. J. Physiol. (London) **397:** 269–278.
20. Woloski, B. M. R. N. J., E. M. Smith, W. J. Meyer III, G. M. Fuller & J. E. Blalock. 1985. Corticotropin-releasing activity of monokine. Science **230:** 1035–1040.
21. Naitoh, Y., J. Fukata, T. Tominaga, Y. Nakai, S. Tami, K. Mori & H. Imura. 1988. Interleukin-6 stimulates the secretion of adrenocorticotropic hormone in conscious freely moving rats. Biochem. Biophys. Res. Commun. **155:** 1459–1468.
22. Del Ray, A., H. Besedovsky, E. Sorkin & C. A. Dinarello. 1987. Interleukin-1 and glucocorticoid hormones integrate an immunoregulatory feedback circuit. Ann. N.Y. Acad. Sci. **496:** 85–92.
23. Kalra, P. S., A. Sahu & S. P. Kalra. 1990. Interleukin-1 inhibits the ovarian steroid induced luteinizing hormone surge and release of hypothalamic luteinizing hormone-releasing hormone in rats. Endocrinology **126:** 2145–2152.
24. Yamaguchi, M., M. Sakata, N. Matsuzaki, K. Koike, A. Miyake & O. Tanizawa. 1990. Induction by tumor necrosis factor-alpha of rapid release of immunoreactive and bioactive luteinizing hormone from rat pituitary in vitro. Neuroendocrinology **52:** 468–472.
25. Spangelo, B. L., R. M. Macleod & P. C. Isakson. 1990. Production of interleukin-6 by anterior pituitary cells in vitro. Endocrinology **126:** 582–586.
26. Yamaguchi, M., N. Matsuzaki, K. Hirota, A. Miyake & O. Tanizawa. 1990. Interleukin-6 possibly induced by interleukin-1b in the pituitary gland stimulates the release of gonadotropins and prolactin. Acta Endocrinol. (Copenhagen) **122:** 201–205.

27. NAKANISHI, S., A. INONE, T. KITA, M. NAKAMURA, A. C. Y. CHANG, S. COHEN & S. NUMA. 1979. Nucleotide sequence of cloned cDNA for bovine corticotropin-β-lipotropin precursor. Nature **278:** 423–430.

28. KRIEGER, D. T., A. LIOTTA & M. BROWNSTEIN. 1977. Presence of corticotropin in brain of normal and hypophysectomised rats. Brain Res. **128:** 575–579.

29. LARSSON, L. I. 1977. Corticotropin-like peptides in central nerves and in endocrine cells of gut and pancreas. Lancet **2:** 1321–1323.

30. LIM, A. T., S. LOLAIT, J. W. BARLOW, O. WAI SUM, I. ZOIS, B. H. TOH & J. W. FUNDER. 1983. Immunoreactive β-endorphin in sheep ovary. Nature **303:** 709–714.

31. SMITH, E. M. & E. J. BLALOCK. 1981. Human lymphocyte production of corticotropin and endorphin-like substances: Association with leucocyte interferon. Proc. Natl. Acad. Sci. USA **77:** 7530–7536.

32. WESTLY, H. J., A. J. KLEISS, K. W. KELLEY, P. K. WONG & P.-H. YUEN. 1986. Newcastle disease virus-infected splenocytes express the proopiomelanocortin gene. J. Exp. Med. **163:** 1589–1599.

33. HARBOUR, M. C., D. MENAMIN, E. M. SMITH & J. E. BLALOCK. 1985. Bacterial lipopolysaccharide induction of leukocyte-derived corticotropin and endorphins. Infect. Immun. **48:** 813–819.

34. ZYRAWSKI, G., M. BENEDIK, B. J. KAMB, J. S. ABRAMS, S. M. ZURAWSKI & F. D. LEE. 1986. Activation of mouse T-helper cells induces abundant preproenkephalin mRNA synthesis. Science **232:** 772–779.

35. MARTIN, J., M. B. PRYSTOWSKY & R. H. ANGELETTI. 1987. Preproenkephalin mRNA in T-cells, macrophages and mast cells. J. Neurosci. Res. **18:** 82–90.

36. KNECHT, M., PEI FENG & K. I. CATT. 1989. Transforming growth factor-beta: Autocrine, paracrine and endocrine effects in ovarian cells. Semin. Reprod. Endocrinol. **7:** 12–20.

37. FEIGGE, J. J., C. COCHET & E. M. CHAMBAR. 1986. Type β transforming growth factor is a potent medulator of differentiated adrenocortical cell functions. Biochem. Biophys. Res. Commun. **139:** 693–701.

38. HOTTA, M. & A. BAIRD. 1986. Differential effects of transforming growth factor type b on the growth and function of adrenocortical cells in vitro. Proc. Natl. Acad. Sci. USA **83:** 7795–7803.

39. FEIGGE, J. J., C. COCHET, W. E. RAINEY, C. MADANI & E. M. CHAMBAZ. 1987. Type b transforming growth factor affects adrenocortical cell differentiated functions. J. Biol. Chem. **262:** 1349–1358.

40. HUME, D. A., D. HALPIN, H. CHARLTON & S. GORDON. 1984. The mononuclear phagocyte system of the mouse defined by immunohistochemical localization of antigen F4/80: Macrophages of endocrine organs. Proc. Natl. Acad. Sci. USA **81:** 4174–4181.

41. LOPKER, A., L. G. ABOOD, W. HOSS & F. J. LIONETTI. 1980. Stereoselective muscarinic acetylcholine and opiate receptors in human phagocytic leucocytes. Biochem. Pharmacol. **29:** 1361–1372.

42. WYBRAN, J., T. APPELBOOM, J. P. FAMAEY & A. COVAERTS. 1979. Suggestive evidence for receptors for morphine and methionine enkephalin on normal human blood T lymphozytes. J. Immunol. **123:** 1068–1077.

43. MANDLER, R. N., W. E. BIDDISON, R. MANDLER & S. A. SERRATE. 1986. β-Endorphin augments the cytolytic activity and interferon production of natural killer cells. J. Immunol. **136:** 934–942.

44. FAITH, R. E., H. J. LIANG, A. J. MURGO & N. P. PLOTNIKOFF. 1984. Neuroimmunomodulation with enkephalins: Enhancement of human natural killer (NK) cell activity in vitro. Clin. Immunol. Immunopathol. **31:** 412–420.

45. KAY, N. E. & J. E. MORLEY. 1983. β-Endorphin enhances human natural killer (NK) cell activity. Clin. Res. **31:** 364A.

46. Fauci, A. S. & D. C. Dale. 1974. The effects of in vivo hydrocortisone on subpopulations of human lymphocytes. J. Clin. Invest. **53:** 240–249.
47. Dale, D. C., A. S. Fauci, I. V. D. Guerry & S. M. Wolff. 1975. Comparison of agents producing a neutrophilic leucocytosis in man. J. Clin. Invest. **56:** 808–813.
48. Dupont, E., K. Huygen, L. Schandene, M. Vandercruys, K. Palfliet & J. Wybran. 1985. Influence of in vivo immunosuppressive drugs on production of lymphokines. Transplantation **39:** 143–151.
49. Carallo, R., M. L. Sartori, G. Gatti & A. Angeli. 1986. Cortisol and immune interferon can interact in the modulation of human killer natural cell activity. Experientia **42:** 177–188.
50. Holbrook, N. J., W. I. Cox & H. C. Horner. 1983. Direct suppression of natural killer activity in human peripheral blood leucozyte cultures by glucocorticoids and its modulation by interferon. Cancer Res. **43:** 4019–4030.
51. Ralston, S. H., R. G. G. Russel & M. Cowen. 1990. Estrogen inhibits release of tumor necrosis factor from peripheral blood mononuclear cells in postmenopausal women. J. Bone Miner. Res. **5:** 983–988.
52. Polan, M. L., A. Danielle & A. Kuo. 1988. Gonadal steroids modulate human monocyte interleukin-1 (IL-1) activity. Fertil. Steril. **49:** 964–968.
53. Bagavadoss, P., S. Kunkel, R. C. Wiggins & P. L. Keyes. 1988. Tumor necrosis factor-α (TNF-α) production and localization of macrophages and T-lymphocytes in the rabbit corpus luteum. Endocrinology **122:** 1185–1187.
54. Kirsh, T. M., A. C. Friedman, R. L. Vogel & G. L. Flickinger. 1981. Macrophages in the corpora lutea of mice: Characterization and effects of steroid secretion. Biol. Reprod. **25:** 629–632.
55. Ben-Rafael, Z. & R. Orvieto. 1992. Cytokines-involvement in reproduction. Fertil. Steril. **58:** 1093–1099.
56. Adashi, E. Y., C. E. Resnick, J. N. Packman, A. Hurwitz & D. W. Payne. 1990. Cytokine-mediated regulation of ovarian function: Tumor necrosis factor-α inhibits gonadotropin-supported progesteron accumulation by differentiating luteinizing murine granulosa cells. Am. J. Obstet. Gynecol. **162:** 889–899.
57. Zolti, M., R. Meirom, M. Shemesh, D. Wollach, S. Mashiach & L. Shore. 1990. Granulosa cells as a source and target organ for tumor necrosis factor-α. FEBS Lett. **261:** 253–255.
58. Shemesh, M., R. Meirom, M. Zolti, Z. Ben-Rafael & D. R. Wellach. 1990. Tumor necrosis factor (TNF-α) and the endogenous prostaglandin inhibitor (PG In) in bovine follicles. *In* Advances in *in Vitro* Fertilization and Embryo Transfer. S. Mashiach, Z. Ben-Rafael, N. Laufer & J. Schenker, Eds.: 129–137. Plenum. New York.
59. Emoto, L. & A. Baired. 1988. The effect of tumor necrosis factor/cachectin on follicle-stimulating hormone-induced aromatase activity in cultured rat granulosa cells. Biochem. Biophys. Res. Commun. **153:** 792–798.
60. Andreani, C. L., D. W. Payne & J. N. Packman. 1991. Cytokine-mediated regulation of ovarian function. Tumor necrosis factor-α inhibits gonadotropin supported ovarian androgen biosynthesis. J. Biol. Chem. **266:** 6761–6766.
61. Roby, K. F. & P. F. Terranova. 1990. Effects of tumor necrosis factor-α in vitro steroidogenesis of healthy and atretic follicles of the rat: Theca as a target. Endocrinology **126:** 2711–2718.
62. Fukuoka, M., T. Tori, S. Taii & K. Yasuda. 1988. Interleukin-1 inhibits luteinization of porcine granulosa cells in culture. Endocrinology **122:** 367–369.
63. Gottschalk, P. E., A. Uehara, S. T. Hoffman & A. Arimura. 1987. Interleukin-1 inhibits follicle stimulating hormone-induced differentiation in rat granulosa cells in vitro. Biochem. Biophys. Res. Commun. **149:** 502–509.

64. KNECHT, M., P. FENG & K. J. CATT. 1987. Bifunctional role of transforming growth factor-beta during granulosa cell development. Endocrinology **120:** 1243–1249.
65. HURWITZ, A., D. W. PAYNE & J. N. PACKMAN. 1991. Cytokine-mediated regulation of ovarian function: Interleukin-1 inhibits gonadotropin induced androgen biosynthesis. Endocrinology **129:** 1250–1256.
66. FUKUOKA, M., K. YASUDA, S. TAII, K. TAKAKURA & T. MORI. 1989. Interleukin-1 stimulates growth and inhibits progesterone secretion in cultures of porcine granulosa cells. Endocrinology **124:** 884–890.

Depression and Suicide in Children and Adolescents

VICTORIA H. BESSEGHINI[a]

Department of Psychiatry
State University of New York
Buffalo, New York 14214

It is only recently in psychiatry that we have come to recognize depression as a condition that can affect children and adolescents. Although the average age of onset is in the late twenties, major depressive episodes may begin at any age, including infancy. The duration of a depressive episode is also variable. Untreated, the episodes may last six months or longer. Usually, there is a complete remission of the symptoms and general functioning returns to the predepression level. But in a large proportion of cases, some symptoms of the episode persist for as long as two years.

In the United States the prevalence of major depression is estimated as 4.7%, and dysthymia, which is what we refer to as chronic or neurotic depression, is found to have a prevalence of 3.3% or, in some studies, as much as 20.8%.

We are also increasingly concerned about attempted and successful suicides, which in some areas have reached nearly epidemic proportions. Among adolescents in the United States, suicide is the third leading cause of death.

A recurrence of suicidal behavior in treated children and adolescents is high. In a study by Kovacs, 26% of recovered patients relapsed within one year, and 40% had relapsed within two years. Prevalence of depression up to age 9 is very low but rises sharply from ages 9 to 19, especially among females.[1]

The transition from childhood to adolescence makes a youngster susceptible to depression as a result of a variety of biological and social familial factors. Many times, it is not easy to distinguish between normal sadness and pathologic depression. If an adverse event has occurred, we must question whether or not we are observing a normal or excessive reaction. Also complicating the diagnosis of depression is the great difficulty that adolescents have in experiencing and controlling depression. They try to protect themselves by acting out through behavioral disruptions in an effort to deny the feeling. They may show their depressive feelings in a number of ways, that is, temper tantrums, disobedience, truancy from school, failing in school and dropping out, stealing, running away from home, getting involved in accidents or engaging in promiscuous sexual involvement, use of drugs, and a wide range of other delinquent behaviors. Depression is sometimes expressed through eating disturbances, particularly anorexia but at times by overeating, weight gain, sleeping too much, or displaying a very low level of energy. Other adolescents may internalize their feelings and present themselves as anxious, withdrawn, and having a variety of somatic complaints, such as excessive fatigue, headaches, and quite often abdominal

[a]Address for correspondence: Victoria H. Besseghini, M.D., 663 Lafayette Avenue, Buffalo, NY 14222.

pain.[2] Most adolescents are unable to contain the depressive feelings. To them anything is better than being depressed. An adolescent will very rarely admit to being depressed, and if confronted will deny it.

During the transition from childhood to adolescence, a variety of biological and social influences make a youngster more susceptible to depression. The biological, social, and psychological transformations of early adolescence may increase susceptibility to moodiness and aggression and stimulate the urge and demands for independence. Yet, the adolescent's capacity to solve problems on the basis of past experiences is limited, and the imbalance between the environmental demands and the adolescent's psychological strengths may generate perceptions of vulnerability. The adolescent battles with feelings of inadequacy, worthlessness, helplessness, and hopelessness and feels lonely and rejected. The adolescent needs to reassess his feelings about his parents in order to move toward a more independent and autonomous self. If there are family problems or intense conflicts with parents and the parent is either not consistently available or is too rigid or oppressive in reaction to the adolescent's attempts toward independence, the adolescent feels hostility toward the depriving parent who is also lost. He or she feels terrible, and depression and guilt are increased. We do not know why one adolescent can contain the depression through acting out behaviors while another needs to expiate his sins by turning his aggression upon himself. Very often, the parents of depressed adolescents have problems of their own. Many have tried to find outlets for their own neurotic and antisocial needs through their children and are unable to perceive and respond to the children's needs. The adolescent ends up with pervasive feelings that his parents do not care for him and have abandoned him. There are four main categories of clues to look for in the clinical assessment of depression. First is the type of behavior the adolescent exhibits and to what extent his or her behavior is self-destructive.

Second is a loss as a precipitating factor. The search is for events that may have triggered the depression and the secondary acting out. It may be an obvious loss like a parent's death, divorce, or remarriage; or it may be that the parents have become, for one reason or the other, preoccupied with their own needs or other family members' needs so that the adolescent has lost their attention. Alternatively, it may be a sibling or another important person in the adolescent's life who has gone off to another state, college, or has gotten married.

Separation from any person who plays an important part in the adolescent's life may be a trigger for depression. At other times, the loss is personal, such as loss of status, a failure to be accepted by peers, loss of self esteem, or any blow to the adolescent's basic narcissism.

A third area to look into is the adolescent's past history regarding the adjustment in school, family, and social areas. Most important is his style of coping with stress. What are the adolescent's interpersonal skills and what are his abilities to generate cognitive and behavioral alternatives to solve problems. Assessments of the adolescent's abilities to control impulses, tolerate frustration, ability to delay reactions, and plan for future events are very important in assessing his or her strengths and weaknesses. The last important area is the parental relationship. In assessing the family environment and parental relationships of many depressed adolescents, one can identify different degrees of emotional deprivation. As a result, the child comes to adolescence with an immature personality substrate, not having achieved the necessary emotional development to be able to cope with the increasing demands of that developmental period.[3]

In treating the depressed adolescent, we use antidepressant medications, but we truly do not have enough rigorous studies to prove that they are effective. We now have better antidepressants in our formulary, at least ones that have fewer side effects, but the most important form of intervention remains psychotherapy. The first step in treatment is to try to get the adolescent to control his behavior by establishing a relationship and developing insight into the self-destructive nature of his actions. Care has to be taken that depression is not introduced too early in the course of treatment as an explanation for the acting out. The adolescent will deny it and may never come back. It is more effective to allow him to first recognize the destructive nature of his actions. Each time he controls some aspect of that behavior, he becomes more depressed. It is at this time that he can acquire more insight into his state of depression. The aim of psychotherapy is to replace the feeling of hopelessness with a sense of hope. One thing that is important in working with adolescents is that they will not respond to treatment unless they become convinced that you understand them and accept them and that you are knowledgeable enough to know what you are doing.

Of course, in working with the depressed adolescent, the ongoing concern is the risk of suicide. Although not all suicides are a result of depression, suicidal attempts frequently indicate a serious degree of depression. Motives for suicides and ways of attempting it are varied, and there are no set rules for preventing it. One thing is certain, any adolescent who talks about committing suicide has to be taken seriously. This does not mean that they have to be hospitalized or even indulged. They need to be assessed individually because the number of those who toy with the idea of committing suicide is many times greater than the number who actually do it. Also the number that attempt suicide is several times larger than the number that succeed. Estimates in the literature are that for every completed suicide there are 6 to 50 attempts. The suicide rate in the United States for adolescents is about 5 to 20 per hundred thousand in the 15 to 24 age group. Statistics for attempts are higher, with an estimate of 2 to 10% of young people attempting suicide, although some statistics go as high as 20 to 25%.[4] Males are more often successful than females. For females, the rate of completed suicide is 20% of all suicides among adolescents with 80% being males. There also some rather interesting data about females in comparison to males who commit suicide. Females are more psychiatrically disturbed than males. They have generally made previous suicide attempts and have had a history of psychiatric care and severe depression. Males exhibit more antisocial behavior, substance abuse disorders, and adjustment disorders. Alcohol abuse seems to be a factor in both males and females. For both groups family problems and interpersonal difficulties are common. Males commit suicide mostly by using firearms and by drowning. Methods used by females are more likely to be overdosing, hanging, or jumping from high places or under trains. The literature concludes that suicide is seldom spontaneous and impulsive. Two-thirds of the adolescents had made previous attempts, and all had seriously considered suicide for a long time as a solution to their troubles. Many of them had cut themselves off from parents, friends, and teachers and had no one to talk to. Many had experienced a romantic attachment that ended in disappointment, and others lost their siblings or close friends. A state of hopelessness and use of drugs or alcohol are the most dangerous combinations. Sometime the suicidal act is an attempt to make a parent or other depriving important person change his way of relating; prove his love; or, in the event of completed suicide, punish the depriver by making him feel sorry, guilty, and responsible for the youngster's death.

A very high percentage of youths who attempt suicide have had a friend or parent who attempted suicide.[5] The phenomenon of contagion may also occur in a particular school system or in other institutional settings.

Suicidal behavior in children has been associated with suicidal behavior among family members. More first-degree relatives of child suicide attempters compared to first-degree relatives of normal children had an antisocial personality disorder such as assaultive behavior and/or substance abuse. Nearly 50% of mothers of suicidal children reported a suicide attempt compared to more than 25% of mothers of children who reported thinking of suicide and a minimal number of mothers of normal children.

In doing a lethality assessment in which we assess the true risk of suicide, what we look for is levels of family support and daily adjustment problems. We also inquire about whether a definite plan exists and whether or not the means for harmful behavior are available. We keep the family alert, and ask them to dispose of guns, poisons, or any other medications that could be potentially harmful. We also direct the family to keep syrup of ipecac in the house because of the possibility of an attempt by the ingestion of drugs.

In treating suicidal youngsters, preventive methods aim at strengthening their defenses (that is the processes that regulate their subjective experiences of painful ideas, affects, and emotions) and by giving them a sense of hope and belief in themselves.

Depression and suicide in adolescents, and in children too, in the United States is a real problem, not a rare event. We need to be on the alert, sensitive to the issue, and be cautious of our own need for denial. Although the prevalence of the problem is different in various parts of the world, no country or city is immune. In the United States, the problem is of epidemic proportion because problems of family disintegration, drug abuse, and other negative sociocultural influences are on the increase.

SUMMARY

Presented here is a review of data regarding depression and suicide in children and adolescents. It covers prevalence, developmental vulnerabilities, defenses specific to adolescence, and symptoms specific to this transitional age.

Psychosomatics, family relations, and societal and moral stresses as they affect psychic stability and identity formation are discussed. Precipitation factors, suicide risk assessment, and review of treatment interventions are included.

REFERENCES

1. SHONFELD, WILLIAM. 1995. Depression in adolescents. Adolesc. Psychiatry Ann. **20:** 31–38.
2. TRAD, J. 1995. Anxiety, depression and psychosomatic disorders in adolescence. Adolesc. Psychiatry Ann. **20:** 179–202.

3. Gould, L. 1965. Suicide problems in children and adolescents. Am. J. Psychother. **19:** 228–246.
4. Teacher, A. & L. Jacobs. 1966. Adolescents who attempt suicide: Preliminary findings. Am. J. Psychiatry **122:** 1248–1257.
5. Miller, Dereck. 1993. Adolescent suicide: Etiology and treatment. Adolesc. Psychiatry Ann. **19:** 361–183.

Estrogen and Progesterone Receptors in the Endometrium

P. MOUTSATSOU[a] AND C. E. SEKERIS[a,b]

[a]*Laboratory of Biological Chemistry,*
University of Athens Medical School
75 Mikros Asias, Goudi 11527
Athens, Greece

[b]*Institute of Biological Research and Biotechnology*
National Hellenic Research Foundation
48, Vas. Constaitinou Avenue
Athens 11635, Greece

INTRODUCTION

Estrogens and progesterone are the principal hormonal regulators of female development and functions of pregnancy. The endometrium is a target of these steroids, which are responsible for the periodic cyclic changes in its anatomy and physiology.[1] The menstrual cycle and pregnancy are complex processes involving cell replication, growth, and differentiation, under the influence not only of the sex hormones, but also of other hormones, growth factors, neurotransmitters, and various regulatory molecules. In all these processes estrogen receptors (ER) and progesterone receptors (PR) play a central role. They receive messages from their own ligands, but also from a whole gamut of other regulatory molecules, transmitting them to genes whose products define the functions of the target tissues.

Most of the genes affected by ER and PR and studied in depth from the molecular point of view either encode the ER and PR themselves or are genes involved in cell cycle control, directly or indirectly, through modulation of the transcription of cell cycle regulatory genes. Many structural components and other specific products of endometrial cells are induced by the sex hormones, but these will not be considered in this review.

As most but not all steroid effects are mediated by the respective hormone receptors, these protein molecules have been subjected to intensive investigation regarding their biochemistry and molecular biology as it relates to the physiology and pathophysiology of the endometrium.

STRUCTURE OF THE ER AND PR

ER and PR are members of the superfamily of nuclear receptors and are modeled on the same principles, with main functional domains for ligand binding, DNA binding, and transcription modulation.[2,3] Cloning of the genes and studies at the protein level have elucidated the primary structure of these proteins.[4,5] FIGURE 1 shows the structure of the ER.

The ER is composed of 595 amino acids and can be divided into six functional regions (A–F). Region E (amino acids 302–552) is responsible for efficient hormone binding, for dimerization of the receptor, its interaction with heat-shock protein 90K (hsp90), and activation of transcription. Region A/B (amino acids 1–185) is involved in transcription modulation and is the most immunoreactive part of the receptor. Region D (amino acids 250–274) is involved in interaction with hsp90 and in nuclear localization of the receptor. Region F, the COOH-terminal region (amino acids 552–595), seems to have a specific modulatory function that affects the transcriptional activity of the liganded ER and also the agonist–antagonist effectiveness of antioestrogens. Region C (amino acids 185–250), the highly conserved DNA-binding domain, is shown in FIGURE 2 as two subregions CI (amino acids 185–215) and CII (amino acids 216–250), each containing four highly conserved cysteine residues that coordinate zinc tetrahedrally to form a zinc finger. The three amino acids within region CI, which are important for the receptor to distinguish between an estrogen-responsive element and a glucocorticoid-response element, are denoted by asterisks.

The human progesterone receptor depicted schematically in FIGURE 3 exists in two sizes, A (768 amino acids) and B (933 amino acids), the B form consisting of the A protein plus 165 additional amino acids at the NH_2-terminus.[5,6]

Regions C and E of ER and PR are highly conserved (100% and 94%, respectively). In their transcriptionally inactive form, ER and PR are associated with other proteins, such as the hsp90, hsp70, p59, p54, p50, and p23,[7] with which they form a heteropolymer complex.

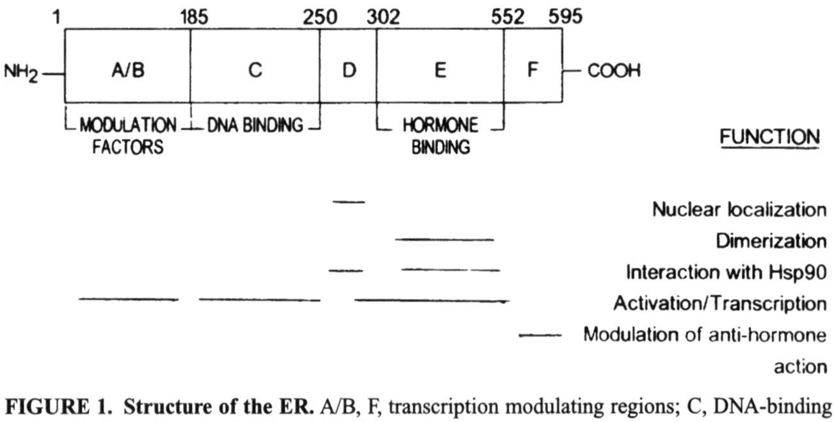

FIGURE 1. Structure of the ER. A/B, F, transcription modulating regions; C, DNA-binding region; D, "hinge" region; E, ligand-binding region.

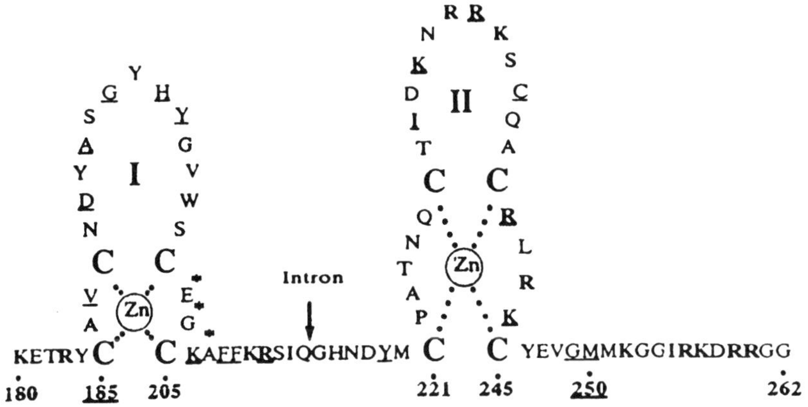

FIGURE 2. The DNA binding domain of the estrogen receptor.

MECHANISMS OF ACTION OF STEROID HORMONES

Interaction of Receptors with the Genetic Material

The mechanism of action of hormonal steroids by way of modulation of transcription is well documented[2,3,8] and is shown schematically in FIGURE 4.

The steroid hormone binds to the receptor and induces a change in its conformation, which leads to dissociation of the hsp and other proteins, dimerization of the receptor, binding of the dimer to specific DNA sequences, the hormone response elements (HRE) (TABLE 1), and formation, in association with other nuclear

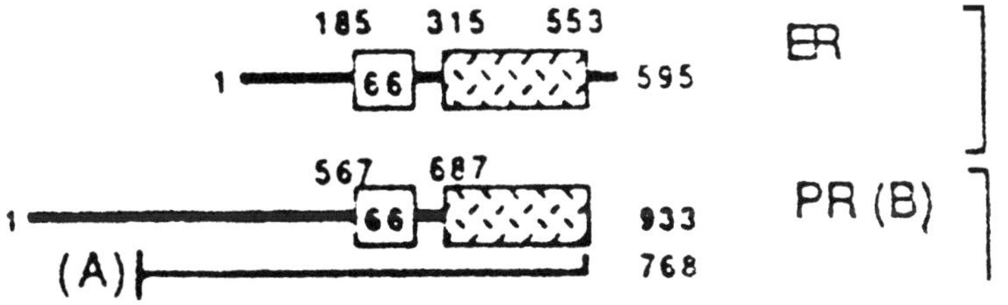

FIGURE 3. Structure of the PR—comparison to ER. Boxes indicate highly conserved domains. The position of each domain boundary is given as the number of amino acids from the amino terminus. Figures in the C boxes indicate the number of amino acids in the DNA-binding domain. Receptors: ER, estrogen; PR, progestin.

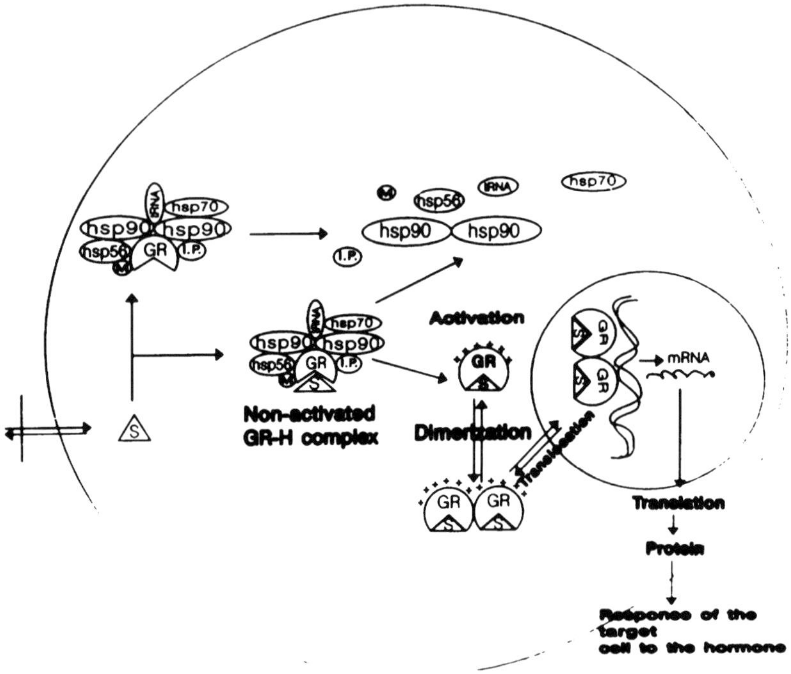

FIGURE 4. The mechanism of action of steroid hormones.

transcription factors, of stable multimeric complexes modulating RNA polymerase activity. This results in changes in mRNA and protein synthesis. Glucocorticoid receptors can modulate the activity of the transcription factor AP-1 or the NF-kB-Rel transcription factors by protein–protein interaction[9–12] or by induction of transcription factor inhibitors,[13] respectively. Recent data concerning the action of estradiol support a model in which the unliganded receptor can dimerize and bind to the respective HRE,[14] whereas the hormone ligand induces conformational changes activating the ligand-dependent transactivation domain.[15] Mechanisms of action of estradiol on gene activation independent of the presence of an ERE have been recently put forward.[16]

TABLE 1. Consensus Responsive Elements for Nuclear Receptors

PRE	GGTACAnnnTGTTCT
ERE	AGGTCAnnnTGACCT

Nongenomic Effects of Steroid Hormones

The action of steroid hormones by way of gene activation requires some hours to be manifest, because of the involvement of the series of steps starting with receptor activation and culminating in protein synthesis. Some of the hormonal effects, however, are manifested within minutes, are independent of protein synthesis and cannot be accounted for by genomic involvement,[17,18] such as the estradiol effects on activation of peptide elongation in the uterus[19] or on endometrium inhibition.[20]

It is still unknown whether the nongenomic effects of steroids are mediated by the nuclear receptors themselves or through other hormone-binding proteins (membrane proteins, ion-channel proteins). The possible involvement of a phosphokinase subunit of the holoreceptor, which upon hormonal activation of the receptor is activated and can phosphorylate proteins involved in the rapid hormone effects, has been discussed.[21]

ANTIHORMONES

Antiestrogens (tamoxifen, 40H-Tamoxifen, ICI 164,384) and antiprogestins (RU486, ZK982999) bind to the hormone-binding site of receptors and consequently compete with the agonist ligands. Antihormones are usually synthetic analogues of steroid hormones, but physiological endogenous steroids may also show such activity. Some antihormones (i.e. tamoxifen) are also partial agonists. The molecular mechanism of antihormone action, especially of those showing agonistic, as well as antagonistic properties, is currently receiving due attention.

Metzger *et al.*[22] present data that suggest both pure antiestrogens and partial agonists permit dimerization and binding of the dimer to DNA, whereas other authors[23,24] described impaired dimerization and binding of the ER to ERE only by the pure antiestrogens (e.g. ICI 164384).

The consequence of binding of the antihormone seems to be conformational changes of the receptor[25] leading, in the case of partial agonists (like tamoxifen), to interference with the transcription activation function of the site located in the hormone-binding domain (AF-2 site), leaving the transcription-modulating domain located at the A/B region (AF-1 site) functionally active.[22] In the case of pure antagonists, like ICI 164384, inactivation of both AF-2 and AF-1 takes place, suggesting cross-talk between the COOH- and NH_2-terminal functional domains of the estrogen receptor.[22] The agonist action of 4-OH tamoxifen has been shown to increase as a result of a mutation in codon 351 of the estrogen receptor, identified in a human breast tumor line.[26]

Recent results by Webb *et al.*[27] show that tamoxifen is a potent activator of ER-mediated induction of promoters regulated by the AP-1 site, in a cell-type-specific manner, the uterus being affected by this antihormone, and suggest that estrogen effects in tissue growth and differentiation could be mediated by the AP-1 pathway.

Antiprogestins can also be classified into pure antagonists, such as ZK98299, and partial agonists, such as RU486.[28] It is generally assumed that the former prevent binding of the receptor to DNA, whereas the latter enable DNA binding of the receptor, but in a form unable to activate the hormone-responsive genes. Tras *et al.*[29] have provided evidence that both categories of antiprogestins are able to bind the HREs in *in vivo* experiments. The precise mechanism of action of antiprogestins remains to be elucidated.

METHODS FOR ASSAY OF STEROID RECEPTORS

Two main methods are used routinely for the assay of steroid receptors, a biochemical and an immuno(cyto)chemical one.[30] The biochemical method is based on the binding of radiolabeled hormone to the respective receptor, elimination of nonbound radiolabel by dextran-coated charcoal, and subsequent measurement of protein-bound hormone (DCC method). The assay performed with different concentrations of hormone and in the presence of competing nonlabeled steroid, gives values, which in Scatchard plots determine the number of binding sites and binding characteristics of the receptor. The amount of receptors is expressed in femtomoles per milligram protein.

Other biochemical methods, such as sucrose gradient centrifugation and isoelectric focusing, are rarely used as routine assays.

The availability of polyclonal and monoclonal antibodies to the steroid receptors[31] led not only to development of related assay methods, that is, immunocytochemical and immunochemical, but also to investigations concerning certain parameters of their biology, such as recycling and intracellular localization. Concerning the latter, it is sufficient to say that using the immunocytochemical method there is a general consensus that ER and PR are localized almost exclusively in the cell nucleus,[31] whereas the GR is mostly localized in the cytoplasm[32] and is mobilized to enter the nucleus upon interaction with the respective ligand, but also by growth factors[33] (see Section 9). The development of the immunocytochemical method has also made the precise cellular distribution of steroid receptors within organs (e.g., ER in endometrium or in brain) possible.

The immunocytochemical assay of ER and PR has certain advantages over the biochemical assay, as it can show possible heterogeneity of a cell population in respect to receptor content and requires small tissue specimens (endometrial scrapings, cell smears, material from needle biopsies), however is inferior as regards the quantitative aspect, as grading is based on subjective criteria. In this aspect the enzyme immunoassay method (EIA) used as a solid-phase "sandwich" method is superior and the results quite comparable to those obtained by the DCC method.

The identification of a series of receptor variants in various tumors lacking regions important for DNA binding, ligand binding, or epitopes potentially recognized by the monoclonal antibodies used in the immunoassays, combined with limitations inherent in the immunocytochemical technique (unavailability of epitope due to the fixative used) has led to further methodologies based on functional tests of the receptor and on the use of fluorescent estrogen analogues (5,6,11,12-tetrachrysene) for the *in situ* visualization of the estrogen receptor, with the additional possibility of studying aspects of ER cell biology (intracellular movements, localization).[34]

REGULATION OF ER AND PR RECEPTORS

The concentration of intracellular receptors can fluctuate in response to various factors, among them the hormones themselves. Estrogens lead to homologous upregulation of ER.[35] This autoinduction of the receptor is inhibited by progesterone. On the other hand, PR levels are increased by estradiol (heterologous upregulation) and decreased by progestins (homologous downregulation).[36]

The pattern of ER and PR at various physiologic states (i.e., normal menstrual cycle) is the result of the ratios of endogenous estrogen to progesterone. States characterized by altered steroid milieu, due either to endogenous or exogenous factors (i.e., pregnancy, induction of ovulation, luteal phase defects) will, as reflection, show altered ER and PR levels.

The molecular mechanism of hormonal regulation of receptor concentrations has been investigated.[35,36] As regards the progesterone receptor gene, an intragenic (+698/+723)ERE has been detected that binds the estradiol receptor and mediates estrogen induction of the gene.[37] Homologous downregulation by progesterone seems to be achieved by the same ERE, not by direct interaction with PR, but by way of protein–protein interaction of PR and ER.

ER AND PR CONCENTRATIONS IN DIFFERENT PHYSIOLOGICAL AND PATHOPHYSIOLOGICAL STATES

The concentration of receptors has been determined in different physiological and pathological states, mainly by immunocytochemical procedures on tissue sections and by ligand-binding assays in cytosol and nuclei.

Menstrual Cycle

Estradiol and progesterone receptor levels change during the menstrual cycle. Binding assays reveal the ER concentrations are high during the proliferative phase (especially the late proliferative phase), peak at the time of ovulation, decline sharply in the secretory phase, and are very significantly lower in late secretory phase. PR levels show a similar pattern of changes throughout the menstrual cycle, increasing in the proliferative phase, peaking at ovulation, and declining gradually in the secretory phase (FIG. 5).[38,39]

Immunohistochemical assays of ER reveal synchrony of the staining intensity of the three cell types (epithelium, stroma, myometrium) throughout the cycle, that is, an increase in late proliferative phase, a maximum at midcycle, and a rapid decline during the secretory phase in all three tissues, in agreement with the biochemical assay results (FIG. 6).[39,40]

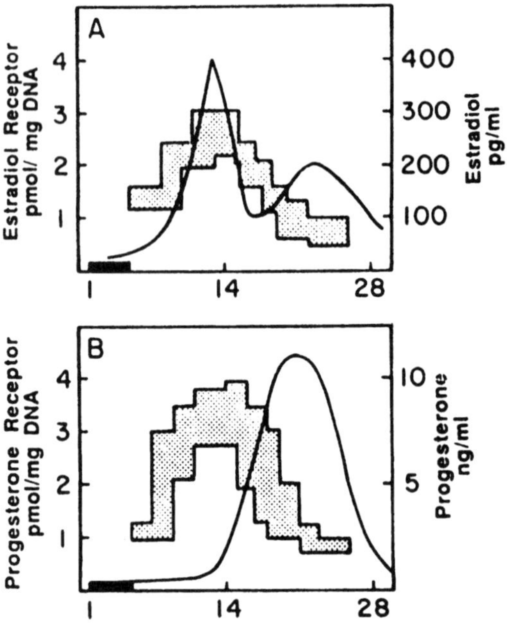

FIGURE 5. Estradiol and progesterone receptors in endometrial cells during the normal menstrual cycle. (**A**) Concentration of estradiol receptor, (**B**) concentration of progesterone receptor (from Ref. 1).

In contrast to ER, PR staining in the three cell types changed in a dyssynchronous pattern throughout the cycle. Although the three cell types show increased staining throughout the proliferative phase, during the secretory phase there is a decline in epithelium PR, but not in stroma or in myometrium (FIG. 6).[39,40]

Pregnancy

In early pregnancy (8–10 weeks of gestation) ER and PR levels are low, similar to those in the late secretory phase of the menstrual cycle. In late pregnancy (38–40 weeks of gestation) ER levels are still low, whereas there is a significant increase in PR levels to those found in the preovulatory period.[41,42]

Abnormal Menstrual Cycle

In anovulatory cycles, a condition characterized by low estradiol levels during the proliferative phase, the ER and PR levels are high, similar to those of the late

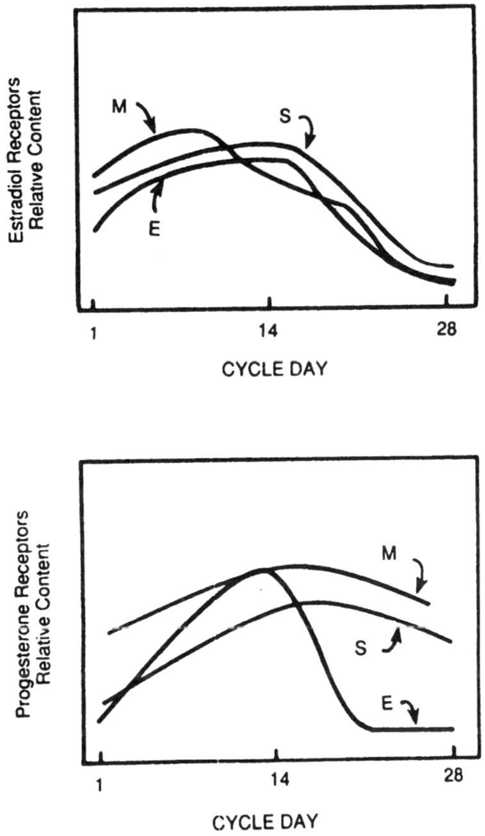

FIGURE 6. Relative levels of uterine estrogen and progesterone receptor immunostaining intensity throughout the menstrual cycle in glandular epithelium (E), stroma (S) and myometrium (M) (from Ref. 1).

proliferative phase in normal cycles.[42] Ovulation induction with anti-estrogens, (clomiphene citrate) despite the high estradiol levels and the anti-estrogenic activity on endometrium, do not affect peri-implantation phase endometrial ER and PR levels.[43]

Analyses of endometrial ER and PR in women diagnosed with luteal phase defects[44] have yielded conflicting results. Some authors find no evidence of a major abnormality in ER and PR levels, whereas others detect very low PR and ER levels. These discrepancies may result from the diverse mechanisms responsible for this disorder and from differences in the methods used for ER and PR assay. The use of oral contraceptives reveals ER and PR levels in the range found in the proliferative phase of the cycle.[45]

Endometrial Cancer

In endometrial cancer, receptors to many steroid hormones, including androgens and glucocorticoids, have been detected.[46,47] The estrogen receptors are invariably found in this cancer, which, at least temporarily, is totally dependent on estradiol. PR, on the other hand, is not always detected, a reverse relation existing between grade and concentration of PR (the higher the grade the lower the concentration).[46]

In recurrent or advanced (clinical stage III and IV) endometrial carcinoma mean total survival time and mean time to recurrence were positively correlated with positive progesterone and estrogen receptor status, which may be used as additional prognostic variables.[48]

ER, PR, AND CANCER

The role of estradiol in cell replication of the endometrium and of other sex steroid–responsive tissues is well known, as is the suppressive effect of progesterone in this process acting as a differentiation agent. The mechanism of action of estradiol on replication involves early effects on transcription of genes encoding key regulatory molecules, such as growth factors (TGF-α) and growth factor receptors (EGFR), or genes encoding transcription factors, involved in secondary gene activation processes.[49] The induction of the *c-fos* and *c-myc* protooncogenes by estradiol soon (30 min and 90 min) after hormone administration, which indicates that they are directly affected by the hormone, has been extensively studied.[50–52] These are tissue-specific effects of the hormone, as they are not observed in all cells. Estradiol also induces *c-jun* expression, directly effecting transcription of the gene, as protein synthesis inhibitors have no effect on *c-jun* gene activation.[53,54] In these genes, HREs to which the ER can bind have been identified. In the *c-fos* gene two sequences upstream of the Cap site have been detected, one of which overlaps with an AP-1-binding site.[55] An ERE has been found within the *jun* gene, identical to the consensus ERE only in the second half-site.[56] Another oncogene, whose expression could be regulated by estradiol but also by corticosteroids, is H-*ras*. In this oncogene, sequences showing strong similarity to EREs and GREs, to which the respective hormone receptors can bind, are present.[57]

Progesterone shows a reverse effect on the expression of some of the protooncogenes involved in DNA replication, inhibiting *c-myc* and *c-fos* (but no *c-jun*) activation.[58] In the avian *c-myc* gene, a possible progesterone regulatory element with strong similarities to the SRE/PRE element of the tyrosine aminotransferase gene has been described.

In addition to the effects related to replication, both estradiol and progesterone induce genes encoding a series of proteins involved in the specific function of the endometrium during the menstrual cycle and at pregnancy. Among the genes stimulated by estradiol in the endometrium are those of the heat-shock proteins, which are not directly affected by the hormone, but are affected indirectly through primary activation of the heat-shock transcription factors.[59]

Estradiol itself is not an initiator of carcinogenesis but can be regarded as a tumor promotor on the basis of its ability to promote cell replication, and hypotheses to explain its promoting action have been proposed.[49,60] The action of estradiol on replication is mediated by regulation of crucial genes, such as the protooncogenes, in a precisely defined temporal and tissue-specific pattern. If the initiating carcinogen has induced mutations in the protooncogenes or changes in gene architecture, aligning protooncogenes to HREs, thus placing them under nonphysiological control, then the link to cellular transformation can be envisaged. Mutation could affect the ER and PR themselves—a series of such mutations in various cancers is known—with possible effects on their specificity of interaction with HREs and their affinity to their DNA binding sites.

CROSS-TALK BETWEEN THE ENDOCRINE SYSTEM AND OTHER REGULATORY SYSTEMS AT THE LEVEL OF THE RECEPTOR PROTEINS

Regulation of cellular processes is always multicomponent and interwined. Transcription regulation is no exception to the rule; and, as mentioned in the section on mechanisms of action of steroid hormones, the ER and PR (and other steroid receptors) can interact at the level of the gene with other regulatory molecules and transcription factors (some, like *c-fos* and *c-jun*, resulting in response to growth factors), modulating their effect on transcription of the various estrogen- and progesterone-inducible genes.

Earlier observations and more recent findings have led to the conclusion that the receptor molecule itself could be a site of the cross-talk of the endocrine system with growth factors and neurotransmitters. It was demonstrated that lectin (PHA)-induced lymph cell proliferation is preceded by translocation of the glucocorticoid receptor into the nucleus in an active form in the absence of steroid hormone,[33] suggesting an indirect effect of growth factor(s) on receptor activation. Inasmuch as growth factors lead, by way of the signal transduction pathways, to receptor phosphorylation and phosphorylation of steroid receptors alters the receptor's transcription modulatory characteristics, this could be a general mechanism of growth factor–steroid receptor interaction.[61,66] More recently, it was shown that progesterone receptor-mediated transcription is activated by phosphokinase A as efficiently as by progesterone.[67]

Cross-talk similar to that between growth factors and steroid receptors has been strongly suggested for neurotransmitters and steroid receptors by the experiments of Power *et al.*[68] These authors showed that dopamine enhances *trans*-activation of chicken progesterone receptor in a ligand-independent manner, by way of phosphorylation of the progesterone receptor at sites different from those phosphorylated by the ligand progesterone. Similar findings have been obtained for the ER. These studies partly explain in molecular terms the observations that neurotransmitters produce marked effects on the endocrine system, that is, on the ovulatory luteinizing hormone surge and prolactin secretion and that catecholaminergic neurotransmitters may increase the ligand-binding activity of ER or that drugs that reduce the levels of noradrenaline reduce the levels of hypothalamic ERs and the ability of estradiol to induce PR.[69]

In this context the serine phosphorylation of the ER by phorbol ester (TPA) should be mentioned, because TPA acts synergistically with estradiol to increase receptor-mediated transcription in MCF-7 cells.[70]

EPILOGUE

The role of estrogen and progesterone receptors in endometrial function is increasingly being understood, because of the amassing of data concerning the molecular biology of the receptors, their molecular mode of action and their interaction with other key regulatory molecules. This interaction is currently in the focus of interest and important new results are to be expected that will further our insights into the mechansims underlying the physiological and abnormal states of the endometrium.

SUMMARY

The endometrium, as a target of estrogens and progestins, possesses the respective receptor proteins. These receptors belong to the superfamily of nuclear receptors, having important functional domains required for steroid ligand binding, for dimer formation, for interaction with HREs of DNA, for transcription modulation, for association with other proteins, for intracellular trafficking, and other activities. The mechanism of action of the steroid hormones involves modulation of gene activity through interaction of the hormone–receptor complex with HREs and with other nuclear proteins, but also encompasses nongenomic effects, which accounts for the rapid effects of the steroids on cellular functions.

Antihormones—antiestrogen and antiprogestins—compete with their respective hormones for binding sites on the receptor molecules. Some antihormones are partial agonists. The molecular mechanisms underlying the dual behavior of antihormones is under consideration.

The concentration of ER and PR in different physiological and pathophysiological states, such as the menstrual cycle, pregnancy, and endometrial cancer, has been determined by biochemical and immuno(cyto)chemical methods. The levels of estrogens and progestins are important regulators of ER and PR gene expression.

Estradiol acts as a cell mitogen, inducing key genes involved in replication, and its tumor promoter effect is discussed in this sense, whereas progesterone has reverse effects when compared to estradiol and acts as a differentiation factor.

The cross-talk between the endocrine system, growth factors, and neurotransmitters can take place both at the receptor level, involving mainly phosphorylation reactions, and at the gene level, mainly through protein–protein interactions.

REFERENCES

1. STRAUSS, F. III & E. GURPIDE. 1991. The endometrium: Regulation and dysfunction. *In* Reproductive Endocrinology. S. S. C. Yen & R. B. Jaffe, Eds. 3rd edit. W. B. Saunders. Philadelphia, PA.
2. EVANS, R. M. 1988. The steroid and thyroid hormone receptor superfamily. Science **240:** 889–895.
3. PARKER, M. G. 1993. Steroid and related receptor. Curr. Opin. Cell Biol. **5:** 499–504.
4. GREEN, S. & P. CHAMBON. 1991. The oestrogen receptor: From perception to mechanism. *In* Nuclear Hormone Receptors. M. G. Parker, Ed.: 15–38. Academic Press. London.
5. MISRAHI, M., M. ATGER, L. D'AURIOL, H. LOOSFELT, C. MERIEL, F. FRIDLANSKY, A. GUIOCHON-MANTEL, F. GALIBERT & E. MILGROM. 1987. Complete amino acid sequence of the human progesterone receptor deduced from cloned cDNA. Biochem. Biophys. Res. Commun. **143:** 740–748.
6. WEN, D. X., Y.-F. XU, D. E. MAIS, M. E. GOLDMAN & D. P. MCDONNELL. 1994. The A and B isoforms of the human progesterone receptor operate through distinct signaling pathways within target cells. Mol. Cell. Biol. **14:** 8356–8364.
7. SMITH, D. F. & D. O. TOFT. 1993. Steroid receptors and their associated proteins. Mol. Endocrinol. **7:** 4–11.
8. BEATO, M. 1989. Gene regulation by steroid hormones. Cell **56:** 335–344.
9. YANG-YEN, H. F., J.-C. CHAMBARD, Y.-L. SUN, T. SMEAL, T. SCHMIDT, J. DROUIN & M. KARIN. 1990. Transcriptional interference between c-Jun and the glucocorticoid receptor: Mutual inhibition of DNA binding due to direct protein–protein interaction. Cell **62:** 1205–1215.
10. SCHULE, R., P. RANGARAJAN, S. KLIEWER, L. J. RANSONE, J. BOLADO, N. YANG, I. M. VERMA & R. M. EVANS. 1990. Functional antagonism between oncoprotein c-jun and glucocorticoid receptor. Cell **62:** 1217–1226.
11. JONAT, C., H. J. RAHMSDORF, K.-K. PARK, A. C. B. CATO, S. GEBEL, H. PONTA & P. HERRLICH. 1990. Antitumor promotion and antiinflammation: Down-modulation of AP-1 (Fos/Jun) activity by glucocorticoid hormone. Cell **62:** 1189–1204.
12. MINER, J. N. & K. R. YAMAMOTO. 1992. The basic region of AP-1 specifies glucocorticoid receptor activity at a composite response element. Genes Dev. **6:** 2491–2501.
13. SCHEINMAN, R. I., P. C. COGSWELL, A. K. LOFQUIST & A. S. BALDWIN. 1995. Role of transcriptional activation of IκBα in mediation of immunosuppression by glucocorticoids. Science **270:** 283–286.
14. METZGER, D., M. BERRY, S. ALI & P. CHAMBON. 1995. Effect of antagonists on DNA binding properties of the human estrogen receptor in vitro and in vivo. Mol. Endocrinol. **9:** 579–591.
15. ZHUANG, Y., B. S. KATZENELLENBOGEN & D. J. SHAPIRO. 1995. Estrogen receptor mutants which do not bind 17β-estradiol dimerize and bind to the estrogen response element in vivo. Mol. Endocrinol. **9:** 457–466.
16. SUKOVICH, D. A., R. MUKHERJEE & P. A. BENFIELD. 1994. A novel, cell-type-specific mechansim for estrogen receptor-mediated gene activation in the absence of an estrogen-responsive element. Mol. Cell. Biol. **14:** 7134–7143.
17. KANAZIR, D. T. 1990. Glucocorticoid receptor and hormonal extragenomic effects. *In* Activation of Hormone and Growth Factor Receptors. Molecular Mechanisms and Consequences. M. N. Alexis & C. E. Sekeris, Eds. Vol. **295:** 269–286. Kluwer Academic Publishers. Dordrecht.
18. MCEWEN, B. S. 1991. Non-genomic and genomic effects of steroids on neural activity. TIPS **12:** 141–147.

19. LABATE, M. E., S. M. WHELLY & K. L. BARKER. 1986. Ribosome-associated estradiol-binding components in the uterus and their relationship to the translational capacity of uterine ribosomes. Endocrinology **119:** 140–151.
20. SZEGO, C. M. & J. ROBERTS. 1953. Steroid action and interaction in uterine metabolism. Rec. Progr. Horm. Res. **8:** 419–435.
21. PERISIC, O., M. RADOJCIC & D. T. KANAZIR. 1987. Protein kinase activity can be separated from the purified activated rat liver glucocorticoid receptor. J. Biol. Chem. **262:** 11688–11891.
22. METZGER, D., M. BERRY, S. ALI & P. CHAMBON. 1995. Effect of antagonists on DNA binding properties of the human estrogen receptor in vitro and in vivo. Mol. Endocrinol. **9:** 579–591.
23. FAWELL, S. E., R. WHITE, S. HOARE, M. SYDENHAM, M. PAGE & M. G. PARKER. 1990. Inhibition of estrogen receptor-DNA binding by the "pure" antiestrogen ICI 164,384 appears to be mediated by impaired receptor dimerization. Proc. Natl. Acad. Sci. USA **87:** 6883–6887.
24. ARBUCKLE, N. D., S. DAUVOIS & M. G. PARKER. 1992. Effects of antioestrogens on the DNA binding activity of oestrogen receptors in vitro. Nucleic. Acids Res. **20:** 3839–3844.
25. MCDONNELL, D. P., D. L. CLEMM, T. HERMANN, M. E. GOLDMAN & J. W. PIKE. 1995. Analysis of estrogen receptor function in vitro reveals three distinct classes of antiestrogens. Mol. Endocrinol. **9:** 659–669.
26. CATHERINO, W. H., D. M. WOLF & V. C. JORDAN. 1995. A naturally occurring estrogen receptor mutation results in increased estrogenicity of a tamoxifen analog. Mol. Endocrinol. **9:** 1053–1063.
27. WEBB, P., G. N. LOPEZ, R. M. UHT & P. J. KUSHNER. 1995. Tamoxifen activation of the estrogen receptor/AP-1 pathway: Potential origin for the cell-specific estrogen-like effects of antiestrogens. Mol. Endocrinol. **9:** 443–456.
28. BAULIEU, E.-E. 1989. RU-486 as an antiprogesterone steroid. JAMA **262:** 1808–1814.
29. TRUSS, M., J. BARTSCH & M. BEATO. 1994. Antiprogestins prevent progesterone receptor binding to hormone responsive elements in vivo. Proc. Natl. Acad. Sci. USA **91:** 11333–11337.
30. MCCARTY, JR., K. S., L. S. MILLER, E. B. COX, J. KONRATU & K. S. MCCARTY, SR. 1985. Estrogen receptor analysis. Correlation of biochemical and immunohistochemical methods using monoclonal antibodies. Arch. Pathol. Lab. Med. **109:** 716–721.
31. GREENE, G. L. & E. V. JENSEN. 1982. Monoclonal antibodies are probes for estrogen receptor detection and characterization. J. Steroid Biochem. **16:** 353–359.
32. PAPAMICHAIL, M., G. TSOKOS, N. TSAWDAROGLOU & C. E. SEKERIS. 1980. Immunocytochemical demonstration of glucocorticoid receptors in different cell types and their translocation from the cytoplasm to the nucleus in the presence of dexamethasone. Exp. Cell. Res. **125:** 490–495.
33. PAPAMICHAIL, M., C. IOANNIDIS, N. TSAWDAROGLOU & C. E. SEKERIS. 1981. Translocation of glucocorticoid receptor from the cytoplasm into the nucleus of phytohemagglutinin-stimulated human lymphocytes in the absence of the hormone. Exp. Cell. Res. **133** 461–465.
34. MIKSICEK, R. J., K. E. CARLSON, K.-J. HWANG & J. A. KATZENELLENBOGEN. 1995. Studies using fluorescent tetrahydrochrysene estrogens for in situ visualization of the estrogen receptor in living cells. Mol. Endocrinol. **9:** 592–604.
35. READ, L. D., G. L. GREENE & B. S. KATZENELLENBOGEN. 1989. Regulation of estrogen receptor messenger ribonucleic acid and protein levels in human breast cancer cell lines by sex steroid hormones, their antagonists, and growth factors. Mol. Endocrinol. **3** 295–304.

36. Milgrom, E., L. Thi, M. Atger & E. E. Baulieu. 1973. Mechanisms regulating the concentration and the conformation of progesterone receptor(s) in the uterus. J. Biol. Chem. **248:** 6366–6374.
37. Savouret, J.-F., M. Rauch, G. Redeuilh, S. Sar, A. Chauchereau, K. Woodruff, M. G. Parker & E. Milgrom. 1994. Interplay between estrogens, progestins, retinoic acid and AP-1 on a single regulatory site in the progesterone receptor gene. J. Biol. Chem. **269:** 28955–28962.
38. Bayard, F., S. Damilano, P. Robel & E.-E. Baulieu. 1978. Cytoplasmic and nuclear estradiol and progesterone receptors in human endometrium. J. Clin. Endocrinol. Metab. **46:** 635–648.
39. Press, M. F., J. A. Udove & G. L. Greene. 1988. Progesterone receptor distribution in the human endometrium. Analysis monoclonal antibodies to the human progesterone receptor. Am. J. Pathol. **131:** 112–124.
40. Lessey, B. A., A. P. Killam, D. A. Metzger, A. F. Haney, G. L. Greene & K. S. McCarty, Jr. 1988. Immunohistochemical analysis of human uterine estrogen and progesterone receptors throughout the menstrual cycle. J. Clin. Endocrin. Metab. **67:** 334–340.
41. Kreitmann, B., F. Bayard. 1979. Oestrogen and progesterone receptor concentrations in human endometrium during gestation. Acta Endocrinol. **92:** 547–552.
42. Levy, C., P. Robel, J. P. Gautray, J. De Brux, U. Verman, B. Descomps, E. E. Baulieu & B. Eychenne. 1980. Estradiol and progesterone receptors in human endometrium: Normal and abnormal menstrual cycles and early pregnancy. Am. J. Obstet. Gynecol. **136:** 646–651.
43. Hecht, B. R., F. S. Khan-Dawood & Y. Dawood. 1989. Peri-implantation phase endometrial estrogen and progesterone receptors: Effect of ovulation induction with clomiphene citrate. Am. J. Obstet. Gynecol. **161:** 1688–1693.
44. Jacobs, M. H., J. Balasch, J. M. Gonzalez-Merlo, J. A. Vanrell, C. Wheeler, J. F. Strauss, III, L. Blasco, J. E. Wheeler & C. R. Lyttle. 1987. Endometrial cytosolic and nuclear progesterone receptors in the luteal phase defect. J. Clin. Endocrinol. Metab. **64:** 472–475.
45. Sanborn, B. M., H. S. Kuo & B. Held. 1978. Estrogen and progestogen binding site concentrations in human endometrium and cervix throughout the menstrual cycle and in tissue from women taking oral contraceptives. J. Steroid Biochem. **9:** 951–955.
46. Prodi, G., C. De Giovanni, M. C. Galli, G. Gola, S. Grilli, R. Rocchetta & C. Orlandi. 1979. 17 Beta-estradiol, 5 alpha-dihydrotestosterone, progesterone and cortisol receptors in normal and neopalstic human endometrium. Tumori **65:** 241–253.
47. Boranzani, G., L. B. Twiggs, B. S. Leung, K. A. Prem, L. L. Adcock & L. F. Carson. 1989. Prognostic significance of steroid receptors measured in primary metastatic and recurrent endometrial carcinoma. Am. J. Obstet. Gynecol. **161:** 1253–1257.
48. Creasman, W. T., J. T. Soper, K. S. McCarty, Jr., K. S. McCarty, Sr., W. Hinshaw & D. L. Clarke-Pearson. 1985. Influence of cytoplasmic steroid receptor content on prognosis of early stage endometrial carcinoma. Am. J. Obstet. Gynecol. **151:** 922–928.
49. Schuchard, M., J. P. Landers, N. Punkay-Sandhu & T. C. Spelsberg. 1993. Steroid hormone regulation of nuclear proto-oncogenes. Endocr. Rev. **14:** 659–669.
50. Murphy, L. J., L. C. Murphy & H. G. Freisen. 1987. Estrogen induction of n-myc and c-myc proto-oncogene expression in the rat uterus. Endocrinology **120:** 1882–1888.
51. Loose-Mitchell, D. S., C. Chiappetta & G. M. Stancel. 1988. Estrogen regulation of c-fos messanger ribonucleic acid. Mol. Endocrinol. **2:** 946–951.

52. WEISZ, A. & F. BRESCIANI. 1988. Estrogen induces expression of c-fos and c-myc proto-oncogenes in rat uterus. Mol. Endocrinol. **2:** 816–824.
53. CHIAPPETTA, C., J. L. KIRKLAND, D. S. LOOSE-MITCHELL, L. MURTHY & G. M. STANCEL. 1992. Estrogen regulates expression of the jun family of proto-oncogenes in the uterus. J. Steroid. Biochem. Mol. Biol. **41:** 113–123.
54. CICATIELLO, L., C. AMBROSINO, B. COLETTA, M. SCALONA, V. SICA, F. BRESCIANI & A. WEISZ. 1992. Transcriptional activation of jun and actin genes by estrogen during mitogenic stimulation of rat uterine cells. J. Steroid. Biochem. Mol. Biol. **41:** 523–528.
55. WEISZ, A. & R. ROSALES. 1990. Identification of an estrogen response element upstream of the human c-fos gene that binds the estrogen receptor and the AP-1 transcription factor. Nucl. Acids Res. **18:** 5097–5106.
56. HYDER, S. M., Z. NAWAZ, C. CHIAPPETTA, K. YOKOYAMA & G. M. STANCEL. 1995. The protooncogene c-jun contains an unusual estrogen-inducible enhancer within the coding sequence. J. Biol. Chem. **270:** 8506–8513.
57. ZACHOS, G., V. ZOUMPOURLIS, C. E. SEKERIS & D. A. SPANDIDOS. 1995. Binding of the glucocorticoid and estrogen receptors to the human H-ras oncogene sequences. Int. J. Oncol. **6:** 595–600.
58. KIRKLAND, J. L., L. MURTHY & G. M. STANCEL. 1992. Progesterone inhibits the estrogen-induced expression of c-fos messenger ribonucleic acid in the uterus. Endocrinology **130:** 3223–3230.
59. YANG, X., E. C. DALE, J. DIAZ & G. SHYAMALA. 1995. Estrogen dependent expression of heat shock transcription factor: Implications for uterine synthesis of heat shock proteins. J. Steroid Biochem. Mol. Biol.**52:** 415–419.
60. SEKERIS, C. E. 1991. Hormonal steroids act as tumor promoters by modulating oncogene expression. J. Cancer Res. Clin. Oncol. **117:** 96–101.
61. IGNAR-TROWBRIDGE, D. M., K. R. NELSON, M. C. BIDWELL, S. W. CURTIS, T. F. WASHBURN, J. A. MCLACHLAN & K. KORACH. 1992. Coupling of dual signaling pathways: Epidermal growth factor action involves the estrogen receptor. Proc. Natl. Acad. Sci USA **89:** 4658–4662.
62. ALI, S., D. METZGER, J.-M. BORNERT & P. CHAMBON. 1993. Modulation of transcription activation by ligand-dependent phosphorylation of the human oestrogen receptor A/B region. EMBO J. **12:** 1153–1160.
63. ARNOLD, S. F., J. D. OBOURN, H. JAFFE & A. O. NOTIDES. 1994. Serine 167 is the major estradiol-induced phosphorylation site on the human estrogen receptor. Mol. Endocrinol. **8:** 1208–1214.
64. CHO, H. & B. S. KATZENELLENBOGEN. 1993. Synergistic activation of estrogen receptor-mediated transcription by estradiol and protein kinase activators. Mol. Endocrinol. **7:** 441–452.
65. DENTON, R. R., N. J. KOSZEWSKI & A. C. NOTIDES. 1992. Estrogen receptor phosphorylation. Hormonal dependence and consequence on specific. DNA binding. J. Biol. Chem. **267:** 7263–7268.
66. DENNER, L. A., N. L. WEIGEL, B. L. MAXWELL, W. T. SCHRADER & B. W. O'MALLEY. 1990. Regulation of progesterone receptor-mediated transcription by phosphorylation. Science **250:** 1740–1743.
67. RANGARAJAN, P. N., K. UMESOMO & R. M. EVANS. 1992. Modulation of glucocorticoid receptor function by protein kinase A. Mol. Endocrinol. **6:** 1451–1457.
68. POWER, R. F., S. K. MANI, J. CODINA, O. M. CONNEELY & B. W. O'MALLEY. 1991. Dopaminergic and ligand-independent activation of steroid hormone receptors. Science **254:** 1636–1639.

69. WOOLLEY, D. E., W. G. HOPE, M. A. THOMPSON-REECE, D. W. GIETZEN & S. B. CONWAY. 1994. Dopaminergic stimulation of estrogen receptor binding in vivo: A reexamination. Recent Progr. Hormone Res. **49:** 383–392.
70. JOEL, P. B., A. M. TRAISH & D. A. LANNIGAN. 1995. Estradiol and phorbol ester cause phosphorylation of serine 118 in the human estrogen receptor. Mol. Endocrinol. **9:** 1041–1052.

Endometrial Corticotropin-Releasing Hormone: Expression, Regulation, and Potential Physiological Implications[a]

A. MAKRIGIANNAKIS,[b] A. PSYCHOYOS,[c] E. ZOUMAKIS,[b]
A. N. MARGIORIS,[d] C. STOURNARAS,[e] AND A. GRAVANIS[b,f]

[b]Department of Pharmacology
[d]Department of Clinical Chemistry
[e]Department of Biochemistry
Medical School
University of Crete
Iraklion 71110, Greece

[c]Gregory Pincus Institute
Hospital Bicetre
Kremlin Bicetre 94270, France

INTRODUCTION

Corticotropin-releasing hormone (CRH) is a 41-amino-acid neuropeptide synthesized in the paraventricular nucleus of the hypothalamus and released in response to stress.[1] Additionally, CRH and its receptors were found widely distributed in various extrahypothalamic sites of the central nervous system (CNS).[2–5] Over the past five years, additional sites expressing CRH have also been detected, such as the resting human white blood cells[6] and various peripheral tissues including those of the reproductive tract.[7–13] Indeed, ovarian theca and stroma cells,[14] testis, and placenta[15,16] express the CRH gene. In particular, CRH is produced at a number of intrauterine sites during pregnancy, including the trophoblast, chorion, amnion, and decidua.[17]

CRH is involved in the inflammatory process, as a proinflammatory regulator detectable at various inflammatory sites.[18] Moreover, immunoneutralization of local CRH attenuates the inflammatory response. In contrast to its systemic indirect immunosuppressive effects via glucocorticoids, it acts as an autocrine or paracrine proinflammatory peptide. CRH has also been shown to induce directly the expression of IL-1, IL-2, and their receptors in leukocytes.[19,20]

In the reproductive tract, ovarian CRH was implicated in inflammatory/apoptosis phenomena such as ovulation, luteolysis, and follicular atresia.[14] Because the reaction of the uterus to the invading blastocyst also has characteristics of aseptic inflammation, we searched for the expression and the regulation of CRH in human and rat

[a]This work was supported by the General Secretariat of Research and Technology, and by Medicon Hellas.

[f]Address for correspondence: Dr. A. Gravanis, Dept. of Pharmacology, Medical School, University of Crete, Iraklion 71110 Greece.

endometrial cells. Specifically, we have studied in both tissues: (1) the presence of CRH mRNA with Northern blot analysis, (2) the localization of immunoreactive material with immunofluorescence and immunohistochemistry, (3) the regulation of CRH gene promoter by studying the effects of steroids and prostanoids, and (4) the content of CRH mRNA and its peptide product in the implantation sites and in the interimplantation regions of the early pregnant rat uterus.

MATERIALS AND METHODS

Human Cell Cultures

Human endometrial epithelial and stromal cells were isolated, as previously described,[21,22] from endometrial specimens obtained from patients undergoing biopsy for fertility evaluation or hysterectomy. Cells were maintained in Dulbecco's modified Eagle's (DMEM)/F12 medium supplemented with 10 mM L-glutamine, 15 mM HEPES, and 1% antibiotic–antimycotic solution to a final concentration of 100 U/ml penicillin and 100 μg/ml streptomycin. Ishikawa cells were established as a permanent cell line from a well-differentiated human endometrial adenocarcinoma.[23,24] They were cultured in DMEM/F12 medium supplemented with 10 mM L-glutamine, 15 mM HEPES, and 1% antibiotic–antimycotic solution.

Animals

Adult female rats of the Sprague-Dawley strain, weighing 220–250 g, were housed at a room temperature of 23–25°C under controlled illumination. Animals were mated with male Sprague-Dawley rats. At 9:00 A.M. of day 6 of pregnancy, the animals received intravenously 0.5 ml of Evans Blue solution (1% of the dye in saline), which allows, by staining blue, visualization of the sites of implantation.[25] Fifteen minutes later the animals were sacrificed by decapitation, and the uteri were removed and placed on ice. Each blue-stained area (implantation site) and unstained (in-between implantation) region was dissected.

Northern Blot Analysis

Normal human glandular endometrial cells, Ishikawa cells, and human placenta as well as the blue-stained implantation sites and the unstained interimplantation uterine regions of three early pregnant rats were harvested and frozen in liquid nitrogen. Total RNA was extracted from frozen tissue by the guanidine thiocyanate method size-fractionated by agarose electrophoresis, transferred to GeneScreen nylon membranes, and hybridized as previously described.[26] A synthetic 48-mer oligonucleotide corresponding to the aminoacids 22–27 of the rat and human CRH sequences was used as a probe.[27] Autoradiographies using Kodak XR film occurred at –70 in the presence of intensifying screens.

Gel Filtration Chromatography

Cellular extracts from normal human glandular endometrial cells, Ishikawa cells, and rat uteri were used. The extraction of hydrophobic peptides was performed using Sep-Pac cartridges, and the extracts were applied on Sephadex G-50 columns (0.9 × 60 cm, bed volume 40 ml). The flow rate was 1.5 ml/hr; 1-ml fractions were collected, dried under vacuum, and reconstituted for RIA. The columns were calibrated with blue dextran and synthetic human CRH. The ir-CRH content of the above Sep-Pac extracts was measured by RIA using a rabbit antiserum raised against r/hCRH which exhibits 100% cross-reactivity to rat CRH and no cross-reactivity to ovine CRH and human ACTH, GnRH, and AVP. The sensitivity of the assay was 1 pg/tube.

Immunofluorescence/Immunohistochemistry

Immunofluorescence microscopy of human endometrial cells was performed as described.[28] The dilution of CRH antiserum was 1:250. Fluorescein isothiocyanate (FITC)-labeled goat anti-rabbit immunoglobulin Gs were used as second antibodies. Fluorescence patterns were analyzed under a Leitz Dialux 2 OEB microscope equipped with epifluorescent illumination. Photographs were taken on Kodak CF 1000 films.

The uterine horns of three rats were removed and divided into areas of the implantation (blue-stained) sites and the inter-implantation (unstained) regions. The thus-obtained uterine sections were prepared for the immunohistochemistry that was performed, as we have already described in detail.[29] For the immunohistochemical localization of ir-CRH, the rabbit polyclonal antiserum TS-2, raised against r/hCRH, was used.

DNA Transfection

The hCRH promoter we have tested was a fragment of the 5′-flanking region of the human CRH gene from the *Hin*d III site at –918 bp to +38 bp of exon 1.[30] The hCRH insert was subcloned in a sense orientation into the promoterless luciferase plasmid pA3luc,[31] which has been shown to exhibit negligible nonspecific luciferase activity. Ishikawa cells were transiently transfected with the hCRH pA3luc construct by lipofectin.[32] The DNAs transfected were hCRH-pA3luc (5 μg) and pRSV-βgal (1 μg) per plate. The latter was used as control for the efficiency of transfection. Luciferase activity was determined in cell lysates as relative fluorescence units using the Promega luciferase assay (Promega Corp., Madison, WI).[33] For the measurement of β-galactosidase activity in cell lysates, we have used the Promega assay, as previously described.[34]

RESULTS

Presence of CRH mRNA in Human and Rat Endometrial Cells

As shown in FIGURE 1**A**, the CRH mRNA was identified in RNA extracts of Ishikawa cells (*lane 1*) and human normal glandular endometrial cells (*lane 2*). The

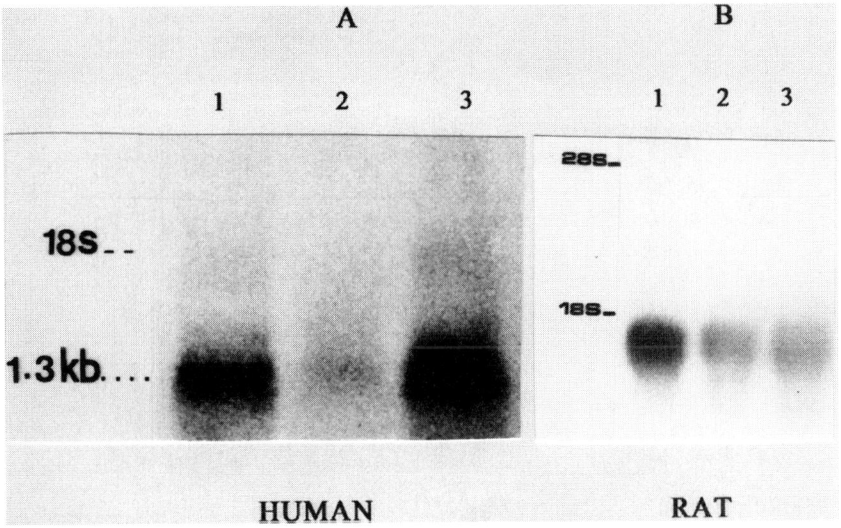

FIGURE 1. Northern blot analysis. (**A**) Human endometrial cells: *Lane 1,* Ishikawa cells; *lane 2,* normal glandular endometrial cells; *lane 3,* human placenta. (**B**) Rat uterus: *Lane 1,* human placenta; *lanes 2* and *3,* rat uterus.

size of the CRH mRNA was about 1.3 kilobases (kb), similar or identical to that present in human placenta (*lane 3*).[35] An approximately 1.3-kb CRH transcript was also identified in RNA extracts from rat uteri, a size similar or identical to that present in human placenta (FIG. 1**B**). The content of CRH mRNA at the implantation sites was 3.5-fold higher than that in the interimplantation uterine regions (FIG. 2).[29]

Chromatographic Characteristics of Endometrial CRH

The bulk of ir-CRH present in extracts from normal human endometrium, Ishikawa cell extracts, and rat uteri had the same chromatographic profile as synthetic 41-amino-acid CRH (FIG. 3), suggesting that endometrial CRH is authentic CRH.[29,35]

Immunohistochemical Localization of CRH in Human and Rat Endometrial Cells

FIGURE 4 depicts the morphology of CRH localization in normal glandular endometrial cells (**a**) and in Ishikawa endometrial adenocarcinoma cells (**b**). Well-demarcated granules positive for ir-CRH were present throughout the cytoplasm. On the other hand, normal stromal endometrial cells were negative for CRH immunostaining (**c**).[35]

Immunoreactive CRH was also detected in the luminal epithelium at the implanta-

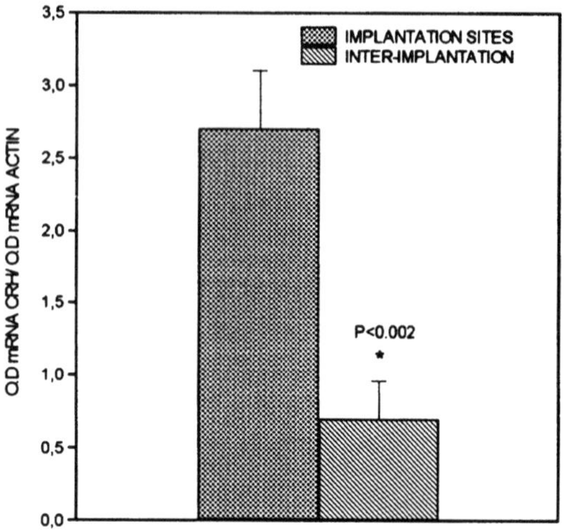

FIGURE 2. Densitometric quantitation of CRH mRNA in the implantation sites and in the inter-implantation uterine regions of three early pregnant rats. Results are expressed as the ratio of optical density (OD) of CRH transcript versus the OD of β-actin transcript. $^*p < 0.002$ by paired *t*-test.

tion sites as well as in the interimplantation regions of the early pregnant rat uterus (glandular epithelium was less intensely stained in both regions) (**d,e**). Stromal decidualized cells were strongly immuno-stained at the implantation sites, whereas they were not or only slightly stained in the interimplantation regions.[29]

Regulation of the Promoter of CRH Gene in Transfected Human Endometrial Cells

Our homologous transfection studies in Ishikawa endometrial cells showed that 8-bromo-cAMP (1 mM), forskolin (20 μM), and EGF (20 U/ml) increased the activity of the CRH promoter (FIG. 5). Estradiol suppressed the activity of the CRH promoter in a dose-dependent manner, an effect that appears to be mediated via estrogen receptors because the addition of a 100-fold molar excess of the antiestrogen 4-hydroxytamoxifen completely abolished it. Progesterone did not affect the activity of the CRH promoter. Dexamethasone suppressed its activity in a dose-dependent fashion, while antiglucocorticoid RU486 exerted agonist effects by also inhibiting its activity. In contrast to estrogens, dexamethasone inhibited in a dose-dependent manner both the FSK- and EGF-induced CRH promoter, suggesting that the inhibitory effect of glucocorticoids on endometrial CRH transcription interferes with both cAMP- and EGF-related pathways. Cyclooxygenase inhibitor indomethacin (1 μM) inhibited the CRH promoter, while exogenously given prostaglandin PGE_2 increased its activity in a dose-dependent manner (FIG. 5).

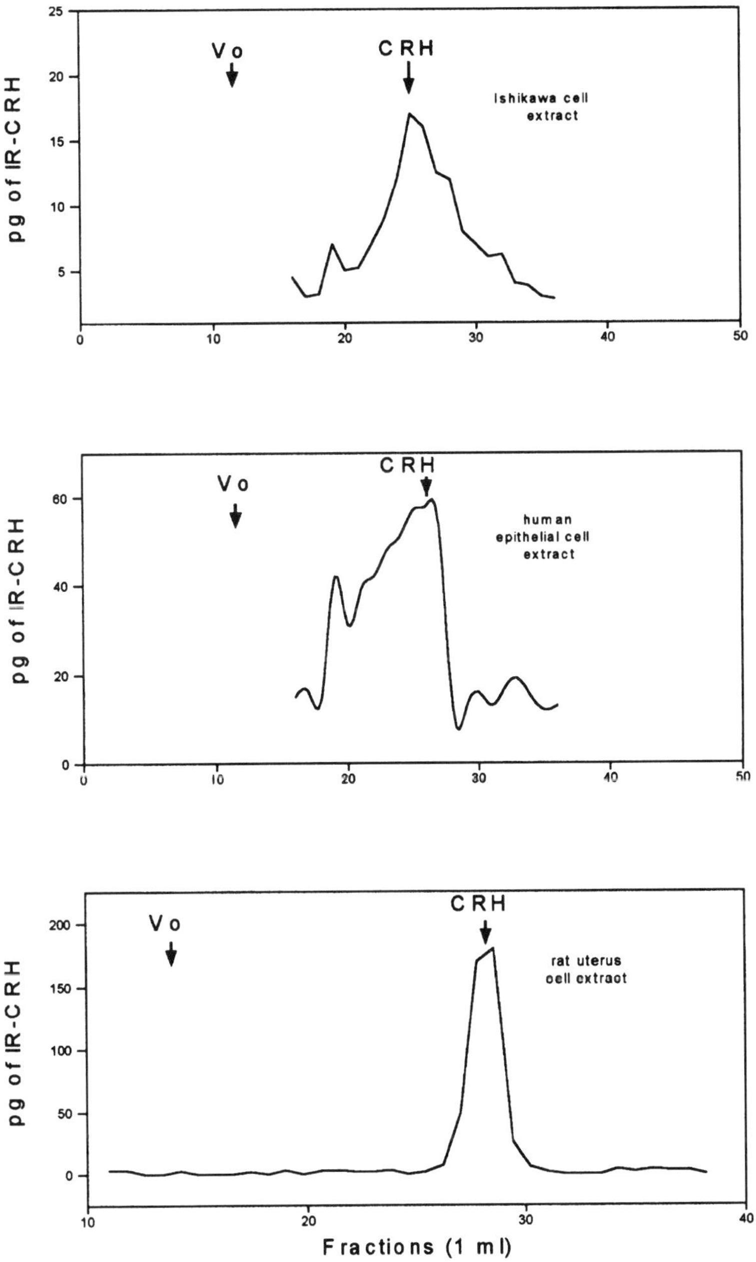

FIGURE 3. Sephadex G-50 gel filtration chromatography of extracts from normal glandular endometrial cells, Ishikawa cells, and rat uterus. One-milliliter fractions were collected. The *arrows* indicate the void volume (Vo) and the elution position of human CRH (hCRH).

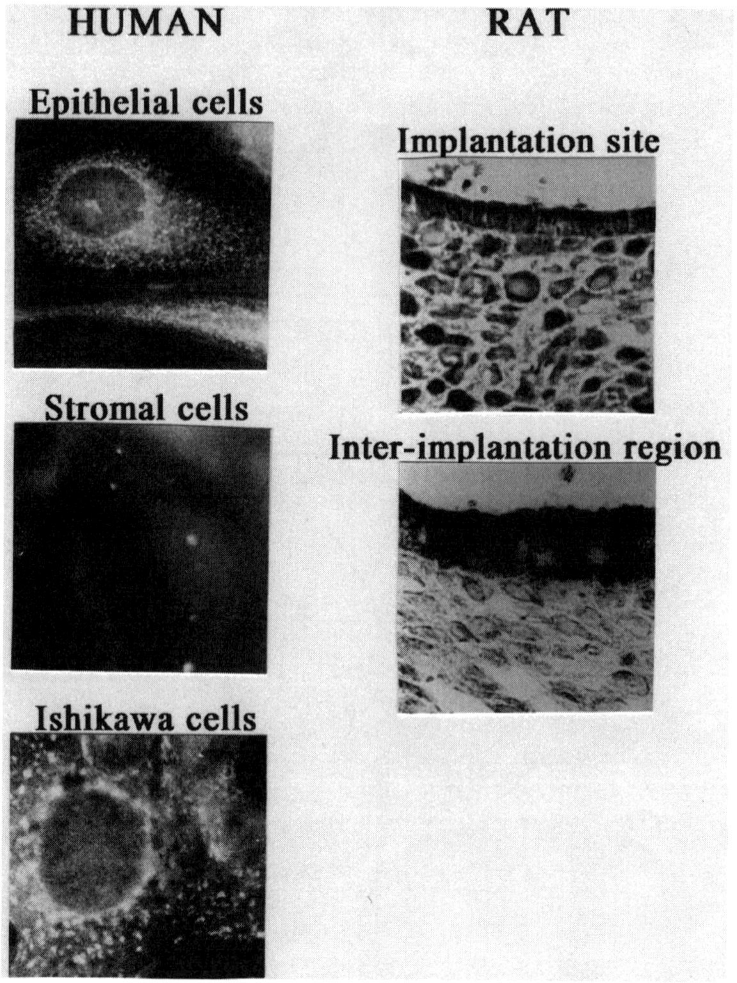

FIGURE 4. (**A**) Immunofluorescence localization of CRH in human normal and tumoral glandular endometrial cells. Normal stromal and glandular endometrial cells and Ishikawa cells grown on coverslips were exposed to hCRH antiserum. The retained anti-CRH antibodies were stained with FITC. Panels demonstrate the staining of glandular, stromal endometrial cells, and Ishikawa cells, respectively, in the presence of CRH antiserum and FITC. (Magnification × 1000.) (**B**) Immunohistochemical localization of IR-CRH in the uterus of the early pregnant rat at the time of implantation. Regions corresponding to the implantation sites and interimplantation uterine zone were determined by the intravenous injection of Evans blue. Tissue was fixed in 4% paraformaldehyde and embedded in paraplast. Immunohistochemical localization was performed using the avidin–biotin peroxidase complex method. Immune rabbit serum against CRH was used at 1:250. The peroxidase activity was revealed with the 3,3′-diamino benzidine reaction, and the sections were not counterstained. (Magnification × 900.)

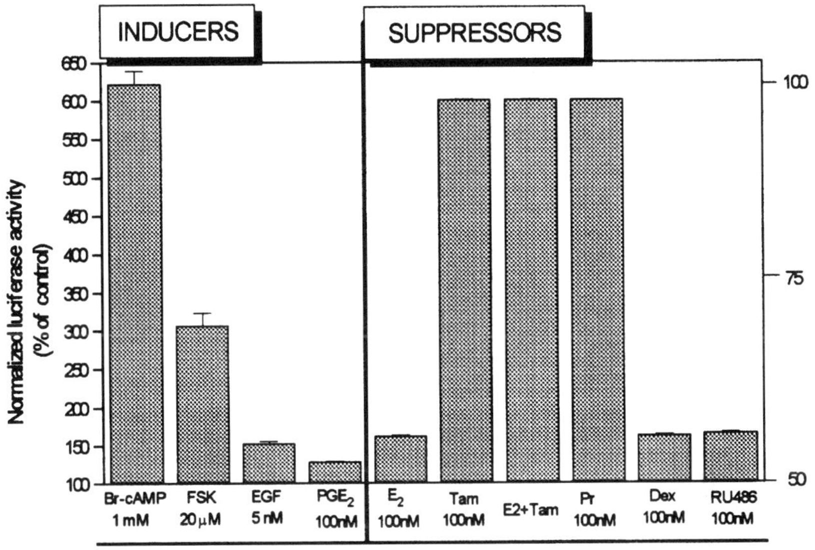

FIGURE 5. Effects on the CRH promoter in transfected human endometrial cells. Transfectants were cultured for 18 hours in the presence of the above compounds, then luciferase activity was measured in cell lysates. Results are expressed as mean ± SEM of percentage of control; that is, transfectants were not exposed to any compound.

DISCUSSION

Our findings show that human and rat uterus express the CRH gene. Epithelial cells of both species are the main source of endometrial CRH, while stroma does not seem to express it, unless it differentiates to decidua.[29,35] Immunoreactive CRH, produced by endometrial cells, has the chromatographic characteristics of authentic hypothalamic CRH while the size of its mRNA in both human and rat uterus is similar or identical with its counterpart, present in placenta and hypothalamus (1.3 kb). Estrogens and glucocorticoids inhibit and prostaglandin E_2 stimulates the promoter of human CRH gene in transfected human endometrial cells, suggesting that endometrial CRH gene expression is under the control of these agents. Moreover, in rats, endometrial CRH expression is significantly higher at the implantation sites, compared to that at the interimplantation uterine regions. These findings point out a significant role for endometrial CRH.

We have recently reported that human endometrial cells also express the proopiomelanocortin (POMC) and prodynorphin (PDYN) genes and synthesize their peptide products.[24,36] Specifically, the secretion of POMC end-product β-endorphin is inhibited by estrogens and glucocorticoids. The co-expression in endometrial epithelial cells of both CRH and POMC suggests that uterine CRH may have an autocrine/paracrine effect on locally produced POMC-derived peptides, as is the case for such other peripheral tissues as the placenta and testes.[37] Thus, the inhibitory effects of estrogens or glucocorticoids on endometrial POMC could be the result of a prior inhibition of endometrial CRH.

It is postulated that CRH participates in inflammatory phenomena, possessing procytokine-like properties. Actually, CRH is detectable in rat and human inflammatory sites, and its immunoneutralization attenuates the inflammatory response.[18] The reaction of uterus to the invading blastocyst has many characteristics of inflammation[38]: Several immune mediators of the inflammatory response, such as IL-1, IL-6, and IL-1, and TNF-α receptors are expressed in endometrial cells.[39,40] It has also been shown that the implanting blastocyst secretes inflammatory mediators, including IL-1 and PGE_2.[41–43] Blastocyst-deriving IL-1 plays an essential role in implantation since, in mice, blockage of its action by the antagonist IL-1ra inhibits it.[44] Furthermore, measurement of IL-1 levels in the periimplantation embryo culture fluid has predictive value for the successful outcome of implantation.[45] It is now known that IL-1 and PGE_2 are major inducers of CRH expression in human placenta and rat hypothalamus.[46,47] Our data show that the implantation sites of the early pregnant rat uterus contain significantly higher concentrations of ir-CRH and CRH mRNA than the uterine tissue between the implantation sites.[29] Additionally, we demonstrated that PGE_2 induced the activity of CRH promoter in endometrial cells.[48] These findings, taken together, suggest that uterine CRH may play a role in endometrial decidualization and egg implantation. Because the blastocyst secretes PGE_2 at the side of nidation, we hypothesize that it might, through the uterine epithelium, induce the local production of pharmacodynamically potent concentrations of CRH, thus facilitating the subsequent endometrial inflammatory reaction associated with egg implantation and the formation of egg nidus. At the same time, the local production of CRH may control the endometrial inflammatory reaction by augmenting the production of uterine β-endorphin, which may induce immunosuppression at the site of nidation. Additionally, blastocyst-deriving estrogens could exert an inhibitory effect on endometrial CRH, thus establishing a local regulatory system of endometrial reaction to the implanting blastocyst.

Uterine CRH, apart from its effects on endometrium, may play a local role in the regulation of myometrial tone. Specifically, CRH receptors have been detected in human myometrium,[49] and CRH may stimulate the release of prostaglandins PGE_2 and $PGF_{2\alpha}$, strong inducers of myometrial tone,[50] and potentiates the stimulatory effect of oxytocin on myometrial tone.[51] CRH may also play a role in the regulation of myometrial tone through its effect on endometrial β-endorphin since β-endorphin has a relaxant effect on smooth muscles.[52] During the peri-implantation period, endometrial CRH and β-endorphin may ensure the necessary uterine relaxation for the efficient implantation of the blastocyst. Thus the blastocyst itself may regulate the myometrial tone, the increase of which, at the moment of implantation, could lead to its expulsion.

Another action of endometrial CRH could be its participation in endometrial vascularization. Peripheral CRH has been found to exert vasodilatory effects. On the other hand, during implantation there is a major increase in vascular permeability surrounding the implanting embryo.[53] Endometrial capillaries adjacent to the primary decidual zone become dilated. It has been suggested that local inflammatory mediators regulate the vascular changes in the endometrium during the implantation process. Thus, endometrial CRH may be part of this sequence of events, which may be under the control of factor(s) originating from the blastocyst.

Finally, a rich network of uterine lymphokines, including interleukin-1 (IL-1), has recently been described. These lymphokines are mainly synthesized from endometrial stromal or epithelial cells, they affect blastocyst attachment and implantation, trophoblast outgrowth or menstruation, and they are inhibited by glucocorticoids including RU486.[39,54,55] Thus, the repressive effects of dexamethasone and RU486 on the activity of the CRH promoter suggest that these molecules could regulate CRH-related intrauterine immune phenomena via the regulation of CRH–cytokine interactions. Further studies are needed to define the exact physiological role of uterine CRH.

SUMMARY

Our findings show that human and rat uterus express the CRH gene. Epithelial cells of both species are the main source of endometrial CRH, while stroma does not seem to express it, unless it differentiates to decidua. Immunoreactive CRH, produced by endometrial cells, has the chromatographic characteristics of authentic hypothalamic CRH, while the size of its mRNA in both human and rat uterus is similar to or identical with its counterpart, present in placenta and hypothalamus (1.3 kb). Estrogens and glucocorticoids inhibit and prostaglandin E_2 stimulates the promoter of human CRH gene in transfected human endometrial cells, suggesting that endometrial CRH gene expression is under the control of these agents. Moreover, in rats, endometrial CRH expression is significantly higher at implantation sites, compared to that at interimplantation uterine regions. Given the proinflammatory/vasoregulatory properties of CRH, we hypothesize that endometrial CRH may participate in the regulation of intrauterine phenomena, such as blastocyst implantation, endometrial vascularization, and myometrial contractility.

REFERENCES

1. Vale, W., C. Rivier, M. R. Brown, J. Spiess, G. Koob & A. Swanson. 1983. Chemical and biological characterization of corticotropin-releasing factor. Rec. Prog. Horm. Res. **39:** 245–267.
2. Fischman, A. J. & R. L. Moldow. 1982. Extrahypothalamic distribution of CRF-like immunoreactivity in the rat brain. Peptides **1:** 149–153.
3. Swanson, L. W., P. E. Sawchenco, J. Rivier & W. Vale. 1983. Organization of ovine corticotropin-releasing factor immunoreactive cells and fibers in the rat brain: An immunohistochemical study. Neuroendocrinology **36:** 165–864.
4. Wynn, P. C., R. L. Hauger, M. C. Holmes, M. A. Millan, K. J. Catt & G. Aguilera. 1984. Brain and pituitary receptors for corticotropin releasing factor: Localization and differential regulation after adrenalectomy. Peptides **5:** 1077–1084.
5. De Souza, E. B. 1987. Corticotropin-releasing factor receptors in the rat central nervous system: Characterization and regional distribution. J. Neurosci. **7:** 88–100.
6. Stephanou, A., D. S. Jessop, R. A. Knight & S. L. Lightman. 1990. Corticotrophin-releasing factor-like immunoreactivity and mRNA in human leukocytes. Brain Behav. Immunol. **4:** 67–73.

7. ORTH, D. 1992. Corticotropin-releasing hormone in humans. Endocrinol. Rev. **13:** 164–191.
8. USUI, T., Y. NAKAI, T. TSUKADA, H. JINGAMI, H. TAKAHASHI & J. FUCADA. 1988. Expression of adrenocorticotropin-releasing hormone precursor gene in placenta and other nonhypothalamic tissues in man. Mol. Endocrinol. **2:** 871–875.
9. SUDA, T., N. TOMORI, F. TOZAWA, T. MOURI, H. DEMOURA & K. SHIZUME. 1984. Distribution and characterization of immunoreactive corticotropin-releasing factor in human tissues. J. Clin. Endocrinol. Metab. **59:** 861–868.
10. PETRUSZ, P., I. MERGHENTHALER, L. MADERDRUT, S. VIGH & A. SCHALLY. 1983. Corticotropin-releasing factor-like immunoreactivity in the vertebrate endocrine pancreas. Proc. Natl. Acad. Sci. USA **80:** 1721–1725.
11. PETRUSZ, P., I. MERGHENTHALER, P. ORDRONNEAU, L. MADERDRUT, S. VIGH & A. SCHALLY. 1984. Corticotropin-releasing factor-like immunoreactivity in the gastro-entero-pancreatic endocrine system. Peptides **5:** 71–72.
12. MASTORAKOS, G., E. WEBSTER, T. FRIEDMANT & G. CHROUSOS. 1993. Immunoreactive corticotropin-releasing hormone and its binding in the rat ovaries. J. Clin. Invest. **92:** 961–968.
13. FABBRI, A., J. C. TINAJERO & M. L. DUFAU. 1990. Corticotropin-releasing factor is produced by rat Leydig cells and has a major local antireproductive role in the testis. Endocrinology **127:** 1541–1543.
14. MASTORAKOS, G., E. L. WEBSTERO & G. P. CHROUSOS. 1993. Corticotropin-releasing hormone and its receptors in the ovary: Physiological implications. Ann. N.Y. Acad. Sci. **687:** 20–28.
15. GRINO, M., G. CHROUSOS & A. MARGIORIS. 1987. The corticotropin-releasing hormone gene is expressed in human placenta. Biochem. Biophys. Res. Commun. **148:** 1208–1214.
16. FRIM, D., R. EMANUEL, B. ROBINSON, C. SMAS, G. ADLER & J. MAJZOUB. 1988. Characterization and gestational regulation of corticotropin-releasing hormone mRNA in human placenta. J. Clin. Invest. **82:** 287–292.
17. PETRAGLIA, F., S. TABANELLI, C. GALASSI, G. C. GARUTI, A. MANCINI, A. GENAZZANI & E. GURPIDE. 1992. Human desidua and in vitro desidualized endometrial stromal cells at term contain immunoreactive CRF and CRF mRNA. J. Clin. Endocrinol. Metab. **74:** 1427–1431.
18. KARALIS, K., H. SANO, J. REDWINE, S. LISTWARK, R. WILDER & G. CHROUSOS. 1991. Autocrine or paracrine inflammatory actions of corticotropin-releasing hormone in vivo. Science **254:** 421–423.
19. KAVELAARS, A., R. E. BALLIEUX & C. J. HEIJNEN. 1989. The role of IL-1 in the corticotropin-releasing factor and arginine-vasopressin-induced secretion of immunoreactive beta-endorphin by human peripheral blood mononuclear cells. J. Immunol. **142:** 2338–2342.
20. SINGH, V. K. 1989. Stimulatory effect of corticotropin-releasing neurohormone on human lymphocyte proliferation and interleukin-2 receptor expression. J. Neuroimmunol. **23:** 257–262.
21. NOYES, R. W., A. T. HERTIG & J. ROCK. 1950. Dating of endometrial biopsy. Fertil. Steril. **1:** 3–25.
22. SATYASWAROOP, P., R. S. BRESSLER, M. DELAPENA & E. GURPIDE. 1979. Isolation and culture of human endometrial glands. J. Clin. Endocrinol. Metab. **48:** 639–641.
23. GRAVANIS, A. & E. GURPIDE. 1986. Effects of estradiol on DNA polymerase a activity in a human endometrial adenocarcinoma cell line (Ishikawa cells). J. Clin. Endocrinol. Metab. **63:** 356–359.
24. MAKRIGIANNAKIS, A., A. MARGIORIS, E. MARKOGIANNAKIS, C. STOURNARAS & A. GRAVA-

NIS. 1992. Steroid hormones regulate the release of immunoreactive β-endorphin from the Ishikawa human endometrial cell line. J. Clin. Endocrinol. Metab. **75:** 584–589.

25. PSYCHOYOS, A. 1993. *In* Implantation in Mammals. L. Gianaroli, A. Campana & A. O. Trounson, Eds.: 49–58. Raven Press. New York.
26. MANIATIS, T., E. F. FRITSCH & J. SAMBROOK. 1989. Molecular Cloning: A Laboratory Manual. Cold Spring Harbor Laboratory. Cold Spring Harbor, NY.
27. SHIBAHARA, S., Y. MOTIMOTO, Y. FUTUTANI, M. NOTAKE, H. TAKAHASHI & S. SHIMIZU. 1983. Isolation and sequence of the human corticotropin-releasing factor precursor gene. EMBO J. **2:** 775–779.
28. FOSTINIS, Y., P. THEODOROPOULOS, A. GRAVANIS & C. STOURNARAS. 1992. Heat shock protein HSP90 and its association with the cytoskeleton: A morphological study. Biochem. Cell Biol. **70:** 779–786.
29. MAKRIGIANNAKIS, A., A. N. MARGIORIS, C. LEGOASCOGNE, E. ZOUMAKIS, G. NIKAS, C. STOURNARAS, A. PSYCHOYOS & A. GRAVANIS. 1995. Corticotropin-releasing hormone (CRH) is expressed at the implantation sites of early pregnant rat uterus. Life Sci. **57:** 1869–1875.
30. VAMVAKOPOULOS, N. & G. P. CHROUSOS. 1993. Structural organization of the 5′ flanking region of the human corticotropin releasing hormone gene. J. DNA Sequence Mapping **4:** 197–206.
31. NORDEEN, S. K. 1988. Luciferase reporter gene vectors for analysis of promoters and enhancers. BioTechniques **6:** 454–457.
32. STAMATATOS, L., R. LEVENTIS, M. J. ZUCKERMAN & J. R. SILVIUS. 1988. Interactions of cationic lipid vesicles with negatively charged phospholipid vesicles and biological membranes. Biochemistry **27:** 3917–3925.
33. SCHENBORN, E. & V. GOIFFON. 1993. A sensitive assay for firefly luciferase activity. Promega Notes **41:** 11–14.
34. ROSENTHAL, N. 1987. Identification of regulatory elements of cloned genes with functional assays. Methods Enzymol. **152:** 704–721.
35. MAKRIGIANNAKIS, A., E. ZOUMAKIS, A. N. MARGIORIS, P. THEODOROPOULOS, C. STOURNARAS & A. GRAVANIS. 1995. The corticotropin-releasing hormone in normal and tumoral epithelial cells of human endometrium. J. Clin. Endocrinol. Metab. **80:** 185–189.
36. GRAVANIS, A., A. MAKRIGIANNAKIS, C. STOURNARAS & A. N. MARGIORIS. 1994. Interaction between steroid hormones and endometrial opioids. Ann. N.Y. Acad. Sci. **734:** 245–256.
37. MARGIORIS, A. N., M. GRINO, P. PROTOS, P. GOLD & G. CHROUSOS. 1988. Corticotropin-releasing hormone and oxytocin stimulate the release of placental proopiomelanocortin peptides. J. Clin. Endocrinol. Metab. **66:** 922–926.
38. PSYCHOYOS, A. 1976. Hormonal control of uterine receptivity for nidation. J. Reprod. Fertil. **25:** 17–28.
39. TABIBZADEH, S. 1991. Cytokine regulation of human endometrial function. Ann. N.Y. Acad. Sci. **622:** 89–98.
40. TABIBZADEH, S., U. SANTHANAM, P. B. SEHDAL & L. T. MAY. 1989. Cytokine-induced production of IFN-β2/IL-6 by freshly explanted human endometrial stroma cells. J. Immunol. **142:** 3134–3139.
41. KASAMO, M., K. ISHIKAWA, K. YAMASHITA, K. SENGOKU & T. SHIMIZU. 1986. Possible role of prostaglandins in blastocyst implantation. Prostaglandins **31:** 321–336.
42. CHIDA, S. & L. METTLER. 1989. Effects of indomethacin, prostaglandin E2 and prostaglandin F2 alpha on mouse blastocyst attachment and trophoblastic outgrowth in vitro. Prostaglandins **37:** 411–416.
43. ZOLTI, M., Z. BEN-RAFAEL, R. MEIROM, M. SHEMESH, D. BIDER, S. MASHIACH & R. APTE. 1991. Cytokine involvement in oocytes and early embryos. Fertil. Steril. **56:** 265–272.
44. SIMON, C., A. FRANCES, G. PIQUETTE, I. DANASOURI, G. ZURAWSKI, W. DANG & M. POLAN.

1994. Embryonic implantation in mice is blocked by interleukin-1 receptor antagonist. Endocrinology **134:** 521–529.

45. SHETH, K. V., G. L. ROCA, S. AL-SEDAIRY, R. PARHAR, G. HAMILTON & F. AL-ABDUL JABBAR. 1991. Prediction of successful embryo implantation by measuring interleukin-1-alpha and immunosuppressive factor(s) in preimplantation. Fertil. Steril. **55:** 952–957.
46. SAPOLSKY, R., C. RIVIER, G. YAMAMOTO, P. PLOTSKY & W. VALE. 1987. Interleukin-1 stimulates the secretion of hypothalamic corticotropin-releasing factor. Science **238:** 522–524.
47. PETRAGLIA, F., G. C. GARUTTI, B. DERAMUNDO, S. ANGIONI, A. GENAZZANI & M. BILEZIKJIAN. 1990. Mechanisms of action of interleukin-1 in increasing CRF and ACTH from cultured human placental cells. Am. J. Obstet. Gynecol. **163:** 1307–1312.
48. MAKRIGIANNAKIS, A., E. ZOUMAKIS, A. N. MARGIORIS, C. STOURNARAS, G. P. CHROUSOS & A. GRAVANIS. 1995. Estrogen and glucocorticoids repress the activity of the 5′-flanking region of human corticotropin-releasing hormone (CRH) gene in transiently transfected Ishikawa human endometrial cells. Abstract in 76th Endocrine Meeting, Washington, DC.
49. HILLHOUSE, E. W., D. GRAMMATOPOULOS, N. G. MILTON & H. W. QUARTERO. 1993. The identification of a human myometrial corticotropin-releasing hormone receptor that increases in affinity during pregnancy. J. Clin. Endocrinol. Metab. **76:** 736–741.
50. LENG, G., R. J. BICKNELL, S. MANSFIELD & R. G. DYER. 1986. Oxytocin, opioids and parturition. J. Endocrinol. **108**(Suppl. Abstr.)**:** 19.
51. FRAIOLI, F., M. CAPPA & A. FABBRI. 1984. Lack of endogenous inhibitory tone on LH secretion in early puberty. Clin. Endocrinol. (Oxford) **20:** 299–303.
52. WIEMANN, J. N., D. K. CLIFTON & R. A. STEINER. 1989. Pubertal changes in gonadotropin-releasing hormone and prooiomelanocortin gene expression in the brain of the male rat. Endocrinology **124:** 1760–1767.
53. ROGERS, P. A. 1992. Early endometrial microvascular response during implantation in the rat. Reprod. Fertil. Dev. **4:** 261–264.
54. HILL, J. A. 1982. Cytokines considered critical in pregnancy. Am. J. Reprod. Immunol. **28:** 123–126.
55. ANTONAKIS, N., V. GEORGOULIAS, A. MARGIORIS, C. STOURNARAS & A. GRAVANIS. 1994. In vitro differential effects of the antiglucocorticoid RU 486 on the release of lymphokines from normal human lymphocytes. J. Steroid Biochem. Mol. Biol. **51:** 67–72.

Uterine Pinopodes in Peri-implantation Human Endometrium

Clinical Relevance

GEORGE NIKAS[a] AND ALEXANDER PSYCHOYOS

Laboratoire de Physiologie de la Reproduction
Hôpital Bicêtre
Bâtiment INSERM Gregory Pincus
80 rue du Général Leclerc
Le Kremlin Bicêtre, France

Research during the last decades has greatly advanced our understanding of mammalian implantation, but many of its cellular and molecular mechanisms still remain obscure. Moreover, the development of assisted reproduction treatments has demonstrated implantation to be of major clinical importance, and the need for methods to assess the uterine receptivity has emerged. This article summarizes data available on the investigation of endometrial pinopodes as markers of the human implantation window and discusses some clinical and scientific implications of these findings.

INTRODUCTION

Mammalian implantation has been a fascinating field of research and discovery for the last century (see Psychoyos[1] for a historical review). After successful fertilization and cleavage, the ovum arrives in the uterine cavity, typically at the morula stage. Soon afterwards it develops into a blastocyst, sheds the zona pellucida, attaches to the uterus, and implants. Implantation begins with apposition, when the free-floating blastocyst ceases moving and comes into close proximity with the folds of the uterine mucosa. Adhesive interactions develop actively between specific molecules on the plasma membranes of trophoblastic and surface endometrial cells, marking the adhesion stage. Adhesion is followed by invasion and development of the placenta. With the beginning of implantation, the early embryonic period ends, a period that is generally similar in all mammals. Subsequent placentation varies greatly among different species, reflecting the specific life conditions of each. However, as comparative studies by Enders[2] suggest, the initial stages of implantation (apposition and adhesion) are common in all species.

Initiation of implantation represents the successful meeting of two separate processes: endometrial differentiation and ovum development. A synchronism between these functions is important, as became apparent from ovum transfer experi-

[a]Address for correspondence: George Nikas, M.D., Human Embryology Laboratory, Institute of Obstetrics and Gynaecology, Royal Postgraduate Medical School, Hammersmith Hospital, Du Cane Road, London W12 ONN, U.K.

ments in rodents (McLaren and Michie[3]). The endometrium, in preparation for implantation, undergoes a sequence of cellular changes leading to the development of uterine receptivity. The hormonal control of implantation in the rat was determined by the pioneer studies of Psychoyos[4,5] during the 1960s and remains a solid model of mammalian implantation. Receptivity in this animal lasts only 12 hours, followed by a refractory state during which the uterus is hostile to the ovum. Blastocyst implantation can start only during this brief phase of receptivity, called the "nidation window" by Psychoyos.

During this phase the endometrial epithelium displays a number of unusual properties, which Denker[6] called "the cell biological paradox." Among other changes, the apical membrane loses its microvilli and becomes adhesive, and a general loss of cell polarization is noticed. Contact of the blastocyst with these cells produced a signal that transmitted to the underlying stroma, triggers the cascade of the implantation reaction. The nature of this signal is as yet unidentified. Research of the last decades has revealed that many factors participate in implantation, and several mechanisms for their action have been proposed.[7,8] It remains to be clarified which component is indispensable and which is not in this complex and precisely controlled process. This article will focus on some clinical aspects of the early stages of implantation.

IMPLANTATION IN WOMEN

The early stages of human implantation remain largely a mystery. The gaps in our knowledge are mostly filled by analogy with information from other species, and recently by *in vitro* human implantation models. From the limited series available from Hertig,[9] Croxatto,[10] Buster,[11] and Formigli,[12] it appears that the human conceptus arrives in the uterus at the morula stage four days after ovulation and fertilization. On the fifth day a blastocyst is present in the uterus. The zona pellucida disappears by a rapid process occurring the same day, and apposition and adhesion start one day after (sixth day of embryonic life—day 20 of a normal 28 day menstrual cycle). No direct information on the morphological relationships between the human blastocyst and the luminal epithelial cells during the apposition and adhesion steps is available. The most precocious specimen of human implantation yet observed concerns a blastocyst (Carnegie No. 8020), which presumably on day 21 is firmly attached and already invading the endometrium.[9] The orientation of this and older Carnegie specimens, as well as the interactions of human blastocysts and endometrial monolayers in culture (described by Lindenberg *et al.*[13]), suggests that apposition and adhesion is initiated at the embryonic pole.

There are no data concerning the success of this step alone during natural conception. If we consider that the overall fecundity of the human is around 25% for the first month of unprotected coitus,[14] and given the known losses occurring during the numerous steps of reproduction (reviewed by Edwards[15]) and because abnormal embryos can implant, we may presume that under physiological conditions and in the presence of a blastocyst, implantation effectively begins.

However, a number of clinical conditions associated with luteal defects and hormonal imbalances[16] may affect the development of endometrial receptivity. Moreover, the progesterone contraceptive minipill and hormonal regimens used as interceptives (next-morning pills) may inhibit implantation at this level.[17] The expansion of human *in vitro* fertilization and embryo transfer (IVF) made the importance of implantation for the final success of these procedures apparent. Indeed, current IVF treatments yield, in most cases, a fair number of normally cleaving ova; yet only a small percentage of them survives implantation if transferred *in utero.* Obviously a defect exists at the endometrial level.

The existence in the human of a short phase of uterine receptivity obeying a precise timing of appropriate hormonal regulation, in analogy to other species, was postulated long ago.[18] Exogenous hormone administration could adversely affect the development of this phase, preventing implantation. During the last decade, accumulated data from IVF programs have produced evidence in support of these suggestions.

Surprisingly, women suffering from primary or secondary amenorrhoea treated with HRT and ovum transfer have shown higher implantation rates compared to patients with functional ovaries who undergo standard IVF.[20–22] This may be attributed to the milder hormonal conditions and because a better timing of ovum-transfer is possible in the HRT cycles. Likewise, in natural cycle IVF, implantation may have a high chance of success.[23]

Clinical experience with ovum donation in patients under hormone replacement therapy (HRT) has shown that the optimal time for ovum transfer is limited (transfer window). Transfer beyond this time (usually three days) results in implantation failure.[19] Evidently, this is due to the limited span of receptivity.

The importance the endometrium bears on implantation commencement led to research for methods to assess the adequate development of endometrial receptivity in women.

THE HUMAN ENDOMETRIUM

Changes in the human endometrium around the peri-implantation period mostly appear spontaneously in every menstrual cycle, independently of the presence of an implanting blastocyst. Such changes can be studied in tissue samples or endometrial fluid.

The classic work of Noyes *et al.*[24] on dating the endometrial biopsy through the menstrual cycle describes distinct morphological events occurring within a 1- to 2-day span during the luteal phase. Alterations during days 16 through 20 mainly affect the epithelial cell and are related to secretion. The abrupt onset of stromal edema occurring on day 21 signals the switching of events to the stroma, whose predecidual differentiation serves for the dating until the end of the cycle. The Noyes histology has been a basis of all studies on the human endometrium and the standard method of assessing the endometrial maturation and the adequacy of the luteal function.[25] Interestingly, Castelbaum[26] suggests that midluteal rather than late luteal endometrial sampling is more informative for this purpose. Seeking a further refinement of histological dating and the establishment of objective criteria, Johannisson[27] proposed morphometric analysis. Although useful, this method cannot really supplant judgment based on experience in the elaboration of a histological diagnosis.

In any case, the specificity of conventional histology in relation to the development of uterine receptivity is apparently low. A large number of physiological signals expressed in the endometrium at certain periods of the luteal phase have been investigated in research on specific markers of uterine receptivity (see Tabibzadeh and Babaknia[8] for a recent review). We will mention briefly some of them that could be of clinical interest.

At the ultrastructural level nuclear channel systems and giant mitochondria are observed from the early luteal phase forward in the epithelial cells. These structures persist in the late luteal phase, and their detection has been used to assess the progestin potency of HRT regimes in menopausal patients.[28]

Progesterone-regulated proteins synthesized by the endometrial and the decidual cells appearing in the serum and uterine fluid have been extensively studied. The most abundantly produced is the placental protein 14 (PP14). Immunostaining of the endometrium through the menstrual cycle showed that this protein starts to increase at the midluteal phase and continues during the late luteal phase and further into the pregnancy.[29] Interestingly, a low level of PP14 was found in retarded endometria.[30]

An estrogen-induced 24K protein was reported by Ciocca *et al.*[31] to show its maximal expression during the mid-luteal phase in the apical protrusions of the luminal epithelium. Rizk *et al.*[32] found intense staining for this protein to be highly correlated with the establishment of pregnancy in cycles with ovum transfer. The function of this protein and the significance of its expression in the pinopodes remain to be clarified.

Another interesting approach is pursued in the studies on integrin molecules present in the endometrium, because some of them show regulated expression during the luteal phase.[33] Lessey *et al.*[34] reported a co-expression of $\alpha 1$, $\alpha 4$ and $\beta 3$ integrin subunits in the glandular epithelium during a 5-day interval, from days 20 to 24 of a normal cycle, and proposed this to reflect the duration of the implantation window.

The cytokine leukemia-inhibiting (LIF) factor is expressed in the mouse endometrium during receptivity. In transgenic animals lacking a functional LIF gene, implantation cannot commence, showing that this molecule is necessary for implantation in mice (Stewart *et al.*[35]). In the human endometrium, LIF is found mainly in the glandular epithelium, and its production increases during the mid- and late-secretory phase.[36] The significance of this cytokine in human implantation remains unknown.

Although highly interesting, these and other studies on human receptivity have not yet been conclusive and little is known about to what extent the expression of these signals is specifically related to receptivity. Most of them last over a long period, and their detection requires sophisticated methods. Therefore, much controversy continues to exist about the human implantation window and the definition of endometrial receptivity in women remains vague.

In our attempts to establish a clinical marker for this purpose, we have taken advantage of studies in other species and, more precisely, of the existence of pinopodes as an ultrastructural marker of uterine receptivity in the rat.

UTERINE PINOPODES

Early morphological studies on the rat and mouse endometrium during the phase of receptivity revealed striking modifications in the ultrastructure of the luminal epithelium. The apical membranes of the secretory cells lose their microvilli and develop large ectoplasmic protrusions resembling sponges.[37,38] Intrauterine administration of tracers showed that these structures are involved in an apico-basal transport of fluid and macromolecules towards the stroma.[39,40] Because of this function, the protrusions were termed pinopodes (from the Greek πινω = drink and ποδες = feet). It was further suggested that the pinopodes are associated with the thinning of the glycocalyx and the reduction of the negative cell surface charge observed during receptivity.[41] Pinocytosis could also be involved in the capture by the epithelial cells of signals from the embryo.

Scanning electron microscopy (SEM) studies in rat pregnancy and during delayed implantation indicated that the development of pinopodes is progesterone-dependent, and their presence coincides strictly with the implantation window.[42,43] Displacement of receptivity in the rat through antiprogestin administration was accompanied by displacement of pinopode formation.[44] High doses of estrogen, which inhibit pinopode formation, also block implantation in this animal.[9,45] Similar protrusions have been described in cows at the time of implantation, but in this case they were found associated with coupled endocytotic-secretory activity.[46] Pinopodes were also observed during the perinidatory period in the baboon (Psychoyos, unpublished data).

In the human endometrium, Nilsson[47] reported the presence of apical protrusions (pinopodes) in midluteal endometrial specimens. Martel *et al.*[48] found pinopodes in samples taken around the 20th day of a normal cycle, which is the presumed day of blastocyst attachment. The appearance of pinopodes was studied further in patients under exogenous hormonal treatments. In patients receiving clomiphene citrate followed by hMG and hCG for ovarian stimulation (OS), endometrial samples were taken on day 2 or day 6 after ovulation. Most of the endometria were found already advanced on day 2, and on day 20 pinopodes were present in only 15% of the specimens, compared to 80% of the control.[49] In another group of patients with ovarian failure under HRT, receiving estradiol per o.s. followed by vaginal progesterone starting from day 15 of the cycle, endometrial samples were taken on days 19 or 21. The majority of specimens on both days showed a retarded maturation, with pinopodes beginning to form on day 21.[50] The displacement of pinopode appearance under these treatments fitted well with other histological studies, which showed accelerated and retarded endometrial maturation under OS and HRT, respectively.[51,52] These results strengthen the possibility that the pinopodes can serve as a marker of receptivity in humans.[53]

RECENT STUDIES ON PINOPODES IN WOMEN

To investigate further the potential of uterine pinopodes to mark the receptive period in women, we examined the kinetics of their formation in sequential endometrial tissue samples taken from the same individuals during the same cycle. Patients participating in these studies, some of them still ongoing, were enrolled in ovum donation programs and had natural, HRT, or OS cycles. Two to four endometrial samples were taken sequentially, usually at 2-day intervals during the early and midluteal phase.

HRT Cycles

In the first study,[54] we examined normally menstruating patients receiving 8 mg/day estradiol valerate per OS starting on day 2 of the cycle and 100 mg of progesterone intramuscularly added from the 8th day of this treatment (day P1). Two endometrial samples per cycle were taken from each patient, either on days P6 and P9 or on days P8 and P10. All showed the presence of epithelial pinopodes in at least one of the two samples. When pinopodes were present in both biopsies, they were found developing in the first biopsy and regressing in the second one, suggesting that their total lifespan does not exceed a period of 48 hours. Fully developed pinopodes, when observed, existed in only one of the two biopsies obtained from the same patient. One could thus estimate that fully developed pinopodes appeared for one day only, but on different days of the artificial cycle. The range of these differences extended to five days, from P6 to P10, with most of them peaking on day P8.

In another study,[55] we examined HRT patients receiving 4 mg daily estradiol valerate per o.s. together with 600 μg Buserelin, starting from day 2 of the cycle. From days 8 to 14 the dose of estrogen was increased to 8 mg daily. On day 15 Buserelin was discontinued, and a daily dose of 50 mg of progesterone in oil intramuscularly was added (day P1). Two endometrial samples were obtained from each patient on days P6 and P8 or P7 and P9 (FIGS. 1, 2, and 3). Again, fully developed pinopodes were found only in one sample, but the time variations between patients

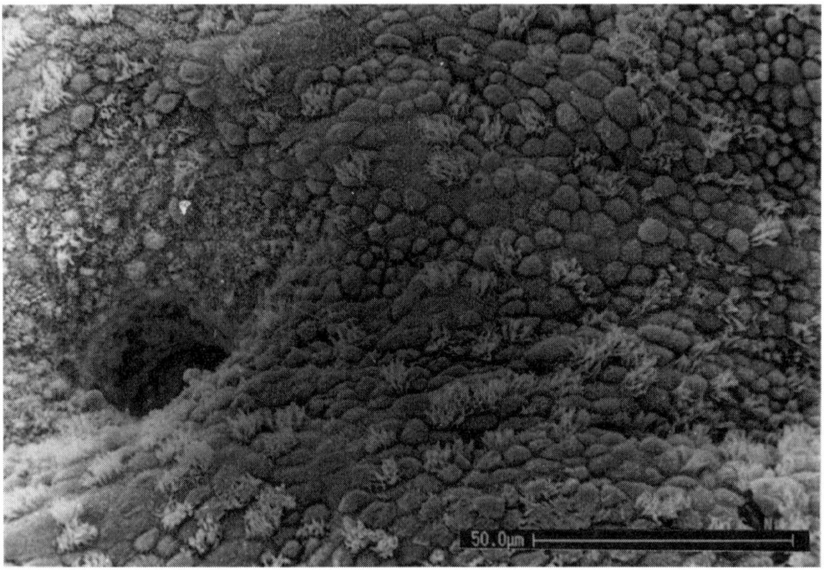

FIGURE 1. Human endometrium on the sixth day of progesterone treatment.

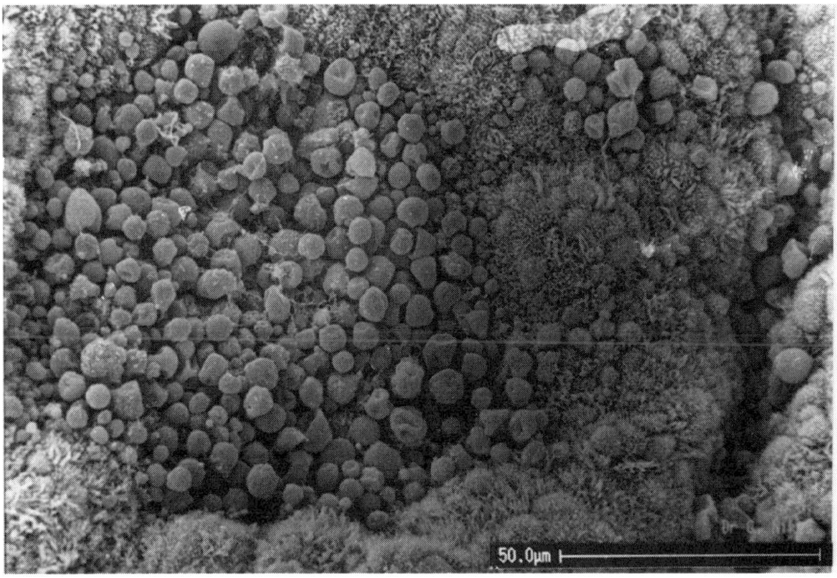

FIGURE 2. Human endometrium on the seventh day of progesterone treatment. Note the presence of pinopodes around the gland opening.

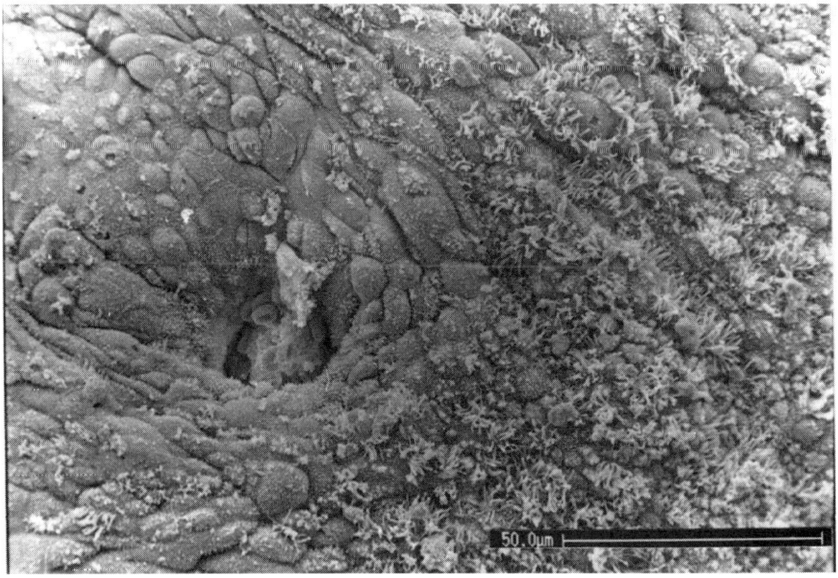

FIGURE 3. Human endometrium on the eighth day of progesterone treatment.

were less pronounced, compared to the previous study, and confined to 3 days, from P7 to P9.

Ovarian Stimulation Cycles

In this study[56] we examined patients undergoing ovarian stimulation for oocyte donation. After pituitary suppression with leuprolide acetate the patients received hMG and FSH (Metrodin/Pergonal; Serono), followed by hCG. Endometrial samples were taken on days of oocyte retrieval (designated day 14) and/or days 17, 19, and 21 (FIG. 4). Pinopodes were detected mainly on days 19 and 21, most of them being developing on day 19 and regressing on day 21.

Natural Cycles

Normal menstruating fertile patients were followed for ovulation detection by serum LH or ultrasound monitoring starting from day 10 of the cycle. The day of LH surge was designated as day 14, and the day the follicle was seen ruptured as day 15. Sequential sampling usually taken every 48 hours during days 17 through 23 revealed that fully developed pinopodes are confined to one sample and this can vary from day 19 to 21 (FIG. 4), from patient to patient (Nikas *et al.*, unpublished data).

This sequential sampling led us to conclude that the pinopodes in all cases have a limited life-span that does not exceed 48 hours. Furthermore, their evolution follow a distinct morphological pattern, allowing to be distinguished developing, fully developed or regressing pinopodes (see also Ref. 57). In addition, according to the numbers of pinopodes present, we can distinguish patients showing good, moderate, or low endometrial response to the treatment.

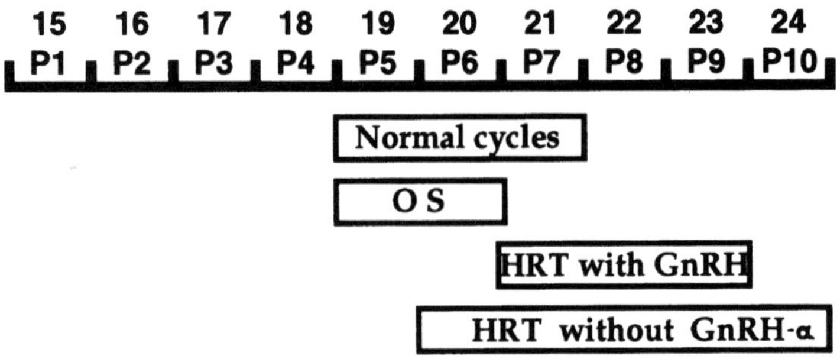

FIGURE 4. Range of variations of the pinopode appearance in natural, stimulated (OS), and artificial cycles (HRT).

DISCUSSION

The significance the uterine pinopodes could bear in relation to the human implantation window was suggested by Psychoyos many years ago.[18] From the amount of evidence existing from other species and following our recent studies in the human, we propose that pinopodes are directly involved in cell-surface changes associated with endometrial receptivity, and therefore their appearance is an accurate marker of the nidation window in women. Investigation of the kinetics of this marker reveals that the window is short, lasting less than 48 hours. Furthermore, the length of the time between ovulation (or progesterone commencement) and the onset of endometrial receptivity varies between women over a range of at least 3 days. This variation is attested to by the following facts: The length of the menstrual cycle, while relatively stable in each woman, ranges between 24 and 32 days in the normal fertile population.[58] The few human conceptuses described *in vivo* show a varying postovulation development, and viable ova ranging from the 8-cell to the blastocyst stage have been recovered from the uterine cavity five days after ovulation.[9–12] Finally, the rate of postinsemination development of human embryos *in vitro* is also variable, and blastocysts can form on days 5, 6, or 7 of culture.

From a clinical standpoint a short duration and a discrete timing of the window could be an important reason for the low implantation rates in IVF programs. In IVF cycles using clomiphene citrate for ovulation induction the pinopodes appeared earlier. This can be detrimental to the IVF embryo, which, in contrast, may be retarded, owing to the *in vitro* conditions. However, when hMG/FSH were used for ovulation induction, the epithelium appeared normal or slightly advanced in SEM, but the stroma in these specimens was greatly advanced.[55] The significance of this finding is unknown, since this protocol results in good implantation rates. Considering the paracrine communication between epithelium and stroma at the beginning of implantation, this phenomenon may compromise uterine receptivity or early trophoblastic invasion. In menstruating patients under HRT without pituitary downregulation, the variation of the nidation window extended to 5 days, from days 20 to 24.[54] A similar length of the transfer window (from days 16 to 20) leading to viable pregnancies was observed in a similar treatment.[59] When GnRH-α is administered, variations are confined to 3 days (from day 21 to day 23), probably owing to the prevention of spontaneous ovulation, which interferes with the HRT. In fact the transfer window for the most clinics is considered to be from day 17 to day 19, for day 2 ova.

Our data imply that the examination of pinopodes could be a very useful tool for the prediction of the implantation window on an individual basis, during infertility treatment. Such a prediction could allow for better timing of the intrauterine transfer of donated or frozen ova to the recipients, because in these cases, and unlike the standard IVF cycles, the endometrium and/or the embryonic age can be manipulated. This effort is already in progress in an ovum donation program: The patients undergo mock HRT cycles with dual 48-hour midluteal endometrial sampling to detect uterine pinopodes. The mock cycle is followed by a transfer cycle in which the ovum is replaced according to the timing of the appearance of the pinopodes during the assessment cycle. Preliminary results are highly encouraging, showing increased pregnancy rates and very strong correlation between the presence of pinopodes and positive pregnancy tests.[55]

Examination of pinopodes may have a place in infertility evaluation, complementary to classical endometrial histology. Because the natural purpose of progesterone action on the endometrium is the preparation for implantation, pinopodes could also be used for the assessment of progestin potential in HRT at menopause. Finally, this marker deserves further investigation in relation to molecular changes occurring during the receptive phase. Pinopodes in this case could assist in precise dating of endometrial tissue in relation to the implantation window. Such a correlative study is already in progress, aiming to reveal the expression of cell adhesion molecules on the endometrial cells before, during, and after the pinopode formation. It is hoped that pinopodes will contribute substantially to our understanding of the beginning of implantation in our species, which is now the "last frontier" in infertility treatment.

CONCLUSIONS

The human implantation window, as determined by the formation of uterine pinopodes, is short and varies with different hormonal treatments and among different individuals. Examination of endometrial samples for pinopodes may assess the timing of uterine receptivity as well as its quality. This can be very useful for better timing of the ovum transfer as part of infertility evaluation, for the assessment of the normality of HRT in menopausal patients, and finally for assisting other studies in human implantation research.

SUMMARY

Current clinical studies indicate the existence in the human of an "implantation/nidation window," similar to that observed in animal models. During this short period of uterine receptivity, the formation of pinopodes on the apical cell membrane of the endometrial epithelium is a consistent morphological event, observed in a number of species studies including the human.

In order to develop a specific marker of the implantation window in clinical practice, we have investigated the kinetics of pinopode formation through sequential endometrial sampling under various hormonal conditions. Our results show that the implantation window in humans, according to this marker, lasts less than 48 hours, and the timing of its opening is dependent on the hormonal treatment applied, occurring earlier in cycles following ovarian stimulation and later in cycles induced by hormone replacement treatment. Furthermore, the timing varies among different individuals under the same treatment. These findings suggest that examination for pinopodes in endometrial samples can be highly useful in infertility treatment and research for the assessment of the nidation window on an individual basis. Our preliminary data strongly support the value of this assessment for better timing of ovum transfer, leading to an increase in implantation rates. Studies are now in progress on the expression of other endometrial signals present in relation to the pinopodes.

ACKNOWLEDGMENTS

Studies described in this article were performed in collaboration with the following institutions: IVF Unit, Alexandra Maternity Hospital, Athens University Medical School, Greece; Service de Gynecologie-Obstetrique, Hopital A. Beclere, Glamart, France; Infertility Unit of the Hammersmith and Royal Masonic Hospitals, London, U.K.; and The Howard and Georgeanna Jones Institute of Reproductive Medicine, Norfolk, Virginia, U.S.A.

REFERENCES

1. PSYCHOYOS, A. 1994. Endocrinology of embryo–endometrial interactions: A hundred years of fascinating discoveries. *In* Endocrinology of Embryo–Endometrium Interactions. S. R. Glasser, J. Mulholland & A. Psychoyos, Eds.: 1–10. Plenum Press. New York and London.
2. ENDERS, A. C. 1994. Contributions of comparative studies to understanding mechanisms of implantation. *In* Endocrinology of Embryo–Endometrium Interactions. S. R. Glasser, J. Mulholland & A. Psychoyos, Eds.: 11–16. Plenum Press. New York and London.
3. MCLAREN, A. & D. MICHIE. 1956. Studies on the transfer of fertilized mouse eggs to uterine foster-mothers. I. Factors affecting the implantation and survival of native and transferred eggs. J. Exp. Biol. **33:** 394–416.
4. PSYCHOYOS, A. 1966. Recent research on egg implantation. *In* Ciba Foundation Study Group on Egg Implantation. W. Wolstenholme & M. O'Connor, Eds.: 4–28. Churchill. London.
5. PSYCHOYOS, A. 1986. Uterine receptivity for nidation. Ann. N.Y. Acad. Sci. **476:** 36–42.
6. DENKER, H. W. 1993. Implantation: A cell biological paradox. J. Exp. Zool. **266:** 541–558.
7. TABIBZADEH, S. & A. BABAKNIA. 1995. The signals and molecular pathways involved in implantation, a symbiotic interaction between blastocyst and endometrium involving adhesion and tissue invasion. Hum. Reprod. **10:** 1579–1602.
8. PSYCHOYOS, A., G. NIKAS & A. GRAVANIS. 1995. The role of prostaglandins on blastocyst implantation. Hum. Reprod. **10**(Suppl. 1): 30–42.
9. HERTIG, A. T., J. ROCK & E. C. ADAMS. 1956. A description of 34 human ova within the first 17 days of development. Am. J. Anat. **98:** 435–491.
10. CROXATTO, H. B., S. DIAZ, B. A. FUENTEALBA, H. D. CROXATTO, D. CARRILO & C. FABRES. 1972. Studies on the duration of egg transport in the human oviduct. I. The time interval between ovulation and egg recovery from the uterus in normal women. Fertil. Steril. **23:** 447–458.
11. BUSTER, J. E., M. BUSTILLO, I. A. RODI, S. W. COHEN, M. HAMILTON, J. A. SIMON, I. H. THORNEYCROFT & J. R. MARSHALL. 1985. Biologic and morphologic development of donated human ova recovered by nonsurgical uterine lavage. Am. J. Obstet. Gynecol. **153:** 211–217.
12. FORMIGLI, L., G. FORMIGLI & C. ROCCIO. 1987. Donation of fertilized uterine ova to infertile women. Fertil. Steril. **47:** 162–165.
13. LINDENBERG, S., P. HYTTEL, S. LENZ & P. V. HOLMES. 1986. Ultrastructure of the early human implantation in vitro. Hum. Reprod. **1:** 533–538.
14. MILLER, J. E., E. WILLIAMSON, J. GLUE, Y. B. GORDON, J. G. GRUDZINSKAS & A. SYKES. 1980. Fetal loss after implantation: A prospective study. Lancet **2:** 554–556.
15. EDWARDS, R. G. 1986. Causes of early embryonic loss in human pregnancy. Hum. Reprod. **1:** 185–198.

16. McNeely, M. J. & M. R. Soules. 1988. The diagnosis of luteal phase deficiency: A critical review. Fertil. Steril. **50:** 1–15.
17. Psychoyos, A., G. Nikas, L. Saranti & A. Gravanis. 1995. Hormonal anti-implantation agents: Antiprogestins. Hum. Reprod. **10**(Suppl. 1): 140–150.
18. Psychoyos, A. 1976. Hormonal control of uterine receptivity for nidation. J. Reprod. Fertil. **25**(Suppl.): 17–28.
19. Navot, D., R. T. Scott, K. Droesch, L. L. Veeck, H. C. Liu & Z. Rosenwaks. 1991. The window of embryo transfer and the efficiency of human conception in vitro. Fertil. Steril. **55:** 114–118.
20. Paulson, R. J., M. V. Sauer & R. A. Lobo. 1990. Embryo implantation after human in vitro fertilization: Importance of endometrial receptivity. Fertil. Steril. **53:** 870–874.
21. Edwards, R. G., S. Marcos, M. Macnamee, J. P. Balmaceda, D. E. Walters & R. Asch. 1991. High fecundity in amenorrhoic women in embryo-transfer programmes. Lancet **338:** 292–294.
22. Psychoyos, A. 1993. The high fertility of agonadal and amenorrhoeic women after oocyte donation. Hum. Reprod. **8:** 498–499.
23. Lenton, E. A., I. D. Cooke, M. Hooper, H. King, A. Kumar, N. Monks, K. Turner & S. Verma. 1992. In vitro fertilization in the natural cycle. Baill. Clin. Obst. Gyn. **6:** 229–245.
24. Noyes, R. W., A. T. Hertig & J. Rock. 1950. Dating the endometrial biopsy. Fertil. Steril. **1:** 3–25.
25. Witten, B. I. & S. A. Martin. 1985. The endometrial biopsy as a guide to the management of luteal phase defect. Fertil. Steril. **44:** 460–465.
26. Castelbaum, A. J., J. Wheeler, C. B. Coutifaris, L. Mastroianni & B. A. Lessey. 1994. Timing of the endometrial biopsy may be critical for the accurate diagnosis of luteal phase deficiency. Fertil. Steril. **61:** 443–447.
27. Johannisson, E., R. A. Parker, B.-M. Landgren & E. Diczfalusy. 1982. Morphometric analysis of the human endometrium in relation to peripheral hormone levels. Fertil. Steril. **38:** 564–571.
28. Ryder, T. A., M. A. Mobberley & M. I. Whitehead. 1995. The endometrial nuclear channel system as an indicator of progestin potency in HRT. Maturitas **22:** 31–36.
29. Waites, G. T., P. L. Wood, R. A. Walker & S. C. Bell. 1988. Immunohistochemical localization of human endometrial secretory protein, "pregnancy-associated endometrial a_2 globulin" (a_2-PEG), during the menstrual cycle. J. Reprod. Fertil. **82:** 665–672.
30. Kletzeris, L. D., J. N. Bulmer, M. Seppala, T. C. Li, M. A. Warren & I. D. Cooke. 1994. Placental protein 14 in cycles with normal and retarded endometrial differentiation. Hum. Reprod. **9:** 394–398.
31. Ciocca, D. R., R. H. Asch, D. J. Adams & W. L. McGuire. 1983. Evidence for modulation of a 24K protein in human endometrium during the menstrual cycle. J. Clin. Endocrinol. Metab. **57:** 496–499.
32. Rizk, B., C. V. Manners, M. C. Davies, C. V. Steer, S. C. Bell, D. Dillon & R. G. Edwards. 1992. Immunohistochemical expression of endometrial proteins and pregnancy outcome in frozen embryo replacement cycles. Hum. Reprod. **7:** 413–417.
33. Tabibzadeh, S. 1992. Patterns of expression of integrin molecules in human endometrium throughout the menstrual cycle. Hum. Reprod. **7:** 876–882.
34. Lessey, B. A., A. J. Castelbaum, C. A. Buck, Y. Lei, C. W. Yowell & J. Sun. 1994. Further characterization of endometrial integrins during the menstrual cycle and in pregnancy. Fertil. Steril. **62:** 497–506.
35. Stewart, C. L., P. Kaspar, L. J. Brunet, H. Bhatt, I. Gadil, F. Kontgen & S. J. Abbondanzo. 1992. Blastocyst implantation depends on maternal expression of leukemia inhibitory factor. Nature **359:** 76–79.

36. CHARNOCK-JONES, D. S., A. M. SHARKEY, A. M. FENWICK & S. K. SMITH. 1994. Leukaemia inhibitory factor mRNA concentration peaks in human endometrium at the time of implantation and the blastocyst contains mRNA for the receptor at this time. J. Reprod. Fertil. **101:** 421–426.
37. POTTS, M. & A. PSYCHOYOS. 1967. Evolution de l'ultrastructure des relations ovoendométriales sous l'influence de l'oestrogène, chez la Ratte en retard expérimental de nidation. C. R. Acad. Sci. Paris **264:** 370–373.
38. POTTS, M. & A. PSYCHOYOS. 1967. L'ultrastructure des relations ovoendométriales au cours du retard expérimental de nidation chez la Souris. Acad. Sci. Paris **264:** 956–958.
39. ENDERS, A. D. & D. M. NELSON. 1973. Pinocytotic activity of the uterus of the rat. Am. J. Anat. **138:** 277–300.
40. PARR, M. B. & E. L. PARR. 1974. Uterine luminal epithelium: Protrusions mediate endocytosis, not apocrine secretion, in the rat. Biol. Reprod. **11:** 220–233.
41. ANDERSON, T. L. 1989. Biomolecular markers for the window of uterine receptivity. *In* Blastocyst Implantation. K. Yoshinaga, Ed.: 219–224. Serono Symposia. Adams Publishing Group. Boston, MA.
42. PSYCHOYOS, A. & P. MANDON. 1971. Etude de la surface de l'épithélium utérin au microscope électronique à balayage. Observation chez la ratte au 4ème et 5ème jours de la gestation. C.R. Acad. Sci. Paris **272:** 2723–2729.
43. PSYCHOYOS, A. & P. MANDON. 1971. Scanning electron microscopy of the surface of the rat uterine epithelium during delayed implantation. J. Reprod. Fertil. **26:** 137–138.
44. SARANTIS, L., D. ROCHE & A. PSYCHOYOS. 1988. Displacement of receptivity for nidation in the rat by the progesterone antagonist RU 486: A scanning electron microscopy study. Hum. Reprod. **3:** 251–255.
45. MARTEL, D., M. N. MONIER, D. ROCHE & A. PSYCHOYOS. 1991. Hormonal dependence of pinopode formation at the uterine luminal surface. Hum. Reprod. **6:** 597–603.
46. GUILLOMOT, M., K. J. BETTERIDGE, D. HARVEY & A. K. GOFF. 1986. Endocytotic activity in the endometrium during conceptus attachment in the cow. J. Reprod. Fertil. **78:** 27–36.
47. NILSSON, O. 1962. Correlation of structure to function of the luminal cell surface in the uterine epithelium of mouse and man. Z. Zellforsch. Microsk. Anat. **56:** 803–808.
48. MARTEL, D., C. MALET, J. P. GAUTRAY & A. PSYCHOYOS. 1981. Surface changes of the luminal uterine epithelium during the human menstrual cycle: A scanning electron microscopic study. *In* The Endometrium: Hormonal Impacts. Plenum Press. New York. pp. 15–29.
49. MARTEL, D., R. FRYDMAN, M. GLISSANT, C. MAGGIONI, D. ROCHE AND A. PSYCHOYOS. 1987. Scanning electron microscopy of postovulatory human endometrium in spontaneous cycles and cycles stimulated by hormone treatment. J. Endocrinol. **114:** 319–324.
50. MASSAI, M. R., C. BERGERON, D. MARTEL, D. DE ZIEGLER, G. MEDURI, A. PSYCHOYOS, R. FRYDMAN & P. BOUCHARD. 1993. Physiological estradiol and progesterone replacement cycles in women with ovarian failure: A model to study endometrial maturation and sex steroid receptors regulation by exogenous hormones. Hum. Reprod. **8:** 1828–1834.
51. COHEN, J., C. DEBACHE, F. PIGEAU, J. MANDELBAUM, M. PLACHOT & J. DEBRUX. 1984. Sequential use of clomiphene citrate, human menopausal gonadotropin and human chorionic gonadotropin in human in vitro fertilization. II. Study of luteal phase adequacy following aspiration of preovulatoru follicles. Fertil. Steril. **42:** 360–365.
52. LI, T. C., M. A. WARREN, P. DOCKERY & I. D. COOKE. 1991. Human endometrial morphology around the time of implantation in natural and artificial cycles. J. Reprod. Fertil. **92:** 543–554.
53. MARTEL, D., R. FRYDMAN, L. SARANTIS, D. ROCHE & A. PSYCHOYOS. 1989. Scanning electron microscopy of the uterine luminal epithelium as a marker of the implantation window. *In* Blastocyst Implantation. Adams Publishing Group. Boston. pp. 225–230.

54. NIKAS, G., P. DRAKAKIS, D. LOUTRADIS, C. MARA-SKOUFARI, E. KOUMANTAKIS, S. MICHALAS & A. PSYCHOYOS. 1995. Uterine pinopodes as markers of the "Nidation Window" in cycling women receiving exogenous oestradiol and progesterone. Hum. Reprod. **10:** 1208–1213.
55. NIKAS, G., N. REDD, & R. WINSTON. 1996. Implantation correlates highly with the expression of endometrial pinopodes in ovum recipients under HRT: A preliminary study. Oral presentation at the IXth World Congress in Human Reproduction, Philadelphia, PA, May 29–June 1, 1996.
56. RAMEY, J., P. HAMACHER, J. HSIU, A. ACOSTA, H. W. JONES, R. POE-ZEIGLER, J. P. TONER, S. OEHNINGER, G. NIKAS & A. PSYCHOYOS. 1995. Effects of superovulation on endometrial maturation: A morphological analysis performed on sequential biopsies obtained from oocyte donor patients. Poster presentation at the 42nd Annual Meeting of the Society for Gynecologic Investigation, Chicago, March 16–18, 1995.
57. PSYCHOYOS, A. & G. NIKAS. 1994. Uterine pinopodes as markers of uterine receptivity. Assist. Reprod. Revs. **4:** 26–32.
58. CHIAZZE, L., F. T. BRAYER, J. J. MASISCO, JR., M. P. PARKER & B. J. DUFFY. 1968. The length and variability of the human menstrual cycle. JAMA **203:** 377.
59. NAVOT, D., P. A. BERGH, M. WILLIAMS, G. J. GARISSI, I. GUZMAN, B. SANDLER, J. FOX, P. SCHREINER-ENGEL, G. E. HOFMANN & L. GRUNFELD. 1991. An insight into early reproductive processes through the in vivo model of ovum donation. J. Clin. Endocrinol. Metab. **72:** 408–414.

Neuroendocrinology of the Menstrual Cycle

ANDREA R. GENAZZANI,[a] FELICE PETRAGLIA,[b]
OMBRETTA GAMBA,[b] LAURA SGARBI,[b] M. MATHILDE GRECO,[b]
AND ALESSANDRO D. GENAZZANI[b]

[a]*Department of Obstetrics and Gynecology*
University of Pisa
Via Roma 35
56100 Pisa, Italy

[b]*Physiopathology of Human Reproduction*
University of Modena
Modena, Italy

INTRODUCTION

The human menstrual cycle is the result of a series of interrelated events that occur simultaneously in the hypothalamus–pituitary–ovarian (HPO) axis. The endometrium is the target organ for estrogens and progesterone secreted from the ovary, which in turn is regulated by pituitary gonadotropins (LH and FSH). Gonadotropin-releasing hormone (GnRH) is the pivot of the HPO axis secreted from the brain. Any change of hormone environment at any level of the system may modify target organ sensitivity, alter hormone secretion at other levels, and produce dysfunctioning of the reproductive cycle.

THE NEUROENDOCRINE CONTROL OF THE HYPOTHALAMUS–PITUITARY AXIS

In the various phases of the menstrual cycle, the secretory pattern of gonadotropins changes in relation to different neuroendocrine mechanisms. The release of GnRH is regulated by the integration of central and peripheral signals. GnRH-secreting neurons are located in the hypothalamic arcuate nucleus, and their axonal projections reach the median eminence of the mediobasal hypothalamus (MBH) where GnRH is released in a pulsatile fashion into the capillary system of the hypothalamic–pituitary portal circulation.[1] GnRH stimulates the pituitary gonadotrophs, binding to specific receptors on the cell surface whose density is regulated by GnRH itself and also by estrogens and progesterone.[2] The intermittent hypothalamic GnRH stimulation of pituitary gonadotrophs promotes episodic LH and FSH release. A close temporal relationship between hypothalamic GnRH release and pituitary LH secretion has been found in monkeys[3] and ewes,[4] as well as in humans.[5] LH changes in peripheral blood reflect the activity of GnRH-secreting neurons.

The GnRH pulse generator works as an independent pacemaker. In fact, the dis-

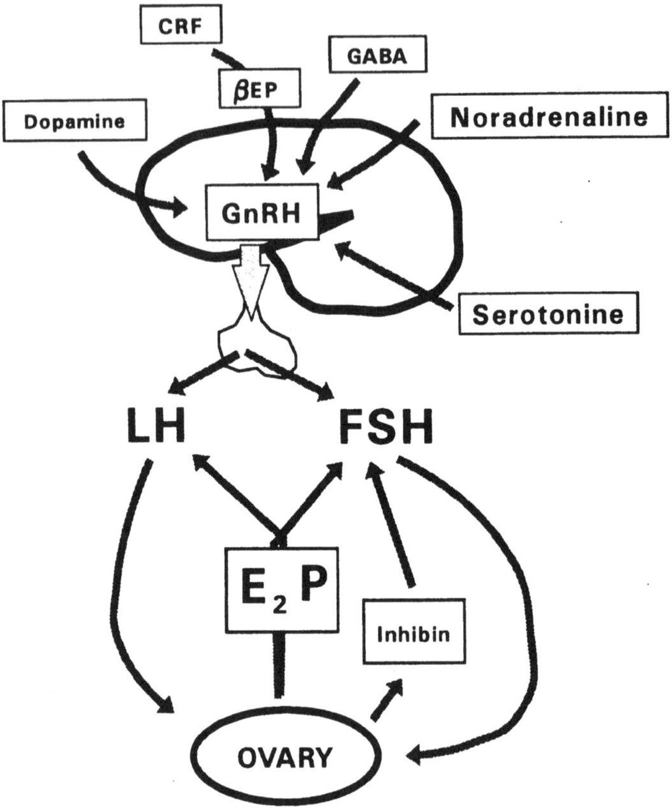

FIGURE 1. Schematic representation of the neuroendocrine modulation of GnRH release from the hypothalamus. The episodic GnRH discharge determines the pulsatile release of both gonadotropins from the pituitary. The ovary participates in the control of the hypothalamus–pituitary unit through the secretion of estradiol (E_2) and progesterone (P) as well as of inhibin.

connection *in vivo* of the MBH does not abolish gonadotropin secretion,[6] whereas the destruction of the arcuate nucleus leads to the complete suppression of GnRH release in monkeys.[6] This intrinsic secretory activity of GnRH-containing neurons has been investigated, and it has been demonstrated to be episodic in the human MBH[7] as well as in rat.[8] This suggests that the median eminence itself may represent the site of action of the neurotransmitters and neuropeptides controlling reproductive function.

Norepinephrine (NE) is the most important neurotransmitter stimulating the release of GnRH. The noradrenergic control seems to be mediated by the suppression of the inhibitory tone exerted by GABAergic interneurons on GnRH-secreting neurons.[9] In the rat the positive feedback on LH secretion by estrogens is mediated by the stimulation of the noradrenergic system.[9] In humans the role of NE in the control of gonadotropin secretion has not yet been clearly defined.

The role of dopamine (DA) on the control of gonadotropin secretion is also still controversial, since both a stimulatory[11,12] and an inhibitory[10,12] influence on GnRH release has been demonstrated. This may depend on the activation of two different dopaminergic pathways: one, located in the dorsal part of the MBH, seems to stimulate the GnRH pulse generator; the other, located in the arcuate nucleus, with axonal projections to the median eminence, the so-called tuberoinfundibular dopaminergic system (TIDA), has an inhibitory effect on the release of GnRH. In addition the existence of an interaction between DA and endogenous opioids in the control of GnRH secretion[14] is demonstrated by the observation that DA infusion inhibits the LH pulsatile release induced by naloxone, an opioid receptor antagonist.

Endogenous opioid peptides (EOPs) play an important role in the control of LH secretion by inhibiting the activity of the hypothalamic neurons releasing GnRH. Naloxone administration increases plasma LH levels in men and women.[15,16] This suggests that in humans EOPs tonically inhibit LH secretion, and their effect is dependent on the steroid hormone milieu. In fertile women, naloxone administration increases LH levels in the late-follicular and in the luteal phase but not in the early follicular phase.[18] The increase in LH is related to circulating estradiol levels.[18] The low frequency of LH pulsatile release during the luteal phase may be ascribed to the activity of EOPs and related to the high progesterone levels.[19] In the postmenopausal period, with the decrease of plasma estradiol levels, naloxone has no effect on LH release, whereas steroid hormone replacement therapy restores a normal response.[20] EOPs have also been suggested to be the key factors of stress inhibition of the hypothalamic–pituitary–gonadal axis. The stress-induced corticotropin-releasing factor (CRF) increase is responsible for the activation of central βEP activity and the decrease of LH secretion in the rat[21,22] and in humans. Recent data demonstrated the efficacy of chronic naltrexone administration in patients with hypothalamic amenorrhea associated with weight loss in restoring both a normal spontaneous episodic LH release and the occurrence of menstrual cyclicity.[23,24]

Many other neurotransmitters and neuropeptides are involved in the control of GnRH secretion. Serotonine and γ-aminobutyric acid (GABA) probably have an inhibitory effect, modulating the circadian rhythm of GnRH release. The action of other neuropeptides, such as neuropeptide Y, neurotensin, substance P, or vasoactive intestinal peptide (VIP), is controversial.

GONADOTROPIN SECRETORY PATTERN

At the beginning of puberty, gonadotropin secretion is selectively activated during sleep, and appreciable gonadotropin secretion can only be detected during the night.[25] Later on, pulsatile gonadotropin secretion extends into the daytime hours, and ovulatory menstrual cycles start shortly after. During the menstrual cyclicity, many differences can be observed in LH episodic secretion. In fact, during the follicular phase, LH pulses show increased frequency and reduced amplitude during the day[26,27] and a slowing of the LH pulse frequency during the night.[28] This last phenomenon is probably mediated by an increase of EOP activity.[28]

At the mid-cycle gonadotropin surge, LH pulses are increased both in frequency and amplitude. During the luteal phase, there is a reduction of LH pulse frequency, probably related to an increase of central opioidergic activity, since naloxone administration increases the frequency of LH peaks.[29] During the early luteal phase, the frequency of LH pulses decreases while the amplitude increases significantly.[26,27] In the follicular phase, each LH pulse is followed by an estradiol (E_2) pulse, with similar characteristics.[30] In the intermediate and the late luteal phase, the ovarian response to pulsatile LH release is represented by the secretion not only of E_2, but also of progesterone (P), whose pulses follow LH peaks.[30,31]

The rise of LH pulse frequency during the follicular phase is probably due to the increase in GnRH activity induced by the estrogenic milieu, whereas the fall of its amplitude may be related to the negative feedback of estrogens on GnRH and/or gonadotropins. The changes of LH pulse frequency and amplitude during the luteal phase are caused mainly by the action of P on the hypothalamic–pituitary system.[19] These effects of gonadal steroids on LH pulsatile secretion may be modulated by changes of the level of activity of EOPs on hypothalamic GnRH release.[32]

At any rate, both the inhibitory and stimulatory effects of sex hormones seem to be largely exerted on the pituitary gonadotrophs. The frequency of the hypothalamic pulse generator, as evidenced by LH pulse frequency, undergoes little changes as estrogens rise during the follicular phase. Furthermore, GnRH pulse frequency is essentially the same in monkeys and women, with or without ovarian function.[33]

FSH is also secreted in an episodic manner, and the finding that an excellent concordance exists between episodic LH and FSH secretion provides additional evidence for a role for GnRH in the physiological control of both gonadotropins.[5,34] FSH release appears to be modulated not only by hypothalamic GnRH, but also by ovarian inhibitory factors (estrogens, inhibin, and follistatin) as well as by pituitary factors acting in a paracrine and/or autocrine way (activin, growth factors). However, recent data demonstrated that other central modulators may control FSH episodic discharge independently from hypothalamic GnRH release in humans.[34]

THE OVARY AS A NEUROENDOCRINE ORGAN

Many ovarian factors are involved in the control of folliculogenesis. They may act both as hormones, modulating the release of gonadotropins (FSH particularly), and as paracrine or autocrine factors, modulating the follicular response to gonadotropins. This is the case with inhibin.

Inhibin is a glycoprotein composed of an α and a β subunit joined by disulfide bonds. It is present as two forms: inhibin A, made of an α and βA subunit, and inhibin B, made of an α and βB subunit. Inhibin has been isolated not only from gonads, but also from placenta, pituitary, adrenal, spleen, kidney, brain, and spinal cord.[35,36] In the ovary inhibin is mainly produced by granulosa and luteal cells. Pituitary is the target organ of inhibin because it inhibits the synthesis and release of FSH by gonadotrophs *in vitro.* Moreover, inhibin decreases gonadotrophic sensitivity to GnRH activity, and so decrease the GnRH-induced secretion of gonadotropins, probably by reducing the number of GnRH receptors.[37] *In vitro* studies have shown that both LH and FSH take part in the control of ovarian inhibin secretion,[38] but also paracrine factors seem to modulate the release of inhibin. GnRH and epidermal growth factor (EGF) inhibit the FSH-induced inhibin secretion, while VIP and insulin-like growth factor 1 (IGF-1) have a stimulatory action.[39] Plasma inhibin levels change throughout the menstrual cycle inversely to FSH levels.[40] It has been proposed that the secretion of inhibin is one of the mechanisms by which the dominant follicle suppresses the further development of the other selected follicles during the follicular phase. Plasma inhibin levels are very low in the follicular phase, but show a periovulatory increase, in parallel with the LH peak. Then they decrease and finally show another peak in the mid-luteal phase, in parallel with progesterone levels.[40] This confirms the production of inhibin by the corpus luteus during the luteal phase. Inhibin may play an important role in the suppression of FSH release during the luteal phase. On the contrary, the fall of plasma inhibin levels and the increase of FSH in the late luteal phase appear to be the signal for the beginning of the folliculogenetic mechanisms of the following cycle.

The physiological role of ovarian inhibin in the control of the hypothalamo–pituitary–gonadal axis *in vivo* is still controversial. However, the modulatory action of inhibin on pituitary FSH release seems to be an important mechanism by which the follicle may control its own development.

Other ovarian factors are involved in the control of FSH secretion. In particular, activin, a dimer of the inhibin β subunit, and follistatin, a glycoprotein isolated from follicular fluid in various molecular forms, appear to have a paracrin action, modulating FSH secretion, and also paracrine/autocrine effects at the ovarian level.[39]

Activin locally stimulates FSH release and increases the response of granulosa cells to FSH. As there is not yet clear evidence for a release of activin in blood, this substance may mainly play the role of a local growth factor. It has been proposed that the release of FSH is induced by pituitary activin. Follistatin, on the contrary, is present in blood in detectable quantities, and so may act as a hormone inhibiting pituitary FSH secretion.

All these ovarian factors, however, have also paracrine/autocrine effects. Inhibin and activin, for example, modulate ovarian production of progesterone and testosterone; inhibin, activin, and follistatin are also regulating factors of FSH-activated aromatase system.[39] CRF is another example of ovarian neuropeptide action on local steroidogenesis and follicular development. It is a stress factor that also has an ovarian source and is bioactive in different modulatory functions. In fact recent data demonstrated that proopiomelanocortin-related peptide (ACTH, βEP, βlipotropin) levels are present in the follicular fluid and that CRF and βEP concentrations change during the menstrual cycle with highest values during the preovulatory days.[40]

CONCLUSIONS

Although the hypothalamus, as an area of integration of central and peripheral signals, still plays a prominent role in the neuroendocrine control of the HPG axis through the release of GnRH, much evidence confirms that ovarian factors can influence the follicular development, acting locally, as paracrine or autocrine factors, or at the hypothalamic or pituitary level, modulating the release of gonadotropins. This suggests that the ovary may be considered "the biological clock" for differential regulation of the reproductive function.

REFERENCES

1. ANTUNES, J. L., P. W. CARMEL, E. M. HOUSEPIAN & M. FERIN. 1978. Luteinizing hormone-releasing hormone in human pituitary blood. J. Neurosurg. **49:** 382–386.
2. CLAYTON, R. N. & K. J. CATT. 1981. Gonadotropin-releasing hormone receptors: Characterization, physiological regulation, and relationship to reproductive function. Endocrinol. Rev. **2:** 186–209.
3. WILDT, L., A. HAUSLER, G. MARSHALL, J. S. HUTCHINSON, T. M. PLANT, P. E. BELCHETZ & E. KNOBIL. 1981. Frequency and amplitude of gonadotropin-releasing hormone stimulation and gonadotropin secretion in the rhesus monkey. Endocrinology **109:** 376–385.
4. CLARKE, I. J. & J. T. CUMMINS. 1982. The temporal relationship between gonadotropin-releasing hormone (GnRH) and luteinizing hormone (LH) secretion in ovariectomized ewes. Endocrinology **111:** 1737–1739.
5. GENAZZANI, A. D., F. PETRAGLIA, C. VOLPOGNI, G. D'AMBROGIO, F. FACCHINETTI & A. R. GENAZZANI. 1993. FSH secretory pattern and degree of concordance with LH in amenorroheic fertile and postmenopausal women. Am. J. Physiol. **264:** E776–E781.
6. KNOBIL, E. 1980. The neuroendocrine control of the menstrual cycle. Rec. Prog. Horm. Res. **16:** 53–88.
7. RASMUSSEN, D. D., M. GAMBACCIANI, W. SWARTZ, V. S. TUEROS & S. S. C. YEN. 1989. Pulsatile gonadotropin-releasing hormone release from the human mediobasal hypothalamus in vitro: Opiate receptor-mediated suppression. Neuroendocrinology **49:** 150–156.
8. RASMUSSEN, D. D. 1991. Pulsatile GnRH release from the male rat isolated median eminence in vitro. 73rd Annual Meeting of the Endocrine Society, San Antonio, TX, June 19–22 (Abstract 1020: 285).
9. LERANTH, C., N. J. MACLUSKY, M. SHANABROUGH & F. NAFTOLIN. 1988. Catecholaminergic innervation of luteinizing hormone-releasing hormone and glutamicacid decarboxylase immunopositive neurons in the rat medial preoptic area. Neuroendocrinology **48:** 591–594.
10. RAMIREZ, B. D., H. H. FEDER & C. H. SAWYER. 1984. The role of brain cathecolamines in the regulation of LH secretion: A critical inquiry. *In* Frontiers in Neuroendocrinology. L. Martini & W. F. Ganong, Eds.: 27–39. Raven Press. New York.
11. POHL, C. R. & E. KNOBIL. 1982. The role of the central nervous system in the control of the ovarian function in higher primates. Ann. Rev. Physiol. **44:** 583–593.
12. RASMUSSEN, D. D., L. H. LIU, P. L. WOLF & S. S. C. YEN. 1986. Gonadotropin-releasing hormone neurosecretion in the human hypothalamus: In vitro regulation by dopamine. J. Clin. Endocrinol. Metab. **62:** 479–483.
13. YEN, S. S. C. 1979. Studies of the role of dopamine in the control of prolactin secretion in humans. *In* Central Regulation of the Endocrine System. K. Fuxe, T. Hokfelt & R. Luft, Eds.: 387–398. Plenum Press. New York.
14. ROPERT, J. F., M. E. QUIGLEY & S. S. C. YEN. 1984. The dopaminergic inhibition of LH secretion during the menstrual cycle. Life Sci. **37:** 2067–2073.
15. ROPERT, J. F., M. E. QUIGLEY & S. S. C. YEN. 1981. Endogenous opiates modulate pulsatile luteinizing hormone release in humans. J. Clin. Endocrinol. Metab. **52:** 583–586.
16. PETRAGLIA, F., S. BERNASCONI, L. IUGHETTI, S. LOCHE, F. ROMANINI, F. FACCHINETTI, C. MARCELLINI & A. R. GENAZZANI. 1985. Naloxone-induced luteinizing hormone secretion in normal, precocious and delayed puberty. J. Clin. Endocrinol. Metab. **63:** 1112–1116.
17. BHANOT, R. & M. WILKINSON. 1983. Opiatergic control of gonadotropin secretion during puberty in the rat: A neurochemical basis for the hypothalamic "gonadostat"? Endocrinology **113:** 596–603.
18. QUIGLEY, M. E. & S. S. C. YEN. 1980. The role of endogenous opiates on LH secretion during the menstrual cycle. J. Clin. Endocrinol. Metab. **51:** 179–181.

19. FERIN, M., D. VAN VUGT & S. WARDLAW. 1984. The hypothalamic control of menstrual cycle and the role of endogenous opioid peptides. Rec. Prog. Horm. Res. **40:** 441–462.
20. PETRAGLIA, F., G. COMITINI, G. D'AMBROGIO, A. VOLPE, F. FACCHINETTI, G. ALESSANDRINI & A. R. GENAZZANI. 1985. Short-term effects of ovariectomy: The opioid control of LH secretion in fertile, climateric and postmenopausal women. J. Endocrinol. Invest. **8:** 325–329.
21. RIVIER, C., J. RIVIER & W. VALE. 1988. Stress-induced inhibition of reproductive functions: Role of endogenous corticotropin factor. Science **231:** 607–609.
22. PETRAGLIA, F., W. VALE & C. RIVIER. 1986. Opioids act centrally to modulate stress-induced decrease of luteinizing hormone in the rat. Endocrinology **119:** 2445–2450.
23. GENAZZANI, A. D., F. PETRAGLIA, M. GASTALDI, C. VOLPOGNI, O. GAMBA & A. R. GENAZZANI. 1995. Naltrexone treatment restores menstrual cycles in patients with weight loss-related amenorrhea. Fertil. Steril. **64:** 951–956.
24. GENAZZANI, A. D., M. GASTALDI, F. PETRAGLIA, C. BATTAGLIA, N. SURICO, A. VOLPE & A. R. GENAZZANI. 1997. Naltrexone administration modulates neuroendocrine control of LH secretion in hypotalamic amenorrhea. Hum. Reprod. In press.
25. BOYAR, R. M., J. W. FINKELSTEIN, H. P. ROFFWARG, S. KAPEN, E. D. WEITZMAN & L. HELLMAN. 1972. Synchronization of augmented luteinizing hormone secretion with sleep during puberty. N. Engl. J. Med. **287:** 582–587.
26. FILICORI, M., N. SANTORO, G. R. MERRIAM & W. F. CROWLEY. 1986. Characterization of the physiological pattern of episodic gonadotropin throughout the human menstrual cycle. J. Clin. Endocrinol. Metab. **62:** 1136–1144.
27. GENAZZANI, A. D., D. RODBARD, G. FORTI, F. PETRAGLIA, G. F. BARAGHINI & A. R. GENAZZANI. 1990. Estimation of instantaneous secretory rate of luteinizing hormone in women during the menstrual cycle and in men. Clin. Endocrinol. **32:** 573–581.
28. ROSSMANITH, W. G. & S. S. C. YEN. 1987. Sleep-associated decrease in luteinizing hormone pulse frequency during the early follicular phase of the menstrual cycle: Evidence for an opioidergic mechanism. J. Clin. Endocrinol. Metab. **65:** 715–720.
29. VAN VUGT, D. A., N. Y. LAM & M. FERIN. 1984. Reduced frequency of pulsatile luteinizing hormone secretion in the luteal phase of the rhesus monkey: Involvement of endogenous opiates. Endocrinology **115:** 1095–1101.
30. BACKSTROM, C. T., A. S. MCNEILLY, R. M. LEASK & D. T. BAIRD. 1982. Pulsatile secretion of LH, FSH, prolactin, estradiol and progesterone during the human menstrual cycle. Clin. Endocrinol. **17:** 29–42.
31. GENAZZANI, A. D., V. GOARDABASSO, F. PETRAGLIA & A. R. GENAZZANI. 1991. Specific concordance index defines the physiological lag between LH and progesterone in women during the midluteal phase of the menstrual cycle. Gynecol. Endocrinol. **5:** 175–184.
32. GENAZZANI, A. R., M. GASTALDI, B. BIDZINSKA, N. MERCURI, A. D. GENAZZANI, R. E. NAPPI, A. SEGRE & F. PETRAGLIA. 1992. The brain as a target organ of gonadal steroids. Neuroendocrinology **17:** 385–390.
33. YEN, S. S. C., C. C. TSAI, F. NAFTOLIN, G. VANDERGERG & L. AJOBAR. 1972. Pulsatile patterns of gonadotropin secretion in subjects with and without ovarian function. J. Clin. Endocrinol. Metab. **34:** 671–675.
34. GENAZZANI, A. D., F. PETRAGLIA, C. VOLPOGNI, O. GAMBA, F. MASSOLO & A. R. GENAZZANI. 1994. Evidence suggesting an additional mechanism regulating LH and FSH episodic secretion in prepuberal and in postmenopausal women. Hum. Reprod. **9:** 1807–1812.
35. MEUNIER, H., C. RIVIER, R. M. EVANS & W. VALE. 1988. Gonadal and extragonadal expression of inhibin α, βA and βB subunits in various tissues predicts diverse functions. Proc. Natl. Acad. Sci. USA **85:** 247–251.
36. PETRAGLIA, F., P. SAWECHENKO, A. T. W. LIM, J. RIVIER & W. VALE. 1987. Localization, secretion and action of inhibin in human placenta. Science **237:** 187–189.

37. Culler, M. D. & A. Negro-Vilar. 1989. Endogenous inhibin suppresses only basal follicle-stimulating hormone secretion but suppresses all parameters of pulsatile luteinizing hormone secretion in diestrous female rat. Endocrinology **124:** 2944–2948.
38. Woodruff, T. K. & K. E. Mayo. 1990. Regulation of inhibin synthesis in the rat ovary. Ann. Rev. Physiol. **52:** 807–821.
39. Ying, H. Y. 1988. Inhibins, activins, and follistatins: Gonadal proteins modulating the secretion of follicle-stimulating hormone. Endocrinol. Rev. **9:** 267–293.
40. MacLachlan, R. I., D. M. Robertson, D. L. Healy, H. G. Burger & D. M. de Kretser. 1987. Circulating immunoreactive inhibin levels during the normal human menstrual cycle. J. Clin. Endocrinol. Metab. **65:** 954–961.
41. Petraglia, F., G. Di Meo, R. Storchi, A. Segre, F. Facchinetti, S. Szalay, A. Volpe & A. R. Genazzani. 1987. Prooppiomelanocortin-related peptides and methionine eukephalin in human follicular fluid: Changes during the menstrual cycle. Am. J. Obstet. Gynecol. **157:** 142–146.

Luteal Function—Luteolysis

I. E. MESSINIS

Department of Obstetrics and Gynecology
University of Ioannina
45332 Ioannina, Greece

INTRODUCTION

The corpus luteum is formed from the remnants of the ruptured preovulatory follicle under the action of the midcycle luteinizing hormone (LH) surge. The principal function of the corpus luteum is the secretion of progesterone, which is required for the preparation of the endometrium in order to support the pregnancy. The latter is achieved through the production of chorionic gonadotrophin (CG) from the implanting embryo that maintains intact the integrity and the secretory capacity of the corpus luteum beyond the time of the missed menstrual period. Although the mechanisms of the formation of the corpus luteum and the support of its functional capacity are well understood, the factors that are responsible for the demise of the human corpus luteum are not clear, and information is mainly derived from studies in primates and other animals.

FORMATION OF THE CORPUS LUTEUM

Before the rupture of the preovulatory follicle under the effect of increasing secretion of pituitary gonadotrophins during the endogenous LH surge, several morphological and biochemical changes take place in the cells of the theca interna and the granulosa cells, a process called luteinization.[1] The main change is hypertrophy of the granulosa cells, which become vacuolated by the accumulation within them of a yellow pigment termed lutein (large luteal cells). After ovulation the basement membrane breaks down, and vascularization occurs by blood vessels that originate from the theca interna and invade the cavity of the ruptured follicle. This is achieved through the effect of an angiogenic factor. In addition to these changes, the cells of the theca interna differentiate into luteal cells (small luteal cells) participating thus in the secretion of luteal hormones. The transformation of the granulosa cells into luteal cells is induced by LH. Receptors of this hormone are located on the membrane of the granulosa cells. During luteinization an increase in the amount of smooth endoplasmic reticulum and the number of mitochondria with lipid droplets takes place, while gap junctions develop between the luteal cells. There are distinct differences in the structure of large and small luteal cells. Apart from the different size, large cells contain numerous mitochondria and abundant endoplasmic reticulum, and the Golgi complex is more pronounced in the large than in the small cells.[2,3]

The receptors of LH in the corpus luteum originate from those in the maturing follicle during the preceding follicular phase. The number of these receptors on the granulosa cells increases dramatically as the follicle grows under the synergistic action of estrogen and FSH.[4] The increasing sensitivity of the preovulatory follicle to LH is important for successful luteinization and normal function of the corpus luteum. In rats, prolactin is also a luteotropic hormone, acting to maintain the normal number of LH receptors in the corpus luteum.

REGULATION OF PROGESTERONE SECRETION

Progesterone is the main steroid product of the corpus luteum. The primary substrate for its synthesis is low-density lipoprotein bound to cholesterol, which is the only form of cholesterol carrier that can enter the luteal cells in any significant quantity by binding to specific receptors. Midcycle LH surge is responsible for the induction of these receptors on the granulosa cells.[5] Within the mitochondria cholesterol is converted to pregnenolone under the effect of LH and via cytochrome P-450.[6] The amount of P-450c17 mRNA is very small in luteinized granulosa cells recovered from patients undergoing *in vitro* fertilization treatment, but increases dramatically under the influence of LH at midcycle along with the expression of the enzyme 3β-hydroxysteroid dehydrogenase.[7] Large and small luteal cells respond to LH or hCG during the early luteal phase in monkeys, although from the midluteal phase only the large cells respond.[8] In general, large cells produce more progesterone than small cells.[9]

It has become clear that circulating LH during the luteal phase, although in low levels, is the single most important luteotropic factor involved in the control of secretion of progesterone regardless of species. For example, in ewes hypophysectomy on the day of ovulation prevents formation of the corpus luteum, while administration of CG restores progesterone levels.[10] In hypophysectomized women treated with gonadotrophins for ovulation induction, normal luteal function occurred after the administration of a single dose of hCG, but not LH, which has a shorter half-life than hCG.[11] Administration of GnRH antagonists to monkeys and women at various stages during the luteal phase induced sustained reductions in progesterone levels and the corpus luteum life span.[12–14] However, hCG in sufficient amounts was able to prevent luteolysis in women induced by a GnRH antagonist even if it was given 72 hours after the administration of the antagonist.[15] Evidence that LH plays a significant role in the support of corpus luteum has been also provided by studies in rhesus monkeys bearing hypothalamic lesions to eliminate endogenous LH secretion and subsequently treated with the pulsatile administration of GnRH.[16] The amount of LH secreted during the midcycle LH surge is also important for the induction of luteinization and normal luteal function. In women undergoing superovulation induction with human menopausal gonadotrophins without the use of a GnRH agonist, the endogenous LH surge is markedly attenuated, and basal LH levels during the luteal phase are significantly reduced.[17,18] In these patients the luteal phase is also shortened, and serum progesterone concentrations significantly reduced. Experiments in rats have shown that although luteinization can be induced even with an LH surge of only 5% of the normal size, follicle rupture and therefore normal luteal function require a threshold greater than 85% of the surge.[19]

In contrast to LH, FSH is not a luteotropic hormone. Data related to the *in vivo* and *in vitro* effects of FSH on steroidogenesis in the human corpus luteum are conflicting. One study has shown an increase in serum estradiol but not progesterone levels following the administration of FSH to women in the early and midluteal phase and aromatization of androgen to estrogen *in vitro* only in large cells,[20] while another study did not show any effect.[21] A more recent study has shown that human corpus luteum during the midluteal phase of spontaneous cycles responds to hCG but not to FSH.[22] In particular, administration of hCG resulted in a significant increase in serum progesterone, estradiol, and inhibin concentrations, whereas administration of FSH resulted in an increase in serum estradiol and inhibin, but not progesterone concentrations. These results suggest that the increase in estradiol and inhibin levels during treatment with FSH in the luteal phase is derived from the stimulation of small antral follicles rather than the corpus luteum. Therefore, a role for FSH in the control of luteal function is restricted to the follicular phase during the recruitment and selection of the dominant follicle and stimulation of its growth to the preovulatory stage. When FSH levels are suppressed during the follicular phase, preovulatory estradiol and midluteal progesterone values are depressed with a decrease in luteal cell mass.[23]

In women, the secretion of progesterone during the midluteal phase of the cycle is episodic. The progesterone pulses are concomitant with the estradiol pulses and temporally related to LH pulses, although some degree of corpus luteum autonomy has been observed.[24] The effect of progesterone during the luteal phase is mainly exerted on the already estrogen-primed endometrium. Progesterone, however, through a negative-feedback mechanism, in which estradiol and inhibin also participate, suppresses FSH secretion and prevents follicle development during the luteal phase.

The corpus luteum, apart from estradiol and progesterone, secretes nonsteroidal substances such as inhibin. The latter is produced by the luteinized granulosa cells under the influence of LH.[25] The levels of inhibin during the luteal phase increase in a pattern similar to that of progesterone, reaching a peak during the midluteal phase and declining towards the end of the luteal phase. The importance of inhibin during the luteal phase of the cycle is not clear. Other substances secreted from the corpus luteum include relaxin, the synthesis of which is stimulated by hCG and oxytocin.[26,27] These substances are mainly secreted by large luteal cells.[9] The concentrations of oxytocin show an increase from the early to midluteal phase and a decline in the late luteal phase.[28] The role of these substances in ovarian physiology has not been fully clarified, although a paracrine action within the ovary is possible.[9]

LUTEOLYSIS

The normal duration of the luteal phase varies from 11 to 17 days.[29] The mechanism, however, of corpus luteum degeneration remains unclear. Although corpus luteum function is LH dependent, the declining LH levels, particularly from the midluteal phase, may not be the only factor responsible for its demise. It has been reported that the number of LH receptors decreases markedly in the late luteal phase of the cycle.[30] However, studies in various animals have shown that the corpus luteum degenerates as a result of the action of various luteolytic factors.

Prostaglandin F2α (PGF2α) produced by the uterus at the end of the cycle serves as the main luteolytic factor in several animals, including sheep, pig, and cow, since hysterectomy prolongs the lifespan of the corpus luteum.[31] In women and monkeys, the uterus does not play any role in luteolysis, since hysterectomy does not affect the duration of the luteal phase.[32,33] This, however, does not exclude the possibility that PGE2a is luteolytic in these species, since a shortening of the luteal phase occurred in women after the direct injection of 500–1000 μg PGF2α into the corpus luteum.[34] The corpus luteum is more sensitive to the luteolytic effect of PGF2α during the late luteal phase.

Another potential luteolytic factor is estrogen. Injection of estradiol into the ovary containing the corpus luteum induced premature luteal regression in both women and monkeys.[35,36] However, in monkeys injection of estradiol into the corpus luteum only produces luteolysis when the secretion of LH is also suppressed.[37] Exogenous administration of estrogen to women during the luteal phase results in decreased progesterone secretion and shortens the luteal phase.[38] In women superovulated with human gonadotropins for *in vitro* fertilization, an inverse relationship between estrogen levels during the follicular and the luteal phase and the length of the luteal phase or the midluteal progesterone levels has been found.[39] In a study, however, in which serum estradiol levels increased markedly during the early luteal phase after the exogenous administration to normal women of a high dose of estrogen during the midcycle LH surge, luteal-phase LH and progesterone concentrations and the duration of the luteal phase were not affected.[18] It is suggested, therefore, that in women either estradiol is luteolytic at its site of ovarian production or in spontaneous cycles the newly formed corpus luteum is refractory to the luteolytic effect of high estradiol concentrations. If estradiol is luteolytic it possibly acts through the production of PGF2α.[40]

A possible role for other intraovarian substances such as LH-releasing hormone, relaxin, and oxytocin in the induction of luteolysis has not been clarified. Oxytocin from the ovary is stimulated by the injection of PGF2α.[41] Low doses of oxytocin added in dispersed human luteal cells *in vitro* stimulate, while high doses inhibit, both the basal and hCG-stimulated production of progesterone.[42] Oxytocin and PGF2α may act synergistically to induce luteolysis.[40] A recent study has shown that progesterone itself may exert an autocrine effect within the ovary, thus regulating the corpus luteum in primates.[43] Also, activin-A significantly decreased basal and hCG-induced progesterone production from small, but not large, luteal cells of human corpora lutea.[44] This suggests the potential involvement of various ovarian products in the maintenance of the integrity of the corpus luteum. Because mRNA levels of the enzyme's cholesterol side-chain cleavage and 3β-hydroxysteroid dehydrogenase are maximal at ovulation, it is possible that the life span of the corpus luteum is established at that time.[45] Therefore, the corpus luteum is destined to regress unless rescued by the hCG of pregnancy.

CONCLUSIONS

The corpus luteum is formed from the ruptured preovulatory follicle under the influence of the midcycle LH surge. Various morphological changes occur in the ruptured follicle that will enable the newly formed corpus luteum to produce and secrete progesterone as well as various steroidal and nonsteroidal substances. Normal follicular development is a prerequisite for optimal luteal function during the normal menstrual cycle. Although FSH is the primary signal for normal folliculogenesis, LH is the single most important luteotropic factor. Progesterone secretion is episodic, and the pulses are temporaly related to those of estradiol and LH. The corpus luteum also secretes nonsteroidal hormones, such as inhibin, which may contribute to the negative feedback effect of progesterone and estradiol on the hypothalamic–pituitary system. The life span of the corpus luteum is probably established at the time of ovulation. Luteolysis is a normal process that occurs in the late luteal phase unless the corpus luteum is rescued by the hCG of pregnancy. The precise mechanism of corpus luteum regression in women is still unclear, although several substances, such as PGF2α and estradiol have been considered as potential luteolytic factors.

REFERENCES

1. Niswender, G. D. & T. M. Nett. 1988. The corpus luteum and its control. *In* The Physiology of Reproduction. E. Knobil & J. D. Neill, Eds. Vol. **1:** 489–525. Raven Press. New York.
2. Enders, A. C. 1973. Cytology of the corpus luteum. Biol. Reprod. **8:** 158–182.
3. O'Shea, J. D., D. G. Cran & M. F. Hay. 1980. Fate of the theca interna following ovulation in the ewe. Cell Tissue Res. **210:** 305–319.
4. Richards, J. S., J. J. Ireland, M. C. Rao, G. A. Bernatii, A. R. Midgely, Jr. & L. E. Reichert, Jr. 1976. Ovarian follicular development in the rat: Hormone receptor regulation by estradiol, follicle stimulating hormone and luteinizing hormone. Endocrinology **99:** 1562–1570.
5. Golos, T. G., E. A. Soto, R. W. Tureck & J. F. Strauss, III. 1985. Human chorionic gonadotropin and 8-bromoadenosine 3′,5′-monophosphate stimulate {125J} low-density lipoprotein uptake and metabolism by luteinized human granulosa cells in culture. J. Clin. Endocrinol. Metab. **61:** 633–638.
6. Marsh, J. M. 1976. The role of cyclic AMP in gonadal steroidogenesis. Biol. Reprod. **14:** 30–53.
7. Ravindranath, N., L. Little-Ihrig, D. F. Benyo & A. J. Zeleznik. 1992. Role of luteinizing hormone in the expression of cholesterol side-chain cleavage cytochrome P450 and 3β-hydroxysteroid dehydrogenase Δ5-4 isomerase messenger ribonucleic acids in the primate corpus luteum. Endocrinology **131:** 2065–2072.
8. Brannian, J. D. & R. L. Stouffer. 1991. Cellular approaches to understanding the function and regulation of the primate corpus luteum. Sem. Reprod. Endocrinol. **9:** 341–351.
9. Mass, S., H. Jarry, A. Teichmann, W. Rath, W. Kuhn & W. Wuttke. 1992. Paracrine actions of oxytocin, prostaglandin F2α and estradiol within the human corpus luteum. J. Clin. Endocrinol. Metab. **74:** 306–312.
10. Hixon, J. E. & M. T. Clegg. 1969. Influence of the pituitary on ovarian progesterone output in the ewe: Effects of hypophysectomy and gonadotropic hormones. Endocrinology **84:** 828–834.
11. Van de Wiele, R. L., J. Bogumil, I. Dyrenfurth, M. Ferin, R. Jewelewicz, M. Warren, T. Rizkallach & G. Mikhail. 1970. Mechanisms regulating the menstrual cycle in women. Rec. Prog. Horm. Res. **26:** 63–103.
12. Fraser, H. M., M. Abbott, N. C. Laird, A. S. McNeilly, J. J. Nestor, Jr. & B. H. Vickery. 1986. Effects of an LH-releasing hormone antagonist on the secretion of LH, FSH, prolactin and ovarian steroids at different stages of the luteal phase in the stumptailed macaque (*Macaca arctoides*). J. Endocrinol. **111:** 83–90.

13. Fraser, H. M., J. J. Nestor, Jr. & B. H. Vickery. 1987. Suppression of luteal function by a luteinizing hormone-releasing hormone antagonist during the early luteal phase in the stumptailed macaque monkey and the effects of subsequent administration of human chorionic gonadotropin. Endocrinology **121:** 612–618.
14. Mais, V., R. R. Kazer, N. S. Cetel, J. Rivier, W. Vale & S. S. C. Yen. 1986. The dependency of folliculogenesis and corpus luteum function on pulsatile gonadotropin secretion in cycling women using a gonadotropin-releasing hormone antagonist as a probe. J. Clin. Endocrinol. Metab. **62:** 1250–1255.
15. Dubourdieu, S., B. Charbonnel, M. R. Massai, J. Marraoui, I. Spitz & P. Bouchard. 1991. Suppression of corpus luteum function by the gonadotropin-releasing hormone antagonist Nal-Glu: Effect on the dose and timing of human chorionic gonadotropin administration. Fertil. Steril. **56:** 440–446.
16. Hutchison, J. S. & A. Z. Zeleznik. 1985. The corpus luteum of the primate menstrual cycle is capable of recovering from a transient withdrawal of pituitary gonadotropin support. Endocrinology **117:** 1043–1049.
17. Messinis, I. E., A. Templeton & D. T. Baird. 1985. Endogenous luteinizing hormone surge during superovulation induction with sequential use of clomiphene citrate and pulsatile human menopausal gonadotropin. J. Clin. Endocrinol. Metab. **61:** 1076–1080.
18. Messinis, I. E. & A. A. Templeton. 1987. Disparate effects of endogenous and exogenous oestradiol on luteal phase function in women. J. Reprod. Fertil. **79:** 549–554.
19. Peluso, J. J. 1990. Role of the amplitude of the gonadotropin surge in the rat. Fertil. Steril. **53:** 150–154.
20. Ohara, A., T. Shunzo & T. Mori. 1989. Stimulatory effects of purified human follicle-stimulating hormone on estradiol production in the human luteal phase. J. Clin. Endocrinol. Metab. **68:** 359–363.
21. Devoto, L., M. Vega, V. Navarro, T. Sir, F. Alba & O. Castro. 1989. Regulation of steroid hormone synthesis by human corpora lutea: Failure of follicle-stimulating hormone to support steroidogenesis in vivo and in vitro. Fertil. Steril. **51:** 628–633.
22. Messinis, I. E., D. Lolis, K. Zikopoulos, S. Milingos, G. Kollios, K. Seferiadis & A. A. Templeton. 1997. Effect of follicle stimulating hormone or human chorionic gonadotrophin treatment on the production of gonadotrophin surge attenuating factor (GnSAF) during the luteal phase of the human menstrual cycle. Clin. Endocrinol. **44:** 169–175.
23. Smith, S. K., E. A. Lenton & I. D. Cooke. 1985. Plasma gonadotrophin and ovarian steroid concentrations in women with menstrual cycles with short luteal phase. J. Reprod. Fertil. **75:** 363–368.
24. Rossmanith, W. G., G. A. Laughlin, J. F. Mortola, M. L. Johnson, J. D. Veldhuis & S. S. C. Yen. 1990. Pulsatile cosecretion of estradiol and progesterone by the midluteal phase corpus luteum: Temporal link to luteinizing hormone pulses. J. Clin. Endocrinol. Metab. **70:** 990–995.
25. McLachlan, R. I., N. L. Cohen, W. E. Vale, J. E. Rivier, H. G. Burger, W. J. Bremmer & M. R. Soules. 1989. The importance of luteinizing hormone in the control of inhibin and progesterone secretion by the human corpus luteum. J. Clin. Endocrinol. Metab. **68:** 1078–1085.
26. Quagliarello, J., L. Smith, B. Steinetz & G. Weiss. 1980. Induction of relaxin secretion in non-pregnant women by human chorionic gonadotropin. J. Clin. Endocrinol. Metab. **51:** 74–77.
27. Wathes, D. C. & R. Swann. 1982. Is oxytocin an ovarian hormone? Nature **297:** 225–227.
28. Dawood, M. Y. & F. S. Khan Dawood. 1986. Human ovarian oxytocin: Its source and relationship to steroid hormones. Am. J. Obstet. Gynecol. **154:** 756–763.
29. Lenton, E. A., B. Landgren & L. Sexton. 1984. Normal variation in the length of the

luteal phase of the menstrual cycle: Identification of the short luteal phase. Br. J. Obstet. Gynaecol. **91:** 685–689.

30. McNeilly, A. S., J. Kerin, I. A. Swanston, T. A. Bramley & D. T. Baird. 1980. Changes in the binding of human chorionic gonadotrophin/luteinizing hormone, follicle stimulating hormone and prolactin to human corpus luteum during the menstrual cycle and pregnancy. J. Endocrinol. **87:** 315–325.
31. Baird, D. T. 1985. Control of luteolysis. *In* The Luteal Phase. S. L. Jeffcoate, Ed.: 25–42. John Wiley. Chichester, England.
32. Beling, C. G., S. L. Marcus & S. M. Markham. 1970. Functional activity of the corpus luteum following hysterectomy. J. Clin. Endocrinol. Metab. **30:** 30–39.
33. Knobil, E. 1973. On the regulation of the primate corpus luteum. Biol. Reprod. **8:** 246–258.
34. Korda, A. R., D. A. Shutt, I. D. Smith, R. P. Shearman & R. C. Lyneham. 1975. Assessment of possible luteolytic effect of intraovarian injection of prostaglandin F2α in the human. Prostaglandins **9:** 443–449.
35. Hoffmann, F. 1960. Untersuchunger uber die hormonale beeinflussung der levensdauer des corpus luteum in zyklus der frau. Gebur. Frauen. **20:** 1153–1159.
36. Karsch, F. J. & G. P. Sutton. 1976. An intraovarian site for the luteolytic action of estrogen in the rhesus monkey. Endocrinology **98:** 553–561.
37. Schoonmaker, J. N., K. S. Bergman, R. A. Steiner & F. J. Karsch. 1982. Estradiol induced luteal regression in the rhesus monkey: Evidence for an extra-ovarian site of action. Endocrinology **110:** 1708–1715.
38. Johansson, E. D. B. & C. Gemzell. 1971. Plasma levels of progesterone during the luteal phase in normal women treated with synthetic oestrogens (RS 2874, F 6103 and ethinyl oestradiol). Acta Endocrinol. **68:** 551–560.
39. Messinis, I. E., A. Templeton & D. T. Baird. 1987. Luteal phase after ovarian hyperstimulation. Br. J. Obstet. Gynaecol. **94:** 345–350.
40. Auletta, F. J. & A. P. F. Flint. 1988. Mechanisms controlling corpus luteum function in sheep, cows, nonhuman primates and women especially in relation to the time of luteolysis. Endocrinol. Rev. **9:** 88–105.
41. Sheldrick, E. L., M. D. Mitchell & A. P. F. Flint. 1980. Delayed luteal regression in ewes immunized against oxytocin. J. Reprod. Fertil. **59:** 37–42.
42. Tan, G. J. S., R. Tweedale & J. S. G. Biggs. 1982. Oxytocin may play a role in the control of human corpus luteum. J. Endocrinol. **95:** 65–70.
43. Duffy, D. M., D. L. Hess & R. L. Stouffer. 1994. Acute administration of a 3β-hydroxysteroid dehydrogenase inhibitor to rhesus monkeys at the midluteal phase of the menstrual cycle: Evidence for possible autocrine regulation of the primate corpus luteum by progesterone. J. Clin. Endocrinol. Metab. **79:** 1587–1594.
44. Di Simone, N., A. Lanzone, F. Petraglia, E. Ronsivalle, A. Caruso & S. Mancuso. 1994. Effect of activin-A on progesterone synthesis in human luteal cells. Fertil. Steril. **62:** 1157–1161.
45. Bassett, S. G., L. L. Little-Ihrig, J. I. Mason & A. J. Zeleznik. 1991. Expression of messenger ribonucleic acids that encode for 3β-hydroxysteroid dehydrogenase and cholesterol side-chain cleavage enzyme throughout the luteal phase of the Macaque menstrual cycle. J. Clin. Endocrinol. Metab. **72:** 362–366.

Dysfunctional Uterine Bleeding

E. DELIGEOROGLOU[a]

Division of Pediatric and Adolescent Gynecology
1st Department of Obstetrics and Gynecology
University of Athens
"Alexandra" Maternity Hospital
Athens, Greece

INTRODUCTION

Dysfunctional uterine bleeding (DUB), defined as "abnormal uterine bleeding in the absence of organic cause," is the most frequent urgent gynecological problem of the adolescent. Organic etiologies of DUB include coagulation defects, pathology involving the reproductive tract, infections, systemic diseases, trauma, and iatrogenic causes. DUB is a diagnosis of exclusion,[1] and thus systemic disease and local lesions must be ruled out first. It is usually secondary to anovulation. In the perimenarcheal adolescent, DUB is the result of an immature hypothalamic–pituitary–ovarian axis.[2] For this reason it is essential to discuss briefly the normal menstrual cycle in order to understand the pathophysiology of dysfunctional uterine bleeding.

NORMAL MENSTRUAL CYCLE

Normal menstrual cycles have been defined as a mean interval of 28 days (±7 days), with a duration of 4 days (±2 to 3 days), and menstrual flow of approximately 30 ml per cycle, with an upper limit of normal at 60–80 ml.[3,4] Any aberration from this normal pattern is considered to be abnormal. For normal cycles to occur, certain conditions must be present: (1) an intact hypothalamic–pituitary system, (2) a normal ovary with normal follicular components, and (3) a normal endometrium, capable of responding to ovarian steroids.

The normal menstrual cycle also depends on an intact internal hormonal milieu. The thyroid and adrenal functions should also be intact, because their aberrations exert deleterious effects on the hypothalamic–pituitary–gonadotropin system.

In addition, weight problems, drugs, and exercise will also affect this system leading to anovulatory cycles.

ABNORMAL MENSTRUAL CYCLE DUE TO DUB: ETIOLOGY

Bleeding that occurs at an interval of 21 days or less for longer than 7 days and greater than 80 ml is considered abnormal.[5] DUB is commonly seen in the adoles-

[a]Address for correspondence: E. Deligeoroglou, M.D., 48, Marathonos Street, 152 35 Vrilissia, Athens, Greece.

cent, and in about 95% of cases it is caused by the slow maturation of the H-P-O axis.

Anovulation is the most frequent cause of abnormal uterine bleeding in this period of life, but other possible causes should be excluded before that diagnosis is established.

Other Causes

Pregnancy complications: The possibility of pregnancy should be considered in any adolescent with abnormal uterine bleeding. A patient having a threatened abortion, an incomplete abortion, or an ectopic pregnancy may present with irregular menstrual periods. Subinvolution of the placental implantation site, retained gestational products, or trophoblastic disease may also result in abnormal uterine bleeding.

Coagulation disorders: Blood loss in a normal menstrual period is self-limited due to the action of platelets and fibrin. Thus, individuals with thrombocytopenia or coagulation deficiencies may have problems with excessive menstrual bleeding. Claessens and Cowell found that 19% of adolescents with menorrhagia requiring hospital admission had a coagulation disorder.[6] Of those who presented with severe blood loss during their first menstrual period, 45% had coagulation disorders. Idiopathic thrombocytopenic purpura (ITP), von Willebrand's disease, Glanzmann's disease (defective platelets), leukemia, and other disorders associated with thrombocytopenia or clotting factor deficiencies can be associated with menorrhagia.

Pathologic conditions involving the reproductive tract: Abnormal bleeding may result from trauma, infection, or neoplasia at any site in the female reproductive tract. Vaginitis, vaginal trauma, a foreign body, or a vaginal neoplasm may cause bleeding that may be assumed by the patient to be irregular menstrual bleeding. Trauma to a vaginal septum may also cause bleeding. Cervical inflammation, erosion, polyps, or neoplasia may similarly present with vaginal bleeding.

Uterine pathology may be responsible for abnormal bleeding. Endometritis, endometrial polyps, submucosal leiomyomata, arteriovenous malformations, and uterine malignancies are potential causes of abnormal uterine bleeding, but these are uncommon in the adolescent age group. Congenital anomalies such as partially obstructed duplications of the mullerian tract may give rise to intermenstrual bleeding.

Endometriosis, the presence of endometrial-like tissue at sites outside the uterus, is most often considered when a patient complains of dysmenorrhea or pelvic pain, but irregular bleeding is a symptom reported in 28–36% of adolescents with endometriosis.[7] Perimenstrual spotting is particularly common.

Systemic diseases: Chronic illness such as hepatic failure, renal failure, or malignancy may also result in abnormal uterine bleeding. However, chronic diseases are, fortunately, rare in adolescents. Patients with liver disease may have deficiencies of the vitamin K-dependent clotting factors (II, VII, IX, X) or of other clotting factors, including fibrinogen and plasminogen.[8] Liver disease may also result in abnormal estrogen metabolism, which may cause endometrial proliferation and estrogen breakthrough bleeding. Renal failure is commonly associated with abnormal bleeding, since most women with chronic renal failure have irregular menses or amenorrhea.[9]

Hyperprolactinemia due to decreased renal clearance of prolactin may contribute to the amenorrhea in some of these patients, but abnormal bleeding also occurs in renal patients with normal prolactin levels. Leukemia and other malignancies may be associated with abnormal uterine bleeding due to thrombocytopenia or decreased fibrinogen levels.

Other endocrine disorders: Other ovarian causes of anovulatory bleeding include abnormal corpus luteum function, steroid-secreting ovarian neoplasms, and impending premature ovarian failure. Adrenal disorders and thyroid abnormalities can also present with abnormal uterine bleeding. Congenital adrenal hyperplasia, Cushing's disease,[10] adrenal insufficiency, and adrenal neoplasia may lead to anovulatory cycles. Hypothyroidism is often associated with menorrhagia.

Iatrogenic causes: Hormonal medications, anticoagulants, neuroleptics, and intrauterine contraceptive devices can all be causes of abnormal uterine bleeding.

PATHOPHYSIOLOGY OF DYSFUNCTIONAL UTERINE BLEEDING

The completion of pubertal changes together with the maturation process of the hypothalamic pituitary system result in menarche. However, it has been found that menstrual cycles following menarche are irregular for a period of 1 to 3 years. This irregularity presents as oligomenorrhea and occasionally as dysfunctional uterine bleeding. This phenomenon is due to the lack of ovulation at this stage, probably due to the lack of positive feedback response by the hypothalamic pituitary system. With the development of that system later on, ovulation occurs, and cycles become regular. However, it seems that this system is very labile and unstable in teenaged girls.[11] Factors such as stress, drugs, and heavy exercise could eventually shut off this system and result in anovulatory cycles. This is why dysfunctional uterine bleeding is common in teenaged girls. In most of these cases there is no ovulation.[12] Lack of ovulation will lead to unopposed estrogen effect on the endometrium. Estrogens, which are produced by the follicles in the ovary and also to a certain extent by extragonadal aromatization of precursors such as androstenedione, will lead to proliferative changes of the endometrium. Endometrial hyperplasia may also be seen. Since the mechanism of ovulation is not fulfilled, the growing follicles will undergo atresia leading to fluctuations in the circulating estrogen levels. Consequently, interruption of the endometrial growth process occurs, resulting in bleeding episodes.[13] The severity of endometrial shedding depends on the amount of the preceding endometrial proliferation. Sampling of this endometrium will show the proliferative process of the endometrium and the lack of any progestational effect.

The imbalance of prostaglandins has also been implicated in the pathophysiology of dysfunctional uterine bleeding. The endometrium is known to synthesize $PGF_{2\alpha}$ and PGE_2. These PGs and their precursors[14] appear to accumulate in the endometrium at about the time of menstruation.[15] An increase in $PGF_{2\alpha}$ and PGE_2 has also been noted at sites with ischemia and necrosis, which is greater in the former (i.e., predominance of vasoconstrictor PGs).[16]

Alterations in the ratio of $PGF_{2\alpha}$ (vasoconstrictor) and PGE_2 (vasodilator) are noted in both anovulatory and ovulatory DUB. In those anovulatory patients, there appears to be decreased availability of arachidonic acid, the precursor for PG synthesis.[17] The $PGF_{2\alpha}/PGE_2$ ratio is also decreased, giving a predominance of vasodilator PG. There is an inverse correlation between the ratio of the endogenous $PGF_{2\alpha}$ to PGE_2 and menstrual blood loss.[16,17] Those patients with ovulatory DUB have an increased bioavailability of arachidonic acid that alters the PG ratios. It has been suggested that the increase of arachidonic acid saturates the $PGF_{2\alpha}$ pathway, thus increasing PGE_2 (and PGI_2) formation. Consequently, the vasoconstrictor to vasodilator ratio lowers due to the action of vasodilating PGs. Interestingly, DUB patients have been shown to have higher PGE_2 receptor concentration.[18,19]

EVALUATION

The initial goal in the diagnostic approach of abnormal uterine bleeding in adolescence is to locate the origin of the bleeding and to rule out organic causes.

1. The first step is to obtain a thorough history from the patient. This should include menstrual history, the severity of the bleeding and the presence of pain, fever, or other associated factors.
2. Family history may suggest the diagnosis of a bleeding disorder such as von Willebrand's disease. A review of systems should include questions regarding pregnancy symptoms, easy bruisability or abnormal bleeding, history of trauma, weight gain or loss, headaches, or central nervous system symptoms.
3. Physical examination should determine the source of bleeding (uterine or elsewhere), as well as the presence or absence of reproductive tract pathology. The patient should also be examined for signs of pregnancy, hyperandrogenism, galactorrhea, thyroid abnormalities, and systemic illnesses.
4. Laboratory studies generally include complete blood count, serum βHCG, coagulation profile, screening of the thyroid function, and serum prolactin. Patients with hirsutism should be evaluated to define the source of the androgen excess, and they should be treated accordingly.
5. Depending on the above findings, pelvic ultrasound, computed tomography, magnetic resonance imaging of the pituitary, or additional tests may be necessary. Hysteroscopy and curettage are necessary in some unusual cases.[20,21]

MANAGEMENT

Endocrine treatment for dysfunctional uterine bleeding is usually indicated in the majority of these cases. Endocrinopathies such as hyperprolactinemia, thyroid problems, or hyperandrogenism have to be treated specifically. The treatment of DUB depends on its severity.

Mild DUB cases do not present therapeutic problems. Reassurance and frank explanation as well as a careful follow-up are usually the only measures to be followed. In certain cases oral contraceptives may be needed.

Moderate DUB is characterized by long, profuse, and irregular bleeding accompanied by anemia (hemoglobin higher than 10 gr). Low-dose oral contraceptives or cyclic progestogens are the treatment of choice. In addition, iron supplements should be prescribed in almost all cases.

Severe DUB cases presenting with heavy bleeding and hemoglobin less than 9 gr usually require hospitalization. Fluid replacement and, in certain cases, transfusion are required to restore hemodynamic balance. Hormonal treatment is immediately initiated with intravenous conjugated estrogens at 25 mg every 6 hours for no more than 24 hours followed by slow reduction of the estrogen dose and a progestogen preparation. Dilation and curettage are not recommended unless hormonal treatment is unsuccessful. High doses of progestogens may be given per os or parenterally, as an alternative treatment. As soon as hemorrhage is reduced, treatment may be substituted by oral contraceptives. Alternative treatment is the use of prostaglandin synthetase inhibitors, LH-RH analogues, and Danazol.[22–24]

Because coagulopathies represent a high proportion of menorrhagia during adolescence, the cooperation of a pediatric hematologist is essential in certain cases. Finally, psychological support and reassurance are recommended both for the patient and for the family.

The management of DUB in the adolescent patient is almost exclusively medical. A D&C is rarely indicated. If medical treatment fails, an organic etiology needs to be reevaluated. The goal of therapy is primarily to regulate menses, correct anemia, and replenish iron stores. Careful follow-up is needed to assure the diagnoses of DUB.

Vaginal bleeding in the pediatric patient requires careful evaluation to diagnose and treat the underlying disorder. In the adolescent patient, the majority of abnormal vaginal bleeding is dysfunctional uterine bleeding. As already emphasized, however, this is a diagnosis of exclusion. Coagulopathies represent the second most common cause of menorrhagia in the adolescent and may present with the first menses. Four years after menarche, about 50% of these adolescents will have normal ovulatory cycles.[25–28]

SUMMARY

Dysfunctional uterine bleeding (DUB) is a frequent gynecological problem during adolescence and the most frequent cause of urgent admission to the hospital over this period of life. In about 95% of cases it is caused by the late maturation of the hypothalamic–pituitary–ovarian axis (HPO), leading to anovulatory cycles. These adolescents lack the E_2 positive feedback on LH. Thus, the continuous production of estrogen with endometrial stimulation is the basic cause of dysfunctional uterine bleeding.

The initial step in the evaluation of DUB includes detailed clinical history, followed by complete physical examination. Laboratory tests should include coagulation profile, complete blood count with platelet evaluation, and sometimes a serum pregnancy test.

The treatment of DUB is related to the severity of symptomatology with the objective of stopping bleeding and preventing recurrences. Modern hormonal and other medical therapies enable physicians to treat DUB effectively, regardless of the cause. Surgical treatment, such as dilatation and curettage, is rarely indicated in the adolescent patient. The importance of continued follow-up in DUB cases should be underlined, until stabilization of ovulatory menstrual cycles.

REFERENCES

1. SANFILIPPO, J. S. & M. A. YUSSMAN. 1985. Gynecologic problems of adolescence. *In* Pediatric and Adolescent Gynecology. J. Lavery & J. S. Sanfilippo, Eds. Springer-Verlag. New York.
2. SPEROFF, L., R. GLASS & N. KASE. 1989. Dysfunctional uterine bleeding. *In* Clinical Gynecologic Endocrinology and Infertility. Eds.: 265–282. Williams and Wilkins. Baltimore.
3. GUILLEBAUD, J. & J. BONNAR. 1978. Longer, lighter menstrual and intermenstrual bleeding with copper as compared to inert IUDs. Br. J. Obstet. Gynecol. **85:** 707.
4. TREOLAR, A. D., R. E. BOYNTON, B. G. BEHN, *et al.* 1977. Variation of the human menstrual cycle during reproductive life. Int. J. Fertil. **12:** 77.
5. HALBERG, L., A. M. HOGDAHL, L. NILSSON, *et al.* 1966. Menstrual blood loss—a population study: Variations at different ages and attempts to define normality. Acta Obstet. Gynecol. Scand. **45:** 320.
6. CLAESSENS, E. A. & C. A. COWELL. 1981. Acute adolescent menorrhagia. Am. J. Obstet. Gynecol. **139:** 277.
7. DURINZI, K. L. & F. D. DELEON. 1993. Endometriosis in the adolescent and teenage female. Adolesc. Pediatr. Gynecol. **6:** 3.
8. MCKEE, P. A. 1985. Disorders of blood coagulation. *In* Cecil's Textbook of Medicine, 17th ed. J. B. Wyngaarden & L. H. Smith, Eds. W. B. Saunders. Philadelphia.
9. LIM, V. S., C. HENRIQUEZ, G. SIEVERTSEN & L. A. FROHMAN. 1980. Ovarian function in chronic renal failure. Ann. Intern. Med. **93:** 21–27.
10. MAGIAKOU, M. A., G. MASTORAKOS, E. H. OLDFIELD, M. I. GOMEZ, J. L. DOPPMAN, G. B. GUTLER, L. K. NEIMAN & G. P. CHROUSOS. 1994. Cushing's syndrome in children and adolescents. N. Engl. J. Med. **331:** 629–636.
11. EVARARD, J. R., B. H. BUSTON, JR. & D. ERICKSON. 1976. Amenorrhea following oral contraception. Am. J. Obstet. Gynecol. **124:** 88.
12. FRASER, I. S., E. A. MICHIE, L. WIDE & D. T. BAIRD. 1973. Pituitary gonadotropins and ovarian function in adolescent dysfunctional uterine bleeding. J. Clin. Endocrinol. Metab. **37:** 407.
13. WORLEY, R. J. 1986. Dysfunctional uterine bleeding: Clarifying its definition, mechanisms, and management. Postgrad. Med. **79:** 101.
14. DELIGEOROGLOU, E. 1988. Prostaglandins: $PGF_{2\alpha}$, PGE_2, 6-keto-$PGF_{1\alpha}$ and TXB_2 serum levels in dysmenorrheic adolescents before, during and after treatment with oral contraceptives. *In* Ph.D. Thesis, Athens. E. Deligeoroglou, Ed.: 15–27.
15. ROSING, J. & A. OLUND. 1989. Endometrial content of prostaglandin precursors during the menstrual cycle. Prostaglandins, Leukotrienes Essential Fatty Acids **36:** 195.
16. RUEDA, R., T. FALCONE, R. HEMMINGS, *et al.* 1991. Dysfunctional uterine bleeding: A reappraisal (monogr). Curr. Prob. Obstet. Gynecol. Fertil. **14:** 3.
17. SMITH, S. K., M. H. ABEL, R. W. KELLY, *et al.* 1982. The synthesis of prostaglandins from persistent proliferative endometrium. J. Clin. Endocrinol. Metab. **55:** 284.
18. ADELANTADO, J. M., M. C. REES, A. LOPEZ, *et al.* 1988. Increased uterine prostaglandin E receptors in menorrhagic women. Br. J. Obstet. Gynecol. **96:** 162.
19. REES, M. C. P., A. B. M. ANDERSON, L. M. DEMERS, *et al.* 1984. Prostaglandins in menstrual fluid in menorrhagia and dysmenorrhea. Br. J. Obstet. Gynecol. **91:** 673.

20. GIMPELSON, R. J. 1984. Panoramic hysteroscopy with directed biopsies vs. dilatation curettage for accurate diagnosis. J. Reprod. Med. **29:** 575.
21. VALLE, R. F. 1981. Hysteroscopic evaluation of patients with abnormal uterine bleeding. Surg. Gynecol. Obstet. **153:** 521.
22. ANDERSON, A. B. M., P. J. HAYNES, J. GUILLEBAUD, *et al.* 1976. Reduction of menstrual blood loss by prostaglandin synthetase inhibitors. Lancet **1:** 774.
23. FRASER, I. S., R. P. SHEARMAN & J. MCILVERN. 1981. Efficacy of mefenamic acid in patient with a complaing of menorrhagia. Obstet. Gynecol. **58:** 543.
24. MCLAUGHLAN, R. I., D. L. HEALY & H. G. BURGER. 1986. Clinical aspects of LHRH analogues in gynecology: A review. Br. J. Obstet. Gynecol. **93:** 431.
25. ALTCHEK, A. 1977. Dysfunctional uterine bleeding in adolescence. Clin. Obstet. Gynecol. **20:** 633.
26. BRUNI, V. 1990. Menometrorragie disfunzionali. *In* Ginecologia dell'infanzia e dell'adolescenza. F. Bellone & V. Bruni, Eds.: 459–470. Societa Editrice Universo. Roma.
27. CREATSAS, G. 1987. Dysfunctional uterine bleeding during adolescence. *In* Pediatric and Adolescent Gynecology. G. Creatsas, Ed.: 180–187. Entopia. Athens.
28. JAFFE, S. B. & R. JEWELEWICZ. 1991. Dysfunctional uterine bleeding in the pediatric and adolescent patient. Adolesc. Pediatr. Gynecol. **4:** 62.

Hormonal Regulation of N-Cadherin mRNA Levels in Rat Granulosa Cells[a]

RIAZ FAROOKHI,[b,c] CHANG-SHAN GENG,[c] COLIN D. MACCALMAN,[d] AND OREST W. BLASCHUK[d,e]

[c]*Departments of Physiology, Obstetrics & Gynecology*
[d]*Department of Surgery*
[e]*Department of Anatomy and Cell Biology*
McGill University
Montreal, Quebec, Canada

INTRODUCTION

The mechanisms regulating the collective cellular organization within follicles of the ovary remain to be defined. It has been well established that cyclical changes in gonadotropins stimulate follicles to develop to either the ovulatory stage or to undergo atresia. Although gonadotropins are required for follicular development, the mechanisms by which these hormones modulate the establishment of follicular cytoarchitecture have not been elucidated. Studies using other systems indicate that cell adhesion molecules (CAMs) play a fundamental role in promoting the formation of cell collectives and the subsequent establishment of intercellular communication.[1–3] On the basis of these observations, we have proposed that gonadotropins regulate folliculogenesis by modulating the expression of granulosa cell adhesion molecules.

We have shown that the CAM known as N-cadherin is expressed by granulosa cells.[4] N-cadherin is a member of the cadherin family of calcium-dependent CAMs.[5] These CAMs are known to be morphogenetic regulators.[6] They have been shown to be capable of regulating the formation of intercellular junctions (e.g. gap junctions), cell sorting, and the establishment of cell polarity.[1,2,7]

N-cadherin is intimately involved in regulating granulosa cell adhesion and responsiveness to gonadotropins.[4,8] Granulosa cell aggregates isolated from diethylstilbestrol (DES)-primed rat ovaries display this CAM.[4] They also respond to FSH by upregulating their LH receptors.[9] In contrast, trypsin-dissociated (disaggregated) granulosa cells do not express N-cadherin, and they do not upregulate their LH receptors in response to FSH.[8,9] We have shown that estradiol is capable of upregulating N-cadherin levels in these disaggregated cells.[4] This estradiol effect is bipha-

[a]This research was supported by grants from the Medical Research Council of Canada to RF and OWB. CDM was the recipient of a Graduate Fellowship from the Royal Victoria Hospital Research Institute.

[b]Address for correspondence: Riaz Farookhi, Ph.D., Departments of Physiology and Obstetrics and Gynecology, F344 Royal Victoria Hospital, 687 Pine Avenue West, Montreal, Quebec, Canada H3A 1A1.

sic.[8] Low concentrations (<100 nM) of estradiol upregulate N-cadherin levels in the disaggregated granulosa cells, thus causing them to aggregate and become responsive to FSH.[10] Antibodies directed against N-cadherin block the estradiol-stimulated aggregation of dispersed granulosa cells and the ability of FSH to stimulate LH receptors in these cells.[8] High concentrations (>100 nM) of estradiol have no apparent effect on the disaggregated granulosa cells. Collectively, these observations have led us to propose that steroids regulate the collective cellular organization and hormonal responsiveness of the follicle by virtue of their ability to modulate N-cadherin levels.

In this study, we have examined the N-cadherin mRNA levels in aggregated and dispersed preparations of hormone-treated rat granulosa cells. Although both preparations were found to contain N-cadherin mRNA transcripts, estradiol and FSH were only capable of stimulating the levels of these transcripts in dispersed granulosa cells. These results demonstrate that the hormonal responsiveness of granulosa cells is dependent on their adhesive state.

METHODS

Preparation and Culture of Granulosa Cells

Dispersed and aggregated granulosa cells were prepared from the ovaries of DES-primed immature rats as described previously.[9] The cells were seeded in 35-mm tissue culture dishes at a density of 2 million cells/dish in serum-free medium (1:1 Ham's F-12/DME). The medium was removed from the cells after 24 hr of culture and replaced with fresh medium containing either estradiol (10, 30, or 100 nM), FSH (30 ng/ml), or estradiol and FSH. Total RNA was prepared from the cells after an additional 24 hr of culture by the phenol–chloroform method of Chomczynski and Sacchi.[11] The experiments were repeated four times.

Northern Blot Procedures

The RNA species were resolved by electrophoresis in 1% agarose gels containing 3.7% formaldehyde.[12] Approximately 20 μg total RNA was loaded in each lane. The fractionated RNA species were then transferred onto charged nylon membranes (GeneScreen Plus, NEN Products, Boston, MA) with the aid of a vacuum blotting system. The Northern blots were probed with radiolabeled N-cadherin cDNA.[13] After washing, the blots were subjected to radioautography, and the resulting radioautograms scanned using an LKB laser densitometer. The Northern blots were also reprobed with a radiolabeled synthetic oligonucleotide specific for 18S rRNA.[14] The blots were again subjected to radioautography to detect the hybridization of the radiolabeled probe to the 18S rRNA. The radioautograms were then scanned by laser densitometry. The absorbance values obtained for the N-cadherin mRNA transcripts were normalized relative to the 18S rRNA absorbance values.

RESULTS

Northern blot analysis revealed the presence of three N-cadherin mRNA species of 5.6, 4.7, and 3.8 kb in the total RNA extracts from the granulosa cells (FIG. 1). The N-cadherin mRNA levels in aggregated granulosa cells did not vary in response to either estradiol or FSH (FIG. 2). In contrast, N-cadherin mRNA levels were significantly higher ($p \leq 0.05$) in dispersed granulosa cells treated with either of these two hormones as compared to the N-cadherin levels in nontreated cultures (FIG. 3). Estradiol stimulated the N-cadherin mRNA levels in a dose-dependent manner. Maximal levels of N-cadherin mRNA were attained by treating the dispersed granulosa cells with 30 nM estradiol. Furthermore, FSH and estradiol used in combination, as opposed to separately, did not significantly increase the cellular N-cadherin mRNA levels. Finally, we compared the levels of the N-cadherin transcripts in aggregated and dispersed granulosa cells cultured in the absence of estra-

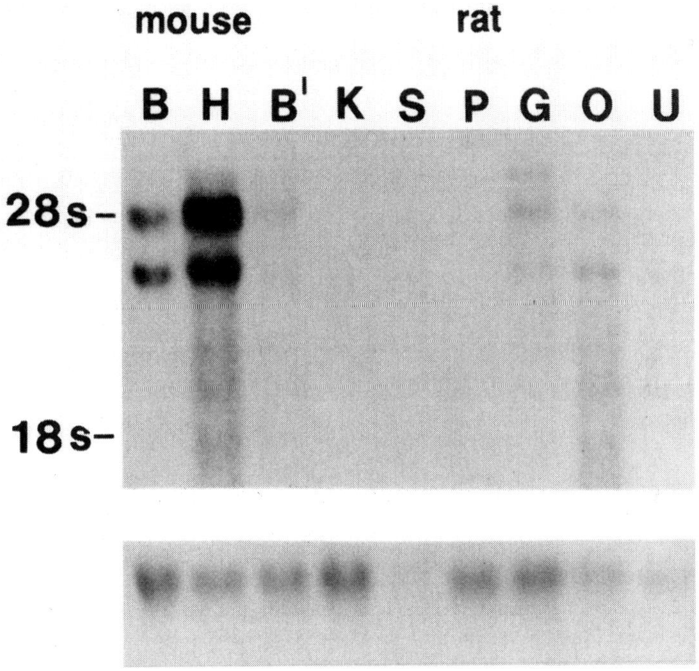

FIGURE 1. Distribution of N-cadherin mRNA transcripts in rat and mouse tissues. Radioautograms of a Northern blot probed with radiolabeled N-cadherin cDNA (*upper panel*) and then reprobed with a radiolabeled synthetic oligonucleotide specific for 18S rRNA (*lower panel*). The blot contains total RNA extracted from the brains (*lane B*), and hearts (*lane H*) of adult mice, as well as the brains (*lane B'*), kidneys (*K*), skin (*S*), placentae (*P*), granulosa cells (*G*), ovaries (*O*), and uteri (*U*) of rats. The position of the 28S and 18S rRNA species are shown on the left-hand side of the upper panel.

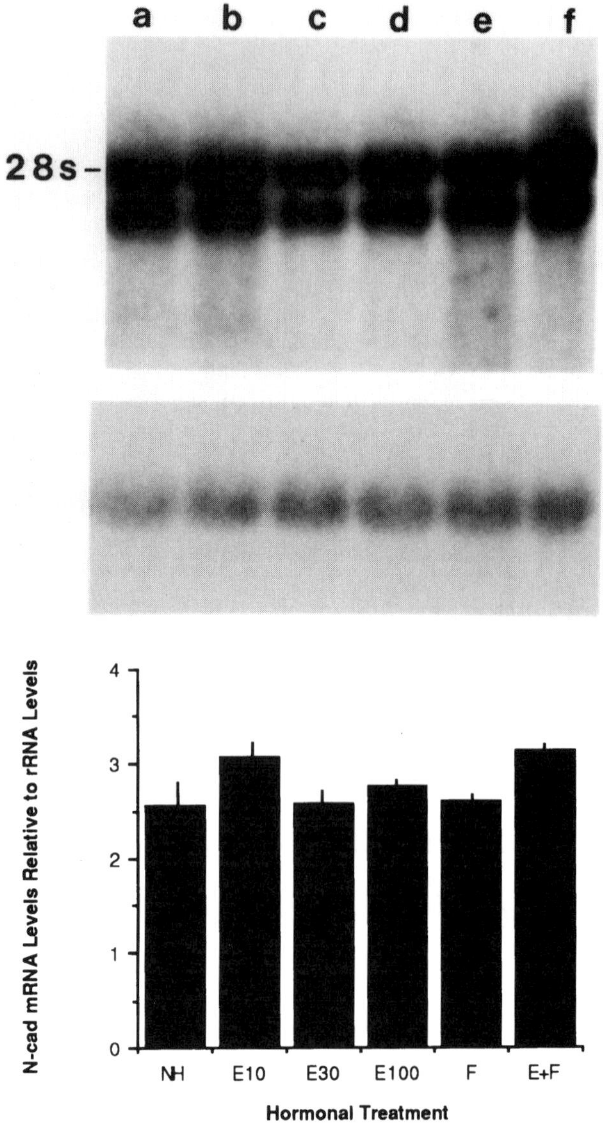

FIGURE 2. Radioautograms of a Northern blot probed with radiolabeled N-cadherin cDNA (*upper panel*) and then reprobed with a radiolabeled synthetic oligonucleotide specific for 18S rRNA (*middle panel*). The blot contains total RNA extracted from *aggregated* granulosa cells cultured in either the absence of hormones (NH), or in the presence of 10 nM estradiol (E10), 30 nM estradiol (E30), 100 nM estradiol (E100), FSH (F), or FSH and 30 nM estradiol (E + F). The position of the 28S rRNA species is shown on the left-hand side of the upper panel. The two radioautograms were scanned using a laser densitometer. The absorbance values obtained from the N-cadherin mRNA transcripts were then normalized relative to the absorbance values for the 18S rRNA. The results derived from this analysis, as well as from three independent studies (radioautograms, not shown) are represented (mean ± SEM; $n = 4$) in the bar graph (*lower panel*).

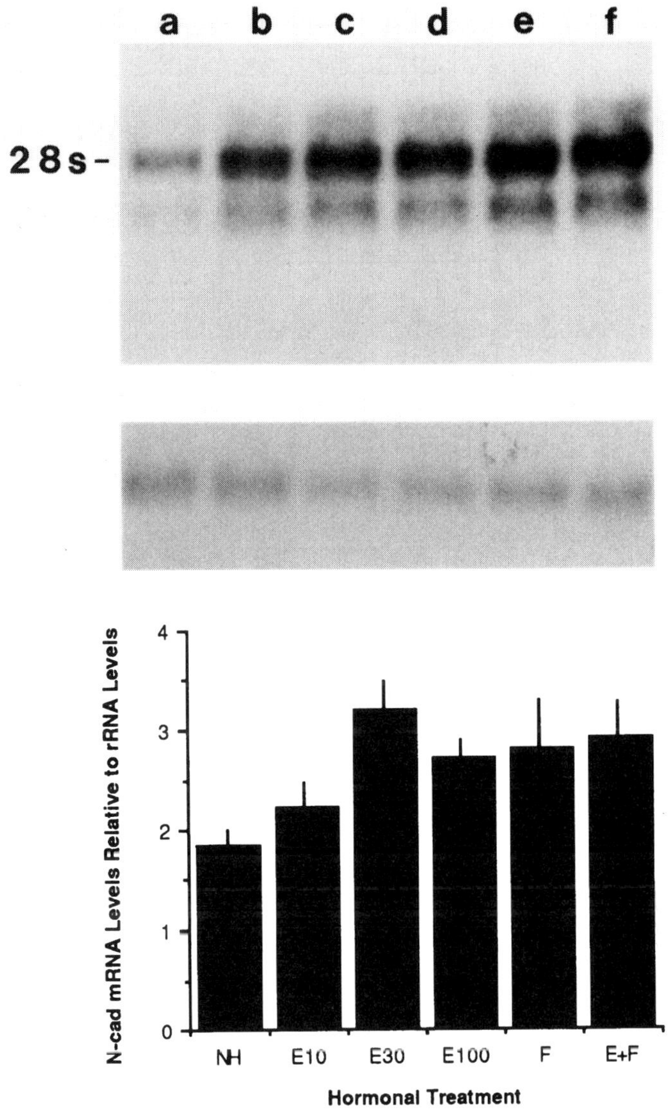

FIGURE 3. Radioautograms of a Northern blot probed with radiolabeled N-cadherin cDNA (*upper panel*) and then reprobed with a radiolabeled synthetic oligonucleotide specific for 18S rRNA (*middle panel*). The blot contains total RNA extracted from *dispersed* granulosa cells cultured in either the absence of hormones (NH), or in the presence of 10 nM estradiol (E10), 30 nM estradiol (E30), 100 nM estradiol (E100), FSH (F), or FSH and 30 nM estradiol (E + F). The position of the 28S rRNA species is shown on the left-hand side of the upper panel. The two radioautograms were scanned using a laser densitometer. The absorbance values obtained from the N-cadherin mRNA transcripts were then normalized relative to the absorbance values for the 18S rRNA. The results derived from this analysis, as well as from three independent studies (radioautograms, not shown) are represented (mean ± SEM; $n = 4$) in the bar graph (*lower panel*).

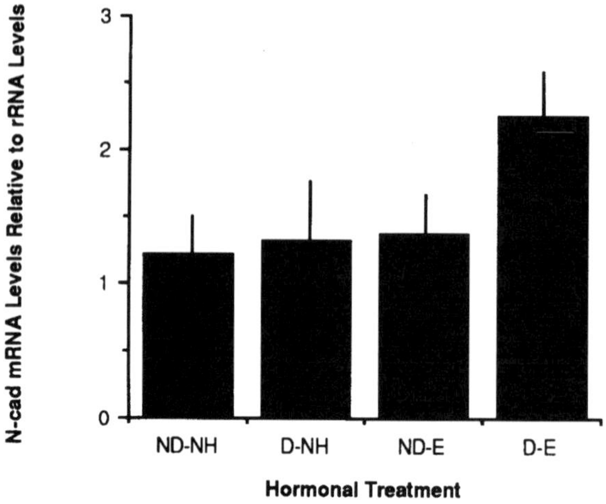

FIGURE 4. Bar graph depicting the N-cadherin mRNA levels in aggregated (ND) and dispersed (D) granulosa cells cultured in either the absence (NH), or presence of 30 nM estradiol (E). Northern blots containing total RNA extracted from these cells were probed with radiolabeled N-cadherin cDNA, and then reprobed with a radiolabeled synthetic oligonucleotide specific for 18S rRNA. Radioautograms of these blots (not shown) were scanned using a laser densitometer. The absorbance values obtained for the N-cadherin mRNA transcripts were then normalized relative to the absorbance values obtained for the 18S rRNA. The results derived from this analysis, as well as from three additional studies, are represented (mean ± SEM; $n = 4$) in the bar graph.

diol (FIG. 4). There was no significant difference between the N-cadherin levels in these two types of cells.

DISCUSSION

Our finding that granulosa cells express N-cadherin is an unexpected observation because N-cadherin is usually found in neural and muscle tissues.[15] Three distinct N-cadherin mRNA transcripts were identified. Miyatani *et al.*[16] and Walsh *et al.*[17] have shown that these three mRNA species exist in brain and heart of embryonic and adult mice but that they are absent from mammalian tissues such as the kidney and placenta. It is not known whether these three different N-cadherin mRNA species encode distinct isoforms of N-cadherin. We have previously demonstrated that antibodies capable of recognizing N-cadherin detect only one granulosa cell cadherin.[5,8,10] Walsh *et al.*[17] speculate that the different transcripts may arise from alternative usage of polyadenylation sites. The nucleic acid sequences of these transcripts must be determined in order to resolve this issue.

Previous studies in our laboratory revealed that N-cadherin levels in dispersed granulosa cells were stimulated by estradiol and, to a lesser extent, by FSH.[4] The results presented here are in accordance with these initial observations. Both estradiol and FSH elevated the levels of N-cadherin mRNA transcripts in dispersed cells. In contrast, the N-cadherin mRNA levels in aggregated (nondispersed) granulosa cells were unresponsive to hormonal treatments. These observations suggest that N-cadherin levels are regulated differently in the two cell preparations.

We speculate that at least some of the diverse morphoregulatory effects that are known to be exerted by steroids may arise from their ability to modulate cadherin levels in developing tissues. Our recent studies have shown that cadherin mRNA levels in other steroid-responsive tissues are also modulated by sex steroids.[13,18,19] Steroid-induced alterations in cadherin levels would have profound effects on morphogenetic processes, since these cell adhesion molecules are directly involved in mediating the ability of cells to form functional collectives.[20] We have proposed that steroid-mediated modulation of cadherins may be involved in tumorigenesis and tumor progression in hormone-responsive tissues.[21,22] Our observation that N-cadherin mRNA levels are regulated in a different manner than those in cell collectives (such as aggregated granulosa cells) further substantiates our hypothesis that the response of cell populations to hormones is dependent on their adhesive state.

SUMMARY

We have examined the ability of hormones to modulate the steady-state levels of N-cadherin mRNA transcripts in aggregated and dispersed rat granulosa cell populations. Estradiol and follicle-stimulating hormone (FSH) had no effect on the levels of N-cadherin mRNA transcripts in aggregated granulosa cells. In contrast, these two hormones stimulated N-cadherin mRNA levels in dispersed granulosa cells. This is the first report that estradiol and FSH are capable of regulating N-cadherin mRNA levels. The results also suggest that the N-cadherin mRNA levels in dispersed and aggregated granulosa cells are regulated by different mechanisms.

REFERENCES

1. MEGE, R.-M., F. MATSUZAKI, W. J. GALLIN, J. I. GOLDBERG, B. A. CUNNINGHAM & G. M. EDELMAN. 1988. Proc. Natl. Acad. Sci. USA **85:** 7274–7278.
2. JONGEN, W. M. F., D. J. FITZGERALD, M. ASAMOTO, C. PICCOLI, T. J. SLAGA, D. GROS, M. TAKEICHI & H. YAMASAKI. 1991. J. CELL BIOL. **114:** 545–555.
3. GEIGER, B. & O. AYALON. 1992. Ann. Rev. Cell Biol. **8:** 307–332.
4. BLASCHUK, O. W. & R. FAROOKHI. 1989. Dev. Biol. **136:** 564–567.
5. TAKEICHI, M. 1990. Ann. Rev. Biochem. **59:** 237–252.
6. TAKEICHI, M. 1991. Science **251:** 1451–1455.
7. NATHKE, I. S., L. E. HINCK & W. J. NELSON. 1993. J. Cell Sci. Suppl. **17:** 139–145.
8. FAROOKHI, R. & O. W. BLASCHUK. 1991. *In* Signalling Mechanisms and Gene Expression in the Ovary. G. Gibori Ed. Springer. New York.
9. FAROOKHI, R. & J. DESJARDINS. 1986. Mol. Cell Endocrinol. **47:** 13–24.
10. FAROOKHI, R. & O. W. BLASCHUK. 1989. *In* Growth Factors and the Ovary. A. N. Hirshfield, Ed.: 257–265. Plenum Press. New York.
11. CHOMCZYNSKI, P. & N. SAACHI. 1987. Anal. Biochem. **162:** 156–159.

12. Davis, L. G., M. D. Dibner & J. F. Battey. 1986. Basic Methods in Molecular Biology.: 143–146. Elsevier. New York.
13. MacCalman, C., D. A. O'Brien, S. Byers & O. W. Blaschuk. 1993. Endocrine **1:** 519–525.
14. Chen, B., O. W. Blaschuk & B. F. Hales. 1991. Teratology **44:** 581–590.
15. Damjanov, I. A., Damjanov & C. H. Damsky. 1986. Dev. Biol. **116:** 194–202.
16. Miyatani, S., K. Shimamura, M. Hatta, A. Nagafuchi, A. Nose, M. Matsunaga, K. Hatta & M. Takeichi. 1989. Science **245:** 631–635.
17. Walsh, F. S., C. H. Barton, W. Putt, S. E. Moore, D. Kelsell, N. Spurr & P. N. Goodfellow. 1990. J. Neurochem. **55:** 805–812.
18. MacCalman, C. D., R. Farookhi & O. W. Blaschuk. 1994. Endocrine **2:** 485–490.
19. MacCalman, C. D., R. Farookhi & O. W. Blaschuk. 1994. Clin. Exp. Metast. **12:** 276–282.
20. Edelman, G. M. 1992. Dev. Dynamics **193:** 2–10.
21. Blaschuk, O. W., S. B. Munro & R. Farookhi. 1994. Can. J. Oncol. **4:** 291–301.
22. Blaschuk, O. W., S. B. Munro & R. Farookhi. 1995. Endocrine **3:** 83–89.

Anovulation and Monophasic Cycles

J. E. H. SPENCE

Department of Obstetrics and Gynecology
University of Ottawa/Ottawa Civic Hospital
1053 Carling Avenue, CPC-536
Ottawa, K1Y 4E9, Canada

Fifty percent of all adolescent gynecological referrals involve abnormal menses. The patient or her mother is often concerned because the periods are too frequent or infrequent, too heavy, or too prolonged. The natural inclination of the physician is to prescribe the oral contraceptive pill, because it regulates and normalizes the menstrual flow. However, there is no evidence that on discontinuation of the pill that the menstrual cycle is improved by this therapy. This is understandable inasmuch as the pill is not a physiological compound and acts by suppressing an awakening hypothalamic–pituitary–ovarian–uterine axis. Earlier studies by Treloar[1] and Vollman[2] have described pubertal menstrual cycles, and many authors have documented the high percentage of these that are anovulatory. It is widely believed, and often stated in textbooks, that anovulatory cycles lead to irregular and variable menstrual flow. However, in clinical experience, most gynecologists recognize that this is not necessarily true because the vast majority of adolescents have few period concerns and don't require any medical advice or management. So what is the basis for the abnormal menses when they present?

In order to appreciate the problem, an understanding of pubertal events is critical. Puberty is not a new endocrine event. The fetus produces both FSH and LH in high amounts, production of which is suppressed after birth and remains at low levels until reactivation occurs at around age ten. What initiates the pubertal hormonal cascade has not been clearly defined, but once activated, pubertal events usually follow in an orderly sequence with the onset of menstrual flow and ovulation the hallmark of maturation. The endocrine events surrounding puberty are extremely complex, not only in the central nervous system, hypothalamus, and pituitary, but also in the ovary. Simultaneously, the reproductive organs mature along with their regulatory systems. It would be unrealistic to think that in each adolescent female, the entire reproductive system could just be switched on with the first period and work perfectly, considering the extensive hormonal interplay that is required to effect an ovulatory response from the ovary. It is a credit to nature that only a few teenage girls actually develop serious menstrual problems.

Endocrinologically, the onset of puberty is first heralded by the increased secretion of LH from the pituitary, first at night, with a concomitant increase in basal LH levels and an increased amplitude. Later in puberty LH pulses occur both day and night but have a lower amplitude and a lower basal level.[3] The ovary is activated because of these changing LH levels, and there is also a concomitant activation of the adrenal gland through its controlling mechanisms. This results in a rise in androstenedione, dehydroepiandrosterone sulfate, and testosterone with a decrease in sex hormone–binding globulin. The picture is very similar to what is seen in classical adult polycystic ovarian disease.[4] This hyperandrogen state, occurring in young post-pubertal females, is quite normal but does lead to menstrual irregularity in a number of adolescents. An ultrasound in these women will demonstrate multifollicularity of the ovaries as well as increased ovarian volume.[5] This phase is transient and is not usually accompanied by obesity, significant acne, or hirsutism. It is interesting to contemplate that persistence of this phase might lead to the full adult polycystic ovarian syndrome. Recent studies have suggested that, although the cycle length in these women may be prolonged and monophasic, ovulation does occur, but after a prolonged follicular phase, and from a smaller follicle. These cycles also have short, insufficient luteal phases. Present wisdom suggests that pubertal menstrual abnormalities are related either to a delayed development of the positive feedback mechanism for the LH surge, or to suppression of the central nervous system, pituitary, or ovary from a normal but fleeting hyperandrogen state.

The actual menstrual flow results from precise hormonal changes, which usually involve falling estrogen and progesterone levels. Ischemic degeneration of the endometrium is an orderly event, progressive, and related to the rhythmic constriction of endometrial arterioles. Vascular stasis occurs by platelet and thrombin plugs, with fibrin deposition, all of which is followed by regeneration and restructuring. Prostaglandins play an important role in normal endometrial shedding, and any abnormal menstrual bleeding is the result of unphysiological sex hormone secretion or deranged prostaglandin interactions.

In order to manage menstrual derangements or dysfunctional uterine bleeding in this age group, it is helpful to understand the estrogen threshold concept. Estrogen is a growth hormone, whereas progesterone is a modifying hormone. In the early post-menarcheal months and years, estrogens are secreted in elevated amounts, often non-cyclically, and can be secreted for long periods without interruption or accompanied by progesterone. Unopposed estrogen leads to endometrial proliferation, and without appropriate conversion to a secretory endometrium, irregular and variable menstrual bleeding occurs, which in some circumstances can be quite profuse with debilitating consequences.

Not all abnormal bleeding problems in this age group are related to dysfunctional uterine bleeding or a hormonal abnormality. Other conditions must be excluded before the diagnosis can be confirmed. Certain systemic diseases such as hematological abnormalities,[6] thyroid dysfunction, or chronic illness can present in this fashion as well as organic reproductive tract disease. Infection, pregnancy, or neoplasm can all cause irregular bleeding. In order to appropriately diagnose dysfunctional uterine bleeding, pregnancy must be ruled out. Hematological abnormalities can be detected by a CBC, platelet count, or bleeding time; and hormonal problems can be confirmed by measuring thyroid-stimulating hormone, prolactin, follicle-stimulating hormone, luteinizing hormone, testosterone, and dehydroepiandrosterone sulfate.

Management is usually quite straightforward and effective if physiological principles are followed. The goal of any treatment is to halt the acute bleeding, correct the anemia, reverse the effects of unopposed estrogen, and allow the development of a hormonal hypothalamic–pituitary–ovarian axis. Progesterone is the key hormone to appropriate management because it limits the growth of the endometrium and converts it from a proliferative to a secretory type. Progesterone also increases the production of arachidonic acid, which enhances prostaglandin production and leads to uniform menstrual shedding. Fortunately, progestins have effects similar to progesterone and are inexpensive, easy to use, have no central suppressive effects and few side effects. If the disturbance is minimal, all that is required is education and reassurance, and time will correct the condition. Menstrual calendars are helpful, and close follow-up can be reassuring to the patient and her family. If the disturbance is more pronounced, the judicious use of progestins given cyclically from day fifteen to twenty-five can be beneficial. The oral contraceptive can be used if the bleeding abnormality persists or if there are any contraceptive concerns. Treatment does not need to be prolonged, but on discontinuation of the medication the patient needs to be carefully followed to treat any recurrences. If, however, the adolescent presents with severe menstrual bleeding or pronounced anemia, she requires the restoration of plasma volume, the correction of the anemia, the arrest of the hemorrhage, and conversion of the proliferative to a secretory endometrium. In these circumstances estrogens are required as well as progestins. The treatment may require many months before tapering with the medication or switching to progestins alone before discontinuing them. Unfortunately, many of the patients that present with menorrhagia and anemia early in their menstrual life have underlying hematological abnormalities. The vast majority of young adolescents with dysfunctional uterine bleeding will do well and can be managed physiologically and expectantly. However, Southam and Richart,[7] in a classical study, followed these patients for 25 years and documented continued abnormalities and poor reproductive performance in a significant number of them over subsequent years. It is hoped, however, that with new understanding and appropriate care some of the persistent abnormalities they innumerated can be anticipated and managed more expeditiously.

SUMMARY

Normal pubertal development is often considered complete when the adolescent experiences her first menstrual period. However, sexual maturity is not attained until the onset of regular ovulatory cycles, which may take a number of months to years to accomplish. This maturation process is orchestrated by a neuroendocrine cascade and modified by autocrine and paracrine events in the ovary. The control of these complex relationships takes time and could not be expected to be fully functional with menarche. During the first menstrual months, the hypothalamic–pituitary–ovarian axis is immature, resulting in the secretion of only estrogens from the developing follicles; positive feedback to trigger ovulation develops later. Consequently, estrogen secretion is variable and unopposed by progesterone, which would normally be produced in ovulatory cycles. Estrogen-only primed endometrium often leads to irregular menstrual cycles with variable flow. Surprisingly, most adolescents do well and have few complaints in spite of these anovulatory cycles. If an abnormality is experienced with the menstrual cycle, once understood physiologically, it can be managed simply, by watchful expectancy or intermittent progestin therapy. Occasionally, severe menstrual bleeding is encountered, and in a proportion of these patients a thorough assessment will delineate an underlying medical problem that needs to be addressed. The management of these patients requires ingenuity from the pediatric reproductive endocrinologist and aggressive hormonal manipulation. Most patients do well, but some require long-term continuing care.

REFERENCES

1. TRELOAR, A., R. E. BOYNTON, B. G. BEHN & W. BROWN. 1967. Variation of the human menstrual cycle through reproductive life. Int. J. Fertil. **12**(1): 77–126.
2. VOLLMANN, R. F. 1956. Degree of variability of the length of the menstrual cycle in correlation with age of women. Gynaecologia **142:** 310.
3. WENNINK, J. M. B., H. A. DELEMARRE-VAN DE WAAL, R. SCHOEMAKER, H. SHOEMAKER & J. SCHOEMAKER. 1990. Luteinizing hormone and follicle stimulating hormone secretion patterns in girls throughout puberty measured using highly sensitive immunoradiometric assays. Clin. Endocrinol. **33:** 333–344.
4. VENTUROLI, S., E. PORCU, R. FABBRI, O. MAGRINI, L. GAMMI, R. PARADISI & C. FLAMIGNI. 1992. Longitudinal evaluation of the different gonadotropin pulsatile patterns in anovulatory cycles of young girls. J. Clin. Endocrinol. Metab. **74**(4): 836–841.
5. VENTUROLI, S., E. PORCU, R. FABBRI, R. PARADISI, L. GAMMI, M. PASSARINI, L. F. ORSINI & C. FLAMIGNI. 1986. Ovarian multifollicularity, high LH and androgen plasma levels, and anovulation are frequent and strongly linked in adolescent irregular cycles. Acta Endocrinol. **111:** 368–372.
6. CLAESSENS, E. A. & C. A. COWELL. 1981. Acute adolescent menorrhagia. Am. J. Obstet. Gynecol. **139**(3): 277–280.
7. SOUTHAM, A. L. & R. M. RICHART. 1966. The prognosis for adolescents with menstrual abnormalities. Am. J. Obstet. Gynecol. **94**(5): 637–645.

The Polycystic Ovary Syndrome

Pathogenesis, Metabolic Implications, and Therapeutic Approach

EVANTHIA DIAMANTI-KANDARAKIS

Endocrine and Metabolic Unit
First Department of Internal Medicine
Laikon General Hospital
School of Medicine
University of Athens
Athens, Greece

Polycystic ovary syndrome (PCOS) is one of the most common endocrinopathies and is probably the most frequent cause of infertility affecting women of reproductive age.[1,2] It is a condition of unknown etiology, characterized by hyperandrogenism and chronic anovulation. It accounts for 75% of anovulatory infertility cases, occurring in 30–40% of women with secondary amenorrhea and 85–90% of those with oligomenorrhea.[3] A reasonably conservative estimate of this disorder is a 5–10% prevalence, although there have been no studies on specific populations.[1]

HISTORY AND MORPHOLOGY

The association of polycystic ovaries with amenorrhea, hirsutism, and obesity was first reported in 1935 by Stein and Leventhal. The initial morphological and histological findings of the ovaries (thickened tunica albuginea, hyperplasia of the theca interna, cortical stroma, multiple subcapsular follicles in various stages of atresia) appeared to be linked with a wide spectrum of biochemical and clinical findings, which subsequently led to the establishment of the term polycystic ovarian syndrome.

There has been much debate about whether it represents a single disorder or several, because its clinical and biochemical features are heterogeneous. Typically, these are the clinical features of hyperandrogenism (hirsutism, acne, alopecia) associated with elevated serum androgens and LH, normal or low serum concentrations of FSH, and polycystic ovaries on the ultrasonography. However, these individual findings are nonspecific. Indeed, women with prolactinomas[4] or virilizing congenital adrenal hyperplasia[5,6] may have polycystic ovarian morphology by ultrasonography and elevated levels of serum LH, indistinguishable from PCOS. These findings support the idea that the polycystic morphology simply indicates a nonspecific response of the ovary to chronic anovulation.

Surprisingly, polycystic ovaries were detected by ultrasound in 40 of 46 women (87%) presenting with hirsutism and regular menses.[7] These findings have been supported by the results of other studies including an analysis of 350 hirsute women among whom polycystic ovarian morphology was detected by ultrasonography in over 50% of those with regular menses.[8,9] Some investigators have required only the presence of oligomenorrhea and hirsutism to make the diagnosis of PCOS.[10] On the other hand, with or without menstrual irregularities or hirsutism, polycystic ovaries are also common in women with hyperandrogenism, whose presenting symptoms are acne, seborrhea, or male-pattern alopecia.[7,8] Interestingly, up to 23% of normal women meet the sonographic criteria for polycystic ovaries.[11]. These criteria are defined by the presence of eight or more subcapsular follicular cysts < 10 mm and increased ovarian stroma.[1] Ironically, despite the fact that the original description of the syndrome was based on the morphology of the ovaries, currently this finding, although consistent with PCOS, is not considered essential for the diagnosis. These changes can be present in women who are entirely endocrinologically normal, thus it is very important to distinguish the ovarian morphologic change from the endocrine syndrome. The current diagnostic criteria for PCOS are hyperandrogenism and chronic anovulation excluding secondary causes of specific disorders, such as nonclassical adrenal 21-hydroxylase deficiency, hyperprolactinemia, or androgen-secreting neoplasms.[1]

PATHOGENESIS

The pathogenesis of the polycystic ovary syndrome remains a controversial subject. Great effort has been devoted to investigation of the pathogenetic role of the endocrine and metabolic abnormalities in PCOS. Typically, these abnormalities are characterized by insulin resistance and hypersecretion of luteinizing hormone (LH) and androgens, particularly testosterone and androstenedione, but with normal or low serum levels of follicular-stimulating hormone (FSH). The issue of whether this elusive syndrome is primarily a hypothalamic or a gonadal disorder has not yet been resolved; however, the body of evidence today favors the ovary as the principal cause.

Neuroendocrine Abnormalities in Polycystic Ovary Syndrome

Gonadotropin Abnormalities

Gonadotropin secretory abnormalities are among the most frequently described in PCOS and include elevated levels of LH or an elevated LH/FSH ratio, an increased LH pulse frequency, and an altered diurnal rhythm of LH secretion. The prevalence of elevated hormone concentrations depends both on the criteria for the diagnosis and on the method of determination, because there is considerable molecular heterogeneity of the LH molecule. The combination of a relatively high LH level, which stimulates theca-interstitial cell secretion of androgens, and a relatively low FSH level, which would not permit efficient aromatization, could clearly cause the ovary to produce more androgens than estrogens. The intraovarian excess of androgens coupled with the poor estrogenic milieu would create an unfavorable environment for the maturation of the follicle, leading to anovulation.[12] The abnormality has been thought to result from inappropriate hypothalamic GnRH secretion as the primary defect. In support of this concept is the correction of ovarian dysfunction by administration of very low doses of FSH *in vivo* and lowering the androgen levels in some PCOS patients.[13] Conversely, LH pulse frequency and the ratio of LH to FSH are normalized when estrogen and progesterone are administered to anovulatory women with PCOS.[13,14] Also, when ovulation is induced by hCG, the gonadotropin response to GnRH is subsequently normalized.[14] Although disturbances of hypothalamic neurotransmitters may exist in PCOS (particularly in patients with high circulating levels of LH) and several neurotransmitters have been implicated as possible mediators, the data do not consistently support this central role.[15–17] In conclusion, a primary hypothalamic defect appears to be unlikely. Taken together, these findings suggest that the gonadotropin dysrhythmia of PCOS is secondary to the altered steroid environment that causes chronic anovulation. The question of whether the gonadotropin abnormality may be secondary to an estrogenic effect on the pituitary has been considered regarding estrone and estradiol. In the estrone hypothesis, it has been postulated that peripheral aromatization of androgens occurs in excess, in particular androstenedione to estrone occurs, and that the elevated estrone sensitizes the gonadotropes to secrete increased amounts of LH, which in turn initiates or maintains the ovarian hypersecretion of androgens.[18] The fact that clomiphene citrate, an antiestrogen, altered the secretion of gonadotropins, has provided supportive evidence.[18] However, neither estrone elevations up to 1.0 nmol/l,[19] nor the peripheral aromatase inhibitor testolactone altered LH levels or the LH response to exogenous GnRH in women with PCOS.[20] Estradiol is unlikely to be directly involved, since high levels have to be reached in order to increase LH responsiveness to GnRH,[21] and estradiol is more commonly low in PCOS.

The second obvious question is whether androgens could play a role in modifying the gonadotropin secretion by a direct action at the level of the pituitary or the hypothalamus, independent of their peripheral aromatization. In various hyperandrogenic disorders, such as in women with androgen-secreting tumors that produce moderate amounts of androgens, mild elevations in basal serum LH and in LH response to GnRH are observed.[18,19] However, gonadotropins are suppressed, as is their response to GnRH, when serum androgens are very high, as in arrhenoblastomas.[22] Pharmacological doses of testosterone in normal women decreased the LH pulse amplitude, its frequency, and the LH response to GnRH.[23] In women with PCOS, modest doses of testosterone had no effect on serum LH levels or LH pulse amplitude and frequency.[24] Treatment with an antiandrogen receptor blocker likewise had no effect on LH response to GnRH.[25,26] Taken together, the above data suggest that the androgen effect on gonadotropin secretion is probably a mild one; and, in particular, modest elevations of plasma testosterone may result in an increase in the ratio of serum LH to FSH, whereas elevations of a greater magnitude have an inhibitory effect. Although a significant proportion of women with PCOS have an elevated level of serum LH and thus meet a common diagnostic criterion, it is now well accepted that elevated serum LH is not necessary for a PCOS diagnosis.[1]

Hyperprolactinemia

Hyperprolactinemia is often associated with infertility and anovulation and occasionally with masculinization. It may be found in the absence of a pituitary neoplasm.[29] Hyperprolactinemia in PCOS may be caused by enhanced estrogen exposure, which is known to stimulate pituitary lactotrophs and possibly to decrease dopaminergic activity.[29] In hyperandrogenic women with an elevated prolactin level, a pituitary adenoma must be excluded.

Ovarian Steroidogenic Abnormalities

The body of evidence favors the ovary as the center of this multifaceted disorder. The *sine qua non* event of PCOS is impaired folliculogenesis. Under normal conditions, this occurs primarily as a result of two interrelated processes, recruitment and selection of the destined single follicle for ovulation. In women with PCOS, the initial steps, recruitment and growth to small antral stages, seem to be intact.[27,28] The next step, selection, is lacking and leads to an accumulation of large numbers of Graafian follicles (cysts).[27]

The key factor in selection of the dominant follicle is the process of acquiring the capacity to synthesize large amounts of estradiol. The process occurs according to the two-cell two-gonadotropin principle.[28] The basis of this principle is that, in response to LH, the theca interstitial cells synthesize and secrete androstenedione (D4A), which diffuses across the basal lamina into the granulosa cells where it is aromatized to E_2 in response to stimulation by FSH. The estradiol is released into both the follicular fluid and the peripheral circulation. In PCOS the selection process does not occur successively, and the follicle produces very little E_2. The major question to be asked is Which are the factors that directly or indirectly lead to this abnormality? The steps of steroidogenesis will be examined in brief as well as whether this is a primary or a secondary defect leading to chronic anovulation in PCOS.

Estrogens

The pattern of estradiol secretion in PCOS differs from that in the normal menstrual cycle because there is no preovulatory or midluteal increase, despite the fact that at the early and mid-follicular phase it remains normal.[31]

If we start working back from the last step of steroidogenesis, aromatase is the first enzyme to be examined. Its activity has been investigated rather extensively, because it is responsible for converting androgen to estrogens. Follicles from PCOS contain high levels of androstenedione and the ratio of androstenedione to estradiol is high, suggesting a defect in aromatization.[32] *In vitro* experiments have shown that when FSH is added to PCO granulosa cells, estrogen production returns to the level of normal granulosa cells.[33–35]

These data suggest that the aromatase defect is not intrinsic to the ovary and may be secondary to inhibition of secretion or action of FSH or secondary to atresia, as atretic follicles have been found to be low in aromatase activity.[35] Recently, however, a P450 aromatase gene mutation has been found to cause a form of PCOS.[36]

The abnormal estrogenic status in women with PCOS is characterized by the acyclical production of estradiol and estrone combined with progesterone deficiency. The unopposed estrogenic effect on the endometrium results in episodes of mennometrorrhagia and an increased risk of endometrial carcinoma in the long term.[37] This uninhibited estrogenic stimulus via LH overstimulation of the interstitial cells also leads to overproduction of estrogens.

Androgens

Intraovarian androgens have been found to be increased, and it appears that they play a significant role in the anovulatory process.[38,39] Whether this is a primary or a secondary event remains to be elucidated.

Defects in different steroidogenic enzymes have been reported to be associated with PCOS and found to lead to intraovarian androgen accumulation. Deficiencies of 17-ketosteroid reductase and 3b-HSD are the most commonly found: The first one is associated with unusually high levels of androstenedione,[40] and the second one results in concordant ovarian and adrenal steroidogenic abnormalities, as this enzyme has equivalent affinity for both C-21 and C-19 steroids.[41]

The biochemical basis of the ovarian androgen excess of this syndrome remains unclear. It has been postulated, based on clinical and *in vitro* studies, that there is a dysregulation of the enzyme P450c that catalyzes both 17-α-hydroxylase and 17,20-lyase activities.[42–44]

According to this view, the polycystic ovary syndrome is equated with functional ovarian hyperandrogenism, characterized by 17-PROG and AD hyperresponsiveness to GnRH agonist (nafarelin test). This pattern of steroid response is unique in women with PCO syndrome, and it has been suggested that it could be used as a marker for PCOS.[45] The authors suggest that one overproduction of 17-PROG in PCOS is caused by either excessive stimulation by LH or via escape from desensitization to LH. The latter situation may result from an intrinsic intraovarian flaw in the paracrine feedback mechanism by which ovarian androgens affect the biosynthesis of estrogens.[46]

Rosenfield and his colleagues provided further evidence to support their hypothesis that PCOS ovaries were functioning as if overstimulated by LH, whether or not there was an excess LH concentration in serum. They compared two types of patients with functional hyperandrogenemia, one group with elevated LH and one with normal levels. There was a remarkably consistent pattern of 17-hydroxyprogesterone hyperresponsiveness to GnRH regardless of the presence of elevated LH levels.[47] In PCO/FOH there appears to be overactive androgen secretion, most prominent in the D4 pathway, and the cultured theca cells from these patients showed that the secretion of 17-hydroxyprogesterone was greater than androstenedione in response to LH.[48]

There may be incipient downregulation of 17,20-lyase activity such that PCOS ovaries seem to escape from normal downregulation production of androgens by LH. These data support the concept that in PCOS thecal steroidogenesis is overactive at the level of 17-hydroxylase and 17,20-lyase, which are possibly activities of the same enzyme (P450c17). Recently, a single base change in the gene coding for this enzyme has been identified in PCOS and is associated with a significant risk of developing the disorder.[46]

Serum concentrations of testosterone and androstenedione are elevated in women with PCOS, but there is a variation among individual women.[49] The presence of hirsutism in PCOS indicates a rather variable sensitivity of the hair follicle, because the degree of hyperandrogenemia is similar among anovulatory hirsute and nonhirsute women.[50] On the other hand, hirsute women with PCOS may have normal serum androgen concentrations, which has been attributed to higher than normal production associated with increased clearance by peripheral tissues.[51] The clearance of testosterone is affected by the concentration of sex hormone–binding globulin, which traditionally has been considered to be the major regulator.[52] Recent data, however, suggest that metabolic factors, in particular insulin, are more important in determining the production of sex hormone–binding globulin.[53]

Adrenal Steroidogenic Abnormalities

The adrenal gland can contribute to the androgen excess in PCOS. DHEAS is elevated in some women with the syndrome. The exact abnormality in the steroidogenic pathway is not clear, but it is unlikely that these abnormalities represent a primary defect in adrenal steroidogenesis, because PCO can occur without any abnormalities in adrenal steroidogenesis.

Metabolic Abnormalities

Important clues to the pathogenesis of PCOS and its substantial metabolic complications have been provided by the finding that the syndrome is associated with a disorder of insulin action. Burghen, Givens, and Kitabchi[54] were the first to report that women with PCOS were hyperinsulinemic and that there were significant positive linear correlations between insulin and androgen levels. Subsequently, a number of studies confirmed and extended the original observation that women with PCOS had hyperinsulinemia that was independent of obesity and secondary to insulin resistance.[1,55] Both lean and obese women with PCOS have evidence of decreased insulin sensitivity, but insulin resistance is most marked when there is an interaction between obesity and the syndrome.[26] In 1987, Dunaif first observed that obese PCOS women had significantly increased glucose levels during an oral glucose tolerance test (OGTT), compared to age- and weight-matched ovulatory hyperandrogenic and control women. Twenty percent of the obese PCOS women had impaired glucose tolerance or frank NIDDM by National Diabetes Data Group criteria,[58] and up to 40% when the less stringent WHO criteria are used. Finally, on the basis of the prevalence of glucose intolerance in women, the prevalence of glucose intolerance in PCOS, and a conservative estimate of the prevalence of PCOS (5%), it can be extrapolated that PCOS-related insulin resistance contributes to approximately 10% of cases of glucose intolerance in premenopausal women.[56–58] It is, thus, clear that PCOS is a major risk factor for NIDDM in women. A decrease of insulin-mediated glucose uptake of similar magnitude, that seen in NIDDM, has been demonstrated by euglycemic glucose clamp studies in PCOS women.[59] This decrease of insulin sensitivity in peripheral tissues, notably muscle and adipose tissue, is independent of the effect of obesity[58,26] and is present in both lean and obese women with the syndrome, but it is most marked when obesity is involved.[1,26] In contrast to the insulin resistance of type II diabetes where hepatic glucose production, basal and insulin mediated, is universally affected, only in obese women with PCOS is hepatic glucose production significantly increased.[1,59] This synergistic negative effect of obesity and PCOS on hepatic glucose production is an important factor in the pathogenesis of glucose intolerance in PCOS.

However, a study from Denmark[60] has failed to find decreased glucose uptake by euglycemic glucose clamp. Both lean and obese women with PCOS with normal insulin sensitivity have also been encountered in other populations.[1] These observations suggest that there are ethnic differences and heterogeneity in the syndrome. In NIDDM both insulin resistance and pancreatic cell dysfunction are present, it is thus essential to examine β-cell function in the presence of peripheral insulin resistance in PCOS.

In PCOS, fasting hyperinsulinemia is present in obese women, and insulin responses to an oral glucose load are increased in lean and obese PCOS women.[58,59] But acute insulin responses to an intravenous glucose load by hyperglycemic clamp demonstrated that first-phase insulin secretion is similar to weight-matched control women.[62,63] When insulin responses were graphed in relation to peripheral insulin sensitivity, however, lean and obese PCOS women fell below the weight-matched control women, and their responses were inadequate for their degree of insulin resistance.[64]

Further evidence for β-cell dysfunction is provided by the elegant studies of Ehrmann, who demonstrated defects in β-cell entrainment to an oscillatory glucose infusion and decreased meal-related insulin secretory responses.[61,65] In summary, the most compelling evidence suggests that β-cell dysfunction, in addition to insulin resistance, is a feature of PCOS.[64]

The cellular and molecular mechanism of insulin resistance in the PCOS remains controversial. Given the multiple steps between insulin binding to its receptor and the ultimate biologic action to increase glucose transport, it is clear that there are many potential levels for false transduction of the insulin message. Studies in adipocytes have not shown decreases in insulin receptor number or changes in insulin binding[59,66] but have revealed markedly decreased sensitivity and responsiveness. The above observations, normal insulin binding and abnormal sensitivity with decreased maximal rates of insulin-stimulated glucose transport, demonstrate that the major defect in insulin action seen in PCOS women is a post-binding defect. This decrease in maximal adipocyte responsiveness was secondary to a reduction of GLUT-4 glucose transporters.[67] Furthermore, it was found that in the absence of insulin the receptor autophosphorylation was normal, although there was a significant decrease in maximal insulin-stimulated autophosphorylation.[66] Studies from cultured fibroblasts from PCOS showed, consistent with our earlier results, no changes in binding or affinity. However, the increased basal autophosphorylation of the insulin receptor was associated with minimal further stimulation by insulin.[68] Phosphoamino acid analysis revealed decreased insulin-dependent receptor tyrosine phosphorylation and increased insulin-independent receptor serine phosphorylation in about 50% of PCOS women. Experimentally, serine phosphorylation of the insulin receptor results in decreased insulin receptor tyrosine kinase activity and a loss of insulin sensitivity similar to that seen in the PCOS serine phosphorylated insulin receptor. Thus, serine phosphorylation of the insulin receptor could function as an off signal, and the abnormal serine phosphorylation observed in some of the PCOS women might explain the concomitant decrease in tyrosine auto- and substrate phosphorylation. In the remainder of PCOS women without the serine phosphorylation defect, a defect further downstream in the signal transduction process may be involved.

Relationship and Molecular Aspects of Ovarian Hyperandrogenism and Hyperinsulinemia

Because the linear relationship between insulin and androgen concentrations has been described in women with PCOS, an ongoing debate has started regarding which is the primary defect. Several syndromes of extreme insulin resistance associated with ovarian hyperandrogenism have been characterized: for example, type A, due to mutations in the insulin receptor gene, and type B, due to anti-insulin receptor antibodies. Because a specific etiology has been identified, the associated hyperandrogenemia would appear to be a consequence of the hyperinsulinemia rather than vice versa.[1,69]

Furthermore, in PCOS women administration of insulin-lowering or -action facilitator agents, like diazoxide, somatostatin analogue, or metformin, results in decreased androgen effects or concentrations,[70,71]

Discrepancies, however, exist among different studies, regarding the effect of antiandrogenic therapy on insulin sensitivity. A 12-week therapy with a long-acting analogue of gonadotropin-releasing hormone (GnRH)[72] and another one of the same duration with an androgen receptor blocker[26] showed no significant change in insulin-mediated glucose disposal, using the same dose of insulin in the clamp studies. However, there is now evidence that androgens directly cause a small degree of insulin resistance in women, and antiandrogen therapy resulted in modest but significant improvement in insulin sensitivity in women with PCOS.[73] The discrepancy between these studies is probably due to the different doses of insulin used in the glucose clamp studies. Androgens decrease insulin sensitivity and amplify insulin resistance without altering maximal response in women, but these effects are sexually dimorphic, because in men estrogens produce insulin resistance.[74]

In the human ovary, insulin-binding sites have been identified, and insulin stimulates androgen production from the ovary *in vitro.*[75] However, because supraphysiologic insulin concentrations have been required to achieve these effects, another possibility has been put forward. Insulin may modify ovarian steroidogenesis by an alternative pathway, via IGF-1 receptors.[76]

Although insulin binds these receptors with low affinity, it is possible that at high concentrations either may stimulate them and/or may upregulate ovarian IGF-1 receptors and cause hyperandrogenism.[76] Furthermore, polycystic ovarian changes would appear to be a prerequisite for these insulin effects, because insulin does not alter androgen secretion in normal women.[77]

Full expression of the syndrome may require the interaction of an insulin abnormality with an underlying disorder of androgen biosynthesis, but an abnormality of insulin action alone is unlikely to cause hyperandrogenism.[77] The precise nature of the interaction of androgens and insulin awaits identification of the gene or genes involved, but this interaction provides a model that may begin to explain the heterogeneity of polycystic ovary syndrome.

GENETIC PREDISPOSITION

A strong familial predisposition exists for the development of PCOS.[1] Moreover, polycystic ovaries (detected by ultrasonography) occur with a striking frequency in the mothers and sisters of PCOS women.[78] The genetic basis of the syndrome remains controversial, because it is a disorder that affects women of reproductive age, and there is no clearly described male phenotype. A recent study of 150 subjects in 10 families of women with the syndrome, in which premature balding was used as the male phenotype, revealed evidence of an autosomal dominant mode of inheritance.[79] Dunaif has found that Caribbean Hispanic women have twice the prevalence of PCOS compared to other ethnic groups.[59,80] These PCOS women are also significantly more insulin resistant than non-Hispanic white women by euglycemic clamp determination of insulin-mediated glucose disposal.[80]

These findings suggest that the increased prevalence of PCOS in this ethnic group may be secondary to an increased prevalence of insulin resistance. However, additional susceptibility factors may be necessary for the development of PCOS. Many Caribbean Hispanic women are not afflicted with PCOS, despite insulin resistance of the same magnitude as non-Hispanic white PCOS women.[80] Two extremely exciting recent findings could explain the association of hyperandrogenemia and insulin resistance in PCOS by a single genetic defect. The first is that in 50% of PCOS women, defects have been found in insulin receptor phosphorylation, a decrease in tyrosine phosphorylation, and an increase in serine phosphorylation resulting in impaired insulin action.[68] The second one is that serine phosphorylation increases its 17,20-lyase activity of human P450c17, the key regulatory enzyme of both ovarian and adrenal androgen biosynthesis, resulting in augmented androgen secretion.[81]

CLINICAL PRESENTATION AND DIAGNOSIS

Hyperandrogenemia causes the peripheral manifestations from the pilocebaceous unit, and their intraovarian excess promotes follicular atresia and chronic anovulation. Hirsutism, acne, or male-pattern alopecia are the most frequent and characteristic clinical signs of PCOS. Anovulation manifests itself as menstrual irregularities, amenorrhea, oligomenorrhea, dysfunctional uterine bleeding, and infertility. Presentation as primary amenorrhea is rare, but menarche may be delayed. Obesity is common, and these obese subjects more frequently present with acanthosis nigricans, the cutaneous manifestations of hyperinsulinemia.

The diagnosis of PCOS is one of exclusion, usually based on the clinical, biochemical, and ultrasonographic criteria.

Biochemical Characteristics

Despite the clinical heterogenity of PCOS, the serum hormone profile in most women shows elevated serum androgens, acyclic estrogen levels in the midfollicular range of the normal menstrual cycle, and inappropriately elevated ratio of LH to FSH.

The principal characteristic of the syndrome is increased androgen production. Androgen elevations are typically mild to moderate. If testosterone levels are consistently >150 to 200 ng/dl when measured in an extraction and chromatography assay, or when DHEAS is >700 μg/dl, an ovarian or adrenal androgen-secreting neoplasm should be excluded. Women with PCOS have low levels of SHBG, and therefore elevated levels of biologically available testosterone. An ACTH stimulation test may be done during the initial visit in order to detect defects in adrenal steroid biosynthesis, which can present with the symptoms characteristic of PCO. A marked rise in 17OHP in response to ACTH is consistent with a diagnosis of adult-onset 21-hydroxylase deficiency. A similar rise in 17OH hydroxypregnenolone and an increase in the ratio of 17OHPreg to 17OHP of greater 4:1 are consistent with a diagnosis of 3β-hydroxysteroid dehydrogenase deficiency. Finally, because these young women are at significant risk of developing impaired glucose tolerance or frank diabetes mellitus, we recommend screening obese PCOS women with an oral glucose tolerance test.

In summary, the presence of hyperandrogenemia, oligomenorrea, or amenorrhea and the exclusion of other disorders is consistent with a diagnosis of PCOS.

TREATMENT

The therapeutic goals for women with PCOS include correcting androgen excess, preventing the manifestations of chronic unopposed estrogens, taking measures to improve insulin sensitivity, and finally overcoming infertility.

Correcting Hyperandrogenemia

Androgen Suppression

The use of an oral contraceptive is the simplest means of suppressing androgen levels. The low-estrogen pills effectively control acne and hirsutism by increasing SHBG level, but higher doses are required to suppress LH-hyperandrogenism. This, however, may exacerbate insulin resistance. Glucocorticoids are generally reserved for the treatment of congenital adrenal hyperplasia, and therapy should not be initiated empirically. Finally, long-acting GnRH agonists reversibly abolish LH-dependent ovarian androgen production by desensitizing pituitary gonadotrophs and decreasing LH secretion. Therapy with GnRH results in medical castration, ablating estrogen as well as androgen secretion, so its use is constrained by the risk of chronic hypoestrogenism.

Antiandrogens

In Europe, the most widely used antiandrogen is cyproterone acetate.[82] It is also progestogenic, and when combined with ethinyl estradiol it provides effective control of menses and contraception.

Cyproterone acetate is not generally available in the United States, but spironolactone, a mineralocorticoid antagonist that is also an antagonist of androgen receptors, has been used extensively.[83] It may be associated with erratic vaginal bleeding and is therefore usually administered with a low-dose oral contraceptive.

More recently there have been reports of the successful use of pure antiandrogens, such as flutamide, where impressive results regarding the improvement of hirsutism and acne have been reported.[26,84] Antiandrogens are the treatment of choice for androgen-dependent alopecia, but complete reversal of it is rare.

Ovulation Induction

Ovarian resection should no longer be considered for the management of fertility. Clomiphene citrate is the first-line therapy for induction of ovulation in PCOS. It is an orally active synthetic nonsteroidal agent with weak biological estrogen effects. Clomiphene inhibits estrogen-binding receptors, causing the hypothalamic–pituitary axis to perceive a low estrogen level.[85] This results in a rise in GnRH and gonadotropin level and subsequent ovulation. Using doses of 50 to 250 mg/day, 80% of women will ovulate, but only 20% of these will conceive. Patients who fail to ovulate or become pregnant while taking clomiphene may benefit from treatment with human menopausal gonadotropin combinations. Preparations exist containing equal amounts of LH and FSH, pure FSH, GnRH agonists, and pulsatile GnRH. There is increased risk of ovarian hyperstimulation and multiple births using these methods.

Endometrial Protection

Patients with PCOS are at risk of developing dysfunctional uterine bleeding and endometrial cancer. In women who have no stigmata of hyperandrogenism or who are not concerned with hirsutism, oral progestins (medroxyprogesterone acetate), 10 mg orally per day for 13 days every 4 to 8 weeks, will induce withdrawal bleeding and protect the endometrial lining.

Management of Metabolic Abnormalities

For many women with PCOS, the associated metabolic abnormalities of NIDDM and dyslipidemia are most important in terms of future health. At the present time, treatment for diabetes mellitus, dyslipidemia, and hypertension in women with androgenic disorders follows the same principles that apply to these conditions when they occur without associated androgenic disorders.[88] However, if insulin resistance could be considered the common denominator of the metabolic abnormalities of the syndrome, theraphentic agents correcting it might be the treatment of choice.

Insulin resistance is the mechanism of glucose intolerance associated with androgenic disorders; oral agents such as glipizide and glyburide are often effective in lowering glucose levels because insulin resistance is mild in most cases. Recently, treatment with troglitasone, of ciglitazone class, an oral hypoglycemic agent, appears to improve glucose metabolism as well as hyperandrogenemia in women with PCOS.[86]

Measures to improve insulin sensitivity should include diet, exercise, and agents that reduce insulin resistance. A reduction in body weight of as little as 15% may restore ovulatory function and reduce hyperandrogenemia in PCOS.[87] Metabolic changes seem to respond best to weight reduction. This can produce improved or normalized glucose tolerance, an increase in HDL cholesterol, a decrease in LDL cholesterol and triglycerides, and a reduction in blood pressure. If diabetes mellitus or obesity are present, or if even in lean anovulatory PCOS women marked insulin resistance is documented, treatment with metformin should be considered. This form of therapy decreases hyperinsulinemia and may thus also decrease androgen concentrations and their bioavailability, probably by decreasing hepatic production of SHBG.[71,89]

REFERENCES

1. Dunaif, A., J. K. Givens, F. Haseltine & Gr. Merriam, Eds. 1992. The Polycystic Ovary Syndrome. Mac Blackwell Scientific. Cambridge.
2. Polson, D. W., J. Wadsworth, J. Adams & S. Franks. 1988. Polycystic ovaries—A common finding in normal women. Lancet 870–872.
3. Petersson, F., H. Fries & S. J. Nillius. 1973. Epidemiology of secondary amenorrhea. Am. J. Obstet. Gynecol. **117:** 80–86.
4. Futterweit, W., & D. T. Krieger. 1979. Pituitary tumors associated with hyperprolactinemia and polycystic ovary disease. Fertil. Steril. **31:** 608–613.
5. Dewailly, D., M. C. Vantyghem, C. Lemaire, F. Duffose, A. Racadot & P. Fossati. 1988. Screening for 21-hydroxylase deficiency among hirsutise women: Lack of utility of the adrenocorticotropin hormone test. Fertil. Steril. **50:** 228–232.
6. Levin, J. H., E. Carmina & R. A. Lobo. 1991. Is the inappropriate gonadotropin secretion of patients with polycystic ovary syndrome similar to that of patients with adult-onset congenital adrenal hyperplasia? Fertil. Steril. **56:** 635–640.
7. Franks, S. 1989. Polycystic ovary syndrome: A changing perspective. Clin. Endocrinol. **31:** 87–120.
8. Conway, G. S., J. W. Honour & H. S. Jacobs. 1989. Heterogeneity of the polycystic ovary syndrome. Clin. Endocrinol. **30:** 459–470.
9. ODriscoll, J. B., H. Mamtora, J. Higginson, A. Pollock, J. Kane & D. C. Anderson. 1994. A prospective study of the prevalence of clear-cut endocrine disorders and polycystic ovaries in 350 patients with hirsutism or androgenic alopecia. Clin. Endocrinol. **41:** 231–236.
10. Pang, S., B. Softness, W. Sweeney & M. I. New. 1987. Hirsutism, polycystic ovarian disease and ovarian 17-ketosteroid reductase deficiency. N. Engl. J. Med. **316:** 1295–1301.
11. Clayton, R. N., V. Ogden, J. Hodgkinson, L. Worswick, D. A. Rodin, S. Dyer & T. W. Meade. 1992. How common are polycystic ovaries in normal women and what is their significance for the fertility of the population? Clin. Endocrinol. **37:** 127–134.

12. VENTUROLI, S., E. PORU, R. FABBRI, O. MAGRINI, L. GAMMI, R. PARADISI, M. FORACCI, *et al.* 1988. Episodic pulsative secretion of FSH, LH, prolactin, oestradiol, oestrone and LH circadian variations in polycystic ovary syndrome. Clin. Endocrinol. **28:** 93–107.

13. CHRISTMAN, G. M., J. F. RANDOLPH, R. P. KELCH & J. C. MARSHALL. 1991. Reduction of gonadotropin-releasing hormone pulse frequency is associated with subsequent selective follicle-stimulating hormone secretion in women with polycystic ovarian disease. J. Clin. Endocrinol. Metab. **72:** 1278–1285.

14. BLANKSTEIN, J., J. RABINOVICI, M. GOLDENBERG, J. SHALEY, A. MEHTA, D. M. SERR & S. MASHIACH. 1987. Changing pituitary reactivity to follicle-stimulating hormone and luteinizing hormone-releasing hormone after induced ovulatory cycles and after anovulation in patients with polycystic ovarian disease. J. Clin. Endocrinol. Metab. **65:** 1164–1167.

15. CUMMING, D. C., R. L. REID, M. E. QUIGLEY, R. W. REBAR & S. S. C. YEN. 1984. Evidence for decreased endogenous dopamine and opoid inhibitory influences on LH secretion in polycystic ovary syndrome. Clin. Endocrinol. **20:** 643–648.

16. BARNES, R. & R. A. LOBO. 1985. Central opioid activity in polycystic ovary syndrome with and without dopaminergic modulation. J. Clin. Endocrinol. Metab. **61:** 779–782.

17. BARNES, R. B., G. N. MIELEIKOWSKY, K. Y. CHA, C. A. SPENCER & R. A. LOBO. 1986. Effects of dopamine and metoclopramide in polycystic ovary syndrome. J. Clin. Endocrinol. Metab. **63:** 506–509.

18. MCKENNA, T. J. 1988. Current concepts: Pathogenesis and treatment of polycystic ovary syndrome. N. Engl. J. Med. **318:** 558–562.

19. CHANG, R. J., F. P. MANFDEL, J. K. LU & H. L. JUDD. 1982. Enhanced disparity of gonadotropin secretion by estrone in women with polycystic ovarian disease. J. Clin. Endocrinol. Metab. **60:** 773–778.

20. DUNAIF, A., C. LOONGCOPE, J. CANICK, T. BADGER & W. F. CROWLY, JR. 1985. The effects of the aromatase inhibitor delta-testosterone on gonadotropin release and steroid metabolism in polycystic ovarian disease. J. Clin. Endocrinol. Metab. **60:** 773–780.

21. YOUNG, J. R. & R. B. JAFFE. 1976. Strength-duration characteristics of estrogen effects on gonadotropin response to gonadotropin-releasing hormone in women. J. Clin. Endocrinol. Metab. **42:** 432–442.

22. ROSENFIELD, R. L. 1985. Congenital adrenal hyperplasia and reproductive function in females. *In* Adolescence in Females. C. Flamigni, S. Venturoli & J. Givens, Eds.: 373–387. Year Book Medical Publishers. Chicago.

23. SERAFINI, P., P. D. SILLV, R. J. PAULSEN, M. EKIND-HERNANDEZ & R. A. LOBO. 1986. Acute modulation of the hypothalamic–pituitary axis by intravenous testosterone in normal women. Am. J. Obstet. Gynecol. **155:** 1288–1292.

24. DUNAIF, A. 1986. Do androgens directly regulate gonadotropin secretion in the polycystic ovary syndrome? J. Clin. Endocrinol. Metab. **63:** 215–221.

25. DIAMANTI, E., N. KAKLAS, E. GEORGIADOU, J. SPINA, D. RANGOU & C. CHLOUVERAKIS. 1992. Intraovarian regulators and polycystic ovary syndrome. The effect of an androgen receptor blocker on gonadotropin release and androgen levels in PCO. Satellite symposium of the 9th International Congress of Endocrinology tr. No. 106.

26. DIAMANTI-KANDARAKIS, E., A. MITRAKOU, M. I. MAGDA, D. P. HENNES, N. KAKLAS, J. SPINA, E. GEORGIADOU, R. G. HOFFMAN, A. H. KISSEBACH & S. RAPTIS. 1995. Insulin sensitivity and androgens therapy in women with polycystic ovary syndrome. Metabolism **44:** 525–531.

27. ERICKSON, G. F. & S. S. C. YEN. 1984. New data on follicle cells in polycystic ovaries: A proposed mechanism for the genesis of cystic follicles. Semin. Reprod. Endocrinol. **2:** 231.

28. ERICKSON, G. 1986. An analysis of follicle development and ovum maturation. Ser. Reprod. Endocrinol. **4:** 233–254.

29. FUTTERWEIT, W. 1984. Hyperprolactinemia and polycystic ovarian disease. *In* Polycystic Ovarian Disease. W. Futterwit, Ed.: 97–111. Springer-Verlag. New York.
30. ERICKSON, G. F., D. A. MAGOFFIN, C. A. DYER & C. HOFEDITZ. 1985. The ovarian androgen producing cells: A review of structure/function relationships. Endocrinol. Rev. **6:** 371–399.
31. POLSON, D. W., S. FRANKS, M. J. REED, R. W. CHENG, J. ADAMS & V. H. JAMES. 1987. The distribution of oestradiol in plasma in relation to uterine cross-sectional area in women with polycystic or multifollicular ovaries. Clin. Endocrinol. **26:** 581–588.
32. ERICKSON, G. F. 1992. Folliculogenesis in polycystic ovary syndrome. *In* Current Issues in Endocrinology and Metabolism: Polycystic Ovary Syndrome. A. Dunaif, J. Givens, F. Haseltine & G. Merrlan, Eds. Blackwell Scientific. Cambridge, MA.
33. ERICKSON, G. F., V. G. GARZO & D. A. MAGOFFIN. 1989. Insulin-like growth factor 1 regulates aromatase activity in human granulosa and granulosa luteal cells. J. Clin. Endocrinol. Metab. **69:** 716–724.
34. ERICKSON, G. F., A. J. HSUEH, M. E. QUIGLLEY, R. W. RADAR & S. S. YEN. 1979. Functional studies of aromase activity in human granulosa cells from normal and polycystic ovaries. J. Clin. Endocrinol. Metab. **49:** 514–519.
35. FRANKS, S. & H. D. MASON. 1991. Polycystic ovary syndrome: Interaction of follicle stimulating hormone and polypeptide growth factors in oestradiol production by human granulosa cells. J. Steroid Biochem. Mol. Biol. **40:** 405–409.
36. CONTE, F. A., M. M. GRUMBACH, Y. ITO, C. R. FISHER & E. R. SIMPSON. 1994. A syndrome of female pseudohermaphroditism, hypergonadotropic hypogonadism, and multicystic ovaries associated with missense mutations in the gene encoding aromatase (P450). J. Clin. Endocrinol. Metab. **78:** 1287–1292.
37. SHERMAN, A. I. & S. BROWN. 1979. The precursors of endometrial carcinoma. Am. J. Obstet. Gynecol. **135:** 947–956.
38. HILLIER, S. G. & G. T. ROSS. 1979. Effects of exogenous testosterone on ovarian weight, follicular morphology and intraovarian progesterone concentration in estrogen-primed hypophysectomised immature female rats. Bil. Reprod. **20:** 61–68.
39. HOFFMAN, F. & C. MEGER. 1965. On the action of intraovarian injection of androgen on follicle and corpus luteum maturation in women. Geburst. Frauenheik. **25:** 1132–1137.
40. PANG, S., B. SOFTNESS, W. SWEENEY & M. I. NEW. 1987. Hirsutism, polycystic ovarian disease and ovarian 17-ketosteroid reductase deficiency. N. Engl. J. Med. **316:** 1295–1301.
41. RHEAUME, E., Y. LACHANCE, H-F. ZHAO, N. BRETON, M. DUMONT, Y. DE LAUNOIT, C. TRUDEL, V. LUU-THE, J. SIMARD & F. LABRIE. 1991. Structure and expression of a new complementary DNA encoding the almost exclusive 3b-hydroxysteroid dehydrogenase/D5-D4 isomerase in human adrenals and gonads. Mol. Endocrinol. **5:** 1147–1157.
42. ROSEFIELD, R. L., R. B. BARNES, J. F. CARA & A. W. LUCKY. 1990. Dysregulation of cytochrome P450c 17 alpha as the case of polycystic ovarian syndrome. Fertil. Steril. **53:** 785–791.
43. WHITE, D., A. LEIGH, C. WILSON, A. DONALSON & C. FRANKS. 1995. Gonadotropin and gonadal steroid response to a dose of long-acting agonist of gonadotropin releasing hormone in ovulatory and anovulatory women with polycystic ovary syndrome. Clin. Endocrinol. **42:** 475–481.
44. VOUTILAINEN, R., J. TAPANAINEN, B-C. CHUNG, K. J. MATTESON & W. L. MILLER. 1986. Hormonal regulation of P450 scc(20- 22-desmolase) and P450c17(17α-hydroxylase/17,20-lyase) in cultures human granulosa cell. J. Clin. Endocrinol. Metab. **63:** 202–207.
45. EHRMANN, D. A., R. L. ROSENFIELD, R. BARNES, D. F. BRIGELL & Z. SHEIKH. 1992. Detection of functional ovarian hyperandrogenism in women with androgen excess. N. Engl. J. Med. **327:** 157–162.

46. ROSENFILD, R. L., R. B. BARNES & D. A. EHRMANN. 1994. Studies of the nature of 17-hydroxyprogesterone hyperresponsiveness to gonadotropin releasing hormone agonist challenge in functional ovarian hyperandrogenism. J. Clin. Endocrinol. Metab. **79:** 1686–1692.
47. ROSENFILD, R. L., R. B. BARNES & D. A. EHRMAN. 1994. Studies of the nature of 17-hydroxyprogesterone hyperresponsiveness to gonadotropin releasing hormone agonist challenge in functional ovarian hyperandrogenism. J. Clin. Endocrinol. Metab. **79:** 1686–1692.
48. GILING-SMITH, C., D. S. WILIS, R. W. BEARD & S. FRANKS. 1994. Hypersecretion of androstenedione by isolated cells from polycystic ovaries. J. Clin. Endocrinol. Metab. **79:** 1158–1165.
49. CONWAY, G. S., J. W. HONOUR & H. S. JACOBS. 1989. Heterogeneity of the polycystic ovary syndrome. Clin. Endocrinol. **30:** 459–470.
50. LOBO, R. A. 1991. Hirsutism in polycystic ovary syndrome: Current concepts. Clin. Obstet. Gynecol. **34:** 817–826.
51. BARDIN, C. W. & M. B. LIPSETT. 1967. Testosterone and androstenedione blood production rates in normal women and women with idiopathic hirsutism or polycystic ovaries. J. Clin. Invest. **46:** 891–902.
52. ADERSON, D. C. 1974. Sex-hormone-binding-globulin. Clin. Endocrinol. **3:** 69–96.
53. PUGEAT, M., J. C. CRAVE, M. ELMIDANI, *et al.* 1991. Pathophysiology of sex hormone binding globulin (SHBG): Relation to insulin. J. Steroid Biochem. Mol. Biol. **40:** 841–849.
54. BURGEN, G. A., J. R. GIVENS & A. E. KITABCHI. 1980. Correlation of hyperandrogenism with hyperinsulism in polycystic ovarian disease. J. Clin. Endocrinol. Metab. **50:** 113–116.
55. DUNAIF, A. 1993. Insulin resistance in polycystic ovarian syndrome. Ann. N.Y. Acad. Sci. **687:** 60–64.
56. KING, H. & M. REWERS. 1993. Global estimates or prevalence of diabetes mellitus and impaired glucose tolerance in adults. Diabetes Care **16:** 157–177.
57. HARRIS, M. I., W. C. HADDEN, W. C. KWOLER & P. H. BENNETT. 1987. Prevalence of diabetes and impaired glucose tolerance and plasma glucose levels in U.S. population aged 20–74 yr. Diabetes **36:** 523–534.
58. DUNAIF, A., M. GRAF, J. MANDELI, V. LAUMAS & A. DOBJANSKI. 1987. Characterization of groups of hyperandrogenic women with acanthosis nigricans, impaired glucose tolerance and/or hyperinsulinemia. J. Endocrinol. Metab. **65:** 499–507.
59. DUNAIF, A., W. FUTTERWEIT, K. R. SEGAL & A. DOBRJANSKY. 1989. Profound peripheral insulin resistance, independentn of obesity, in the polycystic ovary syndrome. Diabetes **38:** 1165–1174.
60. OVESEN, R., J. MOLLER, H. J. INGERSELEV, J. O. L. JORGENSEN, A. MENGEL, Q. SCHMITZ, K. G. M. M. ALBERTI & N. MOLER. 1993. Normal basal and insulin-stimulated fuel metabolism in lean women with polycystic ovary syndrome. J. Clin. Endocrinol. Metab. **77:** 1636–1640.
61. OMeara, N. M., J. D. Blackman, D. A. Ehrmann, R. B. Barnes, J. B. Jaspan, R. L. Rosenfield & K. S. Polonsky. 1993. Defects in b-cell function in functional ovarian hyperandrogenism. J. Clin. Endocrinol. Metab. **76:** 1241–1247.
62. DE FRONZO, R. A., J. D. TOBIN & R. ANDRES. 1979. Glucose clamp technique: A method for quantifying insulin secretion and resistance. Am. J. Physiol. **237:** E214–223.
63. DIAMANTI-KANDARAKIS, E., A. MIRTRAKOU, D. PLATANISSIOTIS, G. SPINA, E. DYTELIS, S. PAPTIS. (Sponsor: S. Nader). 1994. Polycystic ovary syndrome: A model of primary defect of insulin action. First and second Department of Medicine, University of Athens Medical School, Greece. Abstract No. 834. 76th Annual Meeting Endocrine Society, Anaheim, CA.

64. DUNAIF, A. & D. FINEGOOD. 1996. b-Cell dysfunction independent of obesity and glucose intolerance in the polycystic ovary syndrome. J. Clin. Endocrinol. Metab. **81:** 3.942–3.947.
65. ERRHMAN, D. A., R. B. BARNES & R. L. ROSENFILD. 1995. Polycystic ovary syndrome as a form of functional ovarian hyperandrogenism due to dysregulation of androgen secretion. Endoc. Rev. **16:** 322–353.
66. GARALDI, T. P., A. EL-ROEIY, Z. MADAR, D. REICHART, J. M. OLEFSKY & S. S. C. YEN. 1992. Cellular mechanisms of insulin resistance on polycystic ovarian syndrome. J. Clin. Endocrinol. Metabol. **75:** 577–583.
67. ROSENBAUM, D., R. S. HABER & A. DUNAIF. 1993. Insulin resistance in polycystic ovary syndrome: Decreased expression of GLUT-4 glucose transporters in adipocytes. Am. J. Physiol. **264:** 197–202.
68. DUNAIF, A., J. XIA, C-B. BOOK, E. SCHENKER & Z. TANG. 1995. Excessive insulin receptor serine phosphorylation in cultured fibroblasts and in skeletal muscle: A potential mechanism for insulin resistance in the polycystic ovary syndrome. J. Clin. Invest. **96:** 801–810.
69. KAHN, C. R., J. S. FLIER, R. S. BAR, J. A. ARCHER, P. GORDEN, M. M. MARTIN & J. ROTH. 1976. The syndromes of insulin resistance and acanthosis nigricans. N. Engl. J. Med. **294:** 739–745.
70. NESTLER, J. E., C. O. BARLASCINI, D. W. MATT, *et al.* 1989. Suppression of serum insulin by diazoxide reduces testosterone levels in obese women with polycystic ovary syndrome. J. Clin. Endocrinol. Metab. **68:** 1027.
71. VELAZGUEZ, E. M., S. MENTOZA, T. HAMER, F. SOSA & C. J. GLUECK. 1994. Metformin therapy in polycystic ovary syndrome reduces hyperinsulinemia, insulin resistance, hyperandrogenemia and systolic blood pressure, while facilitating normal menses and pregnancy. Metabolism **43:** 647–654.
72. DUNAIF, A., G. GREEN, W. FUTTERWEIT & A. DOBRJANSKY. 1990. Suppression of hyperandrogenism does not improve peripheral of hepatic insulin resistance in the polycystic ovary syndrome. J. Clin. Endocrinol. Metab. **70:** 699–704.
73. MOGHETTI, P., F. TOSI, R. CASTELLO, *et al.* Antiandrogens and insulin action. J. Clin. Endocrinol. Metab. In press.
74. POLDERMAN, K. H., J. K. GOOREN, H. ASSCHERMAN, A. BAKKER & R. J. HEINE. 1994. Induction of insulin resistance by androgens and estrogens. J. Clin. Endocrinol. Metab. **79:** 265–271.
75. BARBIERI, R. L. 1992. Effects of insulin on ovarian steroidogenesis. *In* Polycystic Ovary Syndrome. A. Dunaif, J. H. Givens, F. P. Haseline, *et al.*, Eds. Blackwell Scientific. Cambridge, MA.
76. ADASHI, E. Y. 1993. Intraovarian regulation: The proposed role of insulin-like growth factors. Ann. N.Y. Acad. Sci. **687:** 10–12.
77. NESTLER, J. E., J. N. CLORE & W. G. BLACKARD. 1992. Effects of insulin on steroidogenesis in vivo. *In* Polycystic Ovary Syndrome. A. Dunaif, J. R. Givens, F. P. Halestine, G. R. Merriam, Eds.: 265–278. Blackwell Scientific. Oxford, England.
78. HAGUE, W. M., J. ADAMS, S. T. REEDERS, T. E. A. PETO & H. S. JACOBS. 1988. Familial polycystic ovaries: A genetic disease? Clin. Endocrinol. **29:** 593–605.
79. CAREY, A. H., K. L. CHAN, F. SHORT, D. WHITE, R. WILLIAMSON & S. FRANKS. 1993. Evidence for a single gene effect causing polycystic ovaries and male pattern baldness. Clin. Endocrinol. **38:** 653–658.
80. SORBARA, L., D. WEISS, R. DELSON, C. RICHARDS, A. DOBRJANSKY & A. DUNAIF. 1991. Polycystic ovary syndrome, ethnicity and insulin action. 14th IDF Congress Satellite on Epidemiology of Diabetes. Williamsburg, VA. Abstr.
81. ZHANG, L., H. RODRIGUEZ, S. OHNO, *et al.* 1995. Serine phosphorylation of human

P450c17 increase 17,20 lyase activity: Implications for adrenarche and polycystic ovary syndrome. Proc. Natl. Acad. Sci. USA **92:** 10619–10623.

82. Vermulen, A. & R. Rubens. 1988. Effects of cyproterone acetate plus ethinylestradiol low dose on plasma androgens and lipids in mildly hirsute or acneic young women. Contraception (USA) **38:** 419–428.
83. Barth, J. H., C. A. Cherry, F. Wojnarowska & R. P. Dawer. 1989. Spironolactone is an effective and well tolerated systemic antiandrogen therapy for hirsute women. J. Clin. Endocrinol. Metab. **68:** 966–970.
84. Cusan, L., J. L. Dupond, R. R. Gomez, Tremblay & F. Labrie. 1994. Comparison of flutamide and spironolactone in the treatment of hirsutism: A randomized controlled trial. Fertil. Steril. **61:** 281–287.
85. Adashi, E. Y. 1986. Clomiphene citrate-induced ovulation: Aclinical update. Semin. Reprod. Endocrinol. **4:** 255–275.
86. Hofman, C. A., C. W. Edwards III, R. M. Hilman & J. R. Colca. 1992. Treatment of insulin-resistant mice with oral antidiabetic agent pioglitazone: Evaluation of liver GLUT2 and prosphoenolpyruvate carboxykinase expression. Endocrinology **130:** 735–740.
87. Kiddy, D. S., D. Hamilton Fairley, A. Bush, F. Short, V. Anyakou, M. J. Reed & S. Franks. 1992. Improvement in endocrine and ovarian function during dietary treatment of obese women with polycystic ovary syndrome. Clin. Endocrinol. **36:** 105–111.
88. Geoffrey, P. R. 1995. Androgenic disorders of women: Diagnostic and therapeutic decision making. Am. J. Med. Assoc. **98:** 120–129s.
89. Diamanti-Kandarakis, E., Ch. Kouli & G. Tolis. 1996. Therapeutic effect of Metformin on insulin resistance and hyperandrogenism in the polycystic ovary syndrome(PCO). Abstr. No. P~808. Proceedings of the 10th International Congress of Endocrinology (ICE '96). San Francisco, CA.

Adolescent Polycystic Ovary Syndrome

V. DRAMUSIC, U. RAJAN, P. CHAN, S. S. RATNAM, AND Y. C. WONG

Department of Obstetrics and Gynaecology and Psychosocial Medicine
National University Hospital and School Health Service
Lower Kent Road
Singapore 119074

INTRODUCTION

Adolescent medicine, based on the physiological processes of puberty and general maturation, has developed dramatically over the past few decades. The population of persons in the period of puberty and adolescence has been identified as a healthy population, but one at relatively high risk. This is one of the most dramatic and fascinating periods of human life, when processes of physical, mental, and social maturation take place.

During female puberty and adolescence, the hypothalamo–pituitary–ovarian (HPO) axis matures, resulting ultimately in the capacity for full reproductive potential.[1–4] These processes are gradual, however, and it may take up to five gynecological years for regular ovulatory cycles to get established.[5–7] Menstrual dysfunction and anovulatory cycles are very common, in particular during the first two years after menarche,[8–12] and in most instances are short lived. In some young women, however, these may be early manifestations of persistent menstrual disorder; hence, the importance of detecting in adolescence conditions that may progressively lead into reproductive disorders.

During the process of maturation, not everything goes smoothly, and certain conditions, like acne, hirsutism, menstrual irregularities and polycystic ovary syndrome can occur. In fact such conditions usually have their onset in adolescence, but may influence the entire adult life of a woman.[13,14] For these reasons, in recent years there has been an increased interest in diagnosing polycystic ovarian syndrome (PCOS) in adolescents.[15,16] Many women with PCOS have menstrual disturbances that begin in adolescence. Also, the menstrual irregularities, hirsutism,[17] and acne associated with PCOS may be a source of significant concern for the adolescent female since body image and self esteem are important factors that affect social interaction within peer groups.

MATERIAL AND METHODS

Clinics for Paediatric and Adolescent Gynaecology in National University Hospital (Singapore) and School Health Institute were established in mid-1984, and over 3000 patients were seen. The first 700 girls who had menstrual disorders underwent identical screening, and the majority of them have been under follow-up observation for five or more years. Patients have undergone clinical examinations; endocrinological screening on the level of pituitary, adrenal, and ovary; ultrasound scanning; karyotyping; CT scan and GnRH; or other stimulation tests when necessary.

Endocrine evaluation has been done in our research laboratory. It included plasma levels of FSH, LH, estradiol (E_2), testosterone (T), prolactin (PRL), cortisol, dihydrotestosterone (DHT), androstenedione (A), dehydroepiandrosterone-sulfate (DHEA-S), 17-hydroxyprogesterone (17 OHP), and estrone (E_1), measured by in-house radioimmunoassays. World Health Organization–matched reagents were used for assaying the first six hormones, and those for the DHEA-S, A, and E_1 were purchased from Wien Laboratory (USA). Antisera to DHT and 17 OHP were raised in rabbit models by our laboratory.

Transabdominal ultrasound scanning (U/S) was performed in all cases. The ultrasound and scanning measurements are done with Acuson 128/×P10, and Hitachi 565A. Ovarian volume is calculated using the standard formula for ellipsoid = length × width × height × 0.52.

During the last two years insulin and sex hormone binding globulin (SHBG) were assayed in 50 patients together with psychological screening, including Piers-Harris self-concept scale for self esteem, Eating Attitudes Test,[18] Cattell 16 PF personality questionnaire, and the Hospital Anxiety and Depression Scale.[19]

Major groups of patients were as follows: dysfunctional uterine bleeding (DUB) (167 = 23.9%); primary amenorrhea or delayed puberty (128 = 18.3%); secondary amenorrhea (288 = 41%); and oligomenorrhea (118 = 16.8%). From all these groups emerged important subgroups relating to hyperandrogenic stimulation: PCOS (179 = 25.6%) and the PCOS-like group (some but not all PCOS features; 73 = 10.4%).

Because there is no general consensus on all features that are accepted as typical for PCOS, we developed three levels of parameters to be present for labeling our PCOS cases:

- clinical features: menstrual irregularities and/or acne/hirsutism, often obesity;
- endocrine features: reversed LH/FSH ratio and increase in androgens;
- U/S features: increased volume and morphological changes including dense stroma, subcapsular cysts, and thickened capsule.

All adolescents with PCOS were assessed in an identical manner; however, 150 patients had repeated endocrinologic and ultrasound screening at least once after one year. All figures relate to the group of 150 adolescents with PCOS.

CLINICAL FEATURES

Ages of all patients when first seen ranged between 12 and 22 years of age. The majority were between 15 and 18 years (76.7%, 115 cases). Interestingly, very few (16% or 24) of the patients came to the clinic at the later age, suggesting that symptoms of PCOS usually appear early. Early onset of the disorder is also evidenced by the number of girls seen in their early teens, between 12 and 14 years (7.3%, 11).

Most of the girls came to the Adolescent Clinic between the third and fifth gynecological year (56.8%, 84); fewer waited longer (16%, 24). These data indicate persistence of menstrual disorder. Remaining patients included 14% (21) with primary amenorrhea and another 14% seen already during the first or second gynecological year.

A considerable proportion of girls were early maturers, experiencing menarche between 9 and 12 years of age in 52.8% (79) of the cases. The mean age for menarche for Singapore girls is 12.6 ± 1.3 years, which is later than for PCOS patients. It is important not to forget that primary amenorrhea was the major complaint of 14.0% (21), leaving only 33.2% of girls with PCOS reaching menarche at 12 years or older.

All patients presented with menstrual disorders of some kind. Secondary amenorrhea of up to one year was present in 16% (24), menarche only in 10.7% (16), oligomenorrhea in 19.3% (29), dysfunctional uterine bleeding in 19.3% (29), and primary amenorrhea in 14.0% (21 cases). Girls with primary amenorrhea came to the clinic by the age of 15 to 16, most with hirsutism and/or acne and obesity (FIG. 1).

In addition to menstrual disorders, other clinical features suggestive of PCOS were acne and hirsutism, both seen in 52.6% (79) of cases. Only those cases of moderate acne (64.6%, 51) and severe acne (11.4%, 9) as well as moderate (32.9%, 26) and severe (6.3%, 5) hirsutism are of clinical importance (FIG. 2). These cases correlated well with degree of hyperandrogenism confirmed endocrinologically. Ethnic correlation to excess androgen stimulation showed hirsutism predominantly among Indian girls with acne being predominant among Chinese girls. Both acne and hirsutism were combined among all ethnic groups; yet hirsutism among Chinese girls was presented mainly as long hairs around nipples, along the linea alba, above the upper lip, in contrast to a more generalized and prominent pattern among Indian and Malay girls. Both acne and hirsutism were demonstrated in 29.3% (44) of cases.

To evaluate the possible impact of variations of body weight on the endocrine profiles, patients were categorized into three groups according to ideal body weight (IBW) which was calculated as a percentage of the standard weight for the height for

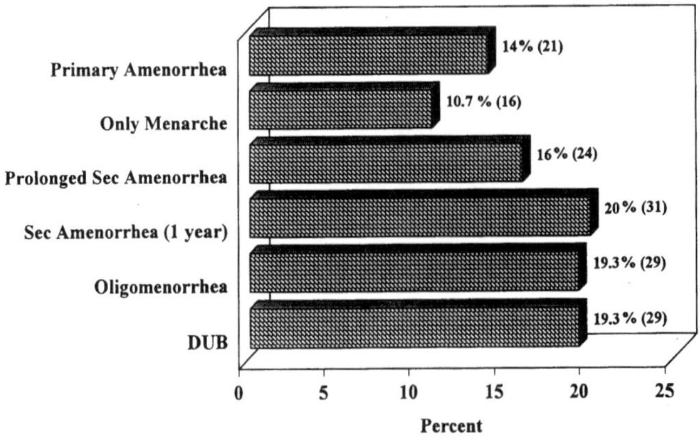

FIGURE 1. Types of menstrual disorder among PCOS patients.

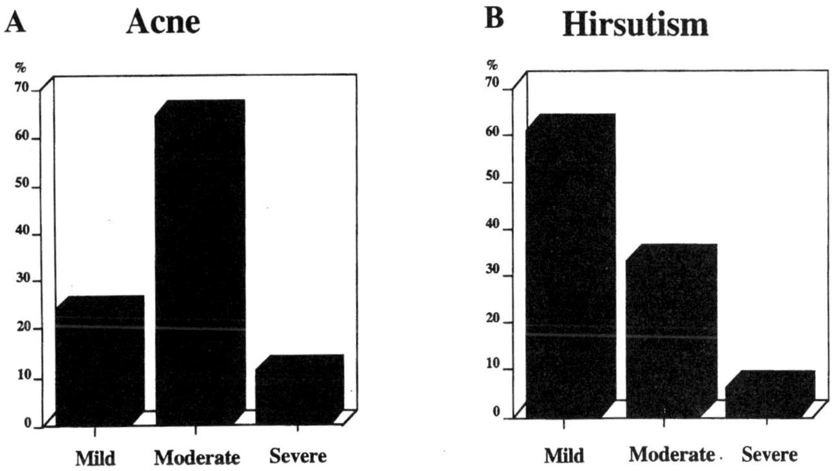

FIGURE 2. Acne (**A**) and hirsutism (**B**) among PCOS patients.

a Singapore population matched for sex and age. Group I: thin (<85% IBW), 9.3% (14); Group II: normal weight (86–120% IBW), 63.3% (95); and Group III: obese (>120% IBW) 27.4% (41). The grossly obese (up to 210% IBW) made up 10.6% (16) of cases.

There is a possible relation between body weight and type/length of menstrual disorder. If the percentage of obese girls is related to type of menstrual disorder, it becomes evident that majority of obese girls belonged to groups with primary amenorrhea (42.9% being obese), menarche only (37.5% obese), or prolonged secondary amenorrhea (33.3% obese). Normal body weight was the predominant feature among cases with DUB, oligomenorrhea, or secondary amenorrhea of shorter duration. The majority of skinny girls had DUB (FIG. 3). Importantly, excessive obesity may not provide an indication of the severity of the endocrine dysfunction in adolescents with PCOS, but it can significantly influence the outcome of treatment among these patients.

ULTRASOUND FINDINGS

We consider ultrasound an important and reliable tool that is most helpful in distinguishing genuine cases of PCOS from those whose clinical and/or hormonal findings are merely suggestive of PCOS. Ultrasound findings typical for PCOS include enlarged ovaries (volume exceeding 6 ml), accompanied in all cases by morphological changes in the ovaries: thickened capsule, multiple subcapsular cysts, and hypoechogenic, dense stroma. The decision to take an ovarian volume of 6 ml as the upper limit of normal was based on our ultrasound standards of normal for our adolescent population.[20] Interestingly, ultrasound findings showed more pronounced changes on

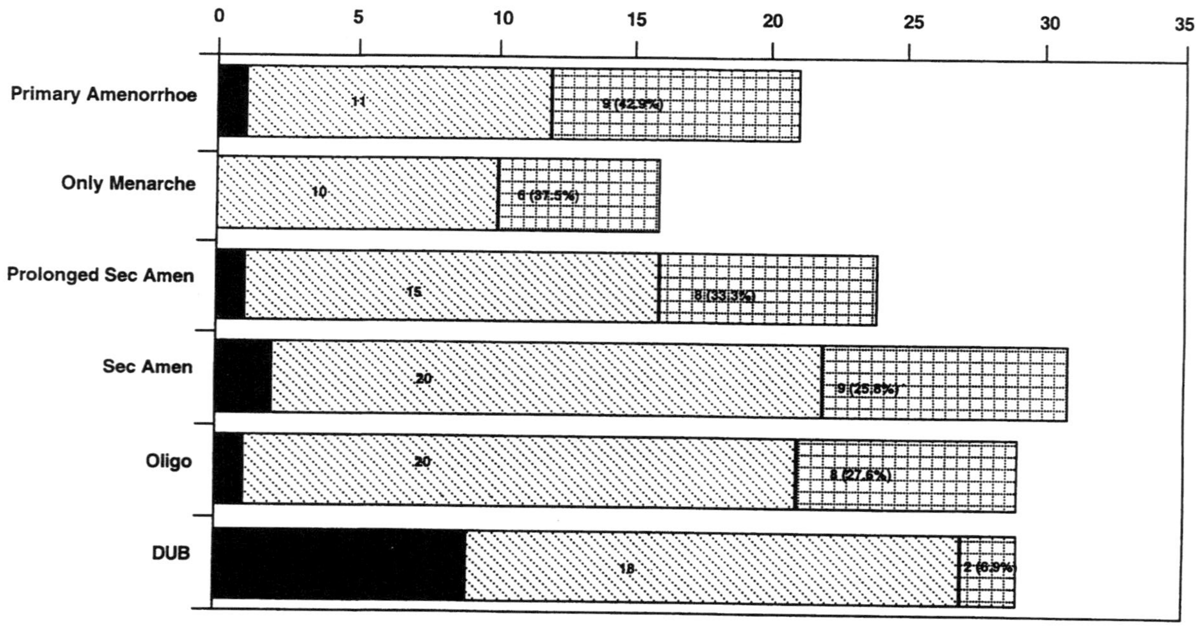

FIGURE 3. Relationship between body weight and type of menstrual disorder. ■ Thin, ▦ obese, ▨ normal.

the right ovary, particularly when volume exceeded 11.0 ml. In extreme cases, the right ovary measured up to 28 ml, whereas the left ovary never exceeded 23 ml.

Among our PCOS patients, right ovary volume was between 8 and 14 ml in the majority of cases (60%); volume was of lesser degree, 6–8 ml, in 16%; above 14 ml was seen in 24%. Left ovary findings were more favorable: less than 8 ml in 31.4%, 8 to 14 ml in 50%, and above that in 18.6%.

ENDOCRINE PROFILES

Endocrine profiles of adolescents with polycystic ovary syndrome were typical of those in adults. Androgen levels were high: 64% had total testosterone levels above 0.8% ng/ml (the upper limit of normal) and dihydrotestosterone (DHT) above 200 pg/ml (the mean of normal women) in 56%. In 31.3% of patients, testosterone levels were greater than 1.0 ng/ml with several as high as >2.0 ng/ml (FIG. 5B). In 2.7% of cases the DHT levels were higher than 500 pg/ml levels, these levels approach the male range. Possible adrenal contribution to hyperandrogenization in PCOS was seen in the form of raised androstenedione (>2,500 pg/ml) in 29.3%. However, plasma concentration of DHEA-S was raised >2,500 μg/ml only in 4.7%

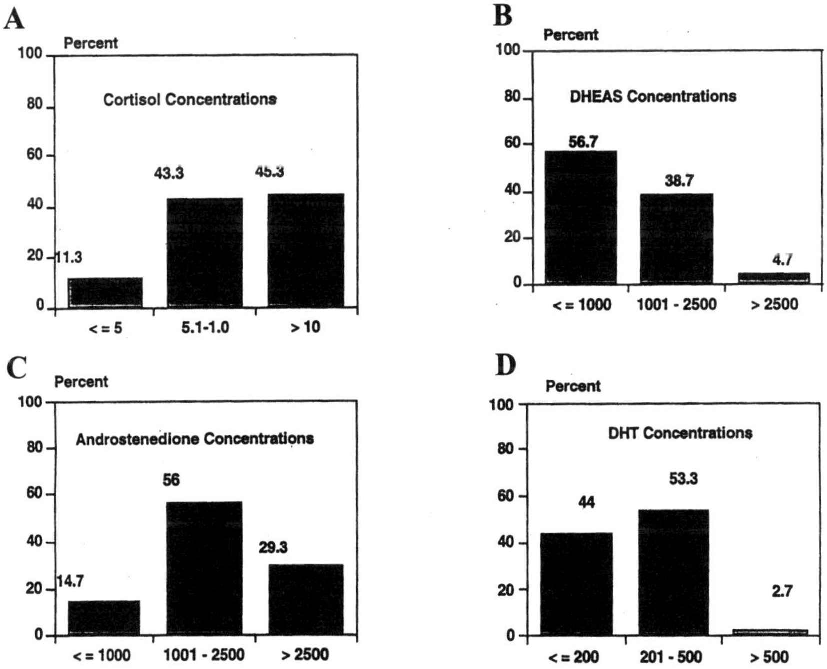

FIGURE 4. Hormonal levels before treatment: (**A**) cortisol concentrations (μg/dl), (**B**) DHEAS concentrations (μg/ml), (**C**) androstenedione concentrations (mIU/l), and (**D**) DHT concentrations (pg/ml).

of patients (FIG. 4). Cortisol was raised in 45.3% of patients. All cases in the study had normal prolactin levels (<500 mIU/l). Estradiol levels in adolescents with PCOS, as in adults, were not characteristic; most had follicular-phase level, and only 6% had levels above 200 pg/ml.

Almost 60% of patients had significantly raised LH levels (57.3%); however, 91.3% had levels that were either high or above normal range. Follicle-stimulating hormone, on the other hand, remained either on the low or within-normal range. This typically resulted in the reversal of the LH/FSH ratio, with 90% having a ratio above 2, of which 63.3% were above 3; only 10% were near a normal ratio of 1.5 to 2 (FIG. 5A).

The endocrine profiles of adolescents with PCOS were not different from adults with PCOS. Similarly, a complex endocrine derangement was seen in this group of adolescents.

PSYCHOLOGICAL SCREENING

All patients were asked to fill in a self-rating questionnaire including basic demographic information, the hospital anxiety and depression scale, and the eating disorder inventory.

The girls were asked about specific concerns regarding the diagnosis of their illness. They were also asked if they would welcome the chance to meet with others suffering PCOS to learn more about it and how to cope with it.

The following results revealed that the patients were from 14 to 22 years old, mean age being 17.6 years. Their educational level ranged from the secondary to the tertiary level, and the mean attainment was "O" level; 71% were students.

Specific concerns of our patients included the following:

- 87.5% were unhappy about their body weight;
- 71% were unhappy about their height;
- 86.6% did not have a boyfriend;

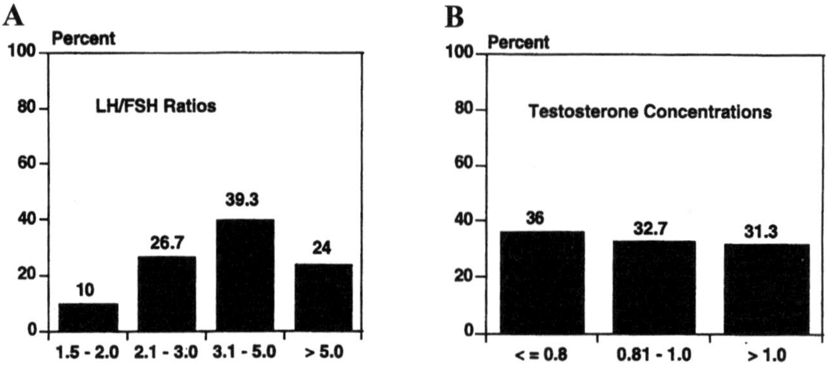

FIGURE 5. Hormone levels before treatment: (**A**) LH/FSH ratios and (**B**) testosterone concentrations (ng/ml).

- 100% were not sexually active;
- 75% were concerned about possible future infertility;
- 33.3% were concerned abut their attractiveness to the opposite sex; and
- 75% were distressed over the diagnosis of PCOS because of irregular menses (83%), effects of being overweight (78%), hair loss (17%), acne (17%), and hirsutism (11%).

Only 17% were able to identify a precipitating life event, schoolwork stress, associated with the onset of menstrual irregularities/obesity.

The Eating Disorder Inventory is an instrument with eight subscales, as well as a total score. The mean subscale scores of our sample group with PCOS were compared with mean from a group of 16-year-old Singaporean girls (n = 654) and a group (n = 64) of American undergraduates.

Our adolescent PCOS group appears to have:

- high "drive for thinness" scores,
- high "body dissatisfaction" scores,
- high "interpersonal distrust" scores.

All mentioned are significantly different from the scores of the Singapore control group. Data is also significantly different from the sample of American undergraduates, showing higher levels of personal ineffectiveness, introspective awareness, and maturity fears among our PCOS adolescents. It is important that 58% of girls expressed a desire to communicate with others with PCOS, although this is lower than the 85% in a similar study done with renal patients undergoing dialysis. Possibly, social support from peers or family is enough for the 42% of PCOS girls who responded negatively, or perhaps the stress of group work may be too great for self-conscious adolescents.

TREATMENTS FOR PCOS IN ADOLESCENCE

Our approach to the treatment of PCOS can be summarized as follows: if the patient is very young, we usually give only gestagens; if marked acne, hirsutism, or persistent menstrual disorder are present, we prescribe antiandrogens (cyproterone acetate); when very marked hirsutism is present, we give high doses of antiandrogens. Body weight correction is a valid adjuvant treatment. Oral contraceptives are not well accepted as a treatment for PCOS among the Asian population and are not often used, except in the case of a few older teenagers who have become sexually active.

Although various treatments were offered to our patients, the majority of them 82.6% (124) were treated with antiandrogen cyproterone acetate (in a preparation containing 2 mg + 35 μg ethinyl estradiol (EE) in a 3-week course per month (the preparation exhibits oral contraceptive properties, but it is not listed as such). Cyproterone acetate is an antiandrogen with progestational behavior; it competes with androgens at the end-organ level and also suppresses the hypothalamus. Added ethinyl estradiol elevates SHBG, thus decreases free androgens, ensures cyclicity, and prevents pregnancy. Treatment was given for a minimum of six months, but is often continued for up to 12 or even 18 months (hirsutism and severe acne) or repeated after a period of nontreatment. Each group made up nearly one-third of the full group with regard to length of treatment. Eleven girls (7.3%) defaulted treatment after an initial period of 1 to 3 months, at times restarting it (off and on). Twelve girls with hirsutism were given higher doses of antiandrogens—50–100 mg of cyproterone acetate daily added to the first 10 days of cycle treatment.

Several months after completion of initial treatment or when recurrences appeared, 1 to 2 cycles of low-dose clomiphene citrate were given in 67 girls, and results were excellent for 68.7% (46). Most of these girls had presented with cases of DUB, oligomenorrhea or secondary amenorrhea of shorter duration, and were nonobese. However, clomiphene failed to trigger hypothalamic–pituitary response in 31.4% (21) of girls principally from groups with primary amenorrhea, menarche only or prolonged secondary amenorrhea, and/or obese. At these early years of our project, clomiphene served as a simple test to judge time of restitution of cyclicity. However, as a result of new information on the possible long-term effects of this treatment, use of clomiphene was discontinued and substituted with gestagens.[21]

Fourteen girls (9.4%) opted for treatment with gestagens, and 12 (8%) defaulted or decided on no treatment except observation, usually at parents' request.

OUTCOME OF THE TREATMENT

Outcome of the treatment and the parameters influencing it may be observed from various angles; for example, one can judge the effect of treatment on acne, hirsutism, and cyclic ovarian function.

Following treatment, acne resolved completely or showed visible improvement in 93.7% of the patients. Remarkably successful outcome of the treatment of acne must be in part due to skin (end organ) response to antiandrogens. A varying degree of improvement in hirsutism was noted in 60.8% of girls.

Importantly, cyclic function either was normalized or improved in 62.7% (94) of girls. However, the situation remained unchanged in 11.3% (17) and in 26% (39) it worsened. Restoration of cyclic function was assessed not only on a clinical basis but also by comparison of repeated hormonal levels and U/S targeted for not earlier than one year from previous investigations and not earlier than three months after discontinuation of treatment. Increasingly, patients are undergoing a third round of follow-up investigations.

The test of proportion comparison was performed for each hormone in both readings. There is a statistically significant difference for testosterone (p value 0.003), with a shift to lower values in those who responded well; however, in 36.7% there was an increase in testosterone correlated with poor outcome of the treatment (FIG. 6).

LH concentration demonstrated a general trend of lowering concentration, particularly among those who had very high levels previous to treatment. FSH increased concentrations in the medium range group (2.1–4.0 IU/liter), thus bringing the LH/FSH ratio nearer to normal, which was statistically significant ($p = 0.001$) compared to pretreatment findings (FIG. 6).

There was some significance ($p = 0.03$) in the change of cortisol concentrations towards medium levels (5–10 μg/dl). DHEA-S had a decrease in high levels; for

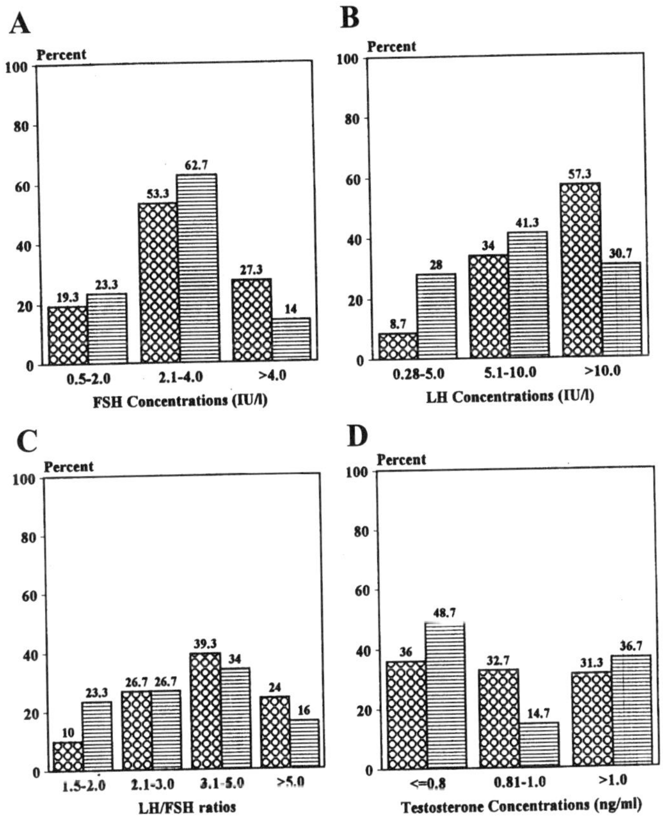

FIGURE 6. Distribution of hormone concentrations in 150 adolescents with PCOS. (**A**) FSH concentrations (IU/l), (**B**) LH concentrations (IU/l), (**C**) LH/FSH ratios, and (**D**) testosterone concentrations (ng/ml). ▩ First reading; ▤ second reading.

DHT, androstenedione, prolactin, and estradiol there were no statistically significant changes.

Ultrasound plays an important diagnostic role, not only in establishing a diagnosis but also for follow-up and monitoring response to treatment. Analysis of ultrasound scan following the treatment in 150 cases showed a reduction of ovarian size in 61.3% (92) cases. Among them, mean volume of the right ovary before and after treatment was 11.4 ml and 9.6 ml, respectively, and for the left ovary 10.7 ml and 8.6 ml. The phenomenon of ovarian volume decrease was bilateral in 87 girls and unilateral in only 5.

Most interesting was the group in which morphologic changes occurred after treatment, reversing into multicystic in 34% (52) of cases (FIG. 7). However, the great majority of these girls (48) had an ovarian volume before treatment of less than 12 ml; only 4 had one or both ovaries of more than a 12-ml volume. In the whole group,

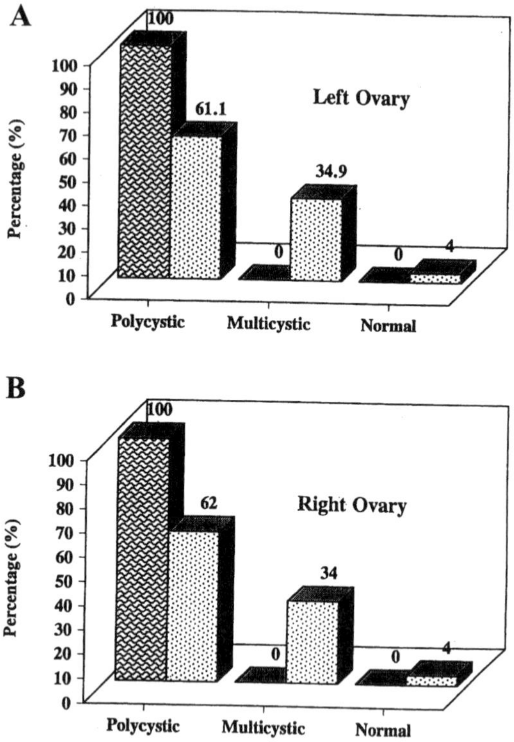

FIGURE 7. Ultrasound morphology before and after treatment: (**A**) Left ovary, (**B**) right ovary. Before; after.

only nine girls were obese, but all decreased body weight during treatment and follow-up. Not all patients with volumes less than 12 ml had morphologic changes; 6 decreased volume only, as well as another 5 who had only one ovary less than 12 ml before treatment. There were 18 girls with larger ovarian volume (more than 12 ml) who decreased volume during treatment (4 patients decreased body weight as well), but no morphologic changes occurred.

A special feature occurred in six girls (4%) in whom normal morphological features were observed after treatment. Ovarian volume before treatment was less than 10 ml (Fig. 7) for each of these girls.

Obviously, reversal of morphological changes in PCOS is limited to ovaries that are not grossly enlarged; similarly, a general decrease in ovarian volume alone is observed. In a follow-up of the cases, apart from clinical symptoms, U/S may be a sufficient parameter to indicate progression or regression of PCOS and may help in making decisions regarding length of treatment or the need to repeat treatment.

H-P-O axis cyclicity has been established or improved in the majority of the cases: 62.7% (94) had good outcome of the treatment, with the patients showing improvement in the following areas: regained cyclicity; lessening of acne and hirsutism;

decreased LH/FSH ratio, androgens, and ovarian volume; often morphologic changes in ovaries. Obesity was noted only in 13.8% (13) of girls in this group.

Among patients who showed little or no improvement after the treatment (11.3%, 17 cases) in repeated hormonal and ultrasound findings, minimal variations or none were observed, and menstrual disorders persisted. A significant proportion of these patients were obese (64.7%, 11).

Twenty-six percent (39) of our patients experienced a worsening of their condition, with visible further increase in ovarian volume noted on ultrasound and more pronounced hormonal imbalance. Obesity was a significant feature in this group; 64.1% (25) were obese.

Our preliminary data on SHBG and insulin will be briefly mentioned and related to 36 PCOS girls who were obese and/or hirsute and for whom the outcome of the treatment was poor or whose condition remained unchanged.

Insulin was found to be elevated in 25% (9) of patients. Fasting glucose was normal in all girls. SHBG was very low (<20 mmol/l) in 38.9% (14). It was at the low end of the normal range (20–45 mmol/l) in 50% (18) and at the medium end of normal range (46–90 nmol/l) in only 12.1% (4). SHBG decreased in 88.9% of patients in this group, consistent with their clinical, hormonal, and ultrasound findings.

In a psychologically screened sample of PCOS adolescents, there were eight identified cases of anxiety and one case of depression, and these should have been referred for treatment at an earlier date. Psychological distress among these patients is highly correlated with dissatisfaction with body shape and weight, which was cited by 91.3% of subjects. Thus, we have proposed a program of group therapy in adolescence that includes the following:

- Dietary advice and exercise regimes for weight and shape management;
- Education about effects of PCOS and treatment strategies; and
- Group therapy in small workshops to increase self-esteem and personal effectiveness, manage anxiety, and prevent depression.

Contact with other "survivors" of chronic medical conditions is known to increase coping skills through various therapeutic factors and vicarious learning from the experiences of others. Irregardless of initial enthusiasm of the patients for the offered program, more time will be needed to assess the results.

DISCUSSION

With advancing puberty a metabolic cascade occurs: significant increases in nutrition, growth hormone (GH), insulin-like growth factor I (IGF-I), and androgens from the adrenal. Possible derangements in these processes that may lead to PCOS were suggested recently by Nobel and co-workers.[22]

Nobel's hypothesis proposes that the transient hyperinsulinemia and the elevated IGF-I levels of puberty induce a PCOS-like state in a substantial number of adolescent girls. After puberty, the insulin and IGF-I levels progressively decline in most patients, resulting in normalization of the clinical and morphological picture. PCOS persists only in a few cases, either because hyperinsulinemia remains or because another pathogenic factor has taken over its role in the meantime. In fact, Nobel *et al.* proposed the hypothesis that PCOS is a state of hyperpuberty, as many of the endocrine changes that occur during puberty are also present in PCOS, but in excess.

PCOS in adolescence attracted our attention because of the significant number of patients we saw in our adolescent clinics and their concerns regarding persistent menstrual irregularities, acne, hirsutism, and obesity. Similarly, we shared patients' concern about their future fertility. Additionally, we have the unique opportunity of access to almost all schoolchildren through our adolescent clinic in School Health Service, thus ensuring a long follow-up.

If we summarize our present data, it becomes evident that adolescent girls with PCOS who responded well to treatment were those with ovarian size <12 ml; testosterone levels of <0.9 ng/ml; body weight ranging from 90 to 120% of ideal body weight; and menstrual disorders consisting of dysfunctional uterine bleeding, oligomenorrhea, or secondary amenorrhea <2 years' duration. Also, later minor variabilities in cycles responded well to gestagen treatment for one to two cycles, particularly in DUB and oligomenorrheic girls.

On the other hand, the treatment outcome was not satisfactory, at least not for a long period of time, in cases with ovarian size >12 ml, testosterone >0.9 ng/ml, body weight over 120% or body weight increasing during treatment, and treatment less than 6 months and in patients with primary amenorrhea or menarche only, or prolonged secondary amenorrhea.

Our previous as well as present data support the general opinion that body composition has an important influence on establishment of the female cyclic function. Early or exaggerated adrenarche leading to increased anabolism (obesity), increased androgen stimulation (acne and hirsutism), and inadequate feedback (chronic anovulation) may lead to PCOS and other menstrual disorders. Persistence of disorder and outcome of treatment is significantly negatively influenced by obesity. Obesity in adolescence clearly favors hyperandrogenic conditions and contributes to poor response to treatment and a high rate of recurrences. The length of the menstrual disorder is an equally important factor for the outcome of the treatment, being negatively correlated. Impact of obesity, length of menstrual disorder, time of its onset, and length of treatment were all variables that influenced outcome considerably.

One of our aims is to pursue our patients until the stage of life when they decide to bear children. So far, fertility performance data are sparse. Singaporean girls generally aspire to high levels of education, which means marriage and reproduction are postponed until the late twenties or even mid-thirties, so our present long-term follow-up results are rather modest. Only 74 of our patients have reached this stage: 5 delivered; 5 terminated their pregnancies; in 18 ovulation was confirmed (ultrasound or hormone testing); another 21 developed pubertal dysmenorrhea when they regained regular cycles; and 15 kept regular cycles and were sexually active, and chose to use oral contraceptives. We can only presume that ovarian function is intact in the last two groups. Unfortunately, few of our obese girls with persistent PCOS are under the care of subfertility unit.

We propose as general conclusions a need for early diagnosis of adolescent PCOS, possibly treatment, and certainly long-term follow-up for the following reasons:

- Immediate concerns about menstrual irregularities, hirsutism, acne, and obesity;
- Possible health hazards in adult life—impaired fertility and, if pregnancy occurs, frequent miscarriages, estrogen-dependent malignancies possible at an earlier age due to persistent chronic anovulation, insulin resistance-related conditions, and lipids imbalances; and
- Chronic psychological distress.

Complete management of adolescent PCOS should include medical correction of hormonal imbalance, body weight correction, and psychological intervention. In adolescents the group therapy model is a useful vehicle to deliver treatment designed to manage anxiety and depression, to raise self-esteem, and to provide education on diet and exercise regimes.

Female cyclic activity, the hallmark of sexual maturity, has its onset in puberty and is definitely established during adolescence, hence the importance of monitoring conditions that may lead to reproductive disorders.

REFERENCES

1. YEN, S. S. C. 1980. The polycystic ovary syndrome. Clin. Endocrinol. **12:** 177–208.
2. GRUMBACH, M. M., J. C. RATH, S. I. KAPLAN & R. O. REITER. 1974. Hypothalamic–pituitary regulation of puberty in man: Evidence and concepts derived from clinical research. *In* The Control of the Onset of Puberty. M. Grumbach, G. Grave & F. Mayer, Eds.: 115–166. John Wiley. New York.
3. THOMAS, M. A. & R. W. REBAR. 1989. The endocrinology of normal and abnormal female puberty. Curr. Opin. Obstet. Gynecol. **1:** 259–265.
4. STEWARD, P. M., R. PENN, R. HOLDER, A. PARTON, J. G. RATCLIFFE & D. R. LONDON. 1993. The hypothalamo–pituitary–adrenal axis across the normal menstrual cycle and in polycystic ovary syndrome. Clin. Endocrinol. **38:** 387–391
5. WHITFIELD, C. R. 1988. Dewhurst's Textbook of Obstetrics and Gynaecology for Postgraduates. 4th edit. Singapore.
6. APTER, D. & I. SIPILA. 1993. Development of children and adolescents: Physiological, pathophysiological and therapeutic aspects. Curr. Opin. Obstet. Gynaecol. **5:** 764–773.
7. DORING, G. K. 1969. The incidence of anovular cycles in women. J. Reprod. Fertil. Suppl. **6:** 77–81.
8. APTER, D. & R. VIHKO. 1990. Endocrine determinants of fertility: Serum androgen concentrations during follow-up of adolescents into the third decade of life. J. Clin. Endocrinol. Metab. **71:** 970–974.
9. DRAMUSIC, V. 1977. Menstrual disorders in adolescence. Doctoral thesis. Belgrade University. Belgrade, Yugoslavia.
10. SIZONENKO, P. C. & J. PAUNILK. 1975. Hormonal changes in puberty III: Correlation of dehydroepiandrosterone, testosterone, FSH and LH with stages of puberty and bone age in normal boys and girls and patients with Addison's disease or hypogonadism or with premature or late adrenarche. J. Clin. Endocrinol. Metab. **41:** 894–904.
11. APTER, D., L. VINIKKA & R. VIHKO. 1978. Hormonal pattern of adolescent menstrual cycles. J. Clin. Endocrinol. Metab. **47:** 944–954.
12. FOX, R. 1990. Polycystic ovarian disease. Curr. Opin. Obstet. Gynaecol. **2:** 3370–3377.

13. FRANKS, S. 1989. Polycystic ovary syndrome: A changing perspective. Clin. Endocrinol. **31:** 87–120.
14. FALCONE, T., Y. BOURQUE, L. GRANGER, R. HEMMINGS & P. MIRON. 1993. Polycystic ovary syndrome. Curr. Probl. Obstet. Gynecol. Fertil. **16:** 65–95.
15. MCCLAMROCK, D. & E. Y. ADASHI. 1992. Polycystic ovarian syndrome and associated hirsutism in the adolescent. Adolesc. Pediatr. Gynecol. **5:** 231–241.
16. DRAMUSIC, V., M. YANG, H. H. GOH, S. S. RATNAM & U. RAJAN. 1994. Long-term follow-up of menstrual disorders. *In* Women's Health Today. Parthenon. New York. pp. 111–118.
17. FERRIMAN, D. & J. D. GALLWEY. 1961. Clinical assessment of body hair growth in women. J. Clin. Endocrinol. Metab. **21:** 1440–1447.
18. AMERICAN PSYCHIATRIC ASSOCIATION. 1987. Diagnostic and Statistical Manual of Mental Disorders. 3rd edit. Revised. American Psychiatric Association. Washington, DC.
19. FAIRBURN, C. G. & S. BEGLIN. 1990. Studies of the epidemiology of bulimia nervosa. Am. J. Psychiatry **147:** 401–408.
20. DRAMUSIC, V. & Y. C. WONG. 1994. The ovary in paediatric and adolescent ages: Place of sonography in ultrasound and the ovary. Parthenon. London. pp. 47–63.
21. ROSSING, M. A. & Y. R. DARLING, *et al.* 1994. Ovarian tumours in the cohort of infertile women. N. Engl. J. Med. **331:** 771–776.
22. NOBELS, F. & D. DEWAILLY. 1992. Puberty and polycystic ovarian syndrome: The insulin/insulin-like growth factor-I hypothesis. Fertil. Steril. **58:** 655–666.

Female Sexual Precocity

C. DACOU-VOUTETAKIS

First Pediatric Department
Athens University
Agia Sophia Children's Hospital
Goudi, 115 27 Athens, Greece

INTRODUCTION

Precocious puberty is defined as the appearance of secondary sex characteristics at an age lower than two standard deviations from the mean expected for a population group.[1] For most Western countries, including Greece,[2] puberty initiation in girls before 8 years of age must be considered precocious. Precocity may involve only breast or pubic hair development or both and must be classified as central or peripheral. This initial distinction is very important for either diagnostic or therapeutic orientation.

Before the theoretical and actual causes of precocious sexual maturation are discussed, it may be appropriate to briefly delineate the known maturational events that normally lead to the onset of puberty.

It has been shown that gonadotropin-releasing hormone (GnRH) neurons originate in the olfactory placode and during early fetal life (first trimester) migrate through a very accurately programmed pathway to the anterior hypothalamus where they lodge.[3]

GnRH is secreted by the hypothalamic neurons in a pulsatile fashion. This oscillation of GnRH secretion seems to represent an intrinsic characteristic of the GnRH neurons (intrinsic oscillator),[4] and it is modified by inhibitory factors or promoters (neuromodulators). These neuromodulators originate from neurons or glial cells in extrahypothalamic areas of the CNS (γ-aminobutyric acid [GABA], transforming growth factor α [TGFα], and others).

The modulators are most likely responsible for the well-known triphasic curve of gonadotrophins and sex steroid secretion. This curve is characterized by an initial active phase (fetal and early postnatal life) with high levels of gonadotrophins and sex steroids, a quiescent phase (the prepubertal years) with very low gonadotrophin and sex steroid values, and a third phase, the fulminating pubertal spurt. The mechanism that underlies these changes is not known. We do know, however, that maturational events in areas distant or neighboring to the hypothalamic GnRH neurons modify the intrinsic attitude of GnRH neurons for oscillation. These factors depress or increase the amplitude and frequency of GnRH pulses. It is well accepted that the increase in the amplitude and frequency of GnRH pulses constitutes the basic underlying hormonal event of the onset of puberty.[5]

PATHOGENESIS OF SEXUAL PRECOCITY

When the time comes to know what factors are responsible for the depressed period (quiescent period) of hormonal secretion and how this period ends, giving ground to the hormonal flood of puberty, then the mysteries of normal, delayed, and precocious puberty will be disclosed.

Theoretically, sexual precocity could be caused by an earlier than normal catastrophe of the inhibitory mechanism (GABA, pineal hormones, TGFα, and others) or by more active facilitators (promoters) of GnRH neuronal activity. Thus, it has been shown that, in female rhesus monkeys, low levels of GnRH release in the prepubertal period seem to be caused by dominant inhibition of GABA, and the removal of this inhibition may lead to an increase in GnRH release and initiation of pubertal development.[6]

Concerning the pineal, studies from different laboratories including ours have shown a progressive decrease in melatonin values with age and low levels of melatonin in children with idiopathic precocious puberty if compared to age-matched controls. On the contrary, in our two cases of precocious puberty associated with hypothalamic hamartomas, the melatonin values were not low. Furthermore, data in our laboratory have shown that children with central precocious puberty, who had previously been irradiated for brain tumors outside the hypothalamus, had lower melatonin values than otherwise would be expected (FIG. 1).[7–9]

We would like to put forward the following hypothesis concerning hamartomas. It is known that hypothalamic hamartomas include GnRH neurons and they may be associated with GnRH-dependent precocious puberty of quite early onset (FIG. 2). We propose that this developmental abnormality[10] is the antipode of Kallman syndrome. During migration the GnRH neurons go beyond their normal destination and form the hypothalamic hamartomas. This defect in migration of GnRH neurons is the opposite of the arrest of GnRH neuronal migration that characterizes the Kallman syndrome.[3]

Hence the GnRH neurons of the hamartomas, being outside their normal position, are unable to receive the normal inhibitory cues, and a premature amplification of LHRH pulses ensues, leading to precocious puberty.

CLASSIFICATION OF PRECOCIOUS PUBERTY

The initial classifications, when dealing with precocious development of secondary sex characteristics, include the following:

i. central or gonadotrophin dependent,
ii. peripheral or gonadotrophin independent, and
iii. incomplete precocity (isolated thelarche, adrenarche, menarche).

The different known models of sexual precocity are briefly described below.

Central Precocity

1. *Pineal tumors* or cysts are associated with either precocious or delayed puberty, and the mechanism involved is not clear.[1]

2. *CNS irradiation.* It has been observed that some children irradiated for in-

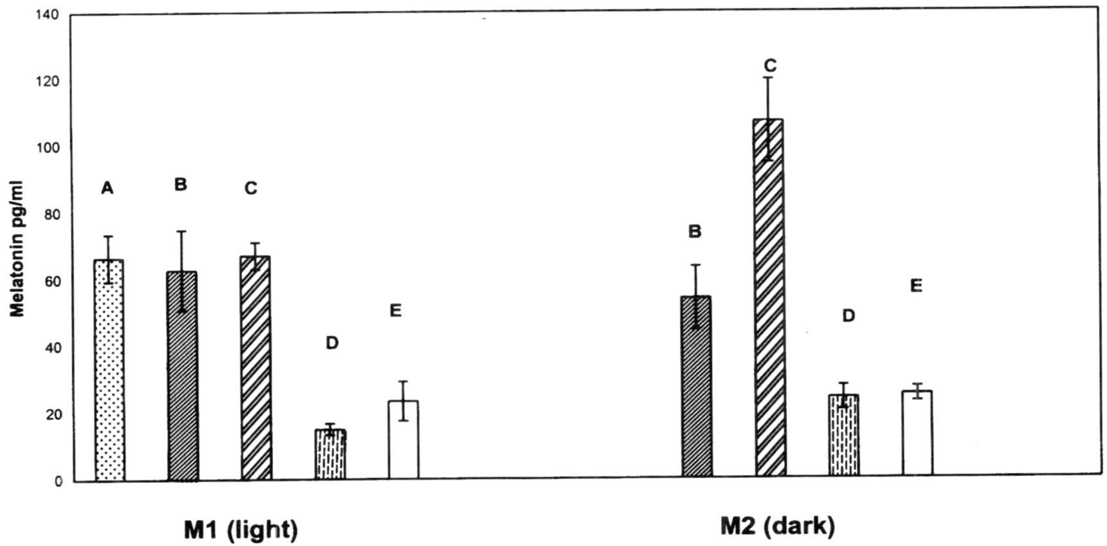

FIGURE 1. Melatonin values (M1: light; M2: dark) **in different diagnostic categories.** (**A**: controls; **B**: irradiated with posterior fossa tumor; **C**: irradiated with tumor in brain areas other than posterior fossa; **D**: idiopathic central precocious puberty; **E**: irradiated posterior fossa tumor with central precocious puberty. Statistically significant differences between groups: In M1 values, A versus E ($p < 0.001$); A versus D ($p < 0.001$). In M2 values, B versus C ($p < 0.01$); C versus E ($p < 0.001$; B versus E ($p < 0.05$). In M1 versus M2 values in group C: $p < 0.01$.

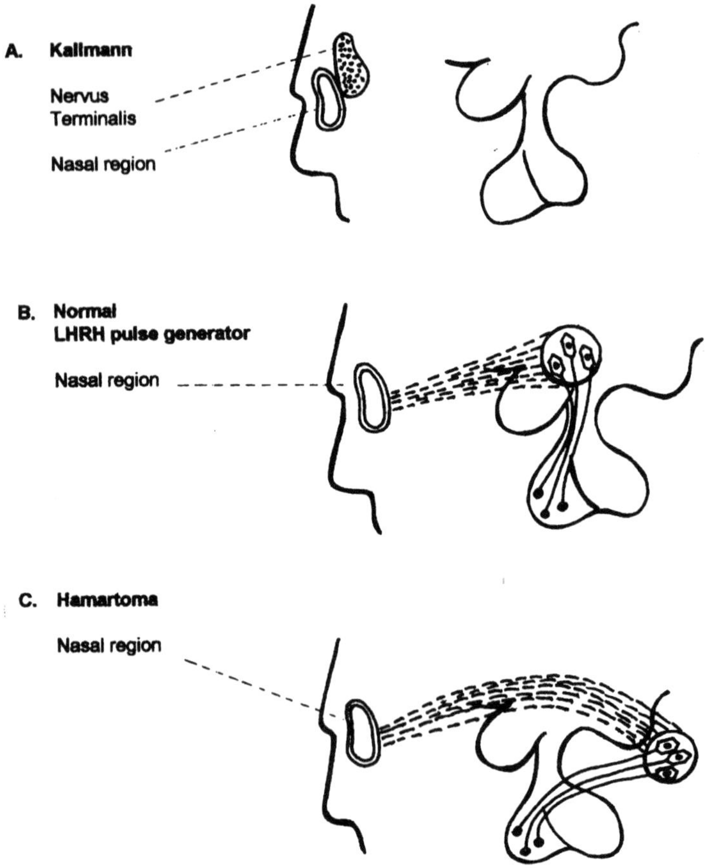

FIGURE 2. Schematic representation of GnRH neuron migration. (**A**) arrested GnRH neurons such as in Kallman syndrome, (**B**) normal pathway from the olfactory placode to the anterior hypothalamus, (**C**) proposed GnRH neuron migration in hamartomas. The GnRH neurons migrate beyond their normal destination and form the hamartoma, a phenomenon opposite to Kallman syndrome.

tracranial tumors, located outside the hypothalamic pituitary area, present with growth hormone (GH) deficiency and central precocious puberty.[9,11,12] The pathogenetic mechanism involved is not apparent. One possible mechanism of precocious puberty could involve destruction of inhibitory mechanisms like GABAergic neurons, glial cells producing TGFα, or pineal secretion.

3. *Specific tumors of the CNS.* Optic gliomas with or without neurofibromatosis, hypothalamic astrocytomas.

4. *Developmental defects.* (**a**) Hypothalamic hamartoma (FIG. 3), (**b**) congenital hydrocephalus, and (**c**) De Morsier syndrome.

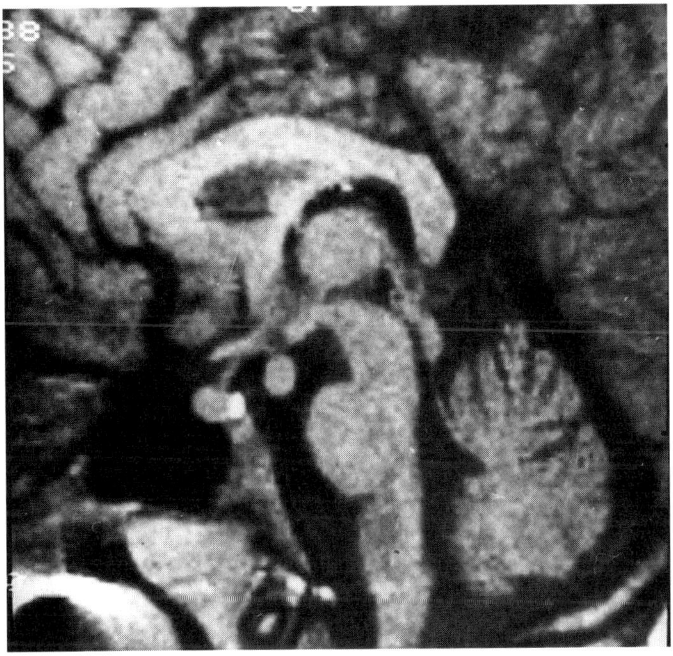

FIGURE 3. Hypothalamic hamartoma in a girl with central precocious puberty.

5. *Severe head trauma.*

6. *Acceleration of energy balance or the events of growth.* This association indicates that there is a hidden link between body composition and/or energy balance to reproductive function and, more specifically, to the maturation of hypothalamic pituitary gonadal axis.[13,14] Central precocious puberty may complicate the peripheral puberty brought about by nonclassical congenital adrenal hyperplasia (CAH), when steroid therapy is started. In such cases central precocious puberty is observed when skeletal maturation (possibly reflecting general maturity of the CNS) reaches a certain level (about 11 years).

7. *Idiopathic central precocious puberty.* Most cases of CPP in girls are idiopathic (about 70%). In our study of 80 cases, using brain magnetic resonance imaging, the diagnosis of idiopathic precocity was made in 75% of the cases. The remaining cases were associated with pineal tumors, tumors of the optic nerves, hypothalamic hamartomas, cranial irradiation, congenital hydrocephalus, or arachnoid cyst.

Peripheral Precocious Puberty

This form of puberty denotes lack of activation of the hypothalamic pituitary axis. The sex steroids causing development of secondary sex characteristics originate in the periphery. The most frequent causes are CAH, ovarian cysts or tumors, and, more rarely, McCune-Albright syndrome, which is caused by mutations of the gene encoding $G_{S}a$ protein.[15]

MANAGEMENT OF PRECOCIOUS PUBERTY

Peripheral

Etiologic management is possible in cases of ovarian cyst or tumor, the removal of which is associated with regression of secondary sex characteristics. As was mentioned above, the late initiation of corticoids in cases of CAH may lead to central precocious puberty and further management with LHRH analogue may be necessary. McCune-Albright syndrome, in early phases, may be managed with testolactone.[16]

Central Precocious Puberty

Etiologic management of central precocious puberty is seldom possible to achieve. Hence, the aim of therapeutic intervention is to arrest pubertal development by acting on the gonadotrophs. Besides the arrest of secondary sex characteristics, which is very important for psychosocial reasons, the goal of our intervention is the improvement of adult height, since short stature is a frequent complication of precocious puberty.

Previous therapies to arrest GnRH-dependent puberty have not given satisfactory results, but the use of GnRH analogues has proven rather effective. More specifically, GnRHa therapy leads to regression or arrest of secondary sex characteristics, and LH values return to prepubertal levels, whereas they become pubertal upon discontinuation of GnRHa therapy (FIG. 4). The effectiveness, however, of GnRHa in substantially improving final height remains a question.

One of the main problems in dealing with this question is methodological. What indices of efficacy are to be used? Changes in predicted height during therapy? Target height versus actual adult height achieved? Most studies do not include a control group, and in a few, which do so, the controls are historical.

If changes in predicted height are used as a criterion of efficacy of therapy, most, if not all, published studies have shown improved growth potentials. When applying the criterion of final height achieved versus target height, there is no uniformity in the published results. Oerter *et al.*[17] showed that adult height was greater than predicted height before initiation of treatment but less than the target height. Brauner *et al.*[18] showed that the adult height in GnRHa-treated subjects was similar to target height.

Using historical controls and combining data from different centers Kletter and Kelch[19] showed that there was no difference in percent of final height achieved between treated and untreated subjects (98.2% versus 98.6%). For those less than 6 years old at the onset of therapy, the percent of final height achieved in the treated group was 98.3% versus 96.3% in the controls.

Recently, Paul *et al.*,[20] using final height as a criterion in 7 children and near final height in 19 children and historical controls matched for the age of pubertal onset,

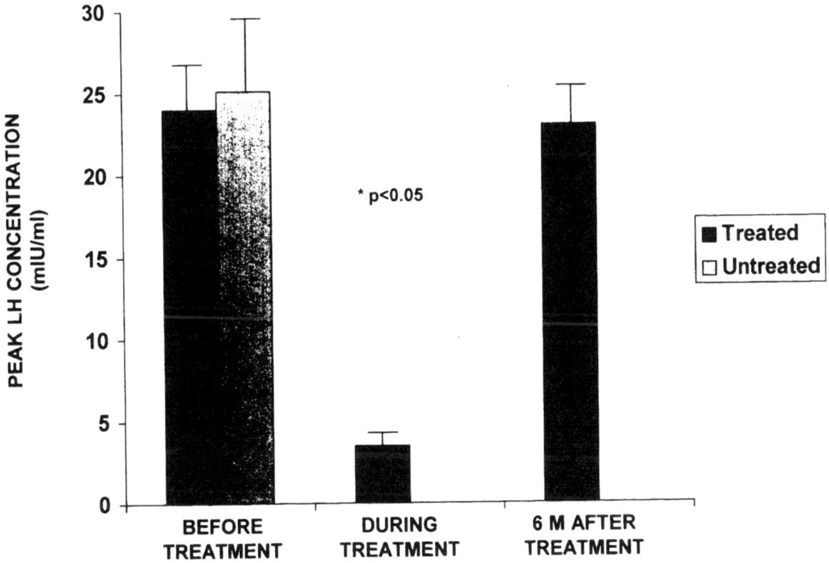

FIGURE 4. Peak values of serum luteinizing hormone after intravenous LHRH administration in subjects treated with LHRH analogue before, during, and after LHRH analogue therapy and in untreated subjects at diagnosis.

showed that mean height of the GnRHa-treated group was 157.6±6.6, whereas in the untreated group it was 152.7±8.6 cm.

Obviously, a parallel, well-matched control group is the best way to prove efficacy, although methodological problems are still present: How is the matching going to be achieved? Chronological age at start of puberty? Bone age at start of therapy? Height SDS for bone age? Predicted height? Even if all these obstacles are overcome, it is rather unethical at this point to randomize patients, considering the fact that there are strong indications of effectiveness in many aspects of precocious puberty problems, including growth.[1]

In our study of 56 children with central precocious puberty, 36 received therapy with a long-acting analogue (TRp^6 LHRH al) injection, given every 25 days in a daily dose of 3 to 6 μg/kg. Twenty of the 56 subjects did not receive therapy and served as controls. The decision for no treatment was dictated primarily by parental denial for therapy and in some cases by lack of drug availability.[21] The two groups were matched for age of first symptoms, bone age, height SDS for BA, and predicted height SDS at treatment initiation.

In our treated group, the height SDS for bone age showed no significant change throughout the observation period, whereas it deteriorated in the untreated, control subjects (FIG. 5).[21]

The final height achieved in the GnRHa-treated group was similar to their target height (154.1±1.6 versus 156.2±1.1 cm, mean ± SEM), whereas it was lower than the target height in the controls (151.0±2.5 versus 157.1±2.6 cm, mean ± SEM). It must

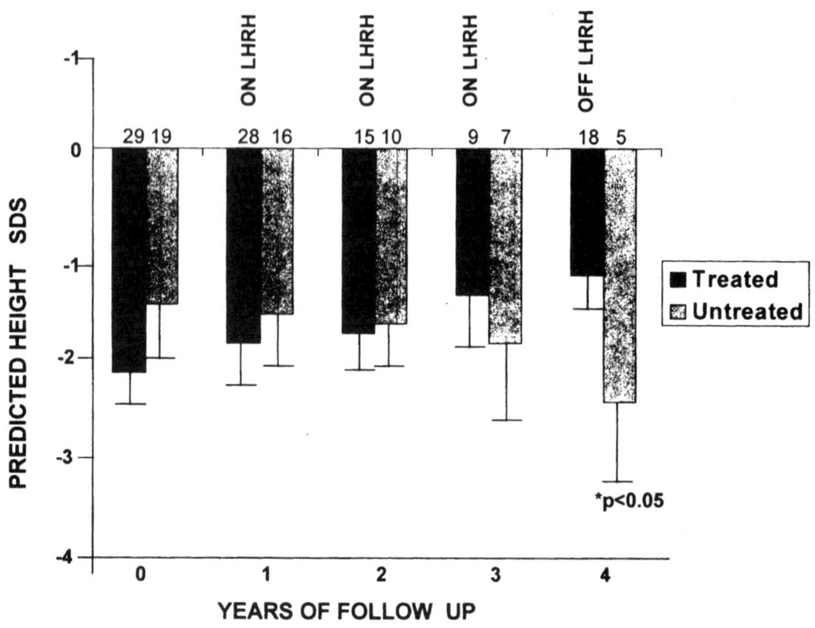

FIGURE 5. Height SDS for bone age in subjects with central precocious puberty treated with LHRH analogue and in untreated controls.

be mentioned, however, that the number of children in the untreated group who reached final height is still small.

CONCLUSION

All studies including ours have shown reversal or arrest of breast development. However, the effect of LHRHa therapy on final height remains controversial. The weak point of most studies is the lack of a parallel control group. Some published reports showed an increase in final height, but others found no improvement. Our data, which include a control group, showed that the height SDS for bone age at therapy initiation did not change throughout the observation period. Hence, the initial growth potential was simply maintained but not increased, whereas it deteriorated in the controls. The actual difference, however, was small. In general, the benefit seems to be higher in children who start GnRHa therapy before age 6 years, and it is accepted that children with puberty initiation before age 6 years, most likely, require therapeutic intervention with GnRHa.

The dilemma of treating or not with GnRH analogue mainly arises in those cases with the so-called "early puberty," namely initiation of breast development close to 8 years. Severely compromised predicted height or possible adverse psychological impact of precocious puberty may indicate intervention. It is uncertain, however, that the gain for final height will be satisfactory.

REFERENCES

1. Kaplan, S. L. & M. M. Grumbach. 1990. Pathophysiology and treatment of sexual precocity. J. Clin. Endocrinol. Metab. **71:** 785–789.
2. Dacou-Voutetakis, C., D. Klontza, P. Lagos, A. Tzonou, E. Katsavou, S. Antoniadis, G. Papazisis, G. Papadopoulos & N. Matsaniotis. 1983. Age of pubertal stages including menarche in Greek girls. Ann. Hum. Biol. **10:** 557–564.
3. Nazimi, M., F. Chigr, D. Jordan, P. Leduque, B. Bloch, M. Jommasi, P. Reband & N. Kopp. 1990. Anatomical distribution of LHRH-immunoreactive neurons in the human infant hypothalamus and extrahypothalamic regions. Brain Res. **516:** 280–291.
4. Wetsel, W. C., M. Valenca, I. Merchenthaler, Z. Liposits, F. J. Lojez, R. I. Weiner, P. L. Mellon & A. Negro-Villar. 1992. Intrinsic pulsatile secretory activity of immortalized luteinizing hormone-releasing hormone secreting neurons. Proc. Natl. Acad. Sci. USA **89:** 4149–4153.
5. Apter, D., T. L. Butzow, G. A. Caughlin & S. S. C. Yen. 1993. Gonadotropin-releasing hormone pulse generator activity during pubertal transition in girls: Pulsatile and diurnal patterns of circulating gonadotropins. J. Clin. Endocrinol. Metab. **76:** 940–949.
6. Mitsushima, D., D. L. Hei & E. Terasawa. 1994 γ-Aminobutyric acid is an inhibitory neurotransmitter restricting the release of luteinizing hormone-releasing hormone before the onset of puberty. Proc. Natl. Acad. Sci. USA **91:** 395–399.
7. Waldhauser, P., P. A. Boepple, M. Schemper, M. J. Mansfield & W. F. Crowley. 1991. Serum melatonin in central precocious puberty is lower than in age-matched prepubertal children. J. Clin. Endocrinol. Metab. **73:** 793–795.
8. Attanasio, A., P. Bowelli & D. Gupta. 1985. Circadian rhythms in serum melatonin from infancy to adolescence. J. Clin. Endocrinol. Metab. **61:** 388–390.
9. Dacou-Voutetakis, C., C. Dascalopoulou-Kefala & M. Dracopoulou. Melatonin values in precocious puberty following cranial irradiation and in other nosologic entities. In preparation.
10. Makachoklertwattana, P., S. L. Kaplan & M. M. Grumbach. 1993. The luteinizing hormone-releasing hormone-secreting hypothalamic hamartoma is a congenital malformation: Natural history. J. Clin. Endocrinol. Metab. **77:** 118–124.
11. Burstein, S. 1994. Growth disorders after cranial radiation in childhood. J. Clin. Endocrinol. Metab. **78:** 1280–1281.
12. Ogilvy-Stuart, A. L., P. E. Clayton & S. M. Shalet. 1994. Cranial irradiation and early puberty. J. Clin. Endocrinol. Metab. **78:** 1282–1286.
13. Van der Spuy, Z. M. 1985. Nutrition and reproduction. Clin. Obstetr. Gynecol. **12:** 579–604.
14. Bourguignon, J. P. 1991. Growth and timing of puberty: Reciprocal effects. Horm. Res. **36:** 131–135.
15. Weinstein, L. S., A. Shenker, P. V. Gejman, M. J. Merino, E. Friedman & A. M. Spiegel. 1991. Activating mutations of the stimulatory G protein in the McCune-Albright syndrome. N. Engl. J. Med. **325:** 1688–1695.
16. Feuillan, P. P., J. Jones & G. B. Gutler. 1993. Long-term testoloctone therapy for precocious puberty in girls with McCune-Albright syndrome. J. Clin. Endocrinol. Metab. **77:** 647–651.
17. Oerter, K. E., P. Manasco, K. M. Barnes, J. Jones, S. Hill & G. B. Cutler. 1991. Adult

height in precocious puberty after long-term treatment with deslorelin. J. Clin. Endocrinol. Metab. **73:** 1235–1240.

18. Brauner, R., L. Adan, F. Malandry & D. Zantleifer. 1994. Adult height in girls with idiopathic true precocious puberty. J. Clin. Endocrinol. Metab. **79:** 415–420.
19. Kletter, G. B. & R. P. Kelch. 1994. Effects of gonadotropin-releasing hormone analog therapy on adult stature in precocious puberty. J. Clin. Endocrinol. Metab. **79:** 331–334.
20. Paul, D., F. A. Conte, M. M. Grumbach & S. L. Kaplan. 1995. Long term effect of gonadotropin-releasing hormone agonist therapy on final and near final height in 26 children with true precocious puberty treated at a median age of less than 5 years. J. Clin. Endocrinol. Metab. **80:** 546–551.
21. Dacou-Voutetakis, C., A. Magiakou, V. Petrou & M. Maniati-Christidi. Growth in children with central precocious puberty treated with LHRHa and in controls. In preparation.

21-Hydroxylase Deficiency

RON S. NEWFIELD AND MARIA I. NEW[a]

Department of Pediatrics
The New York Hospital–Cornell Medical Center
525 East 68th Street, Room N-236
New York, New York 10021

INTRODUCTION

Adrenal hyperplasia is a group of inherited disorders of steroidogenesis, each characterized by a specific enzyme deficiency that impairs cortisol production by the adrenal cortex. Adrenal hyperplasia can be divided into two major forms: (1) congenital adrenal hyperplasia (CAH), or the classical form, and (2) the nonclassical form. In both forms the mode of inheritance is autosomal recessive, but they differ in the degree of enzyme deficiency, and thus in their clinical onset and presentation. Over 90% of CAH cases are caused by 21-hydroxylase deficiency (less frequent causes are 11β-hydroxylase deficiency and 3β-hydroxysteroid dehydrogenase deficiency).[1] When cortisol secretion is diminished, the adrenocorticotropic hormone (ACTH) increases via the negative feedback system of the hypothalamic–pituitary axis (HPA). As a result of ACTH overstimulation, the adrenals become hyperplastic. Each enzyme deficiency acts as a dam, behind which specific steroid precursors accumulate, and those overflow into adrenal biosynthetic pathways unaffected by the block, in particular producing excess androgens (FIG. 1). It is primarily the excess androgens and steroid precursors that determine the clinical presentation.

In CAH due to 21-hydroxylase deficiency (21-OHD) and 11β-hydroxylase deficiency (11β-OHD), prenatal exposure of female urogenital tissues to potent androgens such as testosterone and delta-4 androstenedione at a critical stage of differentiation results in ambiguous external genitalia in genetic females. Up to 75% of cases with classical 21-OHD lack adequate aldosterone production and will be salt wasters.[2]

In the nonclassical form of adrenal hyperplasia, patients are born with normal genitalia; and, with a moderate enzyme deficiency, they present with signs of hyperandrogenism in childhood or later. Classical 21-OHD has an incidence of one in 13,000 live births, and the nonclassical form, which is the most common autosomal recessive human disorder, occurs with a frequency of one in 100 in a heterogeneous population. In certain ethnic groups the frequency is much higher, such as one in 27 in the Ashkenazi Jews.[3] Failing to recognize this readily made diagnosis can result in short stature, acne, hirsutism, menstrual irregularities, and/or infertility. Once the

[a]Corresponding author: Maria I. New, M.D., Professor and Chairman, Department of Pediatrics, Chief, Division of Pediatric Endocrinology, Harold and Percy Uris Professor of Pediatric Endocrinology and Metabolism, The New York Hospital–Cornell Medical Center, 525 East 68th Street, Room N-236, New York, New York 10021.

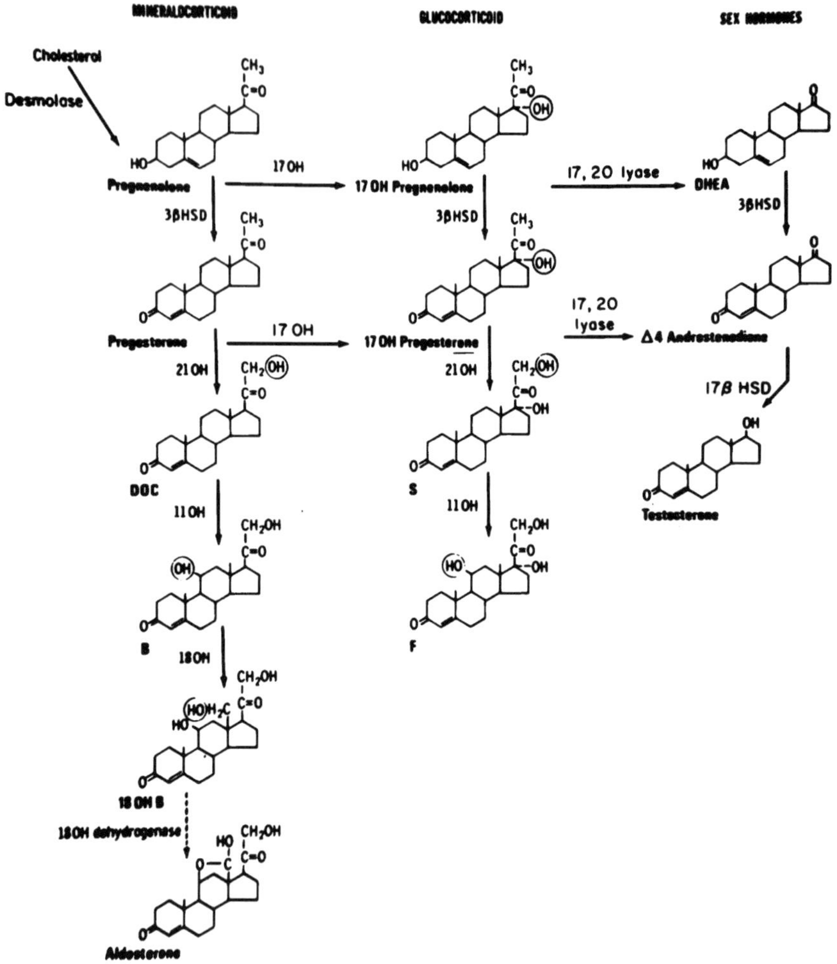

FIGURE 1. Simplified scheme for adrenal steroidogenesis. DOC, deoxycorticosterone; B, corticosterone; S, 11-deoxycortisol; F, cortisol; DHEA, dehydroepiandrosterone; 3β-HSD, 3β-hydroxysteroid dehydrogenase; OH, hydroxylase (for enzymes). The final three enzymatic steps in the mineralocorticoid pathway are performed by aldosterone synthase (CYP11B2) in the zona glomerulosa. (Reproduced from New and Levine.[25] with permission from Plenum Press.)

correct diagnosis is made, appropriate therapy can reverse the symptoms. However, final adult height may be compromised.

This mini-review will concentrate on the gynecologic aspects of 21-OHD and associated therapeutic issues, and will also briefly mention genetic counseling and prenatal diagnosis coupled with prevention of ambiguous genitalia in 21-OHD.

CLINICAL PRESENTATION

Classical Adrenal Hyperplasia

The severity of the 21-hydroxylase enzyme deficiency determines the spectrum of the disease. Severe deficiency results in the congenital or classical form of 21-OHD, which is then clinically divided into salt wasters and simple virilizers. Patients with salt-wasting 21-OHD may present in the first to sixth weeks of life (usually in the second to third week), with vomiting, lethargy, shock, and pronounced hyponatremia, metabolic acidosis and life-threatening hyperkalemia, due to the inability to produce adequate amounts of cortisol and aldosterone. Girls are less likely than boys to die of severe salt-wasting crises, because their ambiguous genitalia usually draws attention to their diagnosis and treatment is initiated. Survivors of extreme electrolyte imbalance may suffer from brain damage. Even though simple virilizers have a milder 21-OH deficiency, the degree of genital masculinization can be as severe as that of salt wasters. Excess adrenal androgens *in utero*, beginning as early as the seventh or eighth week of gestation,[4] cause masculinization of the external genitalia. The degree of virilization in female fetuses is assessed by Prader staging. The most common phenotype consists of clitoromegaly, partial posterior fusion of the labioscrotal folds, and a single orifice representing fusion of the distal urethra and vagina (urogenital sinus). The other enzyme defect that causes masculinized genitalia in female fetuses is 11β OHD. As the females have normal ovaries, fallopian tubes, uterus, cervix, and upper vagina, reproduction is possible.

In untreated simple virilizers, androgen excess will often manifest as initial tall stature, at the expense of marked advancement of skeletal maturation (bone age), and/or premature adrenarche. Such boys typically have small testes, suggesting that the excess androgens are of adrenal source. Hormonal diagnosis will confirm whether it is classical or nonclassical adrenal hyperplasia. These patients, where treatment commences late, usually have the worst height prognosis, and ultimately become short as adults. Poorly controlled patients may also become short as adults. Unfortunately, most patients do not achieve the adult height expected from their parents' height.[5,6,7]

Excess androgens are aromatized peripherally to estrogens. In patients who have an advanced bone age compatible with puberty, starting glucocorticoid treatment suppresses androgens (and their estrogen byproducts), and thus, via the pituitary negative feedback system, gonadotropins are secreted, leading to precocious puberty.

Untreated or poorly treated female patients may develop a masculinized body habitus with poor breast development and primary amenorrhea. True puberty may commence after appropriate therapy has begun. Females treated successfully since early life will have a normal female body habitus, and regular onset of puberty and menarche.[5,6,8] Poor compliance with therapy and hyperandrogenemia may cause secondary amenorrhea or menstrual irregularities due to dysregulation of the cyclical release of gonadotropins.[2,9,10] The disruption in the hypothalamic–pituitary axis, coupled with the direct effect of chronic androgen excess on the ovaries, often results in polycystic ovaries (PCO). One report based on sonographic evidence alone documented polycystic ovaries in 3% of peripubertal girls and 40% of postpubertal girls with CAH.[11] Diagnosis of PCO cannot rely on sonographic appearance of the ovaries alone but should also include a hormonal evaluation of the hypothalamic pituitary ovarian axis.[12]

Other signs of hyperandrogenism in females, alone or in combination, may include hirsutism, oily hair, acne, temporal balding, or infertility.

Psychosexual problems such as gender identity or homosexuality are common among females with classical 21-OHD.[13] Psychoendocrinological counseling is strongly advocated in order to ensure normal gender behavior and gender identity.

Nonclassical Adrenal Hyperplasia

Both boys and girls may present in childhood with premature adrenarche and/or accelerated linear growth velocity. Patients with nonclassical 21-OHD present postnatally.[1] In adolescent females, onset of menarche may be normal or delayed. Hirsutism, menstrual irregularities, and secondary amenorrhea with or without PCO are common in untreated patients. In certain populations, 14–30% of women with hirsutism and oligomenorrhea may have NC21-OHD.[2] Cystic acne that is refractory to conventional therapy with antibiotics and/or retinoic acid or temporal balding have been observed but do not appear to be common presentations of NC21-OHD. Adrenal incidentalomas (hyperplasia or adenoma) may bring attention to the diagnosis of NC21-OHD and are also common in heterozygote patients.[14] Males with NC21-OHD may occasionally have oligospermia and decreased fertility, which improves following glucocorticoid therapy.[15,16] Most males are fertile.

Rare patients with NC21-OHD mutation have symptoms that wax and wane and eventually become symptomatic.

DIAGNOSIS

The hormonal diagnostic test of choice to establish any abnormality in the steroidogenic pathway, including 21-OHD, is the 60-minute ACTH (Cortrosyn, 0.25 mg) stimulation test, which is best performed in the morning (8–10 A.M.). In order to rule out 21-OHD, one should plot the 17-hydroxyprogesterone (17-OHP) levels (baseline versus ACTH stimulated) on the nomogram (FIG. 2). Baseline 17-OHP levels alone can be diagnostic in the classical form; in the nonclassical form, baseline 17-OHP levels may be somewhat elevated or altogether normal. Carriers (heterozygotes) plot the lowest on the nomogram, and they occasionally may overlap with genetically unaffected persons.[17]

A genetic diagnosis for mutations or deletions of the gene for 21-OHD (CYP21), located on the short arm of chromosome 6, is now readily available and has been

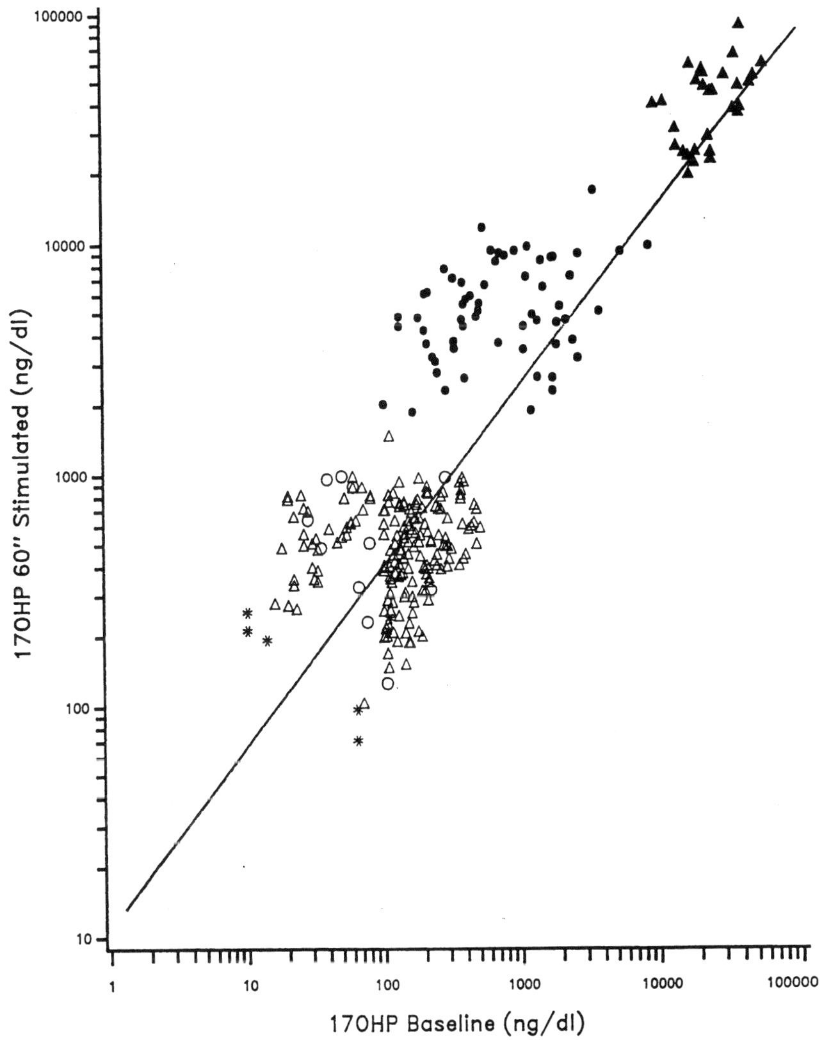

FIGURE 2. Baseline versus ACTH (Cortrosyn)-stimulated 17-hydroxyprogesterone (17OHP) nomogram for the diagnosis of steroid 21-hydroxylase deficiency. Symbols: * genetically unaffected; ▲ patients with classical congenital adrenal hyperplasia; • patients with nonclassical CAH; △ heterozygotes for classical CAH; ○ heterozygotes for nonclassical CAH. The data for this nomogram was collected between 1982 and 1991 at the Department of Pediatrics, The New York Hospital–Cornell Medical Center, New York.

widely used in prenatal diagnosis[18] (see below). It also allows for a quick diagnosis of relatives of an index patient. Genotype does not always predict phenotype,[19] but usually the severe mutations or deletions are associated with salt-wasting classic 21-OHD. On the other end of the spectrum, certain mild mutations correlate with NC21-OHD.

TREATMENT

The goals and modes of treatment of patients with 21-OHD may vary depending on the form of 21-OHD, age, and sex. A recent review of current therapy of 21-OHD describes in full the different aspects of management involved.[20] This mini-review outlines the principles of therapy, and the rationale for life-long therapy.

Prenatal Therapy

Prenatal therapy of female fetuses diagnosed with CAH is made possible by treating their mothers with dexamethasone, which passes the placenta and suppresses fetal ACTH. The aim is to prevent or reduce the genital ambiguity, thus avoiding surgery and some of the psychological complications. This form of therapy has been very successful (see prenatal diagnosis and treatment below).

Postnatal Therapy

In postnatal life, glucocorticoid therapy is essential for all patients with classical 21-OHD. It exerts a negative feedback at the HPA, suppresses further ACTH stimulation, and restores hormonal balance. Patients who are salt-wasters require mineralocorticoid replacement in addition. Preventing hyperandrogenemia in children optimizes their growth potential and chances of undergoing normal pubertal development. Post-pubertally, maintaining good hormonal control protects against infertility (in both sexes) and development of menstrual irregularities, PCO, hirsutism, and other manifestations of hyperandrogenemia. In addition, the harmful effects of ACTH overstimulation on adrenal tissue tumors are avoided.

Corrective surgery of ambiguous genitalia in females is conventionally performed in two stages.[21,22] The first surgery is clitoral recession, performed in early childhood (preferably at 6–18 months of life). The clitoral size is reduced, and the neurovascular bundle is preserved, thus avoiding the loss of sexual sensation associated with clitorectomy, which is no longer performed. The second surgery is vaginoplasty, whereby the vaginal opening is enlarged and urogenital sinus corrected. Vaginal dilations are often required to maintain a patent vagina. In this program, a vaginoplasty is usually performed in late adolescence in females who are sexually active.

In nonclassical 21-OHD patients who are not symptomatic, one may choose to postpone therapy until symptoms occur. However, it is our recommendation that when close follow-up is not feasible, one should definitely treat.

For children still growing, hydrocortisone, taken t.i.d. (or b.i.d.), is advocated as the most physiological replacement. Equivalent doses of longer acting glucocorticoid preparations affect growth adversely. Using excessive hydrocortisone doses may cause growth delay or frank Cushingoid signs. Initial dose is usually 15 mg/M^2 and should be adjusted periodically (usual range of 10–20 mg/M^2), such that the lowest dose possible is used to achieve serum 17-OHP levels grossly between 100 and 1000 ng/dl. Noncompliance should be suspected if doses higher then 20 mg/M^2 are required. Adding 0.1 mg/day of 9α-fludrocortisone (Florinef) to simple virilizers with high renin levels, who require high doses of hydrocortisone therapy, may allow reduction of their daily hydrocortisone dose.[23] Post-pubertally, long-acting glucocorticoids may be used, such as dexamethasone (usually 0.25–0.5 mg at bedtime is sufficient) or prednisone (b.i.d.). Adequacy of treatment should also be judged by serum androgen levels or 24-hour urinary metabolites of 17-OHP (e.g. pregnanetriol) and androgens (e.g. 17-ketosteroids).[2,20] Replacement doses are often lower in NC21-OHD compared to patients with classical 21-OHD.

Mineralocorticoid replacement for infants with salt-wasting CAH may vary between 0.1 and 0.2 mg of Florinef once daily (rarely 0.3 mg/day), coupled with adequate salt (sodium chloride) supplementation of 3–5 mEq/kg per day in 2–4 divided doses. Adequacy of therapy is monitored via plasma renin activity. By early childhood the requirement of Florinef is usually 0.1 mg/day.[20]

Because patients with 21-OHD receive chronic replacement therapy with glucocorticoids, they should carry a medical alert bracelet, alerting health professionals that they require extra doses of glucocorticoids (preferably hydrocortisone) at times of stress. For febrile illnesses, double the regular dose is advocated, but with lethargy or fever above 39.5°C triple doses are taken. In cases of vomiting or diarrhea, parenteral administration of hydrocortisone and intravenous fluids is advised. Surgery imposes greater stress and should always be managed with parenteral hydrocortisone by an experienced anesthesiologist.

Adrenal crisis usually occurs 7 to 10 days after birth but may occur later in life after stress, such as an acute infectious illness. Patients present with hyponatremia, hyperkalemia, acidosis, dehydration, or shock. The crisis is a medical emergency and is best managed in an intensive care facility, where intravenous access is rapidly obtained and close monitoring of electrolyte and cardiac status are possible. Intravenous Dextrose 5%-normal saline infusion coupled with hydrocortisone is given to restore adequate perfusion (5% albumin is rarely needed). If oral intake is feasible, 0.1 mg of Florinef should be administered as well.

PCO syndrome secondary to 21-OHD occurs frequently. If the patient is symptomatic and her adrenal hormones are well controlled for 3–6 months, adjunctive therapies for PCO should be considered.[12]

PRENATAL DIAGNOSIS AND TREATMENT

Congenital adrenal hyperplasia due to 21-OHD is the most common reason for ambiguous genitalia in females. Prenatal diagnosis is sought in families where a previous member has been affected. If 21-OHD is detected, prenatal treatment can pre-

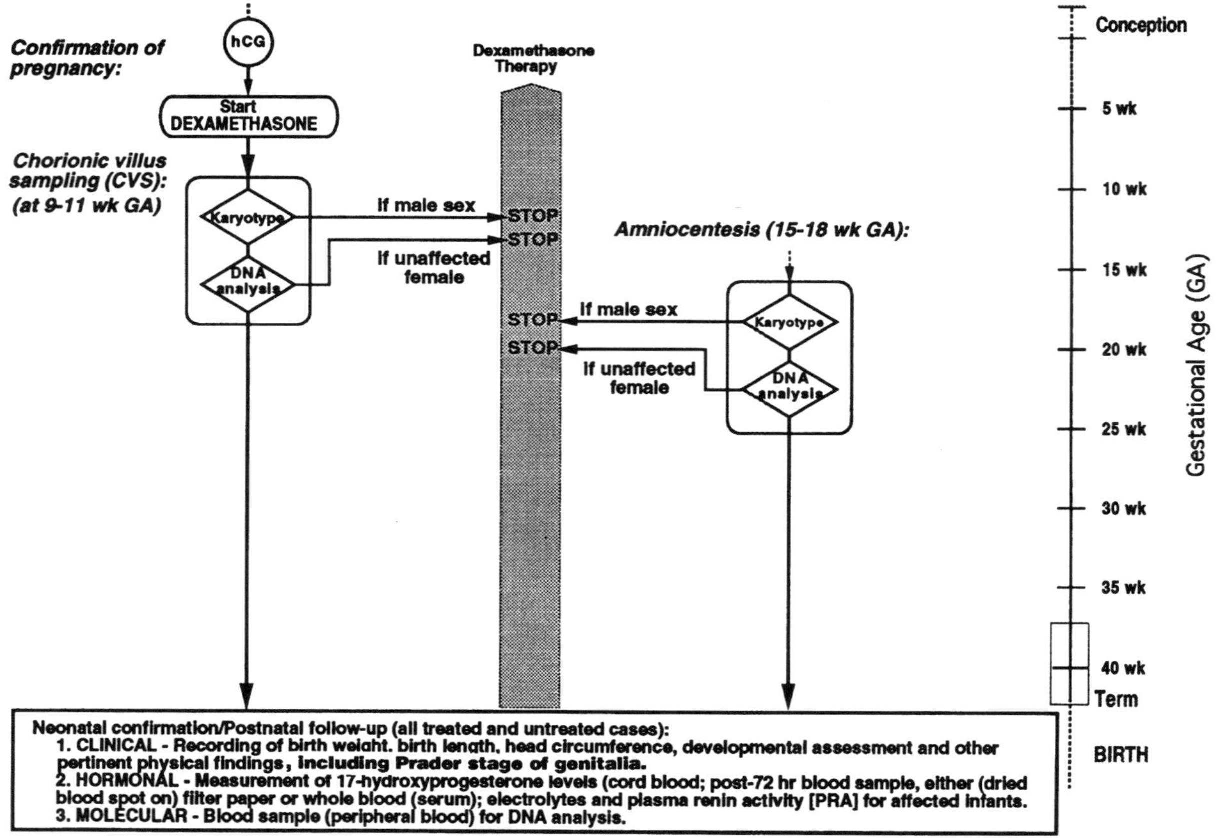

FIGURE 3. Prenatal diagnosis/treatment and postnatal follow-up in pregnancies at risk for 21-OHD CAH.

vent or minimize the ambiguity of the female genitalia, prevent a wrong sex assignment or a salt wasting crisis, and minimize the psychological burden on the patient and family.

Preferably, both parents should be genotyped before conception to determine if they are carriers and whether their mutations predict an offspring who may have classic 21-OHD. Carrier status can also be checked via ACTH stimulation test or by DNA analysis. As soon as the mother realizes she is pregnant, she should be started on dexamethasone therapy (20 μg/kg per day up to 1.5 mg divided in 3 doses) blind to the status of the baby (FIG. 3).[18] After CVS (week 10–11) or amniocentesis, mothers of male fetuses, or female fetuses unaffected by 21-OHD, may stop dexamethasone therapy. The first trimester is the most critical period, requiring strict compliance, in order to avoid or minimize urogenital sinus and labial fusion formation. Therapy started before the 10th week of gestation and carried to term has been shown to be very effective, with minimal side effects to the mother.[18,24] The dose of dexamethasone may be reduced in the second half of pregnancy in women with severe side effects or an underlying condition worsened by dexamethasone treatment.[24] Adequacy of adrenal fetal suppression can be gauged by maternal estriol (E_3) levels. Hormonal prenatal diagnosis is no longer relevant once the mother is receiving dexamethasone, and such therapy should never be stopped for diagnostic purposes before amniocentesis, as it may result in marked virilization. Close cooperation between the obstetrician and a pediatric endocrinologist well versed in this area is crucial for optimal outcome of both mother and offspring.

FUTURE GOALS AND DIRECTIONS:

1. Increased awareness and recognition of 21-OHD among physicians, in particular its reproductive system implications, and availability of prenatal diagnosis and therapy.
2. Alternative therapeutic approaches, aimed at addressing the current limitations of glucocorticoid therapy, are now being investigated. These include solutions such as bilateral adrenalectomies, which may suit a subset of CAH patients, and medical strategies such as the use of antiandrogenic drugs as adjuncts.
3. Genetic or biochemical newborn screening of the general population for 21-OHD, as is done in other neonatal screening programs (for much rarer conditions), is feasible, using filter paper, and represents a cost-effective approach. We believe it would be preferable to the current practice, that is, only testing families in which a prior member is affected with 21-OHD.
4. Gene therapy or transplantation is not likely to be available soon.

ACKNOWLEDGMENTS

The authors wish to express their appreciation to Laurie Vandermolen for her editorial assistance.

REFERENCES

1. NEW, M. I., B. DUPONT, K. GRUMBACH & L. S. LEVINE. 1982. Congenital adrenal hyperplasia and related conditions. *In* The Metabolic Basis of Inherited Disease. 5th edit. J. B. Stanbury, J. B. Wyngaarden, D. S. Fredrickson, J. L. Goldstein, & M. D. Brown, Eds.: 973–1000. McGraw-Hill. New York.
2. NEW, M. I., L. GHIZZONI & P. W. SPEISER. 1995. Update on congenital adrenal hyperplasia. *In* Pediatric Endocrinology. 3rd edit. F. Lifshitz, Ed. Chapter 16: 305–320. Marcel Dekker. New York.
3. SPEISER, P. W., B. DUPONT, P. RUBINSTEIN, A. PIAZZA, A. KASTELAN & M. I. NEW. 1985. High frequency of nonclassical steroid 21-hydroxylase deficiency. Am. J. Hum. Genet. **37:** 650–667.
4. BRANCHAUD, C. L. & B. E. P. MURPHY. 1992. Physiopathology of the fetal adrenal. *In* Hormones and Fetal Pathophysiology. J. R. Pasqualini & R. Scholler, Eds.: 53. Marcel Dekker. New York.
5. KLINGENSMITH, G. J., S. C.GARCIA, H. W. JONES, C. J. MIGEON & R. M. BLIZZARD. 1977. Glucocorticoid treatment of girls with congenital adrenal hyperplasia: Effects on height, sexual maturation, and fertility. J. Pediatr. **90:** 966.
6. PANG, S., F. M. KENNY, T. P. FOLEY & A. L. DRASH. 1977. Growth and sexual maturation in treated congenital adrenal hyperplasia. *In* Congenital Adrenal Hyperplasia. P. A. Lee, L. P. Plotnick, A. A. Kowarski, C. J. Migeon, Eds.: 233. University Park Press. Baltimore, MD.
7. NEW, M. I., J. M. GERTNER, P. W. SPEISER & P. DEL BALZO. 1989. Growth and final height in classical and nonclassical 21-hydroxylase deficiency. J. Endocrinol. Invest. **12:** 91–95.
8. JONES, H. W. & B. S. VERKAUF. 1971. Congenital adrenal hyperplasia: Age at menarche and related events at puberty. Am. J. Obstet. Gynecol. **109:** 292.
9. KLINGENSMITH, G. J., A. C. WENTZ, W. J. MEYER & C. J. MIGEON. 1976. Gonadotropin output in congenital adrenal hyperplasia. J. Clin. Endocrinol. Metab. **43:** 933.
10. GRANOFF, A. B. 1981. Treatment of menstrual irregularities with dexamethasone in congenital adrenal hyperplasia. J. Adolesc. Health Care. **2:** 23.
11. HAGUE, W. M., J. ADAMS, C. RODDA, *et al.* 1990. The prevalence of polycystic ovaries in patients with congenital adrenal hyperplasia and their close relatives. Clin. Endocrinol. **33:** 501–510.
12. GHIZZONI, L., R. VIRDIS, A. VOTTERO, M. CAPRA, M. E. STREET, M. ZAMPOLLI, L. IBANEZ & S. BERNASCONI. 1996. Pituitary–ovarian responses to leuprolide acetate testing in patients with congenital adrenal hyperplasia due to 21-hydroxylase deficiency. J. Clin. Endocrinol. Metab. **81:** 601–606.
13. BAKER, S. W. 1981. Psychological management of intersex children. *In* The Intersex Child. Z. Laron, Ed. Pediatric Adolescent Endocrinology. Vol. 8: 261. S. Karger. Basel.
14. JARESCH, S., E. KORNELY, H. KLEY & R. SCHLAGHECKE. 1992. Adrenal incidentaloma and patients with homozygous or heterozygous congenital adrenal hyperplasia. J. Clin. Endocrinol. Metab. **74:**685–689.
15. WISCHUSEN, J., H. W. G. BAKER & B. HUDSON. 1981. Reversible male infertility in late onset congenital adrenal hyperplasia. Clin. Endocrinol. **14:** 571.
16. AUGARTAN, A., R. WEISSENBERG, C. PARIENTE & J. SACK. 1991. Reversible male infertility in late onset congenital adrenal hyperplasia. J. Endocrinol. Invest. **14:** 237–240.
17. WHITE, P. C., M. I. NEW & B. DUPONT. 1987. Congenital adrenal hyperplasia (Part I). N. Engl. J. Med. **316:** 1519–1524.
18. MERCADO, A. B., R. C. WILSON, K. C. CHENG, J-Q. WEI & M. I. NEW. 1995. Extensive personal experience with prenatal diagnosis of congenital adrenal hyperplasia owing to steroid 21-hydroxylase deficiency. J. Clin. Endocrinol. Metab. **80:** 2014–2020.
19. WILSON, R. C., A. B. MERCADO, K. C. CHENG & M. I. NEW. 1995. Steroid 21-hydroxylase

deficiency: Genotype may not predict phenotype. J. Clin. Endocrinol. Metab. **80:** 2322–2339.

20. NEW, M. I. & R. S. NEWFIELD. 1997. Congenital adrenal hyperplasia. *In* Current Therapy in Endocrinology and Metabolism. 6th edit. C. W. Bardin, Ed.: 179–187. Mosby-Year Book. Philadelphia, PA.
21. HENDREN, W. H. & P. K. DONAHOE. 1980. Correction of congenital abnormalities of the vagina and perineum. J. Pediatr. Surg. **15:** 751.
22. HENDREN, W. H. & J. D. CRAWFORD. 1969. Adrenogenital syndrome: The anatomy of the anomaly and its repair. J. Pediatr. Surg. **4:** 49.
23. ROSLER, A., L. S. LEVINE, B. SCHNEIDER, M. NOVOGRODER & M. I. NEW. 1977. The interrelationship of sodium balance, plasma renin activity and ACTH in congenital adrenal hyperplasia. J. Clin. Endocrinol. Metab. **45:** 500–512.
24. LEVINE, L. S. & S. PANG. 1994. Prenatal diagnosis and treatment of congenital adrenal hyperplasia. J. Pediatr. Endocrinol. **7:** 193–200.
25. NEW, M. I. & L. S. LEVINE. 1973. Congenital adrenal hyperplasia. *In* Advances in Human Genetics. Vol. 4. H. Harris & K. Hirschhorn, Eds.: 251–326. Plenum Press. New York.

Late-Onset Congenital Adrenal Hyperplasia

CH. PANITSA-FAFLIA AND M. L. BATRINOS

Endocrine Unit
Department of Pharmacology
University of Athens Medical School
Athens 115-27, Greece

The finding of biochemical abnormalities suggestive of congenital adrenal hyperplasia (CAH) in subjects who had no clinical manifestation of the disease in childhood has been variously referred to as the postpubertal, delayed-onset, partial, acquired, attenuated, mild, adult-onset, cryptic, nonclassical, and late-onset form of the disease.[1]

At puberty the clinical features of this form of CAH are extremely variable, ranging from totally asymptomatic subjects to patients with moderate to severe hirsutism and menstrual disorders.[2,3] In our series of 18 postpubertal subjects with hirsutism and high basal 17-OH PG levels (>7.5 ng/ml), four presented with primary amenorrhea, seven with primary oligomenorrhea (occurring immediately postmenarche), one with secondary oligomenorrhea (occurring after 1–2 years of postmenarche cycles of normal length), one with secondary amenorrhea, four with ovulatory cycles, and one with anovulation. All of these subjects displayed hirsutism. We had also a case with normal ovulatory cycles without hirsutism; normal serum androgens. ACTH, and cortisol; and 17-OH PG levels of >20 ng/ml.

This condition is distinguished from other etiologies on the basis of an estimate of serum 17-OH PG, which is a marker of the enzymatic defect responsible for the deviation of steroidogenesis in favor of androgen production. Certain authors believe that an increase of basal serum 17-OH PG levels is the hallmark of the diagnosis, whereas others are of the opinion that the most sensitive diagnostic test is the ACTH-induced rise in 17-OH PG.[4–6]

From the point of view of a purely differential diagnosis, the first opinion is more acceptable. In the presence of normal 17-OH PG levels, it would be unreasonable to attribute a hyperandrogenemic state to 21-hydroxylase deficiency, because this steroid is the more sensitive marker of and the first to be affected in this condition. This assumption also stands true for subjects with normal basal serum 17-OH PG in whom a high post-ACTH rise in 17-OH PG is observed, because it is the secretion and serum concentration of androgens in basal conditions that may induce pathophysiological changes and not their episodic increase in the rare case of severe stress, causing an increased release of endogenous ACTH.

This reasoning leads to two assumptions: (a) first, in cases with basal 17-OH PG levels within the normal range, any clinical or biological evidence of androgen excess must arise from causes other than 21-hydroxylase deficiency and should be treated accordingly; (b) second, in cases with high basal 17-OH PG levels, one would expect a parallel between 17-OH PG concentrations and hyperandrogenemia.

In a series of 359 consecutive cases with hirsutism, mostly young subjects, single

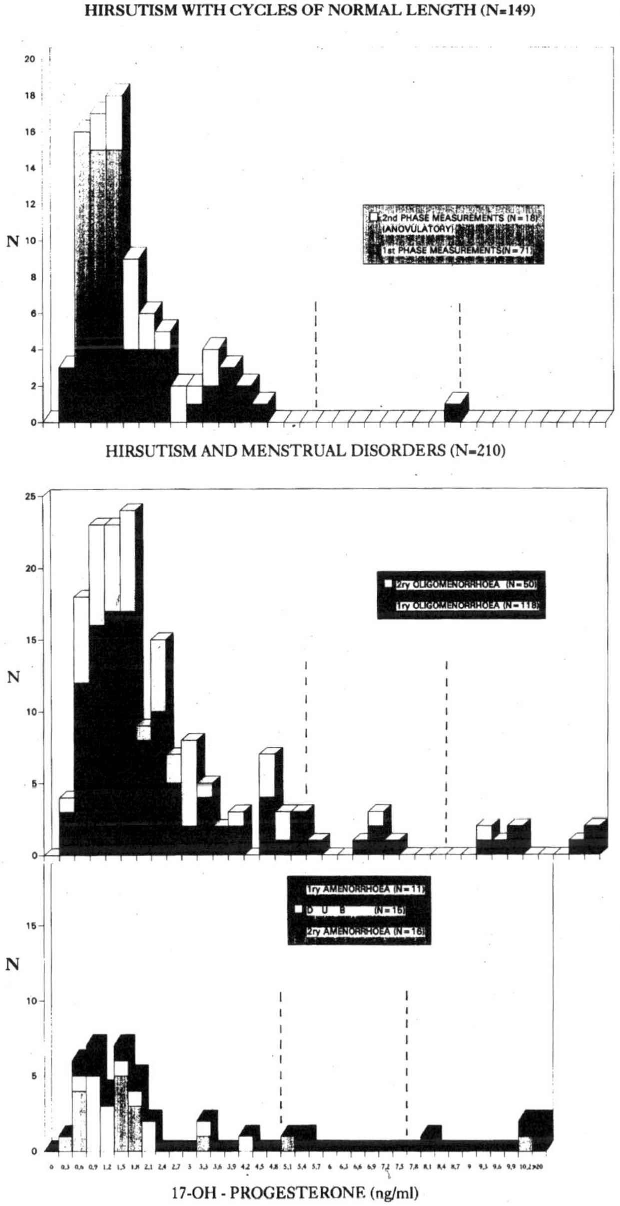

FIGURE 1. Distribution of serum 17-OH progesterone values in hirsute subjects with cycles of normal length in whom the assay was made in the follicular phase or on the 18th through 22nd day of anovulatory cycles and in patients with menstrual disorders.

measurements of serum 17-OH PG, testosterone (T), Δ-androstenedione (Δ_4-A), and dehydroepiandrosterone sulfate (DHEA-S) were made at about 09:00 hours. Of the 359 subjects, 149 (41.5%) had cycles of normal length (NC); and the remaining 210 presented with menstrual disorders, 118 with primary oligomenorrhea (occurring immediately postmenarche), 50 with secondary oligomenorrhea (occurring after 1–2 years of postmenarche cycles of normal length), 16 with secondary amenorrhea, 15 with dysfunctional uterine bleeding (DUB), and 11 with primary amenorrhea. In 71 subjects with NC, the blood samples were obtained in the first phase of the cycle. In the remaining 78 subjects with NC in whom the measurement was made during the luteal phase, progesterone (PG) was also measured. In 60 of them (76.9%), high PG levels (>7 ng/ml) indicated ovulatory cycles, whereas in the remaining 18 the cycles were anovulatory (PG<1.5 ng/ml).

The correlation between 17-OH PG and T, Δ_4-A and DHEA-S was evaluated in the whole group and separately in the subjects with 17-OH PG levels of 0.1–2.4 ng/ml, 2.5–5 ng/ml and >5.1 ng/ml using Spearmans' correlation coefficient.

The distribution of 17-OH PG values is shown in FIGURES 1 and 2. In the patients with menstrual disorders, with the exception of those with primary amenorrhea, as well as in the subjects with cycles of normal length in whom 17-OH PG was measured in the first phase or in the luteal phase of an unovulatory cycle, the distribution

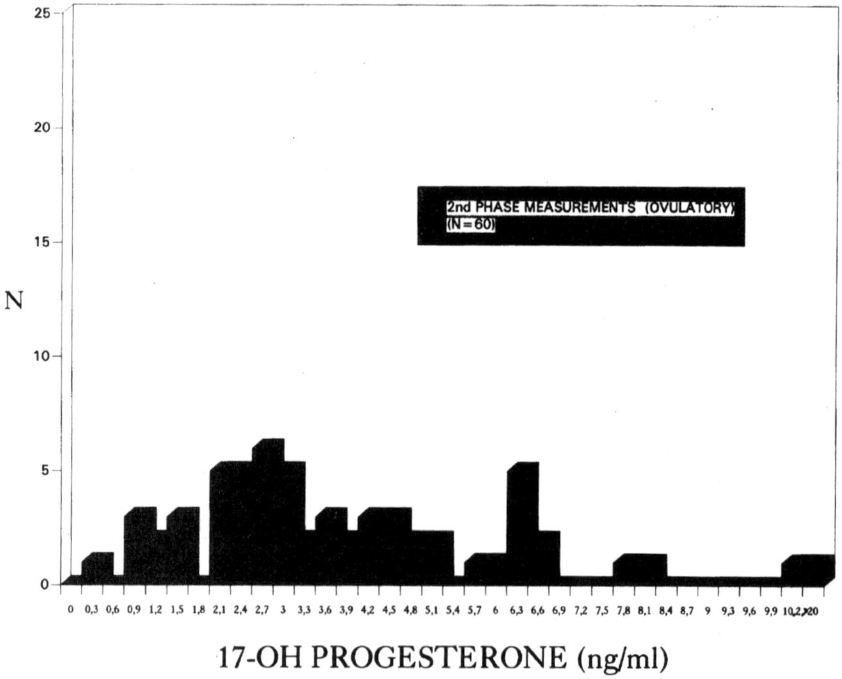

FIGURE 2. Distribution of values of 17-OH progesterone in hirsute subjects with ovulatory cycles in whom the assay was made in the luteal phase.

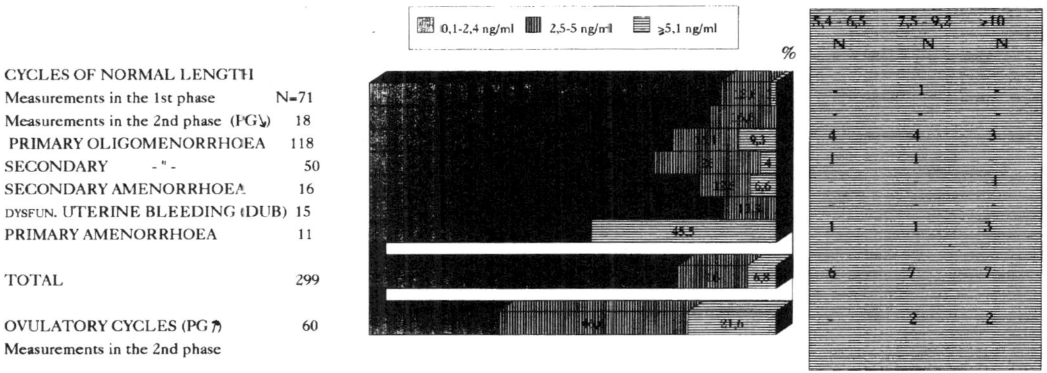
0,1-2,4 ng/ml
2,5-5 ng/ml
≥5,1 ng/ml
%
5,4 - 6,5
7,5 - 9,2
>10
N
N
N
CYCLES OF NORMAL LENGTH
Measurements in the 1st phase N=71
Measurements in the 2nd phase (PG↘) 18
PRIMARY OLIGOMENORRHOEA 118
SECONDARY - " - 50
SECONDARY AMENORRHOEA 16
DYSFUN. UTERINE BLEEDING (DUB) 15
PRIMARY AMENORRHOEA 11
TOTAL 299
OVULATORY CYCLES (PG↗) 60
Measurements in the 2nd phase
9,3
4
6,6
45,5
6,8
21,6

FIGURE 3. The percentage of hirsute subjects having serum 17-OH progesterone levels between 0.1 and 2.4, 2.5 and 5, and > 5.1 ng/ml and the number of patients in each group having 17-OH progesterone values 5.4–6.5, 7.5–9.2 and > 10 ng/ml.

of 17-OH PG values was rather normal, within the range of 1.1–2.4 ng/ml, which included the majority (70–86.6%) of values.

In 12.5–26% of the cases in each group, values between 2.5–5 ng/ml seemed to represent a different population, whereas scattered 17-OH PG values above 5 ng/ml were found in one case in the 82 subjects with cycles of normal length, in 9.3% of those with primary oligomenorrhea (n=118), in 6.6% of those with secondary amenorrhea (n=16), and in 4% of those with secondary oligomenorrhea (n=50). Five of the 11 patients with primary amenorrhea had 17-OH PG values above 5 ng/ml (FIG. 3).

In the subjects with ovulatory cycles (PG>7 ng/ml) in whom blood was obtained in the luteal phase, the greater percentage of values (46.6%) ranged between 2.4 and 5 ng/ml. Values between 0.1 and 2.4 ng/ml were found in 31.6% of the subjects, another 15% had values between 5.7 and 6.5 ng/ml, and four subjects had values over 7.5 ng/ml (FIG. 2).

Statistically significant correlation was found only for 17-OH PG and Δ_4-A (p<0.01) in subjects with 17-OH PG values from 1.2 to 2.4 ng/ml.

The above findings permit the following remarks: (1) The distribution of serum 17-OH PG concentration in hirsutism with cycles of normal length or menstrual disorders shows that values above 5 ng/ml are found in 1.4% and 3.9–9.4%, respectively. When 17-OH PG is measured in the luteal phase, ovarian secretion of 17-OH PG results in a shift of the distribution curve to the right. (2) The degree of the biological hyperandrogenicity, as indicated by serum testosterone, Δ_4-A, and DHEA-S values, is not correlated with the magnitude of the 17-OH PG increase in hirsutism with biochemical evidence of 21-hydroxylase insufficiency.

REFERENCES

1. AZZIZ, R. 1995. 21-Hydroxylase-deficiency nonclassic adrenal hyperplasia. Endocrinologist **5**(4): 297–303.
2. NEW, M. T. 1994. Congenital adrenal hyperplasia. *In* Endocrinology. 3rd edit. L. J. De Groot, Ed. Vol. 2: 1813–1835. W. B. Saunders Co. Philadelphia, PA.
3. KUTTENN, F., P. COUILLIN, F. GIRARD, L. BILLAUD, M. VINCENS, C. BOUCEKKINE, J. C. THALABAR, D. T. MAUDELONDE, P. SPRITZER, I. MOWSZOWICZ, A. BOUE & P. MAUVAIS-JARVIS. 1985. Late-onset adrenal hyperplasia in hirsutism. N. Engl. J. Med. **313:** 224–231.
4. FEUILLAN, P., S. PANG, T. S. CHÜRMEYER, P. C. AVGERINOS & G. P. CHROUSOS. 1988. The hypothalamic–pituitary–adrenal axis in partial (late-onset) 21 hydroxylase deficiency. J. Clin. Endocrinol. Metab. **67:** 154–160.
5. CHETKOWSKI, R. J., J. DEFAZIO, I. SHAMINKI, H. L. JUDD & R. J. CHANG. 1984. The incidence of late-onset congenital adrenal hyperplasia due to 21 hydroxylase deficiency among hirsute women. J. Clin. Endocrinol. Metab. **58:** 595–598.
6. CORBIN, R. H., W. FUTTERWEIT, R. P. FIEDLER & J. C. THORNTON. 1985. Adrenocorticotropic hormone testing in idiopathic hirsutism and polycystic ovarian disease: A test of limited usefulness. Fertil. Steril. **44:** 224–226.

Clinical Syndromes of Primary Amenorrhea

M. L. BATRINOS AND CH. PANITSA-FAFLIA

Endocrine Unit
Department of Pharmacology
University of Athens Medical School
Athens 115-27, Greece

The failure of menses to appear at puberty is a serious cause of anxiety for a girl and her parents because menarche is considered the completion of puberty and the beginning of femininity with a good prospect of future fertility. A delay in the appearance of first menses is also a medical problem of diagnosis and prognosis.

The first medical problem connected with primary amenorrhea is to define the age at which a delay of menarche will be considered pathologic. An objective answer to this problem can only be based on epidemiological studies on the age of appearance of the first menses and of breast development in the general population.

In a study of 1533 Green girls of all socioeconomic classes, it was found that the incidence of menstruation was 98.4% in girls 15 years old and 99.2% in girls aged 16 years.[1] On the other hand, only four of the 217 girls (1.8%) aged 12 years and one of the 241 girls (0.4%) aged 13 years had no breast development. North American statistics give essentially the same results.[2,3]

It is consequently reasonable to regard 15 years as the age beyond which a failure of menses to appear is unphysiological and could, therefore, be considered primary amenorrhea that should be evaluated. The limit of 15 years of age for investigating a subject with lack of menses can be lowered in two cases: (a) in girls with no breast development by the age of 13 and (b) in subjects with clinical signs or stigmata of diseases known to be accompanied by primary amenorrhea such as gonadal dysgenesis.[4]

Patients with chronic systemic diseases and certain dysmorphic syndromes may have delayed menses, but these conditions are diagnosed before the age of puberty, and the failure of menses to appear is only another incident in their long history. Cushing syndrome occurring at puberty may also be associated with primary amenorrhea. Nevertheless, this disease, with its easily recognizable clinical manifestations, does not present a serious problem of differential diagnosis. The same occurs with hypothyroidism, which in order to affect gonadal function has to be severe and, therefore, clinically apparent. Patients with ambiguous genitalia can be recognized by simple inspection and investigated accordingly.[5–7]

With the exclusion of the above cases, the differential diagnosis in primary amenorrhea is confined to subjects with feminine prepubertal or pubertal phenotype. Certain authors believe that the diagnostic consideration in such subjects are the same with those presenting with secondary amenorrhea.[8] However, three important features of primary amenorrhea impose a specific diagnostic strategy in this condition and have an impact on its prognosis:

1. The fact that the majority of causes of primary amenorrhea are organic in origin and seriously affect the fertility or the health of the patients;
2. Many syndromes presenting with primary amenorrhea are not included in the spectrum of secondary amenorrhea etiologies; and
3. Three clinical findings: (a) the failure of breast development, (b) the absence of palpable uterus, and (c) growth retardation, each of which helps orient the diagnosis toward certain etiologies in primary amenorrhea, are nonexistent in secondary amenorrhea.

The aim of this paper is to show that a diagnostic procedure based on a careful evaluation of these clinical findings and assisted by the assay of serum gonadotropins, sonography, and the determination of the karyotype in all the hypergonadotropic subjects can lead, in most cases, to a definite diagnosis or at least can confine the investigation only to certain etiological possibilities.

For diagnostic purposes, the patients with primary amenorrhea can be divided into two categories: (A) those with no breast development and (B) those with spontaneous breast development.

A failure of breast development indicates that there has been no endogenous source of estrogens. Patients in this category can be distinguished into those of normal height and those of short stature or growth retardation and can be further subdivided into a hypogonadotropic group and a hypergonadotropic group (TABLE 1).

TABLE 1. Primary Amenorrhea with No Breast Development

Diagnostic Criteria	*n*
Normal height	
(a) Hypogonadotropic	
1. Idiopathic gonadotropic (or GnRH) deficiency	38
(b) Hypergonadotropic	
1. 46,XY individuals	2
2. 46,XX pure gonadal dysgenesis	5
3. Resistant ovaries	1
4. Autoimmune disease of the ovaries	
5. 17a-hydroxylase deficiency	
Short stature or growth retardation	
(a) Hypogonadotropic	
1. Pituitary dwarfism	2
2. Pituitary tumor (craniopharyngioma)	1
3. Hypothalamic dysfunction(?)	
(b) Hypergonadotropic	
1. Gonadal dysgenesis	16
Insufficient data	25
Total	**90**

HYPOGONADOTROPISM

Hypogonadotropic subjects with no breast development and normal growth belong to the syndrome of isolated idiopathic gonadotropin (or GnRH) insufficiency. This group has an excellent prognosis regarding the hormonal therapy for induction of secondary sexual characteristics and, when required, fertility. Patients with this syndrome constituted the largest group in our cases of primary amenorrhea (38 patients or 23.6%). Among them, there were only two with clinically assessed anosmia.

The differential diagnosis of these patients from simple delay of puberty presents certain difficulties that become less critical with advancing age. At 13 years, the lack of visible follicles at sonography and a negative response to the luteinizing-hormone-releasing-hormone (or LHRH) indicate the syndrome, without excluding delayed puberty. At 14 years, and more confidently at 15 years, these findings confirm the diagnosis. The presence of small follicles at sonography, however, or a weak response of gonadotropins to LHRH stimulation can still cast doubt about the correct diagnosis. Because the establishment of a diagnosis is made with certainty only at an older age, the question is when should treatment be started. We are of the opinion that treatment should commence as soon as possible to avoid unnecessary psychological distress from the lack of secondary sexual characteristics and to achieve a normal peak bone mass and density.

HYPERGONADOTROPISM

Hypergonadotropic subjects with no breast development and normal height are rare and present serious diagnostic and therapeutic problems. Karyotype determination is essential to distinguish 46,XY individuals who require immediate excision of the gonadal areas because of the high frequency (up to 30%) of malignant tumor formation in these patients at a young age.

Hypergonadotropic patients with normal 46,XX karyotype belong to four rare syndromes and necessitate a more elaborate investigation. The diagnosis of 46,XX pure gonadal dysgenesis is based on the laparoscopic finding of streak gonads.

The syndrome of resistant ovaries rarely presents itself without breast development or uterine bleeding. It is believed that it represents an absence of gonadotropic receptors on the follicles or a postreceptor signaling defect. The diagnosis can be made by sonography if follicles are definitely outlined, otherwise ovarian biopsy is necessary.

Patients with ovarian insufficiency due to autoimmune disease rarely present with primary amenorrhea without breast development. However, the detection of this syndrome is necessary because it is usually associated with autoimmune disease of the thyroid and the adrenals that should be evaluated. The diagnosis can only be made by ovarian biopsy, which will show lymphocytic infiltration of the follicles.

PRIMARY AMENORRHEA, LOW SERUM GONADOTROPINS, AND SHORT STATURE

Primary amenorrhea, low serum gonadotropins, and short stature or growth retardation indicating insufficient growth hormone action may be due to the following:

(a) Nontumoral pituitary dwarfism. Insufficiency of the pituitary involving the growth hormone and the gonadotropins may be undiagnosed until puberty, the short stature of the subject being attributed to a familiar factor. We had two such cases in our series.

(b) Pituitary, or suprapituitary, neoplasm that has destroyed the pituitary gland, provoking multiple pituitary insufficiency. Pituitary adenomas are almost nonexistent in childhood and are rare at puberty. In our series we had four cases of prolactinomas with primary amenorrhea all of which, however, had hypoplastic breasts, indicating minimal estrogen secretion by the ovaries. By contrast, craniopharyngiomas occur before or at puberty, usually inducing a complete pituitary insufficiency.

HYPERGONADOTROPIC PRIMARY AMENORRHEA, NO BREAST DEVELOPMENT, SHORT STATURE

Hypergonadotropic primary amenorrhea, no breast development, and short stature are invariably due to the syndrome of gonadal dysgenesis and its variants. The classic form of Turner syndrome with its obvious somatic stigmata is easily recognizable. Patients with chromosomal mosaics or X chromosome abnormalities usually have a milder clinical expression of the syndrome with breast development or menstruation.

PRIMARY AMENORRHEA WITH BREAST DEVELOPMENT PRESENT

The second category of patients with primary amenorrhea are those with breast development of any stage. The presence of mammary tissue in these patients indicates that endogenous estrogens have been produced by the gonads.

For the orientation of the diagnosis on clinical grounds, the patients in this category can be divided into two groups: (a) those with no palpable uterus and (b) those with normal or hypoplastic uterus (TABLE 2).

The first group comprises two syndromes:

1. The syndrome of Müllerian agenesis, in which the entire uterus and the vagina may be absent. Ovarian function is normal in these patients, and the development of secondary sexual characteristics is complete. This syndrome presents no endocrine problem, and its treatment is purely surgical.

2. A complete form of androgen insensitivity syndrome known as testicular feminization. The patients have a male 46,XY genotype with normal testis, but a completely feminine phenotype with excellent breast development. Nevertheless, they have no axillar hair and in the pubis the hair is absent or scanty. This syndrome has a familiar incidence, and its detection demands careful investigation for other affected family members.

The differential diagnosis of patients with breast development and normal or hypoplastic uterus necessitates complementary examinations.

1. The failure of estrogen administration to induce menstruation suggests an obstruction of the uterine cavity, which is a rare condition.

TABLE 2. Primary Amenorrhea with Breast Development

Diagnostic Criteria	*n*
With no palpable uterus	
(a) Müllerian duct agenesis	18
(b) Complete form of androgen insensitivity syndrome (testicular feminization)	5
With normal or hypoplasmic uterus	
(a) Uterine cavity destruction	2
(b) Polycystic ovary syndrome	13
(c) Late-onset CAH	4
(d) Hypergonadotropic group	13
1. Gonadal dysgenesis	4
2. Resistant ovaries	4
3. Unknown cause	5
(e) Pituitary insufficiency	
1. Prolactinomas	4
2. Craniopharyngiomas	4
3. Acromegaly	1
4. Nonsecreting adenomas	2
5. Nontumoral pituitary insufficiency	2
(f) Hypothalamic disorder	21
(g) Simple delayed puberty	6
Insufficient data	23
Total	**118**

2. The presence of acne or hirsutism, indicating hyperandrogenemia, direct the diagnosis to polycystic ovarian disease or to late-onset adrenal hyperplasia.

3. Hypergonadotropic patients should all be karyotyped, and the gonads of those with karyotypes containing a Y chromosome should be removed. Further investigation of the 46,XX subjects is necessary to diagnose resistant ovary syndrome or autoimmune disease.

4. The function of the pituitary must be evaluated in patients who do not belong to the above subgroups. The possibility of pituitary insufficiency, mainly due to pituitary adenomas, should not be ignored at puberty. A prolactin assay, therefore, and a radiologic examination of the sella turcica are the first measures to be taken.

In the presence of a history of retardation of growth rate in recent years or on clinical evidence of hypothyroidism, the thyroid and adrenal function should be assessed.

Our series included a considerable number of girls aged 15, 16, or more years who had a normal rate of growth, breast development of various stages, and no sign of thyroid hypofunction or pituitary insufficiency. These girls were characterized as having a hypothalamic disorder, a diagnosis made by exclusion. In the history of some of them, there were conditions such as an unfavorable psychosocial environment, nutritional factors, or excessive physical exercise that would reinforce this diagnosis. However, six patients in this group ultimately proved to have a simple delay of menses and the follow-up in most of the remaining patients was incomplete.

REFERENCES

1. BATRINOS, M. L., C. PANITSA-FAFLIA, N. COURCOUTSAKIS & V. CHATZIPAVLOU. 1990. Incidence, type, and etiology of menstrual disorders in the age group 12–19 years. Adolesc. Pediatr. Gynecol. **3:** 149–153.
2. ZACHARIAS, L., W. M. RAND & J. R. WURTMAN. 1976. A prospective study of sexual development and growth in American girls: The statistics of menarche. Obstet. Gynecol. Surv. **31:** 325–337.
3. HARLAN, W. R., E. A. HARLAN & G. P. GRILLO. 1980. Secondary sex characteristics of girls 12 to 17 years of age. The U.S. Health Examination Survey. J. Pediatr. **96:** 1047–1978.
4. REINDOLLAR, R. H., J. R. BRYD & P. G. MCDONOUGH. 1981. Delayed sexual development: A study of 252 patients. Am. J. Obstet. Gynecol. **140:** 371–380.
5. MASHCHAK, C. A., O. A. KLETZKY, V. DAVAJAN & D. R. MISHELL. 1981. Clinical and laboratory evaluation of patients with primary amenorrhea. Obstet. Gynecol. **57:** 715.
6. CHRYSSIKOPOULOS, A. & O. GEORGIOU. 1987. The etiology in 77 primary amenorrhea patients. Int. J. Fertil. **32:** 245–249.
7. FEINDOLLAR, R. H., S. P. T. THO & P. G. MCDONOUGH. 1990. Delayed puberty: An updated study of 326 patients. *In* Transactions of the American Gynecological and Obstetrical Society. J. R. Scott, Ed. Vol. 3: 146–160. Mosby Year Book, Inc. St. Louis, MO.
8. YEN, S. S. C. 1991. Chronic anovulation caused by peripheral endocrine disorders. *In* Reproductive Endocrinology. 3rd edit. S. S. C. Yen & R. B. Jaffe, Eds.: 576–630. W. B. Saunders Co. Philadelphia, PA.

Clinical Syndromes of Secondary Amenorrhea

KONSTANTINOS MAVROUDIS[a]

Second Division of Endocrinology
"Alexandra" Hospital
Athens, Greece

INTRODUCTION

Regular menstrual cycles are the result of (a) regulated feedback systems (positive and negative) involving the hypothalamus, anterior pituitary, and ovary and (b) the integrity of the uterus and outflow of the genital tract. After the maturation of the hypothalamic–pituitary–ovarian axis, regular ovulatory cycles are established, and the pattern of menstrual cycles for each person is remarkably constant. The variability in the length of the cycle increases in the decade before the menopause, reflecting a gradual decline in ovarian function. The normal menstrual cycle occurs at intervals of between 21 and 35 days and usually lasts less than 7 days. After the age of 20, there is a decrease in the mean length of the menstrual cycle owing to a shorter follicular phase.[1] Abnormalities of the menstrual cycle may range from amenorrhea to continuous menstrual bleeding. Amenorrhea during the reproductive years is very common. It has been estimated that the prevalence of amenorrhea in the general population during the reproductive years is 1.8% to 3%.[2] In college-aged women it is 2.6%[3] and may reach 20% in patients complaining of infertility.

Conventionally, secondary amenorrhea is defined as the absence of menstrual bleeding for a period of more than 6 months in a woman with previous regular menses.

ETIOLOGY

The physiological causes of amenorrhea are pregnancy and lactation, and these must always be kept in mind before any investigation is carried out. From a diagnostic point of view, the pathologic causes of amenorrhea can be due to (1) disorders of the central nervous system (CNS), secondary hypothalamic amenorrhea syndrome; (2) disorders of the anterior pituitary gland; (3) disorders of the ovary; and (4) disorders of the uterus and the outflow tract (FIG. 1).

DISORDERS OF THE CENTRAL NERVOUS SYSTEM

Hypothalamic amenorrhea syndrome is a common category of hypogonadotrophic hypogonadism and is diagnosed by the exclusion of pituitary lesions. These are due to either hypothalamic destructive lesions (craniopharyngioma, germinoma,

[a]Address for correspondence: Dr. Konstantinos Mavroudis, 30, Ergaton Typou Street, 16346 Illoupolis, Athens, Greece.

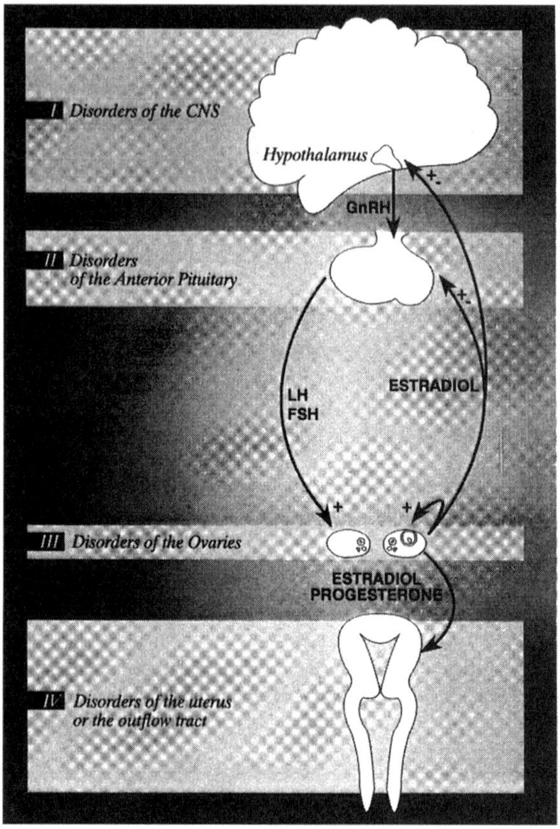

FIGURE 1. Schematic representation of the hypothalamic–pituitary–ovarian axis and disorders leading to secondary amenorrhea.

Hand-Schuller-Christian disease, head injuries, external irradiation) or to hypothalamic dysfunction (psychological stress; exercise; weight loss; anorexia nervosa; drugs, e.g., reserpine, phenothiazine; systemic diseases).[4]

The term "functional hypothalamic amenorrhea" refers to the reversible nature of the cessation of menstrual cycles in young women without organic abnormalities of the pituitary–ovarian axis. It represents one of the most common types of amenorrhea and includes a variety of physiological as well as pathophysiological conditions and is thus nonspecific.[4]

DISORDERS OF THE ANTERIOR PITUITARY GLAND

Lesions of the anterior pituitary gland include the following: (a) hemorrhage and pituitary apoplexy, which are uncommon; (b) infarcts, particularly smaller ones, which are not uncommon. However, hypopituitarism occurs only if more than 90% of the functional adenohypophyseal parenchyma is destroyed. A special form of pituitary infarction, rarely seen today in developed countries, is the postpartum massive adenohypophyseal ischemic infarction resulting in panhypopituitarism (Sheehan's syndrome); (c) various nonneoplasmatic conditions (tuberculosis, syphilis, sarcoidosis, histiocytosis X) may cause destruction of the adenohypophysis; (d) suprasellar granulomas or neoplasms may produce pituitary dysfunction (hypopituitarism or hyperprolactinemia) by interfering with the pituitary stalk; (e) lymphocytic hypophysitis, which is a rare disorder, occurs almost exclusively in women.[5]

Pituitary Neoplasms

Pituitary neoplasms can be primary or secondary, benign or malignant, functional or inactive. Pituitary adenomas are the most common primary tumors of the pituitary gland. According to current classification, based primarily on immunocytochemistry, electron microscopy, and endocrinological investigation, pituitary adenomas can be divided into the following entities (with the corresponding incidence in unselected surgical material of more than 1700 adenomas in parentheses): (1) somatotroph (growth hormone [GH] cell) adenomas (13%–15%); (2) lactotroph (prolactin [PRL] cell) adenomas (25%–28%); (3) mixed somatotroph and lactotroph adenomas (3%–5%); (4) acidophil stem cell adenomas (1%–3%); (5) mammosomatroph adenomas (1%–2%); (6) corticotroph adenomas (8%–10%); (7) silent adenomas (5%–7%); (8) thyrotroph adenomas (1%); (9) gonadotroph adenomas (7%–9%); (10) null cell adenomas (13%–15%); (11) oncocytomas (10%–12%); (12) plurihormonal adenomas (1%–3%).[5] Pituitary adenomas result in different clinical conditions depending on the secreted hormone; for example, GH-secreted adenomas result in acromegaly, the corticotroph adenomas in Cushing's disease and lactotroph adenomas in hyperprolactinemia and galactorrhea.

Hyperprolactinemia

Hyperprolactinemia is the most common cause of secondary amenorrhea. About 15%–20% of women with secondary amenorrhea have PRL concentrations that are persistently elevated above the normal range.[6] Apart from prolactinomas, other causes of hyperprolactinemia are interference with the pituitary stalk (e.g., trauma or tumor); drugs that interfere with dopamine activity (e.g., phenothiazide, metoclopramide, sulpiride, haloperidole, reserpine, methyldopa); diseases of the central nervous system (e.g., craniopharyngioma, sarcoidosis); hyperplasia of lactotrophs (e.g., hypothyroidism); and neural stimulation (e.g., chest wall thoracotomy, herpes zoster, burns, nipple stimulation).[1] Polycystic ovary syndrome (PCOS) may also be associated with increased levels of PRL. If serum PRL is elevated without any demonstrable pituitary or hypothalamic lesions or any other recognized cause, the term idiopathic hyperprolactinemia is applied.

An empty sella refers to an enlarged pituitary fossa resulting from arachnoid herniation through an incomplete sellar diaphragm. An empty sella may be either primary, from a congenital diaphragmatic defect, or secondary, from damage to the diaphragm by pituitary infarction, radiation therapy, or surgery. In addition, pituitary tumors may undergo subclinical hemorrhagic infarction and cause contraction of the overlying suprasellar cistern downward into the sella. Therefore, the presence of an empty sella does not exclude the possibility of a coexisting pituitary tumor. Most of the patients with primary empty sella are asymptomatic, and approximately 15% have mild hyperprolactinemia.[7,8]

DISORDERS OF THE OVARY

Polycystic Ovary Syndrome

Polycystic ovary syndrome (PCOS) is the association of hyperandrogenism with chronic anovulation in women without specific underlying diseases of the adrenal or pituitary glands.[9] Although the pathogenetic mechanism of polycystic ovary syndrome is not clear, it seems likely that the ovary is the principal source of excess androgen secretion. The high level of luteinizing hormone (LH) is a result rather than the cause of ovarian dysfunction.[10]

The typical clinical features of PCOS are hirsutism, acne, or male-pattern alopecia; obesity is also a common symptom. Anovulation is presented as menstrual disturbance (amenorrhea, oligomenorrhea, or dysfunctional uterine bleeding) and infertility. The diagnosis of PCOS is based on a combination of clinical, ultrasonographic, and biochemical criteria. A woman with secondary amenorrhea or oligomenorrhea may have PCOS if she has one or more of the following three features: polycystic ovaries on ultrasonography, hirsutism, and hyperandrogenemia. Many women may have high LH concentrations, but normal LH levels do not rule out the diagnosis of PCOS.

Premature Ovarian Failure

Estrogen secretion demands the presence of oocytes, and the ovary cannot function as an endocrine gland without them. Premature ovarian failure may be defined as the appearance of amenorrhea with raised gonadotropin levels before the age of 40. In the majority of women, the cause is unknown and may be a genetic disorder. Premature ovarian failure may be due to radiotherapy, chemotherapy, infection, or previous pelvic surgery including oophorectomy. Autoimmune ovarian failure is probably the most common cause of premature ovarian failure. Before premature menopause, some women experience an intermittent return of menses, interspersed with variable periods of amenorrhea.[1,7,11] In most cases it is unnecessary to confirm the absence of oocytes by ovarian biopsy. The patients have anovulatory cycles and the plasma follicle-stimulating hormone (FSH) levels are elevated in comparison with the LH in the early follicular phase.

DISORDERS OF THE UTERUS AND THE OUTFLOW TRACT

Secondary amenorrhea of uterine origin may occur because of endometrial synechiae after repeated curettage of the uterus, abortion, myomectomy, or cesarean section or after infection.[7] However, these causes are becoming very rare in developed countries, and hysterectomy is a much more common iatrogenic cause of amenorrhea.

EXTRAOVARIAN DISEASES

The most common extraovarian diseases that may be responsible for secondary amenorrhea are thyroid and adrenal diseases. Both hyperthyroidism and hypothyroidism may be associated with amenorrhea or dysfunctional bleeding. Adrenal hyperplasia (late onset) and adrenal tumors (benign or malignant) through the overproduction of androgens or estradiol, may suppress gonadotropins and disturb the hypothalamic–pituitary–ovarian axis, thereby giving rise to secondary amenorrhea.[1]

Clinical Manifestations and Consequences of Amenorrhea

An amenorrheic woman might present different symptoms and signs depending on the cause of the amenorrhea. The consequences depend on the presence or absence of endogenous estrogen. A detailed description of all the clinical features associated with amenorrhea is, however, beyond the scope of this review.

Estrogen deficiency results in hot flushes, night sweats, insomnia, vaginal dryness, lack of energy, loss of libido, fatigue, depression, thinning and wrinkling of the skin, urogenital atrophy and "urethral syndrome," but the main long-term consequences of hypoestrogenism may be osteoporosis and cardiovascular disease.[11]

Estrogen deficiency induces a dramatic increase in bone turnover, with a greater increase in bone resorption than in bone formation. Osteoporosis results from an imbalance between bone resorption and bone formation. Osteoclast resorption is accelerated in the first 6 months, peaks 1 to 3 years after cessation of ovarian function, and slows down thereafter for the next 8 to 10 years. In its early stages, osteoporosis is predominantly a disease of trabecular bone.[11] The initial rapid bone loss is inhibited by estrogen replacement treatment.

Women with premature loss of ovarian function have been found to be at increased risk of developing cardiovascular disease. All authorities now agree that long-term estrogen replacement therapy is accompanied by a decrease in the incidence of coronary events. High-density lipoprotein is increased, whereas total cholesterol and low density lipoprotein are decreased. Estrogens also have a direct effect on vascular tissue: They reduce lipid deposition, platelet aggregation, smooth muscle proliferation, collagen and elastin production, foam cell formation, endothelin (potent vasoconstrictor) production and increase the production of vasodilating and antimitogenic factors (prostacyclin and nitric oxide).[12]

Amenorrheic patients with normal or high estrogen levels, for example, with

PCOS, are at high risk of developing endometrial hyperplasia and carcinoma because of the unopposed effect of estrogen.

Evaluation of Amenorrhea

The evaluation of an amenorrheic patient starts with a careful history and a physical examination in order to seek evidence of a physiological cause of amenorrhea, emotional stress, signs of a physical problem, nutritional status, galactorrhea, and so forth.[7,13] FIGURE 2 depicts a workup for differential diagnosis of secondary amenorrhea in two steps.

The first step, after ruling out pregnancy and lactation, is the serum measurement of thyroid-stimulating hormone (TSH), PRL, LH, and FSH followed by prescription of medroxyprogesterone acetate, 10 mg daily for 7 days. The purpose of the progestational challenge is to assess the level of the endogenous estrogen and the integrity of the uterus and the outflow tract. If the patient bleeds, the diagnosis of anovulation is reliably established, a reactive endometrium sufficiently prepared by endogenous estrogen, and a patent outflow tract is confirmed. If there is no withdrawal bleeding and the levels of LH and FSH are high, one is dealing with primary ovarian failure. High levels of TSH with high or normal PRL levels indicate the presence of primary hypothyroidism. Elevated PRL with normal or low TSH levels indicates hyperprolactinemia of pituitary or hypothalamic origin.

In the second step both patients with hyperprolactinemia and patients with no withdrawal bleeding, in the presence of low or normal gonadotropins, are asked to

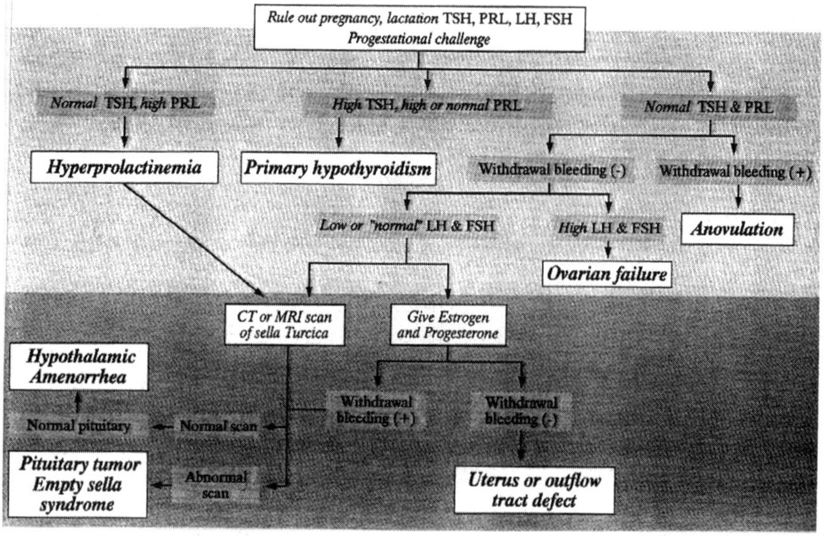

FIGURE 2. Diagnostic evaluation of secondary amenorrhea.

undergo investigation of the sella turcica by means of computed tomography (CT) or magnetic resonance imaging (MRI) scan. A normal scan is compatible with normal pituitary gland and hypothalamic amenorrhea. An abnormal scan indicates the presence of a pituitary tumor or the empty sella syndrome. A patient with normal levels of TSH, PRL, LH, and FSH and negative withdrawal response to progestational challenge is given a combination of estrogen and progesterone (conjugated estrogens, 1.25 mg daily for 21 days, and medroxyprogesterone acetate, 10 mg daily for the last 7 days). In the absence of withdrawal flow, a second course of treatment should be tried. If the patient does not bleed, the diagnosis of a defect in the endometrium or outflow tract is made.

The presented workup is a practical and simple approach to the diagnosis of the cause of secondary amenorrhea. In certain cases further investigation may be needed. For example, in patients with hypogonadotrophic hypogonadism with normal pituitary CT or MRI scanning and clinical suspicion of hypopituitarism, dynamic tests (evaluation) of the anterior pituitary function should be carried out.

Management of Amenorrhea

The management of amenorrhea depends on its specific cause and whether the patient has low or normal estrogen levels.

In the first instance the treatment is targeted at the organic disease. In patients with pathological hyperprolactinemia, the treatment of choice is bromocriptine or another dopamine agonist such as pergolide or lysuride. These drugs interact with the dopamine receptors of the lactotrophs and inhibit the secretion of prolactin. Bromocriptine (2.5–15 mg daily) reduces the levels of prolactin and leads to reduction of adenoma size in the first months of treatment with improvement in clinical symptoms. Bromocriptine has to be stopped as soon as pregnancy is diagnosed, although it does not have a teratogenic effect. During pregnancy if there is evidence of enlargement of the prolactinoma, bromocriptine can be restarted safely and usually results in shrinkage of the tumor.[1]

Other drugs that may be used for the treatment of hyperprolactinemia are depot bromocriptine (Parlodel LAR), terguride, cabergoline, and the nonergot dopamine agonist, quinagolide (CV 205-502).[14]

Rarely in patients with macroprolactinomas not responding to drug therapy is pituitary surgery (transsphenoidal) to remove the adenoma required. Radiotherapy may be used in a patient with a recurrent tumor following surgery or postoperatively to reduce the probability of tumor recurrence.[14,15] The treatment of hyperprolactinemia is individualized for each patient and depends on the presence or absence of a pituitary tumor and its size and on whether or not pregnancy is desired.

In women with anovulation and normal estrogen levels (PCOS), the treatment depends on whether or not the patient wishes to become pregnant. In infertile women, the treatment for induction of ovulation includes the following: (1) clomiphene citrate, (2) gonadotropin preparation (menopausal gonadotropin or purified FSH), (3) pulsatile administration of gonadotropin-releasing hormone (GnRH), (4) ovarian wedge resection, and (5) corticosteroids.

If pregnancy is not desired, the treatment should aim at (1) the prevention of endometrial hyperplasia and (2) the amelioration of hyperandrogenism and its consequences, hirsutism and acne. Low-dose oral contraceptive or cyclical administration of progesterone is the treatment of choice to prevent endometrial hyperplasia. For the treatment of hirsutism, antiandrogens are used, and these include cyproterone acetate, spironolactone, flutamide, and the 5α-reductase inhibitor finasteride. Acne can be treated by antibiotics, retinoic acid derivatives, and antiandrogens. Weight control and regular exercise may reduce the levels of androgens and restore a normal menstrual cycle, particularly in patients with hyperinsulinemia.

Finally, in patients with amenorrhea and hypoestrogenism, the treatment of choice is estrogen replacement. Estrogen replacement therapy (ERT) may improve all the "menopausal" symptoms and protect the patients from developing osteoporosis and cardiovascular diseases with the result of a potential prolongation of life.

In women with an intact uterus, estrogens are usually administered cyclically from day 1 through day 25 each month, and progesterone is added from days 13 through 25 to prevent endometrial hyperplasia. The most popular regimen is to give conjugated oral estrogen, 0.625 to 1.25 mg/day, or transdermal estrogen, 50- to 100-μg patches twice weekly, and medroxyprogesterone acetate (MPA), 5 mg/day in the prescribed cyclical way. Other effective estrogens include mestranol (28 μg/day) and ethinyl estradiol (20 μg/day); instead of MPA, norethindrone can be given. In women who want to avoid withdrawal bleeding, a continuous combined treatment, that is, conjugated estrogen (0.625 mg) and MPA (2.5 mg). In women with hysterectomy, estrogen alone can be given safely. The protective effects on lipids are not seen when estrogen is administered transdermally because the first-pass effect on the liver is lost.[7,12,16] The addition of progestogen tends to attenuate the increase in serum HDL cholesterol levels and the decrease in serum LDL cholesterol levels that occur in women treated with estrogen alone.[17]

The side effects of ERT include uterine bleeding, breast cancer, breast soreness, fibrocystic changes, headaches, lipid effects, gallstones, fluid retention, and thromboembolism.[12]

General measures to minimize the detrimental effects of amenorrhea include discouraging cigarette smoking and alcohol consumption and achieving ideal weight through proper diet (calcium intake) and reasonable exercise.

CONCLUSIONS

Secondary amenorrhea is defined as the absence of menstrual bleeding for ≥6 months in a woman with previous regular menses and merits evaluation. The cause is diagnosed as either of hypothalamic, pituitary, ovarian, or lower genital origin. A specific cause is sought for each case. A "workup" is followed for differential diagnosis, and the appropriate therapy has to be given early. Untreated amenorrhea is associated with significant long-term morbidity, especially in young women. Most of the amenorrheic women are hypoestrogenic and are susceptible to osteoporosis and fractures as well as lipid disorders and are at increased risk from cardiovascular events. Amenorrhea due to anovulation (noncycling estrogen levels, unopposed by progesterone, PCOS) is associated with an increased risk of endometrial hyperplasia and carcinoma even in young patients. The ultimate goal is to prevent the long-term morbidity associated with the hypoestrogenic state (osteoporosis and cardiovascular disease) and that associated with the unopposed estrogen effect (endometrial hyperplasia).

REFERENCES

1. BAIRD, D. T. 1995. Amenorrhea, anovulation, and dysfunctional uterine bleeding. *In* Endocrinology. Leslie J. DeGroot, Eds. Vol. 3: 2059–2079. Saunders. Philadelphia, PA.
2. PETTERSSON, F., H. FRIES & S. J. NILLIUS. 1973. Epidemiology of secondary amenorrhea. Am. J. Obstet. Gynecol. **117:** 80–86.
3. BACHMANN, G. A. & E. KENMANN. 1982. Prevalence of oligomenorrhea and amenorrhea in a college population. Am. J. Obstet. Gynecol. **144:** 98–102.
4. YEN, S. S. C. 1993. Female hypogonadotropic hypogonadism. Endocrinol. Metab. Clin. N. Am. **22:** 29–57.
5. HORVATH, E. & K. KOVACS. 1995. Anatomy and histology of the normal and abnormal pituitary gland. *In* Endocrinology. Leslie J. DeGroot, Eds. Vol. 1: 160–177. Saunders. Philadelphia, PA.
6. JACOBS, H. S., S. FRANKS, M. A. F. MURRAY, *et al.* 1976. Clinical and endocrine features of hyperprolactinemic amenorrhea. Clin. Endocrinol. **5:** 439–454.
7. SPEROFF, L., R. H. GLASS & N. KASE. 1994. Clinical Gynecologic Endocrinology and Infertility. 5th edit. Williams & Wilkins. Baltimore, MD.
8. FINDLING, J. W. & J. B. TYRRELL. 1991. Anterior pituitary gland. *In* Basic and Clinical Endocrinology. F. S. Greenspan, Ed.: 79–132. Lange Medical Publications.
9. ZAWADZKI, J. K. & A. DUNAIF. 1992. Diagnostic criteria for polycystic ovary syndrome: Towards a rational approach. *In* Polycystic Ovary Syndrome. A. Dunaif, J. R. Givens, F. P. Haseltine & G. R. Merriam, Eds.: 377–384. Blackwell Scientific. Oxford, England.
10. FRANKS, S. 1995. Polycystic ovary syndrome. N. Engl. J. Med. **333**(13): 853–861.
11. SCHACHTER, M. & Z. SHOHAM. 1994. Amenorrhea during the reproductive years—is it safe? Fertil. Steril. **62:** 1–16.
12. LUFKIN, E. G. & S. J. ORY. 1995. Postmenopausal estrogen therapy. Trends Endocrinol. Metab. **6:** 50–54.
13. GOLDFIEN, A. & S. E. MONROE. 1991. Ovaries. *In* Basic and Clinical Endocrinology. F. S. Greenspan, Ed.: 442–490. Lange Medical Publications.
14. SERRI, O. 1994. Progress in the management of hyperprolactinemia. N. Engl. J. Med. **331**(14): 942–944.
15. GROSSMAN, A. 1991. The modern management of macroprolactinomas. Trends Endocrinol. Metab. **2:** 163–168.
16. ODELL, W. 1995. The menopause and hormonal replacement. *In* Endocrinology. Leslie J. DeGroot, Ed. Vol. 3: 2128–2139. W. B. Saunders Company. Philadelphia, PA.
17. BELCHETZ, P. E. 1994. Hormonal treatment of postmenopausal women. N. Engl. J. Med. **330**(15): 1062–1071.

Bone Mineral Metabolism in Diet-Induced Amenorrhea

VINCENZINA BRUNI,[a] LUISA BIGOZZI,[a] METELLA DEI,[a]
AND M. LUISA BRANDI[b]

[a]*Department of Obstetrics and Gynecology*
[b]*Department of Endocrinology*
University of Florence
Medical School
Florence, Italy

INTRODUCTION

It is well known that osteopenia of both trabecular and cortical bone is a serious complication of hypoestrogenic amenorrhea. The phenomenon has been extensively studied in subjects with anorexia nervosa; it has been correlated with the age of onset, the duration of the illness, and residual body fat mass.[1–3] The accelerated bone loss is similar to that in post-menopausal osteoporosis; and, especially at the lumbar spine, it is likely to be dependent on estrogen deficiency. Although the role of estrogen replacement therapy in preventing bone loss at menopause has been clearly established, the beneficial effects of estrogen administration in women with anorexia nervosa are still being debates.[3–5] The lack of full protection by estrogen in the latter patients indicates that some factors other than estrogen deficiency have a role in the pathogenesis of this type of osteopenia. These factors could be related to the nutritional status and/or other hormonal influences (e.g., cortisol excess, IGF-1 deficiency) that are known regulators of bone remodeling.

In the present study, clinical and hormonal variables affecting bone density in subjects with hypoestrogenic diet-induced amenorrhea (excluding typical anorexia nervosa) were compared with values obtained from subjects of similar age who were suffering from premature ovarian failure.

SUBJECTS AND METHODS

We studied 41 young women (age range 16–34 years; mean age 22.3 ± 5.0) with diet-induced amenorrhea (DA). All subjects had had amenorrhea for at least 6 months, which occurred in close proximity to the onset of a quantitative and/or qualitative restriction of diet as well as weight loss of more than 10% of basal weight. The response to medroxy progesterone acetate was negative in all 41 patients. Some subjects with partial weight recovery were included in this study, but women with typical anorexia nervosa, as defined by the *Diagnostic and Statistics Manual III-R,*[6] were excluded.

Twenty-two women (age range 16–34 years; mean age 30.0 ± 6.3), affected by premature ovarian failure (POF) with normal karyotype, served as the reference control group. No patient had any illness or was taking estrogens or any medication known to affect bone density or endocrine status at the start of this study. Informed written consent was obtained from all subjects.

The study protocol included a complete clinical history and physical examination to assess weight loss; eventual weight recovery (for subjects with DA); body mass index (BMI); actual weight, height, and menstrual function before amenorrhea; duration of amenorrhea (in months); and physical exercise. All subjects with DA were asked to keep a food diary. We evaluated blood glucose, electrolytes, creatinine, calcium, phosphorus hemoglobin, iron, proteins, transaminases, amylase, cholesterol, and triglycerides. Breast and pelvic ultrasonography was performed.

The endocrine profile was investigated using the following parameters: FSH; LH; PRL in duplicate by IRMA (MAIA CLONE, Serono); E_2 in duplicate by DIRIA (ESTR K, Sorin Biomedica); FT3, FT4, and TSH by IRMA (ARIA HT, Becton Dickinson Immunodiagnostics); IGF-1 by RIA (IL, Nichols); cortisol by RIA (TDX, Abbott); parathyroid by IRMA (IL, Nichols); and 25-hydroxyvitamin D by RIA (INCSTAR, Sorin Biomedica). Bone turnover was investigated by the serum measurement of two markers of bone mineral apposition: osteocalcin (GLA) by RIA (OSTK-PR) and alkaline phosphatase by Granutest 25 (Merck) and by the evaluation of three urinary markers of bone resorption: hydroxyproline (OHP) according to Nordin by HPLC (Biorad) and pyridinoline (PYR) and deoxypyridinoline (DPYR) by HPLC (Biorad). Fasting serum samples were obtained at 8:00 A.M.; early morning urinary samples were collected. Spinal bone density was measured at the L1–L4 level by dual-energy X-ray obsorptiometry (DEXA), using bone densitometer (HOLOGIC QDR 1000). The Z score (number of standard deviations above or below the mean for age) was calculated.

Differences among those patients with DA and those with POF were analyzed using two-tailed *t* tests for unpaired variables. The accepted level of significance was $p < 0.05$. Correlations among the parameters were evaluated by Pearson's test, using a linear model for regression analysis, when appropriate.

RESULTS

Clinical data for both groups are shown in TABLE 1. There were no significant differences between the two groups regarding age, age of onset of menses, and duration of amenorrhea. The BMI values of the DA patients were nearly all in the minimum range or lower for age. All the women had normal values for the routine biochemical parameters investigated, except for a trend toward lower levels of serum iron and hemoglobin in subjects with weight loss.

During a preliminary survey before admittance to the study protocol, we had split the group of DA subjects into two groups: those with no weight recovery and those with a minimal but significant weight recovery (> 3 kg). The spinal bone mass was not significantly different between the two groups. We found a similar result by splitting these DA subjects into three groups according to the levels of physical activity (absent, moderate, vigorous). Given that subjects with POF were mostly sedentary,

TABLE 1. Clinical Features of the Subjects

	DA (n=41)[a]	POF (n=22)[a]
Age (yrs)	22.3 ± 5	30.0 ± 6.3
Age at menarche (yr)	12.7 ± 1.4	12.2 ± 1.5
Gynecological age (yr)	9.5 ± 5.3	17.8 ± 6.9
Menstrual regularity before amenorrhea (months)	85.9 ± 47.4	174.2 ± 79.9
Duration of amenorrhea (months)	32.5 ± 35.4	36.7 ± 49.1
BMI (kg/m^2)	17.3 ± 1.7	22.8 ± 5.2
Weight loss (kg)	11.5 ± 6.4	No significant weight modifications
Weight loss/basal weight	0.2 ± 0.09	

[a]Values are expressed as the mean ± SD.

this protocol was not practicable. As a consequence of the results of the preliminary survey, we evaluated the entire group of subjects with DA and compared them with the POF control group.

Mean bone mass density (BMD) was 0.87 ± 0.10 in the DA group and 0.90 ± 0.11 in the POF group. The coefficients of variation were similar (12.3 and 13.0, respectively). The Z score was 1.67 ± 0.9 in the DA subjects and 1.58 ± 0.9 in the POF patients, without any significant differences between the groups. A significant positive correlation between the Z score and the duration of amenorrhea in the DA population (r=0.50; p<0.01) (FIG. 1) was found when the relationship between the Z score and the clinical parameters was considered. This correlation was scantily evident even in the POF group (r=0.37; p=0.08) (FIG. 2). By separately analyzing the subjects with diet-induced amenorrhea by dividing them into two subgroups, those with amenorrhea that had lasted less than a maximum of 20 months and those for whom the condition had lasted more than 20 months, the correlation was significant only in the second subgroup (r=0.57; 2itp<0.01) (FIG. 3). Subjects with POF did not display any significant variability in relationship between the Z score and the duration of amenorrhea with regard to a temporal threshold (r=0.35 less than 20 months and 4=0.37 more than 20 months).

In all the subjects with DA, weight loss, as expressed by the ratio between the decrease in weight and basal weight, was also considered. A positive correlation with the Z score values (r=0.40; p<0.01) (FIG. 4) was found that displayed a pattern similar to the relationship between duration of amenorrhea and the Z score. This was more significant in subjects without menses for more than 20 months (r=0.46; p<0.05 versus r=0.38; p=0.09). Indeed, the weight loss relative to basal weight was directly correlated to the months of amenorrhea in these subjects.

The BMI was not related to the Z score value, either in girls with DA or in the POF control group, even if a weak negative correlation was demonstrated (r=0.28) in the subgroup of patients with DA of longer duration. It must be noted that among the subjects with POF, only three had a BMI that was higher than the normal range.

The mean hormonal concentrations of our two groups of patients were typical

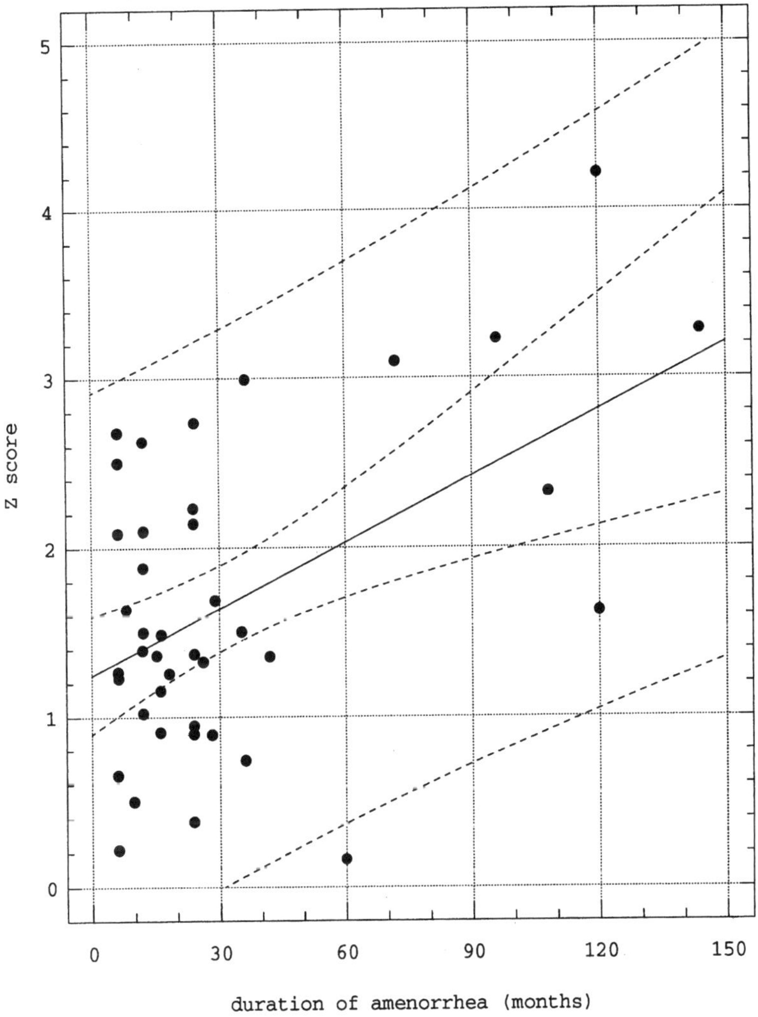

FIGURE 1. DA subjects: relationship between Z score and duration of amenorrhea ($r=0.50$; $p<0.01$).

of these two clinical conditions (TABLE 2). Diet-induced amenorrhea was characterized by low levels of FSH, LH, and 17-beta estradiol; whereas premature ovarian failure showed typically increased FSH and LH concentrations and low estrogen levels.

The mean values of estradiol were not significantly different when the two groups were compared. No relationship was evident between the Z scores and the estradiol levels in the two groups of patients, nor when the two subgroups were considered in relation to duration of amenorrhea.

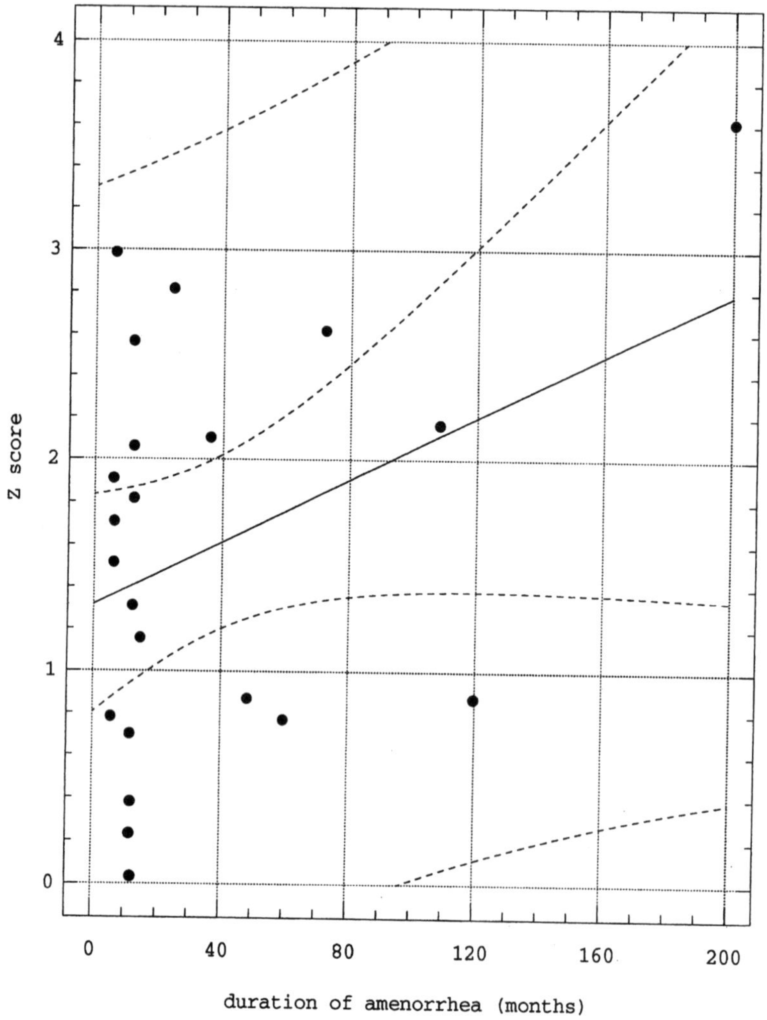

FIGURE 2. POF subjects: relationship between Z score and duration of amenorrhea. (r=0.37; *p*=0.08).

The difference in mean cortisol levels was not significant when the DA and POF control groups were compared. However, a trend toward increasing values in the former was clearly evident. In the POF group, no correlation was found between the cortisol levels and Z score. In patients with weight loss, this correlation appeared significant only in the subgroup with amenorrhea that had lasted less than 20 months (r=0.38) (FIG. 5).

We found no differences between the DA patients and the POF control group re-

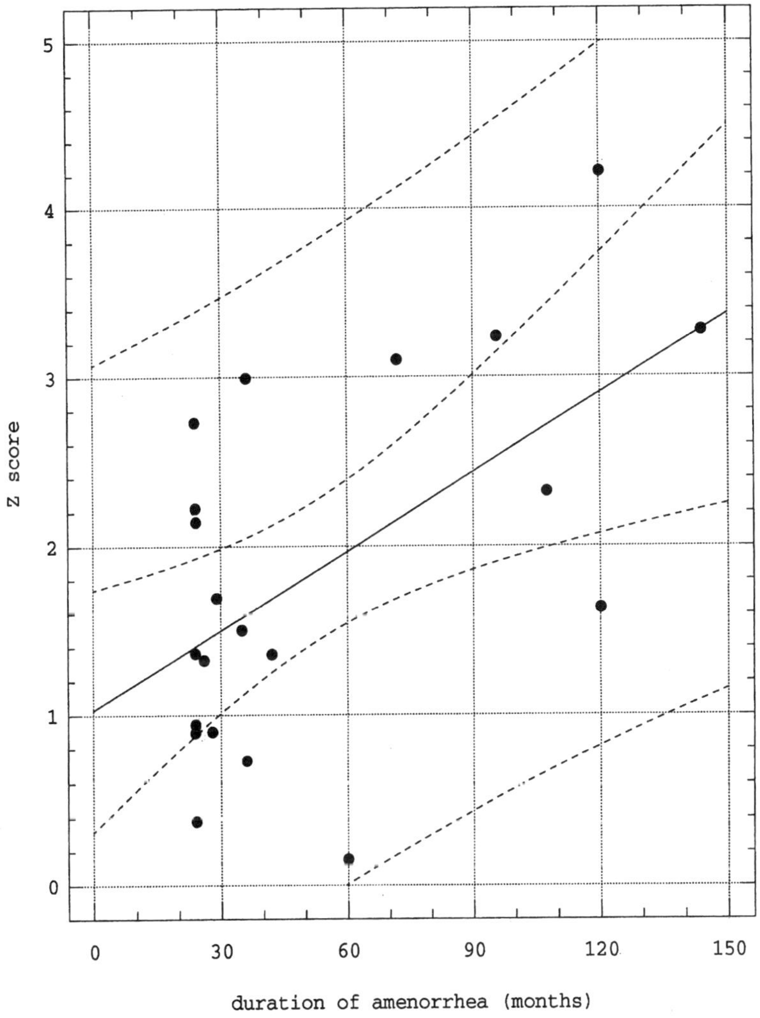

FIGURE 3. DA subjects: relationship between Z score and duration of amenorrhea. (>20 months) (r=0.57; $p<0.01$).

garding parahormone and hydroxyvitamin D. FT3 was also studied as a marker of nutritional status. A highly significant correlation with the Z score in the subjects with amenorrhea lasting more than the threshold of 20 months was found (r=0.50; $p=0.01$) (FIG. 6). IGF-1 concentrations were not correlated to the Z score, even when the two DA subgroups were considered (more and less than 20 months of amenorrhea).

The data concerning the biochemical markers of bone metabolism are shown in

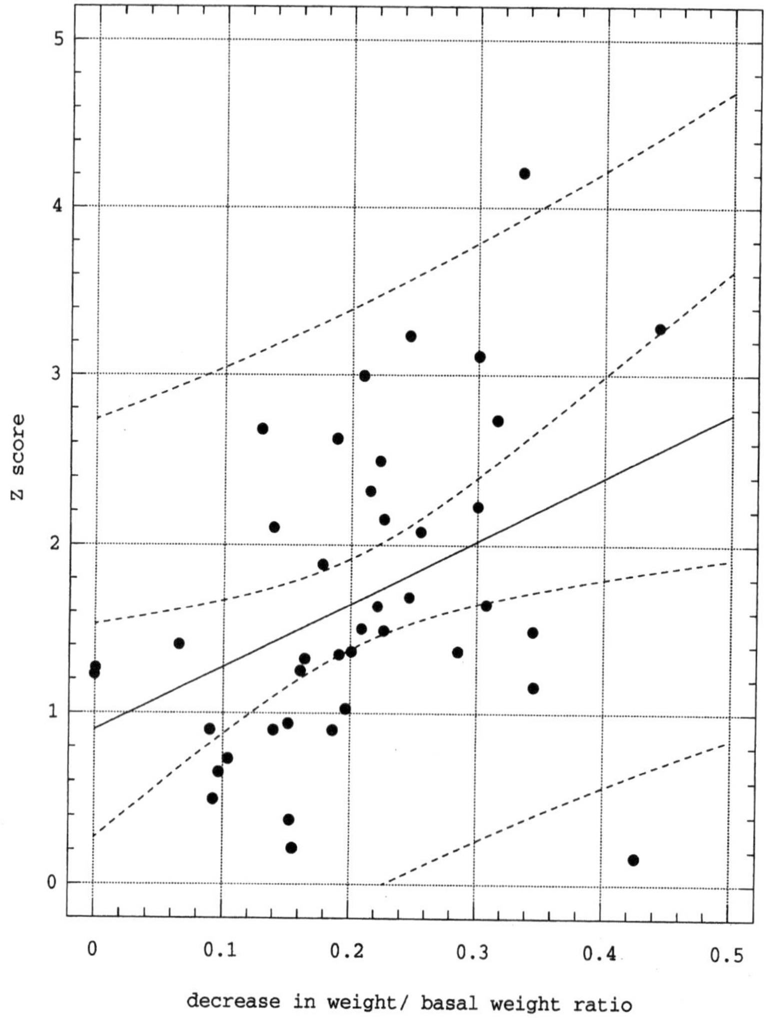

FIGURE 4. DA subjects: relationship between decrease in weight/basal weight ratio and Z score (r=0.40; p<0.01).

TABLE 3. No significant differences were found between the two groups. Upon comparison of the normal values for age range, the urinary excretion of OHP and PYR (markers of bone resorption) clearly showed increases in both DA subjects and the control group. However, the levels of these two markers did not reveal any correlation with the length of amenorrhea.

TABLE 2. Results of the Endocrine Profile

	DA[a]	POF[a]
FSH (mIU/ml)	5.9 ± 3	89.9 ± 35.1
LH (mi/ml)	1.7 ± 0.2	30.5 ± 10.3
PRL (ng/ml)	9.1 ± 5.0	10.4 ± 4.3
E2 (pg/ml)	16.0 ± 13	11.5 ± 8.1
FT3 (ng/ml)	3.8 ± 0.8	4.1 ± 0.9
FT4 (pg/ml)	10 ± 3.3	10.1 ± 3.4
TSH (microU/ml)	1.9 ± 1.2	2.5 ± 3.2
Cortisol (nmol/l)	438.8 ± 136.6	367.6 ± 156.6
IGF-1 (ng/ml)	232.5 ± 89.9	237.4 ± 100.2
Vitamin D (ng/ml)	24.5 ± 11.4	26.6 ± 11
PTH (pg/ml)	33.3 ± 12.9	31.3 ± 12.3

[a]Values are expressed as mean ± SD.

DISCUSSION

The present data confirm the presence of serious bone mass loss in young women with diet-induced amenorrhea, even if there was no important deterioration of the metabolic balance observed in anorexia nervosa. The mean spinal mineral content of our patients was –1.5 standard deviation, that is, below the normal range. Only those subjects with a gynecological age of over 4 years were admitted to the study, in order to minimize the inclusion of subjects with failure to attain peak bone density.[7–10] In fact, recent investigations have established that the attainment of the peak takes place relatively early, that is, from 15 to 18 years.[7,8] Furthermore, no significant increases in bone mineral content at the level of the lumbar spine have been demonstrated in healthy young women with eumenorrhea after those years of pubertal maturation.[9,10]

Because the subjects studied had a period of regular menses for at least 3 years before the onset of amenorrhea, the low bone density found was more likely to have been due to bone loss rather than to low peak done density. The level of physical activity did not seem to influence bone density at the level of the lumbar spine, even if it has been shown to influence bone density at weight-bearing sites such as the femoral neck.[3]

In agreement with other studies,[2,3,5,11] we found that the duration of amenorrhea is a clinical parameter that can predict the severity of osteopenia (independently of minimum partial weight recovery). In a previous work,[12] our group showed how diet-induced amenorrhea is a phenomenon that occurs very soon after caloric restriction (with a mean time of two months from the beginning of the diet to the last menstrual flow). Therefore, the relationship between bone mass density values and the months of amenorrhea reflects the relationship with diet behavior and BMD. It is interesting to consider the trend of bone mass loss over a period of time. From our data, in subjects with less than 20 months of amenorrhea, the variation of the Z score was very rapid and random. Afterwards, the increase appeared to progress steadily. Even if it were not so evident, the POF group showed the same relationship between Z score

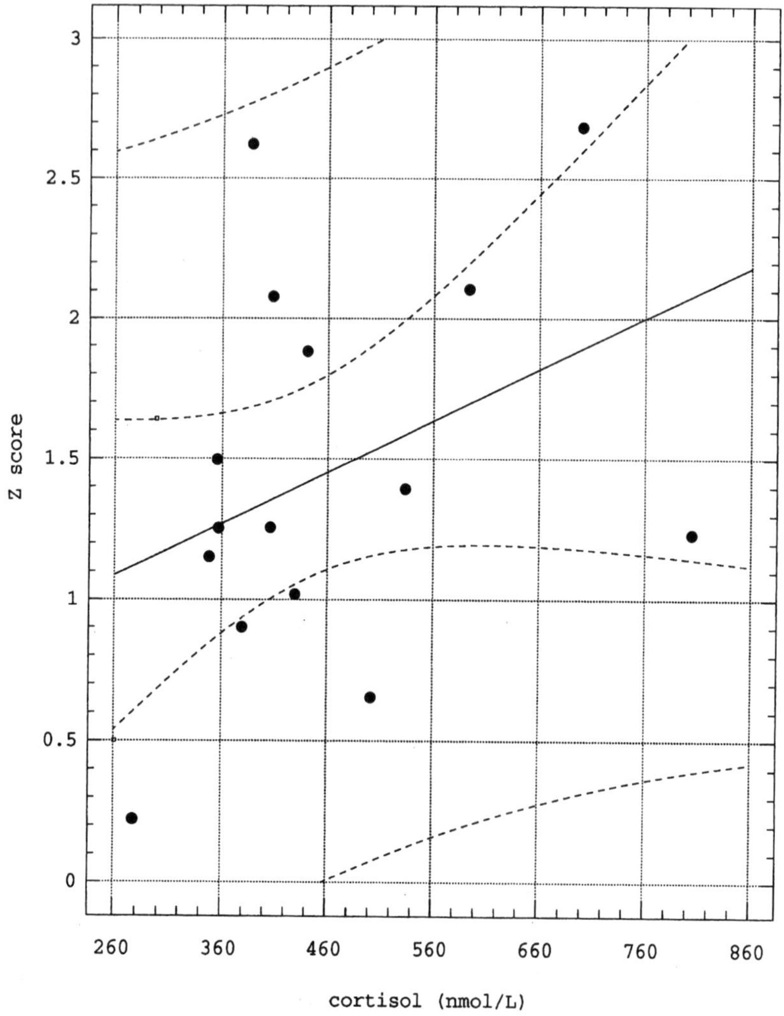

FIGURE 5. DA subjects: relationship between Z score and cortisol (amenorrhea <20 months) (r=0.38).

and duration of amenorrhea as those subjects with diet-induced amenorrhea that had lasted more than 20 months.

These data may indicate that in POF patients the decrease in estrogen production plays the most important role in the modification of bone turnover, whereas in DA subjects other parameters, probably related to metabolic adaptations, act synergistically with hypoestrogenism on bone mineral metabolism. However, a different effect was noted as long as the amenorrhea continued.

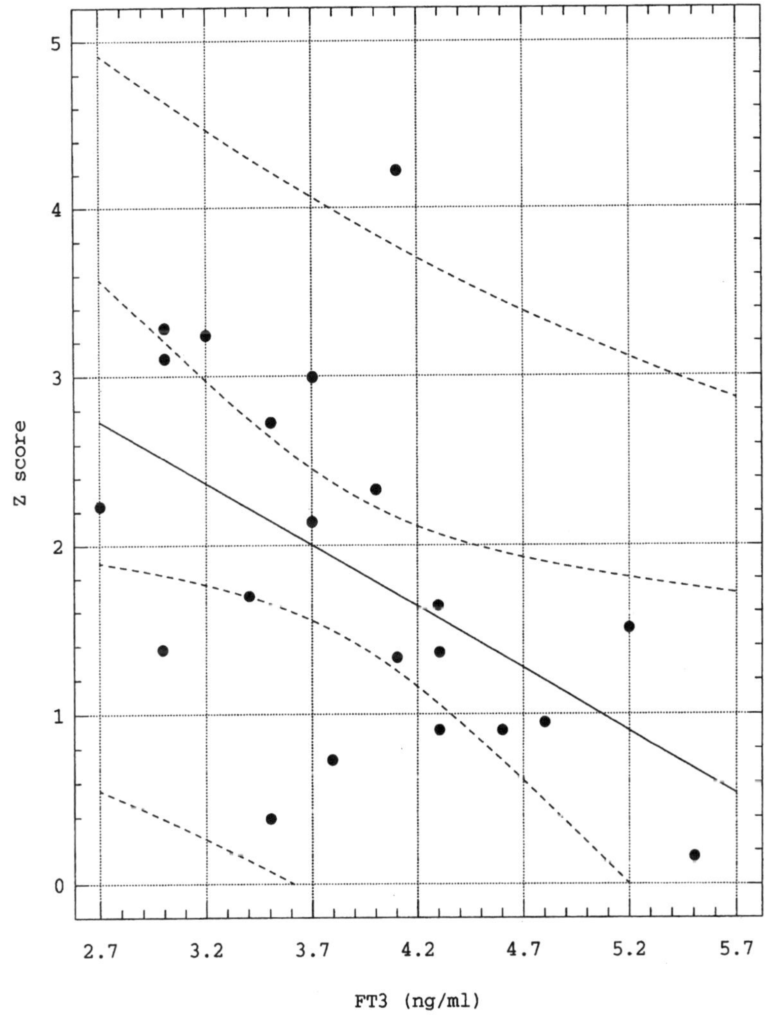

FIGURE 6. DA subjects: relationship between Z score and FT3 (amenorrhea >20 months) (r=0.50; $p<0.01$).

The importance of weight loss in determining bone density in women with anorexia nervosa has also been shown in other studies.[3,5] The BMI at the time of the investigation was not considered a good marker of reduced adiposity in subjects with DA, given that different techniques for the measurements of body composition are better able to characterize the relationships between body fat and lean mass and bone mineral turnover.

The two patient groups studied had comparable mean estrogen levels. The ab-

TABLE 3. Biochemical Markers of Bone Metabolism

	DA[a]	POF[a]
GLA (ng/ml)	21.9 ± 11	23.8 ± 8.9
ALP (U/L)	166.46 ± 46	167.6 ± 45
OHP (mg/g)	24.3 ± 8.5[b]	28.2 ± 8.5[b]
PYR (pmol/μmol)	92.3 ± 44[c]	92.9 ± 41.1[c]
DPYR (pmol/μmol)	16.9 ± 10.3	16.7 ± 7.1

[a]Values are expressed as mean ± SD.
[b]Significantly different from the normal range for age ($p<0.01$).
[c]Significantly different from the normal range for age ($p<0.05$).

sence of a direct correlation between lumbar bone mass and the estradiol concentrations in both populations might reflect the poor reliability of estradiol as a measurement of estrogen status. This may be due to the extraglandular estrogen production and to changes in hepatic sex hormone metabolism, which certainly do play an important role in hypoestrogenism. In amenorrhea related to nutritional deficit, however, other nutritionally dependent variables must be taken into account.

Our results also suggest that there is a clear correlation between changes in bone mass in subjects with long-lasting amenorrhea and FT3 (a sensitive marker of carbohydrate deprivation[13] and metabolic homeostasis[14]). The possibility that increased circulating levels of thyroid hormones—both endogenous and exogenous—play a role in accelerating bone turnover is well known.[15] In our patients, however, an impaired peripheral conversion of the same hormones seemed to be related to a loss of bone mass.

Biller *et al.*[16] found that a correlation exists between urinary cortisol excretion and spinal bone density in women with anorexia nervosa. The present data also raise the possibility of a negative cortisol effect on bone metabolism. Because an increase in the nocturnal cortisol nadir is prevalent in subjects with weight loss,[17] an evening sampling in our protocol would have been better indicated and should be used in future studies to investigate this point. The two hormones, FT3 and cortisol, may have acted at different times, cortisol precociously, FT3 in a delayed manner.

The biochemical markers of bone turnover, extensively studied in the present study, showed an increase in urinary OHP and PYR levels. These data are in disagreement with those dealing with the analysis of bone tissue in subjects with anorexia nervosa,[18] where direct evidence of increased resorption has not been found. A longitudinal evaluation of these markers are necessary to draw any final conclusion.

In summary, the pathogenesis of spinal bone loss in subjects with diet-induced amenorrhea is definitely multifactorial. The effect of the nutritionally dependent hormones (i.e., FT3, cortisol, Gh-IGF 1 complex) together with steroid androgens should be further investigated to understand the role of the timing of the different hormonal actions on bone metabolism and to understand the partial protective effect of hormone replacement therapy at the lumbar spine in patients with anorexia nervosa.[3,5]

SUMMARY

Spinal bone density of 41 girls with diet-induced amenorrhea (DA) was compared with that of the density of 22 subjects with premature ovarian failure (POF) of comparable age. The Z score values, as well as the estradiol levels, were not significantly different in the two groups. The duration of amenorrhea was significantly correlated to bone mass density in the DA population, especially when considering subjects with amenorrhea that had lasted longer than 20 months. A similar correlation between weight loss and BMD was evident. Although estradiol concentrations did not seem to be correlated to the Z score, FT3 and cortisol values exhibited, respectively, a negative and a positive correlation with spinal density. Cortisol seemed to act precociously, whereas FT3 acted later than cortisol.

REFERENCES

1. Bachrach, L., D. Guido, D. Katzman, I. Litt & R. Marcus. 1990. Decreased bone density in adolescents girls with anorexia nervosa. Pediatrics **86**(3): 440.
2. Biller, B. M. K., J. F. Coughlin, V. Saxe, D. Schoenfeld, D. I. Spratt & A. Klibanski. 1991. Osteopenia in women with hypothalamic amenorrhea: A prospective study. Obstet. Gynecol. **78:** 996.
3. Seeman, E., G. I. Szmuckler, C. Formica, C. Tsalamandris & R. Mestrovic. 1992. Osteoporosis in anorexia nervosa: The influence of peak bone density, bone loss, oral contraceptive use, and exercise. J. Bone Mineral Res. **7**(12): 1467.
4. Emans, S. J., G. Estherann, F. A. Hoffer, C. Gundburg, V. Ravnikar & E. R. Woods. 1990. Estrogen deficiency in adolescents and young adults: Impact on bone mineral content and effects of estrogen replacement therapy. Obstet. Gynecol. **76:** 585.
5. Klibanski, A., B. M. K. Biller, D. A. Scoenfeld, D. B. Herzog & V. C. Saxen. 1995. The effect of estrogen administration on trabecular bone loss in young women with anorexia nervosa. J. Clin. Endocrinol. Metab. **80**(3): 898
6. American Psychiatric Association. 1987. Diagnostic and Statistical Manual of Mental Disorders. 3rd edit. American Psychiatric Association. Washington, DC.
7. Gislanz, V., D. T. Gibbens, T. F. Roe, M. Carlson, M. O. Senac, M. I. Boechat, H. K. Huang, E. E. Schultz, C. R. Libanat & C. C. Cann. 1988. Vertebral bone density in children: Effect of puberty. Radiology **166:** 847.
8. Bonjour, J. P., G. Theintz, B. Buchs, D. Slosman & R. Rizzoli. 1991. Critical years and stages of puberty for spinal and femoral bone mass accumulation during adolescence. J. Bone Min. Res. **73:** 555.
9. White, C. M., A. C. Hergendroeder & W. J. Klish. 1992. Bone mineral density in 15 to 21 year old eumenorrheic and amenorrheic subjects. Am. J. Dis. Child. **146:** 31.
10. Slemenda, C. W., T. K. Reister, S. L. Hui, Y. Z. Miller, J. C. Christian & C. Johnston. 1994. Influences on skeletal mineralization in children and adolescents: Evidence for varying effects of sexual maturation and physical activity. J. Ped. **125**(2): 201.
11. Hay, P. J., A. Hall, J. W. Delahunt, G. Harper, A. W. Mitchell & C. Salmond. 1989. Investigation of osteopenia in anorexia nervosa. Austr. N. Z. J. Psych. **23:** 261.
12. Bruni, V., M. Dei, P. Nannalli, R. Perini & A. Verni. 1993. Perdita di peso e funzione mestruale. *In* Nuovi Orientamenti in Fisiopatologia Ginecologica ed Ostetrica. G. B. Melis, A. Volpe & E. Piccione, Eds.: 510. CIC Ed. Intern. Roma.
13. Mathieson, R. A., J. L. Walberg & F. C. Gwazdankskas. 1986. The effect of varying car-

bohydrate content of a very low caloric diet on resting metabolism rate and thyroid hormones. Metabolism **35**(4): 349.
14. Bruni, V., M. Dei, A. Digregorio & A. Verni. 1993. Diet-induced amenorrhea: The effect of moderate recovery of lost weight on endocrine parameters. *In* Recent Developments on Pediatric–Adolescent Gynecology and Endocrinology. G. Creatsas, Ed.: 41. Athens.
15. Benker, G., N. Breuer, R. Windeck & D. Reinwein. 1988. Calcium metabolism in thyroid diseases. J. Endocrinol. Invest. **11:** 61.
16. Biller, B. M. K., V. Saxe, D. B. Herzog, D. Rosenthal, S. Holzman & A. Klibanski. 1989. Mechanisms of osteoporosis in adult and adolescent women with anorexia nervosa. J. Clin. Endocrinol. Metab. **68:** 548.
17. Anderson, I. M., W. S. Crook, S. E. Gartside, C. G. Fairburn & P. J. Cowen. 1989. The effect of moderate weight loss on overnight growth hormone and cortisol secretion in healthy female volunteers. J. Affect. Dis. **16:** 197.
18. Kreipe, R. E. & G. B. Forbes. 1990. Osteoporosis: A new morbidity for dieting female adolescents. Pediatrics **86:** 478.

Luteinizing Hormone Resistance Syndromes

CONSTANTINE TSIGOS, ANA C. LATRONICO,
AND GEORGE P. CHROUSOS[a]

Development Endocrinology Branch
National Institute of Child Health and Human Development
National Institutes of Health
Bethesda, Maryland 20892

INTRODUCTION

Male sexual differentiation is a complex process that requires the sequential activation of several genes and the presence of the hormones human chorionic gonadotropin (hCG) from the placenta, luteinizing hormone (LH) from the anterior pituitary, and testosterone and Mullerian inhibiting hormone from the testis.[1–3] The formation of the male external genitalia is primarily dependent on the active target-tissue metabolite of testosterone, dihydrotestosterone, and, therefore, on the appropriate production and effect of hCG and LH on the Leydig cells of the testes.[3]

In genetic males, several abnormalities in Leydig cell differentiation or function have been reported to result in varying degrees of male pseudohermaphroditism.[4–11] In these patients, Leydig cells were either nonexistent, hypoplastic, or unresponsive to hCG stimulation. *In vitro* studies demonstrated absence of LH-specific binding in testicular biopsy samples examined by autoradiography or membrane binding in genetic male patients with ambiguous genitalia or micropenis, suggesting the possible involvement of the LH receptor (LH-R) in these patients.[9,10]

In normal genetic females, LH plays several roles throughout the menstrual cycle. During the late follicular phase, LH assists with the synthesis of estradiol by stimulating the theca cells to produce androgen precursors for aromatization by granulosa cells, which are under the regulatory influence of follicle-stimulating hormone (FSH).[12] Subsequently, LH, during its midcycle surge, promotes oocyte and follicular maturation, leading to ovulation. In addition, it induces corpus luteum formation by granulosa and theca cells. The corpus luteum, under the influence of luteal-phase LH, secretes progesterone. Embryonic hCG, which also interacts with the LH/hCG receptor, maintains the crucial presence of the corpus luteum of pregnancy. Thus, abnormalities in the LH receptor in females would be expected to result in partial ovarian failure characterized by late defective folliculogenesis, anovulation, absence of a luteal phase, delayed or incomplete feminization at puberty, amenorrhea, and infertility.

Human LH-R belongs to the G-protein-coupled seven-transmembrane domain receptor superfamily.[13] Several groups have reported single, mostly heterozygous point mutations of this receptor, resulting in constitutive activation of the adenylyl cyclase

[a]Address for correspondence: George P. Chrousos, M.D., National Institutes of Health, Building 10, Room 10N262, Bethesda, Maryland 20892.

pathway and the syndrome of familial or sporadic male-limited precocious puberty, an uncommon form of gonadotropin-independent precocious puberty in the male.[14–17] Also, Kremer *et al.* reported a homozygous missense inactivating mutation in the sixth transmembrane domain of the LH-R gene in two male pseudohermaphrodite siblings with a female phenotype and the diagnosis of Leydig cell hypoplasia.[18] We recently described two unrelated kindreds with broadly varying defects in the differentiation of male external genitalia in genetic males and amenorrhea in a genetic female.[19] Three 46,XY siblings presented with female external genitalia, lack of breast development, and primary amenorrhea. A fully developed adult XX sister, who had normal pubertal development, presented with the chief complaint of amenorrhea. A 6-year-old boy from another family presented with micropenis, bilaterally descended testes, and no response to exogenous hCG postnatally. DNA sequencing analysis revealed novel homozygous mutations of the LH-R gene in each of the kindreds, which compromised the LH receptor and prevented it from transmitting the hormonal signal in the testes and ovaries of the affected patients.

FAMILY STUDIES

Family 1

The propositi of this family were two siblings, ages 32 and 23 years old, born to nonconsaguineous parents, that were referred to the Division of Endocrinology, Hospital das Clínicas, University of São Paulo, Brazil, for lack of breast development and primary amenorrhea.[5] A third sibling was seen later, at the age of 15 years. All three patients had a female general appearance, a eunuchoid habitus, absence of breast tissue, and Tanner stage IV (cases 1 and 7) and II (case 14) pubic hair (FIG. 1**A**). Their external genitalia were normal female, with a normal-sized clitoris, absence of posterior labial fusion, and separate urethral and vaginal openings. Gonads of medium size were palpable bilaterally in the inguinal regions, except for the intraabdominal right gonad in case 1. Blood leukocyte karyotypes were 46,XY. Serum gonadotropin levels were elevated (LH was 49, 41, and 36 IU/l, respectively, normal adult males: 7.7 ± 4.7 mean ± SD; FSH was 38, 26, and 30 IU/l, respectively, normal adult males: 6.9 ± 4.9 mean ± SD), while serum testosterone concentrations were <3 ng/ml (<10 nmol/l) and failed to increase after hCG administration. The patients underwent bilateral gonadectomy. Testicular histology showed tubules with thickening of the basal membrane, immature Sertoli cells, and rare spermatogonia in all cases. The interstitium contained fibroblast-like cells but no mature Leydig cells.

Subsequently, one additional sister from this family was referred for evaluation of amenorrhea at the age of 22 years. She had spontaneous gonadarche at age 13 years and a single vaginal bleeding at 20 years. She had a normal height and weight and was normotensive, with Tanner stage V pubic hair and breasts and normal female external genitalia. Hirsutism, galactorrhea, or stigmata of Turner syndrome were absent. Pelvic sonogram revealed the presence of a small-volume uterus (14 ml, normal: 30–90 ml) and unequal size (R: 1.9 cc, L: 7.2 cc) cystic ovaries. Basal LH level was elevated (37.0 IU/l, normal adult midfollicular-phase female: 7.1 ± 3 mean ± SD), whereas serum FSH and prolactin concentrations were normal. After

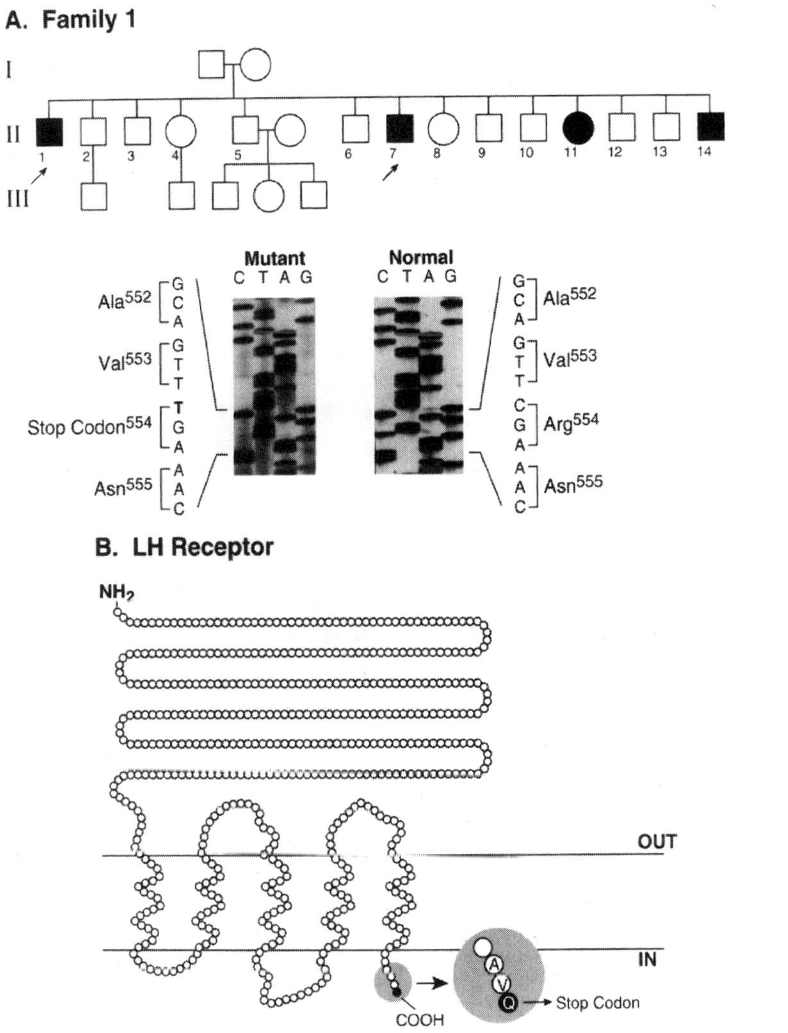

FIGURE 1. (**A**) **Family 1 pedigree.** Direct sequencing showing the homozygous substitution of cytosine by thymine at position 1660 of the cDNA of the LHR gene, resulting in a stop codon TGA within the third cytosolic loop. (**B**) The truncated LH-R shown schematically. (From Latronico *et al.*[19]; used with permission of the *New England Journal of Medicine.*)

GnRH stimulation, peak LH was 81 IU/l. Basal serum estradiol was 32 pg/ml (117.5 pmol/l) (normal adult midfollicular-phase female: 39 ± 15 pg/ml or 143 ± 55 pmol/l, mean ± SD). Basal serum progesterone concentrations were very low on several occasions (<0.36 ng/ml or <1.15 nmol/l). Basal serum testosterone, androstenedione, DHEA, DHEAS, and 17-hydroxyprogesterone concentrations were normal.

Family 2

The only affected member of this family was a 7-year-old boy that was referred as a neonate to the Division of Pediatric Endocrinology, Children's Hospital of New Jersey (Newark, NJ), for evaluation of micropenis (FIG. 2**A**). At birth, his stretched phallus length was 1.5 cm (<2.5 SD below the mean of normal for age). Both testes were descended and measured approximately 1 ml. There was no family history of male pseudohermaphroditism or hypogonadism. There was no history of consanguinity. The blood leukocyte karyotype was 46,XY. The penile response to androgen therapy was assessed by administration of testosterone enanthate i.m. 25 mg every 3 weeks over 3 months. After this treatment, the phallus grew in size to 4 cm. At age 5, an hCG stimulation test was performed with 5,000 U of hCG given i.m. daily for 3 days, and blood was drawn, 24, 48, and 96 hours after the last injection. Plasma testosterone concentrations were undetectable and did not rise after hCG stimulation, while baseline plasma concentrations of 17-hydroxypregnenolone, 17-hydroxyprogesterone, progesterone, Δ4-androstenedione, dehydroepiandrosterone, Δ5-dehydroepiandrosterone sulfate, and estradiol were normal. An ACTH stimulation test (250 μg, i.v.) was also performed at that time. Basal and stimulated concentrations of 17-hydroxypregnenolone, 17-hydroxyprogesterone, progesterone, 11-deoxycortisol, and cortisol were normal. A GnRH test (100 μg, i.v.) demonstrated a normal prepubertal response of both LH and FSH, which rose from 6.3 to 11 IU/l and from 1.3 to 4.2 IU/l, respectively. Baseline serum inhibin was 3.0 IU/ml (normal range: 4–14 IU/ml). A recent hCG stimulation test confirmed the continued lack of testosterone responsiveness and the absence of steroid precursor accumulation.

MOLECULAR BIOLOGY STUDIES

Genomic DNA was isolated from peripheral blood samples, and the entire exon 11, which encodes for all of the receptor molecule except for the long extracellular amino-terminus, was amplified by the polymerase chain reaction (PCR). Direct sequencing of the PCR products from the three XY siblings of the first family with female external genitalia and the diagnosis of Leydig cell hypoplasia revealed a homozygous C to T transition at nucleotide 1660 of the LH-R cDNA (FIG. 1). This mutation changed codon 554 from that of arginine to a stop codon (TGA) within the third cytosolic loop of the LH-R. The XX sister with secondary amenorrhea was also homozygous for this mutation.

Direct sequencing of the entire exon 11 of the LH-R gene from the propositus of the second family with micropenis revealed a homozygous C to A transition at nucleotide 1847 of the LH-R cDNA (FIG. 2). This mutation changed codon 616 from serine to tyrosine within the seventh transmembrane region of the LH-R. The same mutation was carried by the asymptomatic mother and father of the patient, who were heterozygotes for this amino acid substitution.

Cells transfected with the wild-type LH-R cDNA (cloned in pSVL vector) exhibited specific binding for the labeled hLH (Bmax: $4.8 \pm 1.1 \times 10^{-9}$ M/mg, K_D: $7.4 \pm 1.9 \times 10^{-9}$ M). In contrast, no specific hLH binding was found in the tyrosine 616-mutant LH-R cDNA transfected cells (FIG. 3**A**).

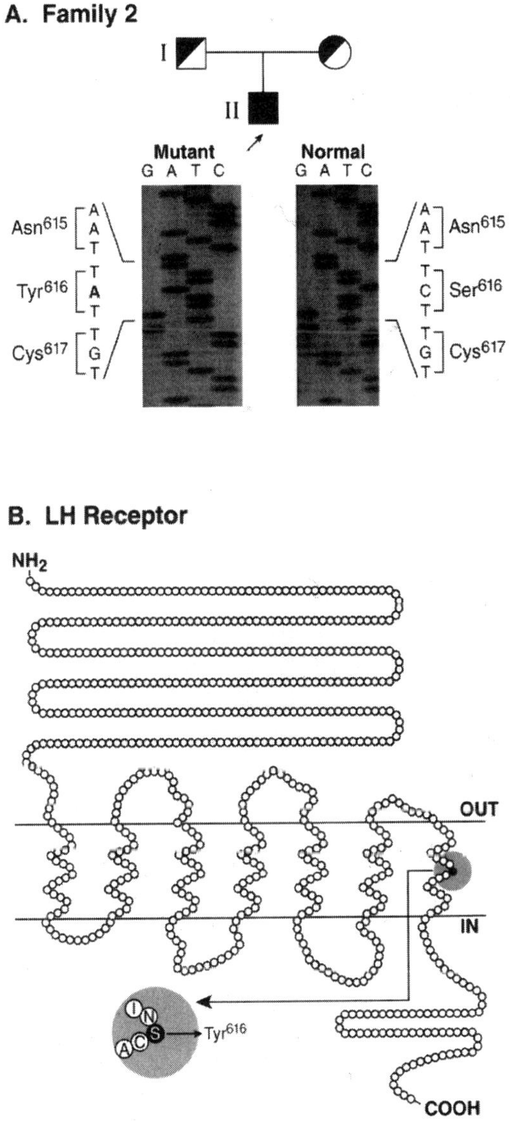

FIGURE 2. (**A**) **Family 2 pedigree.** Direct sequencing showing the homozygous substitution of cytosine by adenine at position 1847 of the cDNA of LH-R gene of the proband, resulting in the exchange of Ser 616 with Tyr at the seventh transmembrane domain. (**B**) The mutant receptor shown schematically. (From Latronico *et al.*[19]; used with permission of the *New England Journal of Medicine.*)

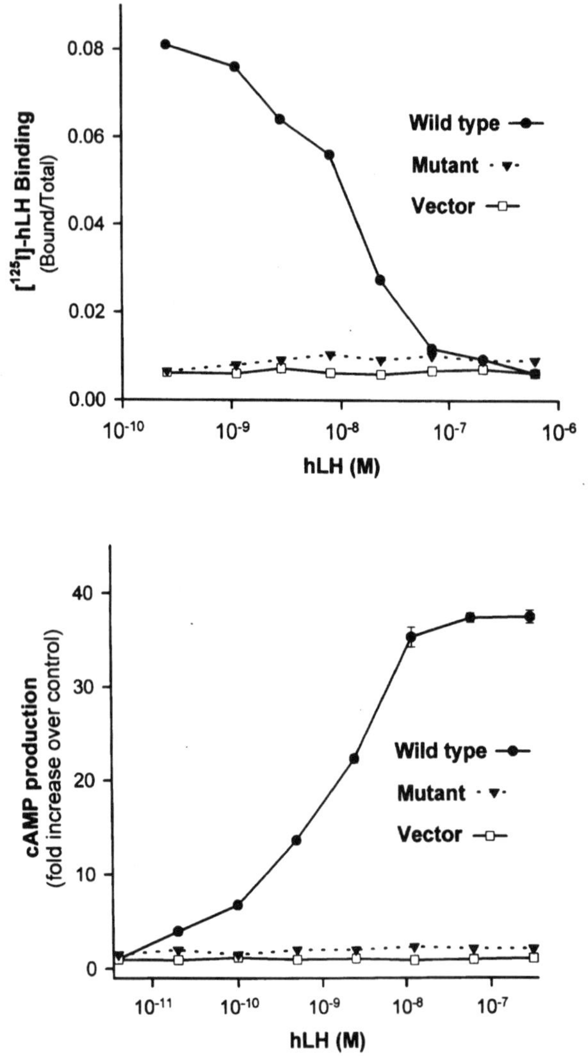

FIGURE 3. **(A) Displacement of ^{125}I-labeled hLH by unlabeled hLH in COS-7 cells transfected with the wild-type LH-R, Tyr^{616} mutant receptor, or vector alone.** Cells transfected with mutant or vector alone demonstrated no specific ^{125}I-labeled hLH binding. Values are mean of duplicates from a representative experiment. (**B**) Extracellular cAMP response to hLH from COS-7 cells transfected with the wild-type LH-R, mutant LH-R cDNA, and vector alone. Cells transfected with mutant or vector alone exhibited no significant increase over basal cAMP levels. Values are mean ± SE of triplicates from a representative experiment. (From Latronico *et al.*[19]; used with permission of the *New England Journal of Medicine.*)

Basal and hLH-induced levels of cAMP in COS-7 cells transfected with Tyr 616 mutant and wild-type LH-R cDNAs were compared to the levels of cells transfected with vector pSVL alone (FIG. 3**B**). Basal levels were similar in all three types of cells. Cells transfected with the wild-type LH-R cDNA responded in a dose-dependent manner, producing a peak increase of 38-fold in cAMP over baseline (EC_{50}: $1.1 \pm 0.5 \times 10^{-9}$ M). However, cells transfected with the tyrosine 616 mutant receptor or vector alone showed no response.

mRNA from both the wild-type and Tyr 616 mutant LH-R was detected in the transfected cells by ribonuclease protection assay (RPA) and reverse-transcriptase PCR. Thus, the Tyr 616 mutant LH-R was normally expressed but apparently unable to bind LH in the transfected cells.

TESTICULAR LH RESISTANCE

Leydig cell hypoplasia is a rare autosomal recessive condition that interferes with normal development of male external genitalia and causes primary hypogonadism in 46,XY individuals. The phenotype of inherited Leydig cell hypoplasia ranges from extremely severe forms, presenting as 46,XY phenotypic females, to mild forms, in which genetic males present with micropenis and hypergonadotropic hypogonadism.[7,8,10] We recently reported two novel homozygous inactivating nonsense and missense mutations (Arg^{554}→Stop codon, TGA; and Ser^{616}→Tyr^{616}) of the LHR gene, respectively, in three pseudohermaphrodite siblings with Leydig cell hypoplasia and a boy with micropenis and primary hypogonadism.[19]

The stop codon found in the third intracellular loop of LH-R of the first family determined a premature interruption of the translation process of the LH-R mRNA, and consequently eliminated a large part of the receptor, which encoded most of the third intracellular loop and the entire intracellular carboxy-terminal tail. Even if properly expressed in the membrane of target cells, this truncated mutant receptor would be unable to transduce the hormonal signal.[19] Interestingly, similar mutations, introducing stop codons in the third cytosolic loop of the adrenocorticotropin receptor, rhodopsin, or vasopressin V2 receptor, were associated with hereditary isolated glucocorticoid deficiency, retinitis pigmentosa, and nephrogenic diabetes insipidus, respectively.[20–23]

Presence of micropenis at birth signifies near-normal testosterone production or effect in the first trimester of pregnancy, when formation of the external genitalia takes place, but suboptimal production or effect in the second and third trimesters, when most penile growth occurs.[24] Our patient with micropenis had clinical evidence of an adequately functioning Leydig cell in the first trimester, which, however, failed during the second and third trimesters of gestation as well as postnatally. Also, this patient had evidence of a properly responsive end-organ, since he demonstrated an adequate penile growth response to exogenous testosterone. These findings could be explained by the defect of the LH-R gene we described, a nonconservative homozygous amino acid substitution in the seventh transmembrane domain of the receptor, which made this receptor unable to properly bind ^{125}I-labeled LH and to respond to LH. Thus, a genetic abnormality of the LH-R appears to be a cause of micropenis and hypogonadism, a suggestion that was made by David *et al.* as early as 1984 in his report of the "syndrome of gonadotropin resistance."[10] The heterozygous parents were reproductively normal, suggesting that one defective LH-R allele causes no overt or subtle clinical disease. This was true for the obligate heterozygote parents of our first family.

Recently, another homozygous missense mutation of the LH-R gene, an alanine to proline substitution at position 593 in the sixth transmembrane domain, was demonstrated by Kremer *et al.* in two XY siblings with female external genitalia and a diagnosis of Leydig cell hypoplasia.[18] Interestingly, this mutation had a milder functional compromising effect in an *in vitro* system than in ours and, yet, its clinical effect was more profound, having influenced the actual formation of male external genitalia, a process that takes place in the first trimester of pregnancy. The *in vivo* pathogenetic properties of these mutations were, thus, quite different from each other and would not have been predicted correctly by the *in vitro* studies performed. The findings of Kremer *et al.*, together with ours, suggest that defects of the LH-R can cause failure of the Leydig cell throughout male prenatal development, underlying the pathology of two ends of a broad spectrum, from phenotypically female external genitalia to micropenis. The presence of normal numbers of Leydig cells in the patient reported by David *et al.*, whose clinical presentation was similar to that of our patient with micropenis, suggested that the term Leydig cell hypoplasia may not be accurate for this condition and LH resistance might be better.

The unusually large extracellular domain of the LH-R is responsible for the recognition and high-affinity binding of LH. Recent evidence from *in vitro* recombinant studies suggested that the carboxy-terminus of the receptor also contributes to hormone binding, albeit not to its specificity, perhaps through a second, low-affinity binding site for the hormone.[25–27] Thus, a truncated form of the receptor demonstrated normal binding specificity, but only a high-affinity site versus the wild-type receptor, which had both a high- and a low-affinity site.[25] In addition, these studies demonstrated that absence of the carboxy terminus, or more specifically the region between residues 616 and 631 of the rat LH-R (corresponding to residues 612 to 627 in the human LH-R), caused trapping of the receptor within the endoplasmic reticulum, precluding its appearance on the outer surface of the cell and binding to the ligand.[25] It is of note that the Tyr^{616} mutation resided within this crucial region of the LH-R and may, thus, have resulted in similar defects in its cytoplasmic traffic and cell membrane expression. The possibility that this mutation might interfere with LH-R gene expression or mRNA stability was unlikely, since both RPA and RT-PCR demonstrated the presence of normal-sized LH-R mRNA in the transfected cells.

The relatively late *in utero* failure and, eventually, complete inability of our patient's Leydig cells to respond to exogenous hCG postnatally, points toward a progressive course, which would at first appear to be inexplicable given the genetic nature of the molecular defect determined. There are, however, two paradigms of progressive loss of function of an end-organ due to G-protein-coupled receptor defects that provide us with precedents. First, a form of hereditary retinitis pigmentosa, caused by mutations of rhodopsin, the photon receptor, is a clearly progressive genetic disease that takes years to attain its final severity.[22] Second, hereditary isolated glucocorticoid deficiency, a syndrome due to abnormalities of the ACTH receptor, may also take months or years to cause complete and symptomatic glucocorticoid deficiency.[20,21]

OVARIAN LH RESISTANCE

Amenorrhea in fully developed genetic females was noted in other families with Leydig cell hypoplasia.[4,11,28] We examined the LH-R gene of the fully developed XX sister of the propositi of the first family, who had secondary amenorrhea and elevated levels of LH, and found the same homozygous mutations (Arg^{554}→Stop codon), as the affected propositi. This LH-R mutation apparently compromised the ovulation and luteinization processes of our patient, while it allowed normal pubertal feminization. An ovarian biopsy, reported in an XX sister of genetic males with Leydig cell hypoplasia who, similarly to our genetic female patient, had amenorrhea, revealed the absence of a corpus luteum or albicans, but a normal number and size of follicles for her age.[28] The normal pubertal feminization and the normal levels of plasma estradiol in our patient suggest that follicular estrogen biosynthesis is not affected in a major fashion by absence of LH effect; neither is pubertal feminization dependent on this hormone.

SUMMARY

Luteinizing hormone (LH) plays its effects on ovarian and testicular cells through binding to a specific cell surface receptor. We recently described two kindreds with LH resistance due to abnormalities of the LH receptor (LH-R) gene. Affected XY members presented with severe or mild fetal undermasculinization (female external genitalia or micropenis) and primary hypogonadism, while an XX affected member showed normal pubertal development, increased plasma concentrations of LH, and amenorrhea.

The first kindred included three XY phenotypic female siblings with Leydig cell hypoplasia and primary hypogonadism and a fully developed XX sister with elevated plasma concentrations of LH and amenorrhea. PCR amplification of genomic DNA and direct sequencing of the entire exon 11 of the LH-R revealed that all four affected individuals had a homozygous mutation (Arg^{554}→Stop codon) in the third cytosolic loop of the LH-R, which resulted in a truncated LH-R unable to transduce the hormonal signal. The second kindred included a 6-year-old XY boy with a micropenis and bilaterally descended testes, who demonstrated no response to exogenous human chorionic gonadotrophin postnatally. This patient had a nonconservative homozygous amino acid substitution (Ser^{616}→Tyr^{616}) in the seventh transmembrane domain of his LH-R gene that was inherited from his heterozygous parents. The mutant receptor expressed in heterologous cells *in vitro* demonstrated no appreciable binding of ^{125}I-labeled hLH, nor did it confer cAMP responsiveness to LH.

Homozygous inactivating mutations of the LH-R cause complete or mild testicular failure in genetic males, resulting in female external genitalia or micropenis and primary hypogonadism. Similar mutations in genetic females may cause failure of ovulation and corpus luteum formation, resulting in amenorrhea. Follicular growth and development are apparently sufficient to allow feminization at puberty.

REFERENCES

1. JOSSO, N. 1981. Physiology of sex differentiation. A guide to the understanding and management of the intersex child. *In* The Intersex Child. N. Josso, Ed.: 1–13. S. Karger. Basel.
2. KAPLAN, S. L., M. M. GRUMBACK & M. I. AUBERT. 1976. The ontogenesis of pituitary hormones and hypothalamic factors in the human fetus: Maturation of central nervous system regulation of anterior pituitary function. Rec. Prog. Horm. Res. **32:** 161–243.
3. SIITERI, P. K. & J. D. WILSON. 1974. Testosterone formation and metabolism during male sexual differentiation in the human embryo. J. Clin. Endocrinol. Metab. **38:** 113–125.
4. ARNHOLD, I. J. P., B. B. MENDONCA, W. BLOISE & S. P. A. TOLEDO. 1985. Male pseudohermaphroditism resulting from Leydig cell hypoplasia. J. Pediatr. **106:** 1057.
5. ARNHOLD, I. J. P., B. MENDONCA, H. BISI, F. O. RUSSO, W. NICOLAU, W. BLOISE & C. A. MOREIRA-FILHO. 1988. Normal expression of the serologically defined H-Y antigen in Leydig cell hypoplasia. J. Urol. **140:** 1549–1552.
6. ARNHOLD, I. J. P., B. B. MENDONCA, S. P. A. TOLEDO, G. MADUREIRA, W. NICOLAU, H. BISI & W. BLOISE. 1987. Leydig cell hypoplasia causing male pseudohermaphroditism: Case report and review of the literature. Rev. Hosp. Fac. Med. S. Paulo **42:** 227–232.
7. SALDANHA, P. H., I. J. P. ARNHOLD, B. B. MENDONCA, W. BLOISE & S. P. A. TOLEDO. 1987. A clinic-genetic investigation of Leydig cell hypoplasia. Am. J. Med. Genet. **26:** 337–344.
8. TOLEDO, S. P. A., I. J. P. ARNHOLD, W. LUTHOLD, E. M. K. RUSSO & P. H. SALDANHA. 1985. Leydig cell hypoplasia determining familial hypergonadotropin hypogonadism. Prog. Clin. Biol. Res. **200:** 311–314.
9. SCHWARTZ, M., J. IMPERATO-MCGINLEY, R. E. PETERSON, E. COOPER, P. L. MORRIS, M. MAC GILLIVRAY & T. HENSLE. 1981. Male pseudohermaphroditism secondary to an abnormality in Leydig cell differentiation. J. Clin. Endocrinol. Metab. **53:** 123–127.
10. DAVID, R., D. J. YOON, L. LANDIN, L. LEW, C. SKLAR, R. SCHINELLA & M. GOLIMBU. 1984. A syndrome of gonadotropin resistance possibly due a luteinizing hormone receptor defect. J. Clin. Endocrinol. Metab. **59:** 156–160.
11. BERTHÈZENE, F., M. G. FOREST, J. A. GRIMAUD, B. CLAUSTRAT & R. MORNEX. 1976. Leydig cell agenesis: A cause of male pseudohermaphroditism. N. Engl. J. Med. **295:** 969–972.
12. MAGOFFIN, D. A., T. J. GELETY & P. C. MAGARELLI. 1994. Follicular development: The role of LH. *In* Ovulation Induction: Basic Science and Clinical Advances. M. Filicon & C. Flamigni, Eds.: 25–36. Excerpta Medica. Amsterdam.
13. MINEGISHI, T., K. NAKAMURA, Y. TAKAKURA, K. MIYAMOTO, Y. HASEGAWA, Y. IBUKI & M. IGARASHI. 1990. Cloning and sequencing of human LH/hCG receptor cDNA. Biochem. Biophys. Res. Commun. **172:** 1049–1054.
14. SHENKER, A., L. LAUE, S. KOSUGI, J. J. MERENDINO, T. MINEGISHI & G. B. CUTLER, JR. 1993. A constitutively activating mutation of the luteinizing hormone receptor in familial male precocious puberty. Nature **365:** 652–654.
15. KREMER, H., E. MARIMAN, B. J. OTTEN, J. W. MOLL, G. B. A. STOELIGNA, J. M. WIT, M. JANSEN, S. L. DROP, B. FAAS, A. ROPERS & H. G. BRUNNER. 1993. Cosegregation of missense mutations of the luteinizing hormone receptor gene with familial male-limited precocious puberty. Hum. Mol. Genet. **2:** 1779–1783.
16. YANO, K., A. HIDAKA, M. SAJI, M. H. POLYMEROPOULOS, A. OKUNO, L. D. KOHN & G. B. CUTLER, JR. 1994. A sporadic case of male-limited precocious puberty has the same constitutively activating point mutation in the luteinizing hormone/choriogonadotropin receptor gene as familial cases. J. Clin. Endocrinol. Metab. **79:** 1818–1823.
17. LATRONICO, A. C., J. ANASTI, I. J. P. ARNHOLD, B. B. MENDONCA, S. DOMENICE, M. C. ALBANO, K. ZACHMAN, B. L. WAJCHENBERG & C. TSIGOS. 1995. A novel mutation of the luteinizing hormone receptor gene causing male gonadotropin-independent precocious puberty. J. Clin. Endocrinol. Metab. **80:** 2490–2494.

18. KREMER, H., R. KRAAIJ, S. P. A. TOLEDO, M. POST, J. B. FRIDMAN, C. Y. HAYASHIDA, M. REEN, E. MILGROM, H. ROPERS, E. MARIMAN, A. P. N. THEMMEN & H. G. BRUNNER. 1995. Male pseudohermaphroditism due to a homozygous missense mutation of the luteinizing hormone receptor gene. Nature Genet. **9:** 160–164.
19. LATRONICO, A. C., J. ANASTI, I. J. P. ARNHOLD, R. RAPAPORT, B. B. MENDONCA, W. BLOISE, M. DE CASTRO, C. TSIGOS & G. P. CHROUSOS. 1996. Testicular and ovarian resistance to luteinizing hormone caused by homozygous inactivating mutations of the luteinizing hormone receptor gene. N. Engl. J. Med. **334:** 507–512.
20. TSIGOS, C., K. ARAI, W. HUNG & G. P. CHROUSOS. 1993. Hereditary isolated glucocorticoid deficiency associated with abnormalities of the adrenocorticotropin receptor gene. J. Clin. Invest. **92:** 2458–2461.
21. TSIGOS, C., K. ARAI, A. C. LATRONICO, A. M. DIGEORGE, R. RAPAPORT & G. P. CHROUSOS. 1995. A novel mutation of the adrenocorticotropin receptor (ACTH-R) gene in a family with the syndrome of isolated glucocorticoid deficiency, but no ACTH-R abnormalities in two families with the triple A syndrome. J. Clin. Endocrinol. Metab. **80:** 2186–2189.
22. DRYJA, T. P., T. L. MCGEE, L. B. HAHN, *et al.* 1990. Mutations within the rhodopsin gene in patients with autosomal dominant retinitis pigmentosa. N. Engl. J. Med. **323:** 1300–1307.
23. MERENDINO, JR., J. J., A. M. SPIEGEL, J. D. CRAWFORD, A. N. O'CARROL, M. J. BROWNSTEIN & S. J. LOLAIT. 1993. Brief report: A mutation in the vasopressin V2-receptor gene in a kindred with X-linked nephrogenic diabetes insipidus. N. Engl. J. Med. **238:** 1538–1541.
24. AARONSON, I. A. 1994. Micropenis: Medical and surgical implications. J. Urol. **152:** 4–14.
25. RODRIGUEZ, M. C., Y. B. XIE, H. WANG, K. COLLISON & D. L. SEGALOFF. 1992. Effects of truncations of the cytoplasmic tail of the luteinizing hormone/chorionic gonadotropin receptor on receptor-mediated hormone internalization. Mol. Endocrinol. **6:** 327–336.
26. SEGALOFF, D. L. & M. ASCOLI. 1993. The lutropin/choriogonadotropin receptor 4 years later. Endocrinol. Rev. **14:** 324–347.
27. THOMAS, D. M. & D. L. SEGALOFF. 1994. Hormone-binding properties and glycosylation pattern of a recombinant form of the extracellular domain of the luteinizing hormone/chorionic gonadotropin receptor expressed in mammalian cells. Endocrinology **135:** 1902–1912.
28. ARNOLD, I. J. P., A. C. LATRONICO, M. C. BATISTA, F. M. CARVALHO, G. P. CHROUSOS & B. B. MENDONCA. 1997. Ovarian resistance to luteinizing hormone: A novel cause of amenorrhea and infertility. Fertil. Steril. In press.

Amenorrhea in β-Homozygous Thalassemia Major

GEORGE TOLIS,[a,b,c] ARTEMIS PAPANDREOU,[c]
AND IOANNIS KARYDIS[c]

[b]Athens University Medical School and
[c]Hippokrateion Hospital
Athens, Greece

The average life-span of β-thalassemia (β-thal) patients has been improved by means of significant progress in β-thal research and improved patient treatment, through frequent blood transfusions and regular iron chelation.[1–3] Before desferrioxamine was employed, therapy was limited to regular transfusions; and patients died, principally, in their twenties or thirties, mainly due to the damaging effects of chronic iron deposition in the myocardium. It is known that every unit of donated blood contains approximately 200 mg iron. In patients with a severe iron overload, a portion of the free iron (not bonded to transferrin) appears in the plasma and may be taken up, by the tissues, to a greater extent than the protein-bonded iron, as shown in *in vitro* studies employing hepatic and cardiac cells.[4,5] Increased iron absorption by the gastrointestinal tract is also reported, which may cause greater harm than the iron accumulation from blood transfusions. The cardiologic, hepatic, and endocrine problems of β-thal patients are the three most common complications. Even though various factors, such as dietary habits (malnutrition), severe chronic anemia, or tissue hypoxia *per se* (due to the disease), may account for some of these problems, many studies lead to the conclusion that chronic iron overload induces significant damage in various organs.

Patients with β-thal exhibit a variety of endocrine abnormalities: growth retardation or failure, pubertal delay or pubertal failure, primary or secondary amenorrhea, infertility, diabetes mellitus, osteoporosis, thyroid dysfunction, and hypoparathyroidism.[6–14] Although problems in sexual development in these patients can exist alone or in combination with other endocrinopathies, they represent the most common endocrine disorder.[13,14] In older times, when the survival rate was low, patients died without attaining normal puberty, development of secondary gender characteristics and sexual maturation.[7,13–16] In a small number of patients, an inverse relationship was found between the degree of iron overload and pubertal development.[17] It is well known that patients with high ferritin plasma concentrations, before iron chelation or with persistent tissue uptake, may be at the highest risk; however, differences in individual susceptibility may account for the observed variation in morbidity. The observation that patients with thalassemia major occasionally achieve normal growth and sexual maturation despite sustained hyperferritinemia is unexplained. It is believed that some endocrine glands are extremely sensitive to the iron toxicity and that

[a]Address for correspondence: George Tolis, M.D., FRCP., Division of Endocrinology, Hippokrateion Hospital, 108 Vas. Sophias Avenue, Athens 115 27, Greece.

even small amounts, if accumulated in the first years of life, may cause irreversible damage, even if intensive iron chelation therapy is employed later; a 50% reduction of iron overload, however, from the first years of childhood may save parenchymatous organs from damage.[18–21]

Disturbances of the hypothalamic–pituitary–gonadal axis are found in 40% of β-thal patients, and this percentage increases dramatically with the advancement of age. Primary amenorrhea appears in 42.9–81% of β-thal women.[20,22] Menarche is usually late, appearing at 14 ± 1.5 years, while secondary amenorrhea is exhibited in almost all the patients, 1 month to 15 years following the onset of menarche, with an average time period of 3.8 years.[18,20,22–24] These phenomena are due to hypogonadotropic hypogonadism.[9,16,18,20,23,24] The latter phenomenon is caused by chronic iron deposition in the pituitary gland, as shown by histopathological findings.[9,24] Iron seems to interact with the cell membrane and other cellular components, for example mitochondria, and therefore may affect the functioning at the receptor and post-receptor levels.[26] Iron deposition may occur in both the pituitary gland and the ovary, although one of the glands may be affected predominantly, and earlier than the second one.[9,26] The high prevalence of ovarian failure in β-thal women with secondary amenorrhea may be age-dependent. Perhaps older women, having been exposed longer to iron overload, are more likely to suffer greater damage to their ovarian tissues or alternatively, the gonadotropin-induced increase in vascularity of post-pubertal ovaries may render them more prone to the deleterious effects of iron infiltration

Delayed onset of puberty, or its absence in β-thal, apart from being due to malfunctioning of the hypothalamo–pituitary–gonadal axis, has also been attributed to abnormal hepatic conversion of steroid hormones to their active metabolites[27] and to a defective hepatic biosynthesis of somatomedins.[28,30]

Somatomedin-C (IGF-I) can be low in the presence of malnutrition or liver failure since there are thalassemic patients with low serum somatomedin activity in the absence of liver disease, and depressed serum somatomedin-C activity is correlated with the extent of iron overload. The mechanism concerned appears to be other than a general impairment of liver production of protein substances. There may be a specific inhibitory effect of iron on somatomedin production, or, perhaps, direct or indirect stimulation of degradation mechanisms.[28] Defective growth and lack of pubertal development are probably strictly correlated; the complex interactions between androgens, estradiol, and somatomedin-C have been reviewed recently,[31] and it was shown that plasma somatomedin-C levels correlated better with pubertal changes than with chronological age. Because there is also an IGF-I–gonadotropin interaction in the gonads, there may be a temporary reduction in their responsiveness to gonadotropins in the absence of IGF-I.[32] IGF-I deficiency is often associated with sexual inflammation and/or amenorrhea.[32,33] *In vitro* studies demonstrated that IGF-I exerts mitogenic activity in granulosa cells; it increases granulosa cell numbers and DNA synthesis in mammalian cell cultures.[34] In cultures of rat and porcine granulosa cells, IGF-I augments FSH-induced estrogen synthesis by accelerating aromatase activity and stimulating progestin synthesis by increasing cholesterol side-chain cleavage.[34] Furthermore, FSH induction of LH receptors is also potentiated up to fivefold the normal value in the presence of IGF-I.[34] IGF-I also plays a role in ovarian thecal-interstitial cell differentiation and enhances the androgen synthetic response of the cells to LH.[32]

The role of chronic anemia in the absence of puberty is particularly evident in patients with hemoglobin levels less than 7g/dl (5.4–6.3 g/dl), in whom spontaneous sexual development never occurred. Transfusion regimen improvement and maintenance of higher hemoglobin levels resulted in spontaneous, though delayed, onset of puberty.[23] Apart from the aforementioned causes, other factors, such as chronic liver disease, diabetes mellitus, and zinc deficiency, may precipitate secondary amenorrhea.[21,22,35] β-Thal patients who had early iron chelation therapy (before they reached their third birthday) showed reduced leukocyte zinc levels, barely significant reduction in hair zinc levels, and reduced levels of the zinc-dependent enzyme LAP (leukocyte alkaline phosphatase).[21] Baseline levels of the adrenal androgens dehydroepiandrosterone (DHEA) and dehydroeriandrosterone sulfate (DHEA-S) were reported to be significantly lower in the patients with β-thalassemia in comparison with age-matched controls; also, their peak stimulated levels of DHEA-S, following prolonged ACTH infusion (0.3 mg i.v. over a period of eight hours), were significantly lower than those of the control group.[36] The extent to which the low adrenal androgen levels contribute to pubertal delay and result from a defective pituitary production of the putative adrenal androgen-stimulating hormone (AASH) is open to speculation. Finally, the finding of a decreased PRL response to TRH, even following sex steroid priming, suggests that patients with thalassemia major appear to have more extensive pituitary involvement than just an isolated gonadotropin insufficiency.[16]

Detailed analysis of diachronic activity of the hypothalamic–pituitary–gonadal–uterine axis in β-thal patients is unavailable; nevertheless, cross-sectional data, including limited studies on the transition from menarche to amenorrhea, allow some valid speculations. Thus, in patients with long-standing secondary amenorrhea and hypoestrogenism, it is unlikely to elicit a normal FSH/LH response to GnRH, whether it is administered as a bolus or in a pulsatile manner over a one-week period. However, a uterine response to exogenously administered sex steroids is almost always seen, albeit in an attenuated fashion. Human gonadotropins may elicit an ovarian response, but it usually requires large amounts for a prolonged period; a failure of properly administered hMG/hCG to induce follicular development may imply the presence of ovarian siderosis/structural damage. With one exception,[37] hMG/hCG therapy has been successful in the induction of ovulation and the achievement of pregnancy.[38,39] Women with β-thal who exhibited menarche but subsequently had scarce cycles, when subjected to studies of their pulsatile FSH/LH secretion patterns and their response to an exogenously administered GnRH bolus, usually exhibited pulses, albeit with attenuated amplitude frequencies and inter-pulse patterns, despite a satisfactory FSH/LH response to GnRH. In a long-term follow-up study of β-thal patients, evaluated while they were experiencing monthly vaginal bleeding, basal and GnRH-stimulated FSH/LH levels were found to be lower than in healthy subjects who were also assessed during the follicular phase of their cycle.[24] These responses deteriorated further within the following two years of amenorrhea, while the pulsatility was lost in two-thirds of the patient population, within five years of amenorrhea; it was of particular interest that, despite the apulsatility, there was still a GnRH-induced pituitary gonadotropin release, even though it was significantly attenuated. The latter has been suggested as being consistent with hypothalamic dysfunction,[24] this is, of course, unproven since no induction of ovulation has ever been reported (upon pulsatile administration of GnRH). In these and other similar cases, the data is greatly in favor of a pituitary FSH/LH reserve deficit. Finally, in relation to β-thal patients with primary amenorrhea, it seems to be important to differentiate between a delay in the maturation of the brain–pituitary–gonad circuits from those linked to pituitary hemosiderosis. The latter concept can be supported by the combination of MRI studies[40] and the demonstration of the absence of an FSH/LH response to GnRH administered as a bolus or infused in a pulsatile manner. In such cases, hormone replacement therapy should be initiated for the prevention of potential sequelae, for example, cardiovascular, immune, metabolic, sexual, osseous, and CNS complications.

SUMMARY

Hemolytic anemias, and, in particular, β-homozygous thalassemia, derange all vital organs. A shift of the survival curve to the right has been achieved, thanks to the intensive programs of blood transfusion; iron chelation; infectious control; and, most recently, bone marrow transplantation. Metabolic and endocrine abnormalities do occur, albeit in less severe forms in comparison to available data from 10 to 20 years ago, for example, osteopenia. The most commonly encountered hormonal disorder is the attenuation of gonadal function on a downstream basis, linked to iron deposition in the hypothalamic–pituitary gonadotropin axis. A transition, from low-amplitude endogenous GnRH pulses to apulsatility of LH patterns, precedes the inability of the pituitary gonadotrope to respond to the GnRH decapeptide administered either as an acute bolus injection or in a pulsatile manner for up to 7 days.

REFERENCES

1. Wolfe, L., N. Olivieri, D. Sallan, *et al.* 1985. Prevention of cardiac disease by subcutaneous desferroxamine in patients with thalassemia major. N. Engl. J. Med. **312:** 1600–1603.
2. Weatherall, D. J., M. J. Pippard & S. T. Callender. 1983. Iron loading in thalassemia—five years with the pump. N. Engl. J. Med. **308:** 456–458.
3. Modell, B., E. A. Letsky, D. M. Flynn, R. Peto & D. J. Weatherall. 1982. Survival and desferrioxamine in thalassemia major. Br. Med. J. **284:** 1081–1084.
4. Hershko, C. & T. E. Peto. 1987. Non-transferrin plasma iron. Br. J. Haematol. **66:** 149–151.
5. Link, G., A. Pinson & C. Hershko. 1985. Heart cells in culture: A model of myocardial iron overload and chelation. J. Lab. Clin. Med. **106:** 147–153.
6. Bannerman, R. M., G. Keutsch, M. D. Birnbaum, V. K. Vance & S. Vaughan. 1967. Thalassemia intermedia with iron overload, cardiac failure, diabetes mellitus, hypopituitarism and porphyuria. Am. J. Med. **42:** 476–486.
7. Canale, V. C., P. Steinberr, M. New & M. Erlandson. 1974. Endocrine function in thalassemia major. Ann. N.Y. Acad. Sci. **232:** 333.
8. McIntosh, N. 1976. Endocrinopathy in thalassemia major. Arch. Dis. Child. **51:** 195.
9. Costin, G., M. D. Kogut, C. B. Hyman & J. A. Ortega. 1979. Endocrine abnormalities in thalassemia major. Am. J. Dis. Child. **133:** 497–502.
10. Kuo, B., E. Zaino & M. S. Roginsky. 1968. Endocrine function in thalassemia major. J. Clin. Endocrinol. Metabol. **28:** 805–808.

11. Masala, A., T. Meloni, D. Gallisai, S. Alagna, P. P. Rovasio, S. Rassu & A. F. Milia. 1984. Endocrine functioning in multitransfused prepubertal patients with homozygous β-thalassemia. J. Clin. Endocrinol. Metab. **58:** 667–670.
12. Lassman, M. D., R. T. O'Brian, H. A. Pearson, J. K. Wise, R. K. Donatedian, R. Felig & M. Genei. 1974. Endocrine evaluation in thalassemia major. Ann. N.Y. Acad. Sci. **232:** 226–237.
13. Vullo, C., V. De Sanctis, M. Katz, B. Wonke, A. V. Hoffbrand, B. Bagni, T. Torresani, G. Tolis, M. Masiero, A. Di Palma, *et al.* 1990. Endocrine abnormalities in thalassemia. Ann. N.Y. Acad. Sci. **612:** 293–310.
14. Kattamis, C., N. Touliatos, S. Haidas & N. Matsaniotis. 1970. Growth of children with thalassemia: Effect of different transfusion regimens. Arch. Dis. Child. **45:** 502–509.
15. Landau, H., I. M. Spitz, G. Gividalli & E. A. Rachmilewitz. 1978. Gonadotropin, thyrotrophin and prolactin reserve in β-thalassemia. Clin. Endocrinol. (Oxford) **9:** 163–173.
16. Kletzky, O. A., G. Costin, R. P. Marrs, G. Bernstein, C. M. March & D. R. Mishell, Jr. 1979. Gonadotropin insufficiency in patients with thalassemia major. J. Clin. Endocrinol. Metab. **48:** 901–905.
17. Economidou, J. 1982. Problems related to treatment of beta-thalassemia major. Pediatrician **11:** 157.
18. Borgna-Pignatti, C., P. De Stefano, L. Zanta, C. Vullo, V. De Sanctis, C. Melevendi, A. Naselli, G. Masera, S. Tarzoli, V. Gabutti & A. Pige. 1985. Growth and sexual maturation in thalassemia major. J. Pediatr. **106:** 150–155.
19. Flynn, D. M., A. V. Hoffbrand & D. Polidis. 1982. Subcutaneous desferrioxamine: The effect of three years treatment on liver, iron, serum ferritin and comments on echocardiography. *In* Thalassemia: Recent Advances in Detection and Treatment. A. Cao, U. Carcassi & P. T. Rowley, Eds. Birth Defects **18:** 347.
20. Bronspiegel-Weintrob, N., N. F. Olivieri, B. Tyler, D. F. Andrews, M. H. Freedman & F. J. Holland. 1990. Effect of age at the start of iron chelation therapy on gonadal function in β-thalassemia major. N. Engl. J. Med. **323:** 713–719.
21. De Virgiliis, S., M. Congia, F. Fran, *et al.* 1988. Desferrioxamine-induced growth retardation in patients with thalassemia major. J. Pediatr. **113:** 661–669.
22. De Sanctis, V., C. Vullo, M. Katz, B. Wonke, A. V. Hoffbrand & B. Bagni. 1988. Hypothalamic–pituitary–gonadal axis in thalassemic patients with secondary amenorrhea. Obstet. Gynecol. **72:** 643.
23. Landau, H., V. Gross, I. Dagan, Z. Palti, E. Rachmilewitz & I. M. Spitz. 1984. Growth and sexual development before and after sex steroid therapy in patients with thalassemia major. *Arch. Intern. Med.* ***144:*** 2341–2346.
24. Chatterjee, R., M. Katz, T. F. Cox & J. B. Porter. 1993. Prospective study of the hypothalamic–pituitary axis in thalassemic patients who developed secondary amenorrhea. Clin. Endocrinol. **39:** 287–296.
25. Bergeron, C. & K. Kovacs. 1978. Pituitary siderosis: A histologic, immunologic and ultrastructural study. Am. J. Pathol. **9:** 295–309.
26. De Sanctis, V., C. Vullo, M. Katz, B. Wonke, R. Tanas & B. Bagni. 1988. Gonadal function in patients with β-thalassemia major. J. Clin. Pathol. **41**(2): 133–137.
27. Baker, H. W. G., H. K. Burger & D. M. de Kretser. 1976. A study of the endocrine manifestations of hepatic cirrhosis. Q. J. Med. **45:** 145.
28. Saenger, P., E. Schwartz, A. L. Markenson, J. H. Graziano, L. S. Levine, M. I. New & M. W. Hilgartner. 1980. Depressed serum somatomedin activity in beta-thalassemia. J. Pediatr. **96:** 214–218.
29. Werther, G. A., R. N. Matthews, H. G. Burger & A. C. Herington. 1981. Lack of response of nonsuppressible insulin-like activity to short term administration of human growth hormone in thalassemia major. J. Clin. Endocrinol. Metab. **53:** 806–809.

30. HERINGTON, A. C., G. A. WERTHER, R. N. MATTHEWS & H. G. BURGER. 1981. Studies on the possible mechanism for deficiency of non-suppressible insulin-like activity in thalassemia major. J. Clin. Endocrinol. Metab. **52:** 393–398.
31. ROSENFIELD, R. L., R. FURLANETTO, R. SYKES & D. BOCK. 1983. The relationship of somatomedin C to puberty, pubertal growth and sex hormones. Pediatr. Res. **17**(suppl. 171A): 1.
32. CARA, J. F. & R. L. ROSENFIELD. 1988. Insulin-like growth factor I and insulin potentiate luteinizing hormone-induced androgen synthesis by rat ovarian thecal-interstitial cells. Endocrinology **123:** 733–739.
33. RAMALEY, J. A. & C. K. PHARES. 1980. Delay of puberty onset in females due to suppression of growth hormone. Endocrinology **106:** 1989.
34. ADASHI, E. V., C. E. RESWICK, A. J. D'ERCOLE, M. E. SVOBODA & J. J. VAN WYK. 1985. Insulin-like growth factors as intraovarian regulators of granulosa cell growth and function. Endocrinol. Rev. **6:** 400.
35. TOLIS, G., G. POLITIS, I. KONTOPOULOU, N. POULATZAS, G. RIGAS, C. SARIDAKIS, V. ATHANASIOU, A. MORTOGLOU, S. MALACHTARI & N. LING. 1987. Pituitary somatotropic function in patients with β-thalassemia on iron chelation therapy. Birth Defects **23**(5a): 449–452.
36. SKLAR, G. A., Z. Q. LEW, D. J. VOON & R. DAVID. 1987. Adrenal function in thalassemia major following long-term treatment with multiple transfusions and chelation therapy. AJDC **141:** 326–330.
37. REUBINOFF, B. E., A. SIMON, S. FRIEDLER, J. G. SCHUKER & A. LEWIN. 1994. Defective oocytes as a possible cause of infertility in a β-thal major patient. Hum. Reprod. **9:** 1143–1145.
38. DANESI, L., M. SCACCHI, A. M. MIRAGOLI, A. I. PINCELLI, A. DUBINI, A. T. MAIOLO, F. CAVAGUINI & E. E. POLLI. 1994. Induction of follicle maturation and ovulation by gonadotropin administration in women with β-thalassemia. Eur. J. Endocrinol. **131:** 602–606.
39. SERRACHIOLI, R., E. PORCU, C. COLOMBI, P. CIOTTI, R. FABRI, V. DE SANCTIS & C. FLAMIGNI. 1994. Transfusion dependent homozygous β-thalassemia major: Successful twin pregnancy following *in vitro* fertilization and tubal embryo transfer. Hum. Reprod. **9:** 1964–1965.
40. FUJISAWA, I., M. MORIKAWA, V. NAKANO & J. KONISHI. 1988. Hemochromatosis of the pituitary gland: MR imaging. Radiology **168:** 213–214.

Disturbances of Menstruation in Thyroid Disease

DEMETRIOS A. KOUTRAS

Athens University
Department of Clinical Therapeutics
80, Vas. Sofias Avenue
GR-115 28 Athens, Greece

INTRODUCTION

Both hyper- and hypothyroidism may result in menstrual disturbances, although the hormonal and other biochemical aberrations are not the same in these two disorders. Furthermore, both hyper- and hypothyroidism are associated with reduced fertility.

The frequency of menstrual irregularities in the more recent studies are not the same as in the older "classic" series. This is because now both hyper- and hypothyroidism are diagnosed at an earlier stage than before, thanks not only to the better diagnostic tests available, but also to greater awareness in the public and easier access to medical care.

Nevertheless, even in several recent studies of women with menstruation or fertility problems, a substantial proportion have been shown to have various endocrine disturbances, especially hypothyroidism but also hyperthyroidism, increased androgen production, hyperprolactinemia, and other disorders.[1–7] The high prevalence of these endocrine disorders in fertility and menstruation abnormalities are probably due to the sensitivity of modern diagnostic tests. Now subclinical hyper- and hypothyroidism can be diagnosed, whereas these would pass unnoticed a few decades ago. Clearly, then, thyroid function should be checked in every case of unexplained menstrual disorder or fertility problems.

In this short review some recent studies are summarized and compared to the older ones, and, additionally, several excellent reviews are mentioned.

HYPERTHYROIDISM

Increased sex hormone–binding globulin (SHBG) is characteristic of hyperthyroidism[8]—so much so that this globulin is used as a test of thyroid function, reflecting the tissue response to the thyroid hormones. Serum levels of estradiol and testosterone should thus be interpreted with this fact in mind because the total amounts are increased out of proportion to the free levels. Serum luteinizing hormone (LH) and follicle-stimulating hormone (FSH) may also be increased.[9,10]

In prepubertal girls menstruation has been reported to be delayed,[10,11] and in women of fertile age with hyperthyroidism oligomenorrhea (decreased menstrual flow) is the most common abnormality.[11] This may progress to amenorrhea, first described in the classic study by von Basedow.[12] Polymenorrhea (increased menstrual flow) is distinctly less frequent, in comparison to its occurrence in hypothyroidism. The frequency of these menstrual disorders varies in different series. Benson and Dailey[13] found that out of 221 hyperthyroid patients 58% had oligomenorrhea or amenorrhea and 5% polymenorrhea. This is in general agreement with other older studies such as those of Goldsmith *et al.*[14] More recently, in India Joshi *et al.*[15] found menstrual irregularities in 64.7% of hyperthyroid women, compared to 17.2% of healthy controls. These irregularities sometimes preceded thyroid dysfunction. However, Krassas *et al.*[16] found irregular cycles in only 21.5% out of 214 thyrotoxic patients. These discrepant results may be attributed to either genetic and other factors or to more delayed diagnosis in India[15] than in Greece.[16]

Anovulation and reduced fertility are common in hyperthyroidism,[10] but not so much in mild or subclinical cases.[17] I have seen several infertile hyperthyroid patients become pregnant as soon as thyroid hyperfunction had been controlled with antithyroid drugs. If, in spite of these abnormalities, a thyrotoxic woman becomes pregnant, there is an increased chance of maternal morbidity (toxemia of pregnancy, etc.), of fetal loss, and of underweight newborn.[17,18] Before antithyroid drugs became available, a fetal loss of about 50% had been reported.[19]

HYPOTHYROIDISM

In hypothyroidism, the serum prolactin (PRL) level may be increased.[10,20–22] This may be due to the fact that the hypothalamic-releasing hormone (TRH) increases the secretion of both thyroid-stimulating hormone (TSH) and PRL. Galactorrhea may occur. These disturbances usually disappear after thyroxine treatment.[20]

In some cases of juvenile hypothyroidism, precocious puberty has been reported.[23,24] This is probably due to a "spillover" effect: TSH, FSH, and LH are all glucoproteins, and they may have interlapping actions. However, because of decreased stature and delayed maturation in general, delayed puberty is more common than a precocious one.[21]

In women of fertile age, hypothyroidism causes several abnormalities, mainly polymenorrhea and menorrhagia, but also anovulation and more rarely amenorrhea.[10,14,17,21,25] In an Indian study, 68.2% of hypothyroid women had menstrual abnormalities, compared to 12.2% of healthy controls.[15] As stated before for hyperthyroidism, in India the diagnosis of hypothyroidism may be delayed, and so the disease may progress to a more severe degree before the diagnosis is made and effective treatment started. The causes of polymenorrhea may be multiple. The defects in hemostasis reported in hypothyroidism such as decreased levels of factors VII, VIII, IX, and XI[26] may contribute. Some cases of menorrhagia may be due to breakthrough bleeding following anovulation.

Pregnancy is rare in hypothyroidism, but when it occurs it is presently abnormal: abortions, stillbirths, and prematurity are quite common.[10,17,27] Older studies had reported perinatal mortality around 20%, congenital abnormalities in the offspring of 10 to 20%, and neurologic dysfunction in about 50%.[27–30] Early treatment of the mother improves the outcome of pregnancy and probably reduces the incidence of congenital abnormalities as well. For this reason, now that hypothyroid patients are diagnosed earlier and become pregnant while euthyroid on thyroxine, the overall picture is much brighter.

GOITER AND MENSTRUATION

In areas with a low or moderate iodine intake, the thyroid gland enlarges during pregnancy, because of the higher iodine requirements of pregnant women and the thyrotrophic activity of chorionic gonadotrophin.[31–34]

It has long been a belief in folklore that the thyroid gland also enlarges during the second half of the menstrual cycle. This has recently been confirmed by modern ultrasonographic techniques. Hegedus *et al.*[35] found in 11 healthy women a mean thyroid volume of 15.4±3.1 ml on day 9 of the cycle and of 24.4±4.8 ml on day 23 ($p<0.01$). Obviously, some old observations have a grain of truth!

SUMMARY

Both hyper- and hypothyroidism may result in menstrual disturbances. In hyperthyroidism, amenorrhea was described as early as 1840 by von Basedow. The most common manifestation is simple oligomenorrhea (decreased menstrual flow). Anovulatory cycles are very common. Increased bleeding may occur, but is rare in hyperthyroidism. Nowadays hyperthyroidism is diagnosed earlier than it once was, and so the clinical picture is generally milder. So, menstrual disorders are less common than in previous series. In a recent paper, 21.5% of 214 patients had disturbances in their cycle, compared to 50% in some older series. In hypothyroidism, on the contrary, polymenorrhea (increased menstrual bleeding) is more common. Defects in hemostasis may contribute to this. Anovulation may be present. Fertility is reduced in both hyper- and hypothyroidism, and the outcome of pregnancy is more often abnormal than in euthyroid women. It is of interest that in juvenile hypothyroidism precocious puberty has been described. This is probably due to a "spillover" effect of the glucoprotein hormones: TSH, which is markedly increased in hypothyroidism, has a small FSH- and LH-like effect. Galactorrhea may also be present in hypothyroidism, possibly because TSH, the hypophyseal TSH-releasing hormone, increases the secretion of both TSH and PRL.

REFERENCES

1. Moltz, L., M. Trapp, G. Bispink & F. Leidenberger. 1987. Rational hormonal diagnosis of secondary amenorrhea. Geburtshilfe-Frauenheilkd. **47**(4): 228–239.
2. Bispink, L., W. Brandle, C. Linder & G. Bettendorf. 1989. Preclinical hypothyroidism and disorders of ovarian function. Geburtshilfe-Frauenheilkd. **49**(10): 881–888.
3. Weise, H. C., L. Moltz, G. Bispink & F. Leidenberger. 1989. Rational hormonal diagnosis of oligomenorrhea. Geburtshilfe-Frauenheilkd. **49**(8): 694–700.
4. Gerhard, I., T. Becker, W. Eggert-Kruse, K. Klinga & G. Runnebaum. 1991. Thyroid and ovarian function in infertile women. Hum. Reprod. **6**(3): 338–345.

5. Moltz, L., F. Leidenberger & C. Weise. 1991. Rational hormone diagnosis in normocyclic functional sterility. Geburtshilfe-Frauenheilkd. **51**(9): 756–768.
6. Blum, M. & G. Blum. 1992. The possible relationship between menorrhagia and occult hypothyroidism in IUD-wearing women. Adv. Contracept. **8**(4): 313–317.
7. Bals-Pratsch, M., O. Schober, J. P. Hanker, C. de Geyter & H. P. Schneider. 1993. Disorders of thyroid function and sterility in the woman. Zentralbl. Gynakol. **115**(1): 18–23.
8. Rosner, W. 1990. The functions of corticosteroid-binding globulin and sex hormone-binding globulin: Recent advances. Endocrinol. Rev. **11:** 80–91.
9. Akande, E. O. & T. R. Hockaday. 1975. Plasma concentration of gonadotropinns, oestrogen and progesterone in thyrotoxic women. Br. J. Obstet. Gynaecol. **82:** 541–551.
10. Thomas, R. & R. L. Reid. 1987. Thyroid disease and reproductive dysfunction: A review. Obstet. Gynecol. **70:** 789–798.
11. Longcope, C. 1991. The male and female reproductive systems in thyrotoxicosis. *In* Werner & Ingbar's The Thyroid: A Fundamental and Clinical Text. 6th edit. L. E. Braverman & R. D. Utiger, Eds.: 828–835. Lippincott. New York.
12. von Basedow, C. A. 1840. Exophthalmos durch Hypertrophie des Zellgewebes in der Augenhohl. Wochenschrift Heilk **6:** 197.
13. Benson, R. C., & M. E. Dailey. 1955. Menstrual pattern in hyperthyroidism and subsequent post-therapy hypothyroidism. Surg. Gynaecol. Obstet. **100:** 19–26.
14. Goldsmith, R. E., S. H. Sturgis, J. Lerman & J. B. Stanbury. 1952. The menstrual pattern of thyroid disease. J. Clin. Endocrinol. Metab. **18:** 846–855.
15. Joschi, J. V., S. D. Bhandarkar, M. Chandha, D. Balaiah & R. Shah. 1993. Menstrual irregularities and lactation failure may precede thyroid dysfunction or goitre. J. Postgrad. Med. **39**(3): 137–141.
16. Krassas, G. E., N. Pontikides, Th. Kaltsas, Ph. Papadopoulou & M. Batrinos. 1994. Menstrual disturbances in thyrotoxicosis. Clin. Endocrinol. **40:** 641–644.
17. Daniels, G. H. 1995. Thyroid disease and pregnancy: A clinical overview. Endocrinol. Pract. **1:** 287–301.
18. Davis, L. E., M. J. Lucas, G. D. V. Hankins, M. L. Roark & F. G. Cunningham. 1989. Thyrotoxicosis complicating pregnancy. Am. J. Obstet. Gynecol. **160:** 63–70.
19. Gardner-Hill, H. 1929. Pregnancy complicating simple goitre and Grave's disease. Lancet **i:** 120–124.
20. Edwards, C. R. W., I. A. Forsyth & G. M. Besser. 1971. Amenorrhea, galactorrhea and primary hypothyroidism with high circulating levels of prolactin. Br. Med. J. **3:** 462–464.
21. Longcope, C. 1991. The male and female reproductive systems in hypothyroidism. *In* Werner & Ingbar's The Thyroid: A Fundamental and Clinical Text. 6th edit. L. E. Braverman & R. D. Utiger, Eds.: 1052–1055. Lippincott. New York.
22. Tolino, A., M. Nicotra, L. Romano, A. Petrone & L. Langella. 1991. Subclinical hypothyroidism and hyperprolactinemia. Acta Eur. Fertil. **22**(5): 275–277.
23. Kendle, F. 1905. Case of precocious puberty in a female cretin. Br. Med. J. **1:** 246–248.
24. van Wyk, J. & M. M. Grumbach. 1960. Syndrome of precocious menstruation and galactorrhea in juvenile hypothyroidism: An example of hormonal overlap pituitary feedback. J. Pediatr. **57:** 416–435.
25. Camargo, C. A. 1989. Hypothyroidism and goiter during pregnancy. *In* Endocrine Disorders of Pregnancy. S. A. Brody & K. Ueland, Eds.: 165–176. Appleton & Lange. Norwald, CT.
26. Ansell, J. E. 1991. The blood in hypothyroidism. *In* Werner & Ingbar's The Thyroid: A Fundamental and Clinical Text. 6th edit. L. E. Braverman & R. D. Utiger, Eds.: 1022–1026. Lippincott. New York.

27. Davis, L. E., K. J. Leveko & F. G. Cunningham. 1988. Hypothyroidism complicating pregnancy. Obstet. Gynecol. **72:** 108–112.
28. Man, E. B., W. S. Jones, R. H. Holden & E. D. Mellitis. 1971. Thyroid function in human pregnancy. VIII. Retardation of progeny aged 7 years: Relationships to maternal age and maternal thyroid function. Am. J. Obstet. Gynaecol. **111:** 905–916.
29. Man, E. B. 1975. Maternal hypothyroxinaemia: Development of 4 and 7 year old offspring. *In* Perinatal Thyroid Physiology and Disease. D. A. Fisher & G. N. Burrow, Eds.: 117–129. Raven Press. New York.
30. Balen, A. H. & A. B. Kurtz. 1990. Successful outcome of pregnancy with severe hypothyroidism. Case report and literature review. Br. J. Obstet. Gynaecol. **97:** 536–539.
31. Crooks, J., M. I. Tulloch, A. C. Turnbull, D. Davidsson, T. Skulasson & G. Snaedal. 1967. Comparative incidence of goitre in pregnancy in Iceland and Scotland. Lancet **2:** 625–627.
32. Bauch, K., W. Meng, F. E. Ulrich, *et al.* 1986. Thyroid status during pregnancy and postpartum in regions of iodine deficiency and endemic goiter. Endocrinol. Exp. **20:** 67–77.
33. Glinoer, D., P. de Nayer, P. Bourdoux, M. Lemone, C. Robyn, A. van Teirteghem, J. Kinthaert & B. Lejeune. 1990. Regulation of maternal thyroid during pregnancy. J. Clin. Endocrinol. Metab. **71:** 276–287.
34. Glinoer, D. & M. Lemone. 1992. Goiter and pregnancy: A new insight into an old problem. Thyroid **2:** 65–70.
35. Hegedus, L., S. Karstrup & N. Rasmussen. 1986. Evidence of cyclic alterations of thyroid size during the menstrual cycle in healthy women. Am. J. Obstet. Gynecol. **155**(1): 142–145.

Sports-Related Problems in Reproductive Function

JUDIT ÖRLEY

Pediatric Gynaecological Ward and Outpatient Department
Department of Obstetrical Gynaecology
Haynal Imre Health Science University
Budapest, XIII. Ker.
Szabolcs u. 35, Hungary

INTRODUCTION

The last third of our century created a fascinating question for all participants in sports programs for youth—and especially for specialists dealing with such youth: is the exercise and competition harmful for the girls before or during the process of puberty or not? Title IX of the U.S. Federal Education Assistance Act which in 1972 mandated equal access to endurance training and sports in schools for young girls—represented a great challenge for parents, coaches, and physicians who all faced this acute problem because of the large number of girls actively participating in sports. Two distinct opinions arose, or perhaps it would be more accurate to say, two conflicting interests became apparent. On one side are those who deny any deleterious effect of sports on the development of reproductive function; on the other side are those who contend that strenuous physical activities are causing dysfunction of the initial period of sexual hormone production. I have been working with children as a pediatric and adolescent gynecologist since 1966 and have had ample opportunity to observe the effect of competitive physical training among girls under 16 years of age in Hungary. I have become convinced that excessive participation in sports can impede growth and development and can delay the initiation and stabilization of reproductive function during puberty. My task is to demonstrate this danger for developing girls, to call attention to it, and to examine its temporary or reversible nature after the endurance training ceases. The dysfunction caused by sports indeed disappears to some extent if the excessive training is diminished and the concommitant dietary deprivation ceases. The risk of hazardous effect is greater in this age group than in adulthood. Therefore, we must warn our patients about all kinds of sports that overwhelm the maturing organism and encourage them to limit their participation sufficiently that harmful effects are avoided.

SUBJECTS AND METHODS

Our routine work as gynecologists with young girls has been assisted since 1977 by a diagnostic method called functional somatometry. At every medical visit, each girl is carefully measured by this applied form of anthropometry. The measurements are performed according to the Martin-Saller technique.[1] This technique consists of taking 30 body measurements, including eight skinfolds on both sides, using 10 calculated indices; and applying equations. We measure height and weight and circumference of the chest, waist, and hips. The bulkiest part of the left upper arm and left calf are also measured in centimeters. Length measurements are done on the left upper and lower extremities. The width of the humerus and the femurs serve to determine body composition determination. Since 1986, we have increased the accuracy of our skinfold measurements (until this time they had been measured by Lange caliper only) by using ultrasonographic technique, and we have extended our measurements bilaterally and symmetrically on the trunk. We measure four skinfolds on the limbs (tricepts, bicepts, gastrocnemius, and triceps surae). The most important skinfolds are on the trunk (subscapular, suprailiacal, spinal, and umbilical). They provide information not only on the nutritive condition of the individual, but also on endocrine–genetic function. The geographical distribution of the subcutaneous fat in the trunk guarantees a quick, painless, and simple diagnostic tool for the developing girl. Our department at the Haynal Imre Health Science University, because of its huge number of patients, made it possible to establish an atlas with one-year intervals for all ages from birth to 16 years of age including all endocrine-genetic disorders within our speciality. 13,500 new patients have been measured, and each patient has had a minimum of four follow-up visits. The atlas comprised basic data on healthy Hungarian girls at each age. These girls represent the controls and are compared to peers experiencing health problems. The measurements are registered on a computer system, which facilitates the calculation of the adapted equations or indices (TABLE 1). We take body composition into account; we calculate body mass index and percent body fat as well as total body water, lean body mass, body surface area, and so forth. Our database is always growing, which makes the utilization of the registered data easier. In 1985 cluster and discriminant analyses were performed on a selected sample of our recorded data: it involved 924 persons with 1522 individual measurements. This provided statistically significant evidence that the skinfolds characterized specific endocrine disorders. In defining our optimal statistical distances for the whole sample, we applied the nearest neighbor decision rule method.[2] A very close relationship was proven between the individually interpreted skinfolds and the examined menstrual or endocrinological disorders. For those girls who are in pubertal development, we use the Tanner's classification.[3] It is divided into five phases according to specified criteria. The functional somatometry method made it possible to differentiate the girls as being of normal weight, lean, or obese. After menarche the body composition plays an important role in the maintenance of the hypothalamo-pituitary-ovarian axis. Too much fat or less than normal, especially at the navel, is an indication of dysfunction in ovarian hormone production. The skinfolds around the hip can provide information about the dermatomes X and XII. The sympathetic innervation of the ovaries—originating from the spinal cord—is found in these dermatomes. The skinfolds indicate subsequent hormonal production. There are typical skinfold-lines for menstrual disturbances. The difference is statistically significant with a confidence limit of 0.01.

TABLE 1. Indices and Equations for Functional Somatometry Calculations

1. Index of Kaup $$\frac{\text{weight (g)}}{\text{height (cm)}^2}$$

2. Index of Hirata $$\frac{\text{height (cm)}}{\sqrt[3]{\text{weight (kg)}}}$$

3. Robusticity index of Pignet-Verwach

$$\frac{\text{weight (kg)} + \text{chest circumference (cm)}}{\text{height (cm)}}$$

4. Density index of Durnin-Rahaman

$$D = 1.1369–0.0598\times\text{Log(B+T+Sc+Si skinfolds)}$$

5. Body fat percentage of Siri

$$\% = \left(\frac{4.95}{D} - 4.5\right) \times 100$$

6. Lean body mass (weight – body fat %)

7. Body surface area, according to Boyd's equation

$$BSAm^2 = weight\ (g)^{0.7285–0.0188\ \log Wt} \times height\ (cm)^{0,03\times3,207\times10} – 4$$

8. Body total water according to Mellits and Cheek's equation

$$BTW=–10.313+0.154\ height\ (cm)+0.252\ weight\ (kg)$$

9. Fat body mass according to Dugdale and Griffith's equation

$$FBM=6.629+0.64Wt–0.14Ht–0.118T+0.035Sc+0.2.68B+0.059Si$$

10. Fat body mass calculated to the body surface area according to Dugdale and Griffith's equation, multiplying the skinfold with the body surface area.

RESULTS

The study of young athletes dates back to 1977. The general medical practice (blood sample for sexual hormones FSH, LH, PRL, E_2, urinary estrogens, etc.) was complemented by the functional somatometry method. In 1979, we first reported on 36 top gymnasts with athletic amenorrhea and oligo-amenorrhea.[4] They all belonged to the lean body composition group with less than normal percentages of body fat. They were forced to maintain a strict diet together with a high level of extensive physical activities. We studied these gymnasts for the duration of this restrictive period and have proven that the correlation between the lean body/high activity combination and amenorrhea is linear. If a female child started serious athletic training in early childhood, her somatic development—including the process of pubertal development—was retarded. This result corresponds well with the observations of the early authors in sports medicine, for example, Malina (TABLE 2). Malina's view proposed

TABLE 2. Surveys on Athletic Oligo-amenorrhea

Reference	Type of Sport	No. of Women	Oligo-amenorrhea
Erdélyi, 1962	Athletes	577	70 (12%)
Foreman, 1967	Long distance runners	46	20 (43%)
Dale, 1979	Runners	23	6 (50%)
	Joggers	10	3 (30%)
Russel, 1984	Swimmers	6	6 (100%)
	Runners	7	0 (0%)

an open question, whether being an athlete promotes delay in first menses or whether the linear physique associated with being an athlete is the result of a delayed menses.[5–7] Frisch[8] and Warren,[9] having studied ballet dancers, found similar loss in weight and/or in percent body fat. Later, Frisch[10] evaluated runners and swimmers as she attempted to correlate premenarcheal training with the age of menarche. She found a delay of approximately 5 months per year of excessive premenarcheal training. The statement corresponded well with our findings. TABLE 3 shows the hormone levels observed in long-term and short-term athletic girls. The urinary estrogens were very low in long-term practicing athletes, but with normal LH/FSH ratios, whereas short-term (6–22 months) exercising girls had LH/FSH ratios typical for anovulation with normal urinary estrogens.

Between 1980 and 1983, we studied 43 athletes with abundant and irregular bleeding. They had been admitted to our ward with significant blood loss. Their mean age at the first medical visit was 13.35 years. Most of them suffered from dysfunctional uterine bleeding, 14 had a short luteal phase, and 12 were polymenorrheics. They were top gymnasts and generally exercised 3 to 5 hours or more daily and attended competitions on weekends. Their hormone levels showed an exaggeratedly high LH and low FSH with a normal level of PRL (prolactine). These admitted athletes were regularly measured for these hormone levels during and after recovery. The calculations were based on 124 measurements following the functional somatometry method. The results were compared first to gynecologically healthy peers and then to nonathletic patients suffering from the same type of menstrual disorder (TABLE 4). When we regard the mean values of the skinfolds measured on the trunk, the athletes and the nonathletes showed the same local loss of fatty tissues in comparison to normally menstruating healthy girls—although the lack of fat was even more pronounced in athletes. This difference was statistically highly significant and representative for the given menstrual disturbance. When the skinfold results of athlete patients were compared to other athletes with a menstrual disturbance, a statistically significant difference existed only between the skinfold results of those with dysfunctional uterine bleeding and the skinfold results of polymenorrheics (TABLE 5). There is also no difference between the skinfold results of nonathletic patients with dysfunctional uterine bleeding and short luteal phase bleeding. Therefore, we have to suspect that these kinds of bleeding disorders reflect only anovulation and subsequent luteal insufficiency, but in milder (short luteal phase) or serious form (dysfunctional uterine bleeding). A lack of progesterone is the common problem in hormonal pro-

TABLE 3. Hormone Results in Chronically and Short-Term Exercising and Dieting Athletic Girls

Group		FSH	LH	PRL	Urinary Estrogens	TSH	T_3	T_4	LH:FSH	No.
Chronic	$\overline{X}$	9.5 mU/ml	20.1 mU/ml	12.1 ng/ml	$\overline{X}$ 4.5 mg/24^h	$\overline{X}$ 1.9	0.9	8.0	2.11	5
Short-term	$\overline{X}$	9.7 mU/ml	62.6 mU/ml	14.8 ng/ml	$\overline{X}$ 19.1 mg/24^h	$\overline{X}$ 2.5	1.0	8.6	6.45	34

TABLE 4. Skinfold Line for Healthy Peers, Athletes, and Nonathletic Patients[a]

Control Peers		Athletes			Nonathletes		
		DUB	Polymenorrh.	Pollakymen.	DUB	Polymenorrh.	Pollakymen.
sc	13.71	12.78	13.67[b]	11.69[b]	13.71	11.5[b]	13.71
si	15.94	13.82	13.53[b]	13.40	15.85	12.08[b]	15.47
sp	12.52	9.48[b]	9.03[b]	9.00[b]	11.21	8.21	10.47
umb	20.31	15.68[b]	14.75[b]	14.48[b]	16.70[b]	13.03[b]	16.60[b]
Kaup i:	2.04	Kaup i: 1.87	Kaup i: 1.91	Kaup i: 1.76	Kaup i: 1.81	Kaup i: 1.77	Kaup i: 1.90
Hirata i:	42.25	Hirata i: 44.16	Hirata i: 44.26	Hirata i: 44.27	Hirata i: 44.5	Hirata i: 44.82	Hirata i: 44.06
BF%:	22.27	BF%: 20.76[b]	BF%: 20.62[b]	BF%: 19.94[b]	BF%: 21.63	BF%: 19.51[b]	BF% 22.28

[a]Abbreviations and definitions: Sc, subscapular skinfold; Si, suprailiacal skinfold; Sp, spinal skinfold; U, umbilical skinfold; BF%, body fat %; DUB, dysfunctional uterine bleeding/irregular bleeding; Polymenorrhea, 28/20 days bleeding; Pollakymenorrhea, short luteal phase 18/8–10 days bleeding.

[b]Indicates a statistically significant difference for a confidence limit of 0.01.

TABLE 5. Statistically Significant Differences among the Different Clinical Symptoms in Athletic and in Nonathletic Patients

	Athletes				Nonathletes		
	DUB	Polymenorrh.	Pollakymen.		DUB	Polymenorrh.	Pollakymen.
Sc	12.78	13.67	11.69	Sc	13.71	11.60[a]	13.71
Si	13.82	13.53	13.40	Si	15.85	12.08[a]	15.47
Sp	9.48	9.03	9.03	Sp	11.21	8.21	10.47
U	15.68	14.74[a]	14.48	U	16.70[a]	13.03[a]	16.60
	Progesteron deficiency syndromes				Progesterone deficiency syndromes		
serious form		mild form		serious form		mild form	

NOTE: Abbreviations and definitions same as for TABLE 4.
[a]Indicates a statistically significant difference for a confidence limit of 0.01.

duction, and this is expressed in patients' skinfold lines. We must add to this observation the fact that the athletes suffer from iron deficiency after menarche. This may impair the heavy bleeding. The loss of subcutaneous fatty tissue at specific sites (umbilical, spinal, and suprailical) was also demonstrated in body fat percent.[11, 12]

From 1983 until 1987, we studied 44 athletes who suffered amenorrhea or oligoamenorrhea. We compared them by using functional somatometry as a diagnostic tool, in the same way as for the earlier group. Their data was compared to healthy peers and to nonathletic oligo-amenorrheic patients. The comparison first divided them according to their body composition into lean or obese groups. The athletes had high LH and low FSH levels with low estrogen. In the skinfolds measured on the trunk, the normal-weight athletes had less body fat in suprailiac and umbilical regions compared to controls. As had been proven earlier, the skinfold line of amenorrheics/oligo-amenorrheics displayed a statistically significant difference in suprailiacal skinfold. Now, this difference was found even in obese athletes with this particular menstrual disturbance (TABLES 6 and 7).[13]

It seems clear that the absolute amount of (in dermatomes) deposited fat in different areas of the body can be demonstrated by functional somatometry. If we regard

TABLE 6. Statistically Significant Differences in Skinfolds of Normal Weight Athletic and Nonathletic Patients

		Athletic Patients		Nonathletic Patients	
	Control Peers	Oligomenorrhea	Amenorrhea	Oligomenorrhea	Amenorrhea
Sc	13.71	13.85	13.90[a]	15.4	17.0[a]
Si	15.94	14.23[a]	12.71[a]	17.7[a]	18.7[a]
Sp	12.52	12.33	12,25	12.9	13.3
U	20.31	17.85	17,96[a]	18.8	19.6

NOTE: Abbreviations same as TABLE 4.
[a]Indicates a statistically significant difference for a confidence limit of 0.01.

TABLE 7. Statistically Significant Differences in Skinfolds of Obese Athletic and Nonathletic Patients

		Athletic Patients		Nonathletic patients	
	Control Peers	Oligomenorrhea	Amenorrhea	Oligomenorrhea	Amenorrhea
Sc	26.00	23.0	22.50	28.10	28.00
Si	28.00	21.0[a]	21.50[a]	30.2	31.3
Sp	21.3	20.5	19.5	24.9	24.8
U	31.3	29.5	28.5	32.5	34.9

NOTE: Abbreviations same as TABLE 4.
[a]Indicates a statistically significant difference for a confidence limit of 0.01.

the measurements as a possible diagnostic tool, we have a gauge for controlling sexual hormone metabolism in young girls. The competition and excessive sports exercise "drain energy," and this is represented in skinfolds. The local loss or excess of subcutaneous fat can be monitored in this way. After recovery, when we measure the healthy, hormonally normal "fat-cover" on the trunk, we can verify that the menstrual problem has ceased. The cessation of training and competition quickly restores a healthy level of body fat. The change can be easily read by functional somatometry. This diagnostic tool, by means of body measurements, provides a simple, low-cost means of monitoring hormone metabolism.

DISCUSSION

Exercise training is being used increasingly to prevent and/or treat diseases, therefore, it is desirable for young or elderly people to participate in sports. In spite of this, we must be aware of the fact that the endocrine functions are more vulnerable both before and after puberty than at any time later in adulthood. Young girls should be warned about potentially damaging physical and mental stress during training and competition while they are in the pubertal developmental process. The position statement approved by the Executive Council of the International Federation of Sports Medicine in 1990[14] includes a recommendation that young children *not* participate extensively in strenuous physical activities because this has become an obvious risk factor—together with the abuse of steroids and other anabolic drugs—for the development of normal reproductive function. The most serious and long-lasting consequences are related to the initial or developmental phase of puberty. Puberty is characterized by changes in the constituents of the fat-free mass.[15] The body's water content decreases, and the bone density increases. The fact that the percentage of osseous minerals and the density of the fat-free mass are lower for late adolescents than for adults indicates that chemical maturity proceeds very slowly and is not complete until adulthood. It is well known that fat is important to the development of bones. Reduction of the fat mass, as has been proven in athletes, could lead to menstrual disorder by altering the feedback mechanism of the hypothalamic–pituitary system. Bone mineral loss is a well-known complication of hypoestrogenism (i.e., Turner syndrome). Therefore, exercise-induced amenorrhea or dysfunctional uterine bleeding must be viewed against the backdrop of skeletal metabolism during childhood and also with respect to the normal function of the reproductive system.

During our studies, we have demonstrated that our athletes suffered iron deficiency. Iron deficiency affects work capacity by impairing oxygen delivery to the muscles. This is a vicious circle that is often overlooked in teenagers, whose rapid growth process requires a constant supply of iron. Iron is important in the activity of thyrosine hydroxylase, a key enzyme in catecholamine synthesis. Epinephrine and norepinephrine are essential for normal chronotropin and inotropin response to exercise. The athletes often engage in strict control of nutrition, in both senses: qualitative regulation together with caloric restriction. The so-called "energy-drain" can impair the menstrual rhythm. If the intensity of exercise is so high that it has an impact on the menstrual cycle, the risks outweigh the possible benefits in sports, and the training must be stopped. This danger is extremely high for young girls before and during puberty. The damage to the endocrine reproductive function will be temporary, if the girl ceases the exercises, gives up competition, and mitigates her dietary deprivation. The health of the individual should be paramount among specialists in pediatric and adolescent medicine, and we should recommend against the type of intense training currently undergone by top athletes because of the abundant evidence that it is deleterious to the development of reproductive function.

REFERENCES

1. Martin, R. & K. Saller. Lehrbuch der Antropologie I–IV. Third edit., 1957–1966) Gustav Fischer Vlg. Stuttgart 2999 pp.
2. Coiver & Hart. 1970. Nearest Neighbour Decision Rule. London Publishing Company. London, England.
3. Tanner, J. M. 1962. Growth at adolescence. Oxford, England.
4. Örley, J. 1979. Late consequences of voluntary fasting in adolescence. V. FIGIF World Congress. Tokyo. Pp. 163–172.
5. Malina, R. M., A. N. Harper, H. H. Avent & D. E. Campbell. 1975. Age at menarche in athletes and non-athletes. Med. Sci. Sports **5:** 11–15.
6. Malina, R. M., W. W. Spirduso, C. Tate & A. M. Baylor. 1978. Age of menarche and selected menstrual characteristics in athletes at different competitive levels and in different sports. Med. Sci. Sports **11:** 218–231.
7. Malina, R. M., C. Bouchard, R. F. Ahoup, A. Demirjian & G. Yriviere. 1979. Age at menarche, family size and birth order in athletes at Montreal Olympic Games 1976. Med. Sci. Sports **11:** 354–365.
8. Frisch, R. E., G. Wyshak & L. Wincent. 1980. Delayed menarche and amenorrhoea in ballet dancers. N. Engl. J. Med. **303**(19): 1424–1426.
9. Warren, M. P. 1981. The effect of exercises on pubertal progression and reproductive function in girls. J. Clin. Endocrinol. Metab. **51:** 1130–1132.
10. Frisch, R. E., A. V. Gotz-Walbergen & H. V. McArthur. 1981. Delayed menarche and amenorrhoea of college athletes in relation to age of onset of training. JAMA **246:** 1159.
11. Örley, J. 1984. Competitive sports and juvenile menstrual disorders. Paper presented at World Congress of "Child and Sport" Urbino.

12. Örley, J. 1984. Body fat deposition and sexual maturation. Pediatr. Ed Adolesc. Gynecol. **2**(2): 145–172.
13. Örley, J. 1988. Athletic amenorrhoea. Proceedings of the IV. European Congress of PAG. Rhodes. pp. 341–348.
14. 1991. Position statement from the FIMS 1990. Hungar. Rev. Sports Med. **32**(2): 141–145.
15. Hergenroeder, A. C. & W. J. Klish. 1990. Body composition in adolescent athletes. Ped. Clin. N. Am. **37**(5): 1057–1083.

Athletic Amenorrhea

A. S. WOLF,[a,b] K. MARX,[c] AND U. ULRICH[b]

[b]*Gynecological Practice of Dr. Wolf & Partners*
Frauenstraße 51
89073 Ulm, Germany
[c]*Gynecological Practice of Drs. Verhoeven, Scholtes & Marx*
Düsseldorf, Germany

The participation of female children and teenagers in competitive sports has appreciably changed the image of women's sports. In several sports disciplines, such as gymnastics, rhythmic sport gymnastics, ballet dancing, swimming, and ice skating, medals are frequently won by adolescent girls. This development has raised criticism as well as admiration. The idea of young girls and adolescents participating in sports was developed in eastern European countries, where participation of children was promoted for special sport disciplines under to the slogan "children for champions." This rationale is based on the early accomplishment of physical body functions with maximum development of vital capacity, static strength, and several neurophysiologic faculties, such as rhythmic movement, jumping adaptation, power of reaction, and skillfulness between the ages of 13 and 15.

Obviously, young girls are especially qualified for gymnastics, rhythmic gymnastics, and ballet dancing because of the extreme flexibility and elasticity of their ligaments and joints. Their boyish and infantile stature with low body weight, long legs, and narrow hips provides ideal levers at low body resistance.

At the same time, a large number of publications have appeared in the past few years that draw attention to the association of competitive sports for children and adolescents with orthopedic lesions, delay of puberty, menstrual cycle disorders, and, consequently, juvenile osteoporosis.

DELAYED PUBERTY AND MENARCHE

In young girls beginning competitive sports before their menarche, a delay of both puberty and menarche can frequently be observed. The question arises whether this is a consequence of the extreme exercise, or rather of an inherited late maturation. Frisch *et al.*[1] speculated that amenorrhea may result if the body fat content is reduced below 22% by means of exercise and/or restrictive diet. The lean-fat hypothesis generated by Frisch and Revelle[2] is based on data from 181 girls and was recalculated using height and weight as an approximation formula for total body water content. The investigators postulated a constant body water content of 72% throughout puberty, which is actually reduced by 0.38% each year from prepuberty to adulthood. The

[a]Address for correspondence: Alfred S. Wolf, M.D., Gynecological Practice and Private Institute of Gynecological Endocrinology, Frauenstrasse 51, D-89073 Ulm, Germany.

data obtained, however, seemed to lack reliability and therefore have been criticized by several authors.[3–5]

Percent body fat estimations show variabilities according to the method used: Increasing values are found when skinfold thickness was measured at two to six sites and were even highest using height and weight for prediction.[3]

In a retrospective analysis, Marx[6] reported on findings in 329 teenaged girls from former East German competitive sports before 1989. All girls had been selected early for their sports discipline according to their specific anthropomorphic measurements and their specific capabilities. Weekly training of all girls was exactly documented and considerably more intense and time consuming than in Western countries. The documented mean age of menarche was slightly higher (13.57 ± 1.3 yr) compared to sedentary controls, but the increase of this mean was mainly due to girls competing in acrobatic sports disciplines (14.8 ± 1.6 yr compared to 13.1 ± 1.2 yr in other disciplines) (FIG. 1). Two hundred and one girls who began exercising before menarche experienced a delay of menarche by 0.88 years (i.e., 13.86 versus 12.98 years). These data suggest that late menarche occurs more frequently in esthetic disciplines (such as floor ballet, gymnastics, ballet dancing, and long distance running). The disciplines mentioned are preferably *chosen* by skinny girls with boyish stature who then exhibit a delay of puberty that is perhaps genetically programmed, and who are *selected* early for optimum performance.[6–8] By contrast, girls with early sexual maturation tend to choose an unathletic lifestyle without exercise exposure more often than late maturers.[8]

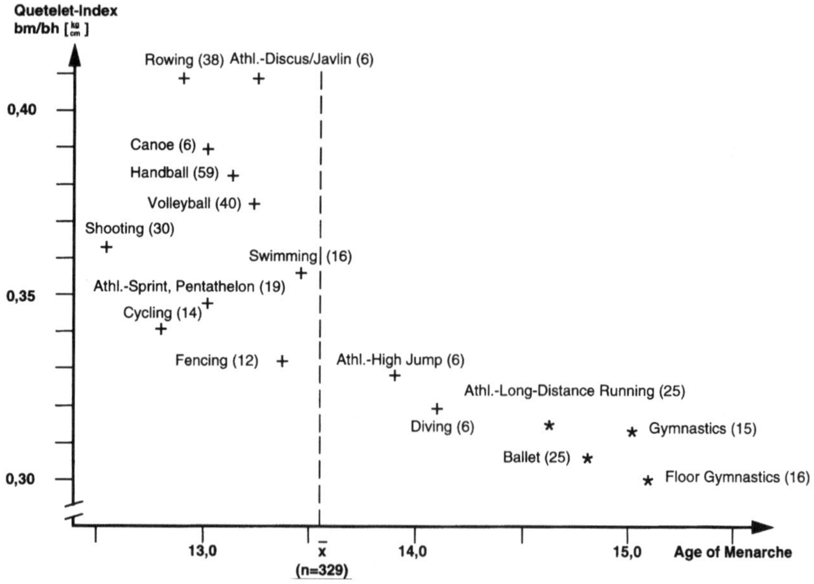

FIGURE 1. Age of menarche plotted against Quetelet index specified for different sports disciplines in 329 high-performance athletes (Marx[6]).

There is an association between body weight and menarche, but it is doubtful whether this association is causal. Warren[9] found reduced bone age in ballet dancers; however, their mothers had experienced delayed menarche as well. These data suggest genetic factors as the main cause for a constitutional delay of puberty.[8] These data also elucidate the multicausal interrelationship of early selection, genetically programmed late puberty, and constitutional factors as the cause of delayed menarche. Observations of a small group of 18 college-aged swimmers and runners by Frisch *et al.*[10] suggest that exercise exposure before menarche delays it by five months for each year of exercise, which may be considered ballpark estimate in view of the complex interrelationships. Finally, if a delay of puberty occurs, this exclusively affects the gonadal maturation, while pubic and axillary hair growth as a sign of adrenarche remain virtually unaffected.

MENSTRUAL CYCLE DISORDERS (OLIGOMENORRHEA)

The incidence of oligomenorrhea among female athletes ranges between 1 and 43%. The different incidences reported may be explained by different groups of athletes being looked at, variable sports disciplines, different intensities of exercise, the variety of analytical methods used in the studies, as well as ambiguous definitions of amenorrhea.

Low incidences of oligomenorrhea were reported from hobby runners and joggers,[11] whereas an increased frequency was found in top athletes, owing to their exercise program and energy drain.[12] The incidence rate of 30% of functional amenorrhea among endurance athletes is markedly higher than the number of 1.8 to 2.6% in the normal female population.[13,14]

PREDISPOSING FACTORS FOR THE DEVELOPMENT OF DELAYED PUBERTY AND MENSTRUAL CYCLE DISORDERS IN FEMALE ATHLETES

From our experience, five factors are more or less associated with gonadal disorders in female athletes:

- Type of sport;
- Genetic predisposition, specific selection of individuals for certain sports disciplines;
- Beginning of competitive sports and menstrual history;
- Intensity of exercise;
- Metabolic alterations and change in the body composition;
- Psychological and emotional factors, stress.

Type of Sports Discipline

The majority of adolescent and women athletes suffering from cycle disorders participate in esthetic disciplines and strenuous endurance sports, with extended and continuous energy drain. In esthetic disciplines, genetic predisposition and distinct eating behaviors lead to cycle and developmental disorders. In both groups, interindividual thresholds for cycle disorders are apparently due to the different—partly genetically determined—influences of sports discipline, specific metabolic characteristics, respiration, distribution of muscle fibers, different training methods, different adaptation, inadequate nutrition, and coping with stress.[6] The energy drain caused by exercise is not the sole factor or influence in producing menstrual cycle disorders.[4] The related disciplines are:

- Esthetic–acrobatic disciplines: gymnastics, ballet dancing, floor ballet, dancing;
- Long distance running (>800 m); cross-country running, jogging (>30 km/week); cross-country skiing, downhill skiing.

Genetic Predisposition and Specific Selection of Individuals

Many girls are selected because of their special anthropomorphic types and discipline-specific capabilities. These girls are more often genetically late matures with constitutional developmental delay or pubertas tarda.[7] They have a reduced bone age and low body height and weight, with low estradiol levels and a sonographically reduced uterine length.

Beginning of Competitive Sports and Menstrual History

Commencement of endurance sports before menarche may result in a delay of both pubertal development and menarche as described above. On the other hand, adolescent girls with oligomenorrhea who begin competitive sports after menarche may experience long-standing oligomenorrhea, indicating underlying labile hypothalamic–pituitary regulation.

Intensity of Exercise

The incidence of amenorrhea is higher in sports requiring intense physical effort. Cycle disorders are positively correlated with the weekly mileage of running, jogging, or cycling, and hours of intense exercise exposure per week, respectively.[7,15,16] Menstrual cycle disorders are worse at the end of an athletic season[13] and show an increasing frequency and duration the longer and faster a woman is running.[12] However, apparently there is not a causal relationship but rather an association.[4]

Metabolic Alterations and Change of Body Composition

Reduced body fat and weight loss associated with an altered lean-to-fat ratio have been reported to cause oligomenorrhea. Frisch and McArthur[1] suggested a minimum critical level of body fat required for menarche and the onset of regular menstrual cycles. This theory has been widely contradicted (see above). Amenorrhea frequently occurs during an acute loss of weight of more than 10 to 15% of normal weight for height (1/3 of body fat[3,25]). The body fat of women runners is reduced to 7 to 8% of their body weight, as compared to 20% in sedentary controls. These data reflect the problems of inappropriate eating behavior and food restriction in an athlete population rather than problems associated with reducing the absolute body fat content. In many sports disciplines, the outward appearance is meager, lean, and scrawny. These girls are easily distinguishable from women performing short-term exhaustive exercises, such as short distance running and throwing the javelin or discus. The latter appear more feminine, with normal proportions and well-developed female characteristics. However, the lean/fat theory of oligomenorrhea has been criticized and called into question, because, especially in scrawny girls, the early awareness of an inherited body image, eating disorders, and emotional problems are frequently associated. The contradiction of the lean/fat theory is supported by several observations. Warren[9] reported on young ballet dancers becoming amenorrheic during exercise and consequent weight loss and experiencing return of menses when they stopped their exercise because of injuries—although weight loss continued. Furthermore, even in amenorrheic girls with anorexia nervosa, normal cycles can be reestablished by pulsatile GnRH replacement therapy.[18] These data indicate that weight loss and decreased body fat are coincidental rather than causative factors contributing to oligomenorrhea.

Eating and nutritional habits seem to play a key role in the scenario of oligomenorrhea. There is a continuity from normal eating to restrained eating or dieting to eating disorders (anorexia, bulimia) with many transitions. The most significant consequences of these disorders are the possibility of amenorrhea with hypoestrogenism plus nutritional deficits of calories and calcium.[19]

Psychological and Emotional Factors: Stress

Adolescent athletes are exposed to several endogenous and external influences. Physical faculty and motivation are the main prerequisites and are mostly acquired during adolescence through friends, parents, and sports idols. In 1993, an article appeared, entitled "Running, an analogue of anorexia?" in which Yates *et al.*[20] described the emotional characteristics of obligatory runners as resembling those of anorectic women in terms of the family background; socioeconomic class; personality factors such as inhibition of anger, high self expectations, and tolerance of physical discomfort and depression associated with having a mania for certain low-calorie diets. Many young athletes feel a serious desire to reduce their body weight (that is, fat) for the best performance and fitness. This striving for a minimum body fat together with the stress of competition and calorie waste through enormous energy expenditure often leads to an excessive weight loss, associated with a partially pathologic aversion to food and fat. These self-generated aversions are often reinforced by persons who play a dominant role in an athlete's life, for example, coaches, teammates, and parents. Parents especially often exert extreme demands for success, dietary practice, and weight control. Daily weight loss of one kilogram and even more is not rare.[21] More and more cases of severe anorexia nervosa have been reported among athletes, especially among gymnasts. Therefore, any physician should be prepared for counseling athletes at risk, and should not only investigate physical features but also use the opportunity to talk about emotional problems.

Unrealistic expectations must be replaced by realistic arguments. Instead of inhuman demands for more and harder training plus deprivation, the aim must be adjusted to the training results. In view of physical fitness, the reduction of body fat in conjunction with muscle increment must be programmed, avoiding "crash programs" and weight loss of more than 1 to 2 kg per week.[22] Physical and emotional stress has been reported to be a contraproductive event, especially in competitive sports. Amenorrheic runners score higher figures in stress rating scales.[22,23] Stress-coping strategies, therefore, are important tools for stress reduction.

ENDOCRINE CHANGES DURING EXERCISE

The data published on hormonal patterns before, during, and after exercise are inconsistent with respect to the duration of performance. Especially during exercise, the dynamics of hormones are not only influenced by their secretion rate, but also by altered vascular transport, reduced metabolism (due to reduced liver circulation), and lowered renal excretion.

Short-term (Acute) Exhaustive Exercise (15–20 min)

The sex steroid hormones estradiol and testosterone rise rapidly because of reduced liver circulation[24–26] with constant levels of SHBG.[26] Prolactin (PRL) responds according to the physical fitness. Increases in PRL are noted in well-trained subjects, and decreasing values in untrained women.[20,27,28] The net increase in PRL is less during short-term exercise than in prolonged exercise, and it is higher during running compared to cycling,[29] probably due to breast movements.

Prolonged (Chronic) Exercise

During prolonged or repetitive nonexhaustive exercise (measured in kilometers or miles per week), the endocrine changes are of greater value in view of the underlying processes. Endocrine analyses have been performed either once before, during, and after prolonged exercise, or repeatedly during a season. Repeated exercise during a season suppresses the menstrual cycle function stepwise within a pathophysiologic continuity from luteal phase defect (low progesterone[30]) to oligomenorrhea (low FSH, LH, and estradiol) being caused by hypothalamic dysfunction with subsequent altered episodic release of LH.[15] The decline of the peripheral sex steroids is a consequence of decreasing gonadotropins. The LH pulsatility depends on the athlete's condition.

In untrained women, the LH episodes decrease or even disappear, while well-trained women show an unaltered increase in both frequency and amplitude of LH pulses with unchanged or increased PRL levels.[17,27,31,32] It is well known that the function of the hypothalamic pulse generator is disturbed in hypothalamic amenorrhea. However, even in eumenorrheic sportswomen, the LH pulsatility may be reduced during the training season.[15]

PATHOPHYSIOLOGIC CAUSES FOR THE HYPOTHALAMIC-PITUITARY-OVARIAN DYSFUNCTION

Athletic oligomenorrhea as well as delay of puberty represent a complex interplay of several factors.

1. The increment of β-endorphins[32,33] and change of catecholamine metabolism with increasing dopamine (simultaneous decrease of PRL and LH episodes). Norepinephrine and epinephrine[32] are the main stress-induced causes for an altered, dysfunctional hypothalamic GnRH pulsatility.
2. Less important is the increase of androgens[28] and PRL,[20,27] as PRL seems more likely to be an endocrine marker than a causative agent.

LONG-TERM CONSEQUENCES: JUVENILE OSTEOPOROSIS

Physiological mineralization and development of mature bone matrix microarchitecture (peak bone mass) seem to be completed 2 to 4 years after menarche. There is a marked reduction of bone mass accumulation after age 15 in girls, but not in boys.[34,35] Exercise, in general, may increase bone mass compared to sedentary subjects.[35]

The main predisposing factors for the development of osteoporosis in athletes are amenorrhea and eating disorders with low calcium uptake, leading to the "female athlete triad," that is, anorexia, amenorrhea, and osteoporosis.[19] Interestingly, girls maturing late who have not primarily developed an appropriate endogenous estrogen synthesis in time, that is, who have primary amenorrhea, may reach a normal bone mineral density for age, whereas a secondary decrease in estradiol due to secondary hypothalamic dysfunction after menstrual cycles had primarily been established may develop osteoporosis (Wolf *et al.*, unpublished data). Girls with eating disorders and amenorrhea are extremely prone to bone demineralization leading to a reduced peak bone mass and a higher risk for stress fractures and scoliosis. There are conflicting data as to whether or not bone density may still reach a normal peak after return of menses.

Additionally, low vitamin D_3 levels have been found in young gymnasts as a result of the indoor exercise and reduced sunlight exposure leading to a low calcium balance. Several authors have reported crash fractures of the lower extremities in athletes due to pathologic demineralization.[29,36]

To prevent overlooking osteoporosis among amenorrheic girls with—perhaps hidden—eating disorders, screening with the use of urinary markers of bone resorption, such as pyridinoline cross-links or cross-linked N-telopeptides, as well as bone densitometry utilizing dual-energy X-ray absorptiometry are highly recommended.

CONCLUSION AND FINAL REMARKS

Delayed puberty and oligomenorrhea in adolescent or adult female athletes seem to result from a complex interplay of physical, nutritional, emotional, and hereditary factors, exerting various impacts upon the hypothalamic regulation of the menstrual cycle at the level of the median eminence and the nucleus arcuatus. Several inhibiting factors seem to interfere with the hypothalamic function, probably depending on their turnover rate. Nevertheless, gonadal dysfunction in adolescent or adult athletes are of hypothalamic origin with an excellent prognosis after cessation of strenuous exercise and with the normalization of eating behavior and caloric uptake. Competitive sports are frequently associated with delayed puberty and oligomenorrhea. Chronic estrogen deficiency, especially when associated with anorexia and amenorrhea, has a long-term impact on bone mineralization, potentially resulting in juvenile osteoporosis.

In the last five years, scandalous reports on "children's sports" have been published. Young girls have spoken out publically about having been hit by their coaches. Romanian gymnasts were tortured with razorblades and nails in order to improve their performance at the stepbar. Deaths of gymnasts due to anorexia have been reported. German radiologists have published alarming numbers of spine deformities in about 80% of the former East German gymnasts. Trainers and coaches have been sentenced to jail for having used criminal training methods. Repulsively, mental and sexual abuse of young athletes show the dark side of today's sports activities. Obviously, there is a widespread problem involving young female athletes being unscrupulously exploited in terms of both commercial profit and media excitement by their coaches and teams, and, last but not least, their ambitious parents or home countries. At the moment, society does not seem to be able to solve the problem. We adolescent gynecologists should be advocates for the sake of children and therefore should propose an international panel to prepare recommendations, or even an obligatory code, for competitive sports among young girls. Otherwise, sports will not stand for "mens sana in corpore sano."

REFERENCES

1. Frisch, R. E. & J. W. McArthur. 1974. Menstrual cycles: Fatness as a determinant of minimum weight for height necessary for their maintenance or onset. Science **185:** 949–951.
2. Frisch, R. E. & R. Revelle. 1971. Height and weight at menarche and a hypothesis of critical body weights and adolescent events. Science **169:** 397–401.
3. Cumming, D. C. & R. W. Rebar. 1984. Lack of consistency in the indirect methods of estimating percent body fat. Fertil. Steril. **5:** 739–742.
4. De Cree, C., M. Ostyn & A. Vermeulen. 1989. Amenorrhea and athletic menstrual irregularities, a state of the art. Geneeskunde en sport (ND) **22:** 2–16.
5. Scott, T. E. C. & F. E. Johnston. 1982. Critical fat, menarche and the maintenance of menstrual cycle. J. Adolsc. Health Care **2:** 249–260.

6. MARX, K. 1996. Sport-Risiko für die endokrine Entwicklung von Adoleszentinnen. *In* Die eßgestörte Athletin. D. Clasing, F. Damm, K. Marx & P. Platen, Eds.: 79–88. Sport und Buch, Strauß-GmbH. Cologne.
7. BAXTER-JONES, A. D. G., P. HELMS, J. BAINES-PREECE & M. PREECE. 1994. Menarche in intensively trained gymnasts, swimmers and tennis players. Ann. Hum. Biol. **5:** 407–415.
8. MALINA, R. M., W. W. SPIRDUSO, C. TATE & A. M. BAYLOR. 1978. Age at menarche and selected menstrual characteristics in athletes at different competitive levels and in different sports. Med. Sci. Sports Exer. **10:** 218–222.
9. WARREN, M. P. 1980. The effects of exercise on pubertal progression and reproductive function in girls. J. Clin. Endocrinol. Metab. **51:** 1150–1157.
10. FRISCH, R. E., A. V. GOTZ-WELLBERGEN, J. W. MCARTHUR, T. ALBRIGHT J. WITSCHI, B. BULLEN, J. BIRNHOLZ, R. B. REED & H. HERMANN. 1981. Delayed menarche and amenorrhea of college athletes in relation to age of onset of training. JAMA **246:** 1559–1563.
11. SPEROFF, L. & D. B. REDWINE. 1980. Exercise and menstrual function. Phys. Sportsmed. **8:** 42–52.
12. FEICHT, C. B., T. S. JOHNSON, B. J. MARTIN, K. E. SPRAKES & W. W. WAGNER, JR. 1978. Secondary amenorrhoea in athletes. Lancet: 1145–1146.
13. BACHMANN, G. A. & E. KEMMANN. 1982. Prevalence of oligomenorrhea and amenorrhea in a college population. Am. J. Obstet. Gynecol. **114:** 98–102.
14. PETTERSON, F., H. FRIES & S. J. NILIUS. 1973. Epidemiology of secondary amenorrhea. Incidence and prevalence rates. Am. J. Obstet. Gynecol. **117:** 80–86.
15. CUMMING, D. C., M. M. VICKORIC, S. R. WALL & M. R. FLUKER. 1985. Defects in pulsatile LH release in normally menstruating runners. J. Clin. Endocrinol. Metab. **60:** 810–812.
16. SCHWARTZ, B., D. C. CUMMING, E. RIORDAN, M. SELYE, S. S. C. YEN & R. W. REBAR. 1981. Exercise-associated amenorrhea: A distinct entity? Am. J. Obstet. Gynecol. **141:** 662–670.
17. PRIOR, J. C. 1982. Endocrine "conditioning" with endurance training. A preliminary review. Can. J. Appl. Sports Sci. **7:** 148–157.
18. BAKER, E. R. 1981. Menstrual dysfunction and hormonal status in athletic women: A review. Fertil. Steril. **36:** 691–696.
19. NATTIV, A., R. AGOSTINI, B. DRINKWATER & K. YEAGER. 1994. The female athlete triad. The inter-relatedness of disordered eating, amenorrhea, and osteoporosis. Clin. Sports Med. **13:** 405–418.
20. YATES, A., K. LEEHEY & C. M. SHISSLAK. 1983. Running—an analogue of anorexia? N. Engl. J. Med. **308:** 251–255.
21. SMITH, N. J. 1980. Excessive weight loss and food aversion in athletes simulating anorexia nervosa. Pediatrics **66:** 139–142.
22. MARSHALL, J. C. & R. P. KELCH. 1979. Low dose pulsatile gonadotropin-releasing hormone in anorexia nervosa: A model of human pubertal development. J. Clin. Endocrinol. Metab. **49:** 712–718.
23. GALLE, P. C., E. W. FREEMAN, M. G. GALLE, G. R. HUGGINS & S. T. SONTHEIMER. 1983. Physiologic and psychologic profiles in a survey of women runners. Fertil. Steril. **39:** 633–639.
24. BOYDEN, T. W., R. W. PAMENTER, P. STANFORTH, T. ROTKISS & J. H. WILMORE. 1983. Sex steroids and endurance running in women. Fertil. Steril. **39:** 629–632.
25. JURKOWSKI, J. E., N. L. JONES, W. C. WALKER, E. V. YOUNGLAI & J. R. SUTTON. 1978. Ovarian hormonal responses to exercise. J. Appl. Physiol. **44:** 109–114.
26. WOLF, A. S., G. KECKSTEIN, K. STERZIK & R. BENZ. 1989. Alteration of episodic LH-release during exercise due to β-endorphin and norepinephrine. *In* Recent Research on Gynelogical Endocrinology. A. R. Genazzani, F. Petraglia, A. Volpe, F. Facchinetti, Eds.: 94–100. The Parthenon Publishing Group. Carnforth.
27. BRISSON, G. R., M. A. VOLLE, D. DECARUFEL, M. DESHARNAIS & M. TANAKA. 1980. Exer-

cise-induced dissociation of the blood prolactin response in young women according to their sports habits. Horm. Res. **12:** 201–205.

28. Shangold, M. M., M. L. Gatz & B. Thysen. 1981. Acute effects of exercise on plasma concentrations of prolactin and testosteron in recreational women runners. Fertil. Steril. **35:** 699–702.
29. Warren, M. P., J. Brooks-Gunn & L. H. Homek. 1986. Scoliosis and fractures in young ballet dancers: Relationship to delayed menarcheal age and secondary amenorrhea. N. Engl. J. Med. **314:** 1348–1353.
30. Shangold, M. M. & H. S. Levine. 1982. The effect of marathon training upon menstrual function. Am. J. Obstet. Gynecol. **143:** 862–869.
31. Veldhuis, J. D., W. S. Evans, L. M. Demers, M. O. Thorner, D. Wakat & A. D. Rogol. 1985. Altered neuroendocrine regulation of gonadotropin secretion in women distance runners. J. Clin. Endocrinol. Metab. **61:** 557–563.
32. Wurster, K. G., M. Zwirner, E. Keller, A. E. Schindler, M. Schrode & H. Heitkamp. 1984. Discipline specific differences in the responses of pituitary, gonadal and arenal hormones to maximal physical exercise in female top athletes. Int. J. Sports Med. **5:** 203–205.
33. Russel, J. B., D. E. Mitchell, P. J. Musey & D. C. Collins. 1984. The role of β-endorphines an catechol estrogens on the hypothalamic–pituitary axis in female athletes. Fertil. Steril. **42:** 690–695.
34. Lindholm, C., K. Hagenfeldt & H. Ringertz. 1995. Bone mineral content of young female former gymnasts. Acta Paediatr. **84:** 1109–1112.
35. Theintz, G., B. Buchs, R. Rizzoli, D. Slosman, H. Clavien, P. C. Sizonenko & J. P. Bonjour. 1992. Longitudinal monitoring of bone mass accumulation in healthy adolescents: evidence for a marked reduction after 16 years of age at the levels of lumbar spine and femoral neck in female subjects. J. Clin. Endocrinol. Metab. **75:** 1060–1065.
36. Drinkwater, B. L., K. Nilson, C. H. I. Chesnut III, *et al.* 1984. Bone mineral content of amenorrheic and eumenorrheic athletes. N. Engl. J. Med. **311:** 277–281.

Etiopathology of Endometriosis

JOHN N. BONTIS[a] AND DIMITRIOS T. VAVILIS

Second Department of Obstetrics and Gynecology
Aristotelian University of Thessaloniki
Hippokration Hospital, Greece

Endometriosis is a common, invasive but non-neoplastic, disease of women during the reproductive period and is defined as the presence of endometrial epithelium and stroma in an ectopic site excluding the myometrium.[1] It is characterized by pelvic pain, dysmenorrhea, and subfertility.

Endometriosis is one of the most enigmatic and mysterious gynecological diseases. Despite all the research performed over the years, there is virtually no agreement concerning any aspect of this disease. The first question asked was about the etiology and pathogenesis of endometriosis. Since Von Rokitansky[2] provided the first detailed description of endometriosis in 1860, many theories of pathogenesis have been proposed. Unfortunately, despite many theories its pathogenesis remains controversial and poorly understood. Because the disorder is primarily a human disease and rare in other animal species, the accumulation of factual information has been difficult and slow.

Three theories of the pathogenesis of endometriosis dominate current thinking. The original theory was that of metaplastic transformation of mesothelial cells lining the pelvic peritoneum forming typical endometrial-like glands and stroma (celomic metapalsia).[3] Metaplastic changes could occur secondary to inflammatory processes or hormonal influences. This view of the pathogenesis of endometriosis had wide support in the early part of the century, and it continues to be popular today.[1] This theory could explain endometriosis in women with Mullerian agenesis, who have an absent uterus or a hypoplastic, nonfunctioning uterus, or the occasional presence of endometriosis in men. There are, however, several problems with this concept. First, if peritoneal cells can easily undergo metaplastic transformation, the disease should be observed more frequently in men. Although there are several case reports of finding histologic endometriosis in men, these occurred in men with prostatic carcinoma undergoing high-dose estrogen treatment.[4] Second, one would anticipate that metaplasia would increase with advancing age. On the contrary, the disease is almost entirely limited to menstruating women. Third, ectopic endometrial implants are not uniformly distributed within the peritoneum. If metaplasia represents the pathophysiologic process for development of the disease, one would have anticipated a fairly uniform distribution on peritoneal surfaces. Finally, endometriosis mainly affects the pelvic organs. Given that the celomic membrane contributes both to the peritoneal cavity and the thoracic cavity, one would anticipate endometriosis would be present in the chest as well.

[a]Address for correspondence: Assoc. Prof. John Bontis, M.D., Ph.D., Obstetrician Gynecologist, 4 Sintrivaniou Square, 54621 Thessaloniki, Greece.

A second theory of pathogenesis is that uterine endometrium is transplanted to ectopic sites. Many mechanisms have been proposed: lymphatic dissemination, hematogenous dissemination, iatrogenic dissemination, and retrograde menstruation. The most widely accepted transportation theory, proposed by Sampson,[5] suggests that viable endometrial cells reflux through the fallopian tubes during menstruation and implant and grow on the surrounding pelvic structures and peritoneum. The reflux implantation theory of Sampson is supported by the presence of viable endometrial cells in the menstrual debris as has been demonstrated in tissue cultures of endometrial cells[6]; by the topographic distribution of lesions in the abdominal cavity[7]; by the demonstration of the presence of endometrial cells in the peritoneal cavity, as has been shown by cytologic evaluation[8]; by epidemiological data suggesting that women who menstruate more frequently, more heavily, or for a longer duration of time, and therefore have increased exposure to retrograde menstruation, have a higher risk of developing the disease[9]; by the high prevalence of endometriosis in women with Mullerian duct anomalies resulting in an obstructed genital outlow tract and thus increased retrograde menstruation[9]; by the immunohistochemical characteristics of retrogradely shed endometrium and by its similarities to *in situ* endometrium[10]; and by animal experiments in which endometriosis was induced by the creation of uteropelvic fistulas. These data suggest that any exposure of the pelvic peritoneum to menstrual reflux would result in an increased risk of endometriosis. This single cause and effect relationship is weakened by the observation that in most women with patent tubes, viable endometrial cells reach the abdominal cavity during menstruation, but only a small number of menstruating women suffer from endometriosis.[11] Whether the sheer volume or the tissue properties of the retrograded menstrual debris determines that endometriosis will develop in some patients and not in others and whether differences in their peritoneal local defense systems contribute to the problem still remain unclear.

Other transport theories include dissemination of endometrial fragments via lymphatics[12] and vascular channels[13] and inadvertent iatrogenic dissemination during abdominal or pelvic surgery.[14] These routes do provide an attractive explanation for extra pelvic endometriosis.

The third theory, proposed for the first time by Levander[15] and known as the induction theory, is a combination of the first two. This theory is based on the assumption that unknown substances released from shed endometrium induce undifferentiated mesenchymatic cells to form endometriotic tissue. Merril implanted filters containing viable endometrial tissue intraperitoneally in the rabbit.[16] This study offers suggestive evidence that substances from endometrium are capable of inducing endometrial metaplasia in mesothelium.

Regardless of which theory of histogenesis is correct, additional factors must be responsible for the expression of the disease. The possibility that the development and progression of endometriosis is associated with abnormal immune function is the most recent hypothesis for the cause of this disease. Over the past 15 years, numerous data have suggested alterations in both cell-mediated and humoral immunity in the most endometriotic patients.

Dmowski proposed in 1981 that deficient cellular immunity or inability to recognize endometriotic tissue may be responsible for the development of endometriosis.[17] In another early study by Weed and Arquembourg, complement deposition was noted surrounding endothelial glands within the uterus in women with endometriosis.[18] The implication is that the explanted endometrial tissue stimulates an immune response that reduces the probability of implantation. Further support of this concept came when Badway and co-workers demonstrated the apparent presence of antibodies to endometrial cell antigen and elevated concentrations of complement components C_{3c} and C_4 in the serum and peritoneal fluid of women with endometriosis.[19] In more recent studies the increased immunoglobulin levels and a high frequency of autoantibodies found in women with this disease indicate polyclonal activation of B cells.[20] These data, together with the fact that other characteristics of autoimmune diseases such as female preponderance, familial occurrence, tissue damage, and multi-organ involvement are also present, support the view that endometriosis is possibly an autoimmune disease.[20]

Alternatively, it is possible that changes in humoral immunity in endometriotic patients are secondary to deficient cellular mechanisms.[20] In healthy women the regurgitated menstrual debris is destroyed by the monocytes, and those retrograde endometrial cells that survive are destroyed by activated macrophages, natural killer cells, and cytotoxic lymphocytes. This peritoneal response prevents the adhesion of viable endometrial cells to the peritoneal lining and their subsequent development into endometriotic lesions. If this defense mechanism fails and/or if the aggression is too voluminous or too strong, viable active endometrial cells will implant and develop into clinical endometriosis. In women with endometriosis a local, sterile inflammation occurs in the peritoneal cavity. Drake and co-workers have reported increased volumes of peritoneal fluid in endometriotic women and have interpreted this as a sign of inflammation.[21] Increased activation of peritoneal macrophages in mild endometriosis has been found.[22] Proteolytic enzymes, interleukins-1 and -2, lysozyme, tumor necrosis factor, and growth factors are among the secretory products of activated macrophages. According to recent studies, the adhesion and outgrowth of viable endometrial cells may be facilitated by some of these secretory products, for example, fibronectin and growth factors.[23] More recently, defective natural killer cell activity has been found in women with endometriosis.[24] Thus, a defect in the peritoneal defense system permits or even facilitates implantation of the retrograde endometrial debris and results in the development of the disease. Whether the immunological factor is a separate cause or an additional synergistic factor still remains to be elucidated. There is, however, little doubt that the immunological process does play an important role in the development and progression of endometriosis.

SUMMARY

Although endometriosis is one of the most frequent problems in gynecology, its pathogenesis remains controversial and poorly understood. Many theories relating to the etiopathology of this disorder have been proposed. The celomic metaplasia hypothesis states that peritoneal mesothelium undergoes metaplasia, forming typical endometrial-like glands and stroma. The transplantation theory suggests implantation and subsequent growth of retrogradely shed, viable endometrial cells. The induction theory states that unknown substances released from shed endometrium induce undifferentiated mesenchyma to form endometriotic tissue. Regardless of which theory is correct, additional factors may be responsible for the expression of the disease. The possibility that the development and progression of endometriosis is associated with abnormal immune function and an inadequate response of the peritoneal defense system is currently the most recent hypothesis for the etiopathology of this disease.

REFERENCES

1. NAKAMURA, M. H., T. KATABUCHI, Y. TOHYA, K. FUKUMATSU, A. MATSUURA & H. OKAMURA. 1993. Scanning electron microscopic and immunohistochemical studies of pelvic endometriosis. Hum. Reprod. **8**(12): 2218–2226.
2. VON ROKITANSKY, C. 1860. Ueber Uterusdrusen—Neubildung in Uterus und Ovarial—Sarcomen. Ztschr. KK Gesellsch. Aerzte Wien **37:** 577–581.
3. MEYER, R. 1903. Ueber eine adenomatose. Wucherung der serosa in einer Banchuabe. Zeit Geburt. Gynak. **49:** 32–38.
4. SCHRODT, G. R., M. D. ALCORN & J. IBANEZ. 1980. Endometriosis of the male uterine system: A case report. J. Urol. **124:** 722–726.
5. SAMPSON, J. A. 1927. Peritoneal endometriosis due to menstrual dissemination of endometrial tissue into the peritoneal cavity. Am. J. Obstet. Gynecol. **14:** 422–469.
6. TE LINDE, R. W. & R. B. SCOTT. 1950. Experimental endometriosis. Am. J. Obstet. Gynecol. **60:** 1147–1173.
7. JENKINS, S., D. L. OLIVER & A. F. HANEY. 1986. Endometriosis: Pathogenetic implications of the anatomic distribution. Obstet. Gynecol. **67:** 335–338.
8. MANNING, J. O. & E. F. SHAVER. 1959. The demonstration of endometrial cells by Papanicolaou and supravital techniques obtained by culdocentesis. Bull. Tulane Univ. Med. Fac. **18:** 193–199.
9. ROCK, J. A. & S. M. MARKHAM. 1992. Pathogenesis of endometriosis. Lancet **340:** 1264–1267.
10. VAN DER LINDEN, P. J. Q., A. F. P. M. DE GOEIJ, G. A. J. DUNSELMAN, E. P. M. VAN DER LINDEN, F. C. S. RAMAEKERS & J. I. H. EVERS. 1994. Expression of integrins and E-cadherin in cells from menstrual effluent, endometrium, peritoneal fluid, peritoneum, and endometriosis. Fertil. Steril. **61:** 85–90.
11. WHEELER, J. M. 1989. Epidemiology of endometriosis associated infertility. J. Reprod. Med. **34:** 41–46.
12. JAVERT, C. T. 1952. The spread of benign and malignant endometrium in the lymphatic system with a note of coexisting vascular involvement. Am. J. Obstet. Gynecol. **64:** 780–788.
13. JAVERT, C. T. 1949. Pathogenesis of endometriosis based on endometrial homeoplasia direct extension, exfoliation and implantation, lymphomatic and hematogenous metastasis. Cancer **2:** 399–406.
14. RIDLEY, J. H. 1968. The histogenesis of endometriosis: A review of facts and fancies. Obstet. Cynecol. Surv. **23:** 1–5.
15. LEVANDER, G. & P. NORMANN. 1955. The pathogenesis of endometriosis. An experimental study. Acta Obstet. Gynecol. Scand. **34:** 366–398.
16. MERRILL, J. A. 1966. Endometrial induction of endometriosis across millipore filters. Am. J. Obstet. Gynecol. **94:** 780–790.
17. DMOWSKI, W. P., R. W. STEELE & G. F. BAKER. 1981. Deficient cellular immunity in endometriosis. Am. J. Obstet. Gynecol. **141:** 377–380.
18. WEED, J. C. & P. C. ARQUEMBOURG. 1980. Endometriosis: Can it produce an autoimmune response resulting in infertility? Clin. Obstet. Gynecol. **23:** 885–892.
19. BADWAY, S. Z. A., V. GUENCA, A. STITZEL, R. D. B. JACOBS & R. H. TOMAR. 1984. Autoimmune phenomena in infertile patients with endometriosis. Obstet. Gynecol. **63:** 271–275.

20. DMOWSKI, W. P., H. M. GEBEL & D. P. BRAUN. 1994. The role of cell-mediated immunity in pathogenesis of endometriosis. Acta Obstet. Gynecol. Scand. **159:** 7–14.

21. DRAKE, T. S., S. A. METZ, G. M. GRUNERT & W. F. O'BRIEN. 1980. Peritoneal fluid volume in endometriosis. Fertil. Steril. **34:** 27–31.

22. HALME, J., M. G. HAMMOND, J. F. HULKA, S. G. RAJ & L. M. TALBERT. 1984. Retrograde menstruation in healthy women and in patients with endometriosis. Obstet. Gynecol. **64:** 151–154.

23. ZHANG, R. H., R. A. WILD, D. MEDDERS & S. R. GUNUPUDI. 1991. Effects of peritoneal macrophages from patients with endometriosis on the proliferation of endometrial carcinoma cell line Ecc-1. Am. J. Obstet. Gynecol. **165:** 1842–1846.

24. OOSTERLYNCK, D. J., C. MEULEMAN, M. WAER, M. VANDEPUTTE & P. R. KONINCKX. 1992. The natural killer activity of peritoneal fluid lymphocytes is decreased in women with endometriosis. Fertil. Steril. **58:** 290–295.

Endometriosis

Laparoscopy—Diagnostic and Therapeutic Approaches

JOSEPH S. SANFILIPPO

Department of Reproductive Endocrinology
University of Louisville School of Medicine
Ambulatory Care Building
550 South Jackson Street
Louisville, Kentucky 40292

INTRODUCTION

Endometriosis is considered to be a disease of women usually in their twenties or thirties, who have postponed childbearing, and not a disorder commonly found in teenagers. This should be of significant concern to the clinician, because endometriosis can affect a young woman's fertility potential. Symptoms of endometriosis must first be differentiated from other causes of pelvic pain such as gastrointestinal problems, genitourinary complaints, and infections of the reproductive tract (TABLE 1). Clinical presentation and treatment of endometriosis is similar for adolescents and older women. Although adolescents are seldom concerned with fertility, however, they should be questioned extensively about associated symptoms and their interest in future fertility. In most cases, treatment for adolescents should be directed toward forestalling the progress of the disease.

INCIDENCE OF ADOLESCENT ENDOMETRIOSIS

Although endometriosis has been a recognized disorder for years, the exact rate of occurrence of endometriosis in adolescents is difficult to establish. However, prevalence of this disorder in young women may not differ greatly from that in older women. Ranney has suggested that between 4% and 17% of all menstruating women have pelvic endometriosis.[3] The incidence, in part, depends on the patient population. In the adolescent age group, Meigs reported a 6% incidence at laparoscopy.[4] In adolescents presenting with chronic pelvic pain, Goldstein *et al.*[5] reported 47% with endometriosis.

Endometriosis is often thought to occur rarely in indigent women and in young black women, but racial differences in the prevalence of the disease are unlikely. Chatman found endometriosis in 21% of black women undergoing laparoscopy for various symptoms. Of those patients with endometriosis, 12.5% were 15 to 19 years of age. Why the incidence appears to be less in the lower socioeconomic class is not thought to be related to disease immunity but rather to malnutrition, poor living conditions, high rates of pelvic inflammatory disease, early marriage, early and frequent childbearing, and inability to obtain medical attention. Adolescents at increased risk

TABLE 1. Causes of Acute and Chronic Abdominal Pain in the Adolescent[a]

Hematometra	Meckel's diverticulum with abscess
Intussusception	Ulcerative colitis
Peritonitis	Constipation
Perforation of a viscus	Urinary tract infection
Urinary calculus	Porphyria
Hematosalpinx	Sickle cell anemia
Pelvic inflammatory disease	Mesenteric lymphadenitis
Imperforate hymen	Hydronephrosis
Vaginal septum	Liver cysts (oral contraceptive related)
Blind pouch of the vagina with hematometra	Bowel obstruction
Ectopic pregnancy	Splenomegaly
Chronic pancreatitis	Neuroblastoma
Regional enteritis	Urachal cysts

[a]Reprinted with permission: Lavery, J. P. & J. S. Sanfilippo, Eds. 1985. Pediatric and Adolescent Obstetrics and Gynecology. Springer Verlag. New York..

for endometriosis are those with genital tract anomalies. TABLE 2 is a review of publications addressing endometriosis in the adolescent.

The exact mechanism of development of endometriosis is not clearly understood. Thus, the current theories of origin apply to adults and to adolescents alike. These theories include (1) Sampson's theory of retrograde menstruation; (2) Meyer's theory of totipotential cells undergoing metaplasia; (3) hematogenous dissemination; and (4) lymphatic spread. No one theory provides a complete answer.

A genetic or familial influence on the occurrence of endometriosis has been demonstrated. A polygeneic multifactorial mode of inheritance for endometriosis has been reported by Simpson *et al.*[27] who found a 6.9% rate of endometriosis in first-degree relatives of women with the disease compared to only 1% in control relatives. Thus, endometriosis should be suspected in symptomatic adolescents who have a family history of the disease.

The major distinction between adolescents and older women in the development of endometriosis is its association with anomalies of the reproductive system. Several anomalies associated with the reproductive tract and development of endometriosis have been reported, including imperforate hymen, vaginal septum, hematocolpos, hematometra, uterine anomalies, and associated urinary tract abnormalities such as renal agenesis. Any obstruction of the outflow tract seems to be associated with the formation of endometriosis. Examples of reproductive tract anomalies that may cause endometriosis are presented in FIGURE 1. In a series reported by Schifrin *et al.*,[8] 6 of 15 endometriosis patients (40%) under age 20 had a genital tract anomaly. Goldstein and coworkers[5] found congenital abnormalities of the reproductive tract in 11% of 74 teenagers with endometriosis.

The clinical course of endometriosis when associated with a reproductive tract abnormality appears to be different from that in which endometriosis is not associated with outflow obstruction. In such cases, when a patent outflow tract is established, reversal of extensive pelvic cavity endometriosis results.

Endometriosis has been reported to be associated with mature ovarian teratomas

TABLE 2. Endometriosis in Adolescents[a]

Meigs[4]	Endometrial cysts in 13- to 19-year-old adolescents.
Goldstein *et al.*[5]	Endometriosis was found in 74 (52%) of 140 adolescents with pelvic pain; 11% had genital anomalies.
Schifrin[8]	Fifteen cases of endometriosis in patients 12 to 20 years old and presenting with epigastric, lower quadrant abdominal pain, or dysmenorrhea. There was an associated increased incidence of GI and GU anomalies.
Fallon[10]	Four percent of teenage females (9 of 225) had endometriosis. Four of the 9 had endometriosis at the time of preoperative diagnosis of acute appendicitis.
Derryberry and Bonney[11]	Endometrioma in a 15-year-old black female with a normal vagina, introitus, and a stenotic cervical isthmus.
Bullock *et al.*[12]	Symptomatic endometriosis in teenagers. Wilford Hall, USAF Medical Center, four cases, 17 to 19 years old.
Hanton *et al.*[13]	Sixty-eight young patients (62 menarche, 5 to 10 years before the diagnosis, and 6 congenital obstruction to menstrual flow) in a 30-year-review of cases at the Mayo Clinic.
Hanton *et al.*[14]	Case report of endometriosis associated with complete or partial obstruction of menstrual egress.
Moore *et al.*[15]	Seven of 127 patients with ovarian masses had endometriosis; age range: birth to 17.
Bruser[16]	Appendectomy with inability to relieve symptoms. Twelve patients, 19 to 31 years old. Subsequently each was found to have endometriosis.
Depp and Pope[17]	Of 233 patients between 10 and 19, 2.3% had endometriosis.
TeLinde[18]	Of 8,789 pelvic laparotomies, 1.2% had microscopically diagnosed endometriosis within 10 years of menarche.
Sutton[19]	Etiological factors in endometriosis—case of reflux
Sutton[20]	menstruation with a bicornuate uterus. Intense distended left horn.
McDonald[21]	Endometriosis associated with didelphic uterus.
King[22]	Metastatic endometriosis in abdominal scars of a 17-year-old female. Pain and tenderness with right lower quadrant abdominal pain noted with a preoperative diagnosis of acute appendicitis.
Mittal *et al.*[23]	Endometriosis of the appendix, presenting as acute appendicitis. Patients were 14 to 62 years old. Forty percent (20 of 50) incidence of GI tract involvement with endometriosis.
Chatman and Ward[24]	Endometriosis was found in 65% of 43 black teenagers.

[a]Reprinted with permission: Wilson, E. A., Ed. 1987. Endometriosis. Alan R. Liss, Inc. New York.

and gliomatosis peritonei in a 10-year-old patient. Endometriosis also has been associated with "smooth muscle metaplasia," hemangiomas, and leiomyomas and adenomyosis of the gastrointestinal tract in adolescent girls. In addition, metastatic endometriosis in abdominal scars has been reported. The endometriosis associated with these disorders is likely to be incidental and not specifically related to the disorder.

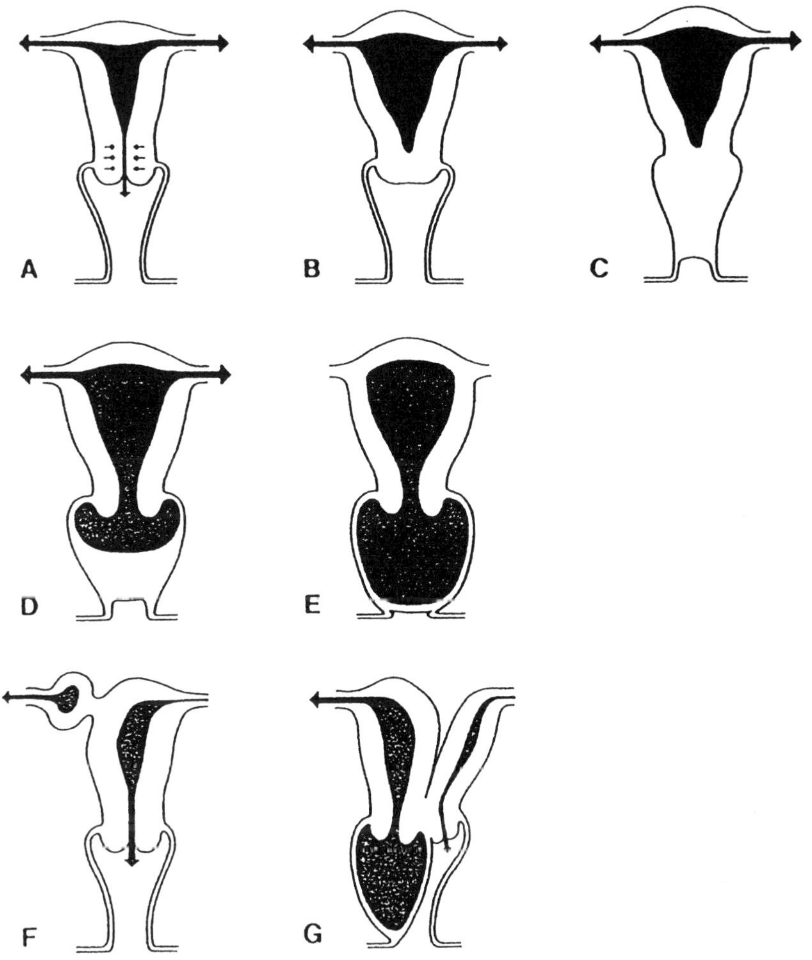

FIGURE 1. Endometriosis in adolescents. Anomalies of the reproductive tract that could result in adolescent endometriosis. **(A)** Cervical stenosis, **(B)** cervical agenesis, **(C)** vaginal agenesis, **(D)** transverse vaginal septum, **(E)** imperforate hymen, **(F)** rudimentary uterine horn, and **(G)** unilateral vaginal obstruction.

CLINICAL PRESENTATION

The characteristic symptoms associated with endometriosis are pelvic pain and infertility. Since fertility is usually not a concern, adolescents usually complain of chronic pelvic pain or dysmenorrhea. In a study of teenagers with documented endometriosis, Chatman and Ward found that the most common complaint was dysmenorrhea in 78% of patients, followed by abnormal bleeding in 35%, bowel symptoms in 37%, and dyspareunia in 14%.[24] Similar presenting symptoms were reported by Goldstein *et al.*[5] in 66 adolescent girls with endometriosis (see Table 3). The dysmenorrhea is usually acquired and increases in severity with age.

The typical presentation is that of dysmenorrhea refractory to nonsteroidal antiinflammatory agents and, in some cases, oral contraceptive therapy. However, although some relief can be obtained with these agents initially, it is usually not long-lasting. Furthermore, endometriosis may cause further ovarian dysfunction and abnormal bleeding. Bowel symptoms include rectal pressure, pain on defecation, and urgency, especially during the late luteal and menstrual phases. The high percentage of young patients with bowel symptoms (21–37%) is somewhat surprising, but it emphasizes how endometriosis can progress symptomatically even in adolescents. Dyspareunia is another common form of pelvic pain associated with endometriosis that teenagers may also begin to experience but may be reluctant to report. The dyspareunia is likely related to the presence of tender endometriosis implants in the cul-de-sac.

Preoperative pelvic findings in teenagers with endometriosis are similar to those found in older patients. Chatman and Ward found that tenderness in the cul-de-sac could be elicited in 78% of adolescents with documented endometriosis, and nodularity with tenderness in 36%.[24] Adnexal masses were present in 11% of teenagers. When Goldstein *et al.*[5] evaluated adolescents with endometriosis, 76% were noted to have pelvic tenderness, 22% cul-de-sac nodularity, and 27% a distinct adnexal mass. Eleven percent of patients had a fixed, retroverted uterus.

Often the pelvic examination is normal even in patients with endometriosis. In the series by Goldstein and coworkers, 17% of young women had a normal examination.[5] These authors emphasized that the examination should be performed during menses or the late luteal phase in order to enhance the pelvic findings.

DIAGNOSIS

A diagnosis of endometriosis is common in adolescents who are experiencing pain. A careful history of symptoms characteristic of endometriosis is helpful in di-

TABLE 3. Presenting Symptoms in 66 Adolescents with Endometriosis[a]

Symptom	No.	Patients (%)
Pain	66	100
Cyclic	42	64
Acyclic	24	36
Abnormal Bleeding	18	28
Dyspareunia	17	25
Gastrointestinal symptoms	14	21

[a]Reprinted by permission of Elsevier Science Publishing Co., Inc., from Goldstein, D., *et al.*: 1980. Adolescent endometriosis. J. Adolesc. Health Care **1:** 37.

agnosing this disorder as well as distinguishing it from other causes of pelvic pain (TABLE 1).

Pelvic examination in an adolescent may be difficult, and rectal examination may be the only means to evaluate the pelvis for tenderness, nodularity, retrodisplaced uterus, or adnexal masses. Anomalies of the hymen, vagina, and cervix can be detected during pelvic examination; and a search should be made for these and other congenital abnormalities that are more likely to cause adolescent endometriosis. Conscious sedation or even general anesthesia may be required for adequate evaluation of the pelvis.

Ultrasonography may be helpful, particularly in adolescents difficult to examine, or when documenting the presence or size of adnexal masses. Ultrasonography can also be used to monitor the size of ovarian cysts in response to therapy. However, endometriosis cannot be distinguished from other pelvic masses by ultrasound, and a persistent mass requires surgical evaluation.

Preoperative evaluation of patients presenting with chronic pelvic pain should also include a complete blood count, urine analysis, cervical cytology, and sedimentation rate. Cervical and urethral cultures, including those for chlamydia, can be performed to identify those patients with acute or chronic inflammatory processes.

Laparoscopy (diagnostic and/or operative) is an integral part of the assessment of pelvic pain and diagnosis of endometriosis in adolescent patients. As stated above, in 140 patients between the ages of 10.5 and 19 presenting with chronic pain, Goldstein and associates confirmed endometriosis in 52%.[5] Early endometriosis usually does not appear as the characteristic "blue-black" lesions. Hemorrhagic areas have been noted by Goldstein *et al.* to be "biopsy-proven" endometriosis. Furthermore, 20% of biopsied lesions were not grossly typical of endometriosis. Consequently, the clinician must be aware that early endometriosis may present with a hemorrhagic or petechial appearance.

When endometriosis is evidenced at laparoscopy, the American Society for Reproductive Medicine (formerly The American Fertility Society) Revised Classification should be utilized, not only to determine the extent of disease but also to aid in the choice of therapy. Using the Acosta classification, Chatman and Ward reported that in their series of patients, 50% had mild disease, 39% had moderate disease, and 11% had severe disease.[24] A similar distribution was seen by Goldstein *et al.*[5] At present, there is no clear correlation between age and severity of disease. Endometriosis in the adolescent is more likely to be severe when it is associated with outflow obstruction. In the author's experience, although early diagnosis in the adolescent is recommended, aggressive treatment unfortunately does not change the course of the disease in adulthood.

TREATMENT

For an adolescent who has no immediate interest in fertility, treatment centers primarily on control of pain. When pelvic pain is encountered in an adolescent, nonsteroidal antiinflammatory agents should be prescribed with the initial onset of pain or before anticipated pain and continued on a regular basis until the pain has completely subsided. All antiprostaglandins basically inhibit prostaglandin synthesis and/or inhibit prostaglandin binding to its receptors to alleviate dysmenorrhea. For the adolescent with cyclical pelvic pain who does not respond to nonsteroidal antiprostaglandins, the next step is to suppress ovulation with an oral contraceptive. A high-progestin, low-estrogen (35–50 μg) preparation should be prescribed in the usual cyclical manner. Failure of these primary measures to alleviate symptoms indicates a need for further evaluation.

Diagnosis of endometriosis primarily involves operative assessment of the pelvic organs. Endometriosis is often an unexpected surgical finding in an adolescent, and there are usually questions regarding intraoperative and postoperative management. Before scheduling any surgical intervention, the physician should counsel the patient and parent (guardian) about the possible need for intraoperative therapeutic alternatives such as laparoscopic fulguration or laser vaporization of the endometrial foci. Improvement in symptoms is greater when fulguration of implants and lysis of adhesions is performed during laparoscopy than when laparoscopy is performed for diagnosis alone. Rarely, conservative surgery (laparotomy) may be necessary at the same operative setting. Persistent endometriomas should be excised, leaving as much functional ovarian tissue as possible. If a laparotomy is performed, uterine suspension and approximation of the uterosacral ligaments should be considered, particularly when endometriosis is present in the cul-de-sac or partial obliteration of the cul-de-sac has occurred. At this setting, presacral neurectomy may also be considered, especially if pelvic pain is severe. Hemostasis and care with handling of tissues is of primary importance in the prevention of subsequent adhesion formation.

The patient should be carefully evaluated for congenital anomalies of the reproductive tract that may obstruct menstrual outflow. The cervix should be probed and/or dilated to assure patency of the cervical canal and to alleviate any element of stenosis. It is important for the clinician to correct obstruction and retrograde menstruation promptly in order to prevent or reverse endometriosis. Vaginal splinting or continued dilations may be required to maintain a patent outflow tract. If these initial measures are unsuccessful, removal of the involved müllerian structures should be considered. A didelphic or rudimentary uterus with unilateral obstruction also can be surgically corrected by lateral anastomosis of the obstructed horn to the unobstructed horn.

Postoperative management of the adolescent patient with endometriosis is a unique challenge. In addition to pain control, the major concern is the preservation of subsequent fertility. Patients interested in fertility usually would be advised to attempt pregnancy as soon as possible. For most teenagers, however, pregnancy in the immediate postoperative period is not an alternative. In these young women, the issue is how to preserve fertility by preventing further progression of the endometriosis. No well-designed studies have been conducted on the treatment of endometriosis in adolescents. The postoperative management of these patients is based on our knowledge of endometriosis, which is inadequate; use of medical therapy, some actions of which are theoretical; and clinical experience, which is anecdotal.

Following laparoscopic or conservative surgery, some form of medical therapy usually is advised to prevent progression of the disease and preserve childbearing function. Not all of these patients will have difficulty achieving pregnancy, but the clinical presumption is that most patients do. In any event, the types of medical therapy for adolescents are the same as for all patients with endometriosis.

The choice of medication and dosage regimen may differ when childbearing is to be delayed for several years. For example, danazol is frequently used for 3 to 6 months, but prolonged administration is not advised because it is reported to have adverse effects on steroid enzymatic pathways and plasma lipids, liver function, and thyroid function. Methyltestosterone may cause masculinization. Even GnRH agonists may cause osteoporosis or other side effects of estrogen depletion when administered for prolonged periods.

Most clinicians use one of the following postoperative medical regimens: (1) danazol, 400–800 mg daily for 3 to 6 months with no subsequent therapy; (2) progestin-dominant oral contraceptive therapy continuously for 6 to 9 months; (3) medroxyprogesterone acetate 20–30 mg daily for 6 to 9 months; (4) cyclic progestin-dominant oral contraceptives administered indefinitely until childbearing is desired; (5) danazol for 3 to 6 months followed by cyclic oral contraceptive therapy; and (6) depo-medroxyprogesterone acetate (Depo-Provera®, the UpJohn Company), 100 mg i.m. monthly.

Theoretically, progestin-dominant oral contraceptives (e.g., LoOvral containing ethinyl estradiol and norgestrel) prevent progression of endometriosis by suppressing endometrial growth and reducing the amount of menstrual reflux, but the therapeutic value of contraceptive steroids given cyclically has never been substantiated. However, their theoretical efficacy and relative safety provide impetus for their long-term use in these patients. Finally, medroxyprogesterone acetate in depo form may be the best alternative for adolescents who wish to delay childbearing. Goldstein *et al.* reported that when compared with danazol and continuous use of oral progestins, depo-medroxyprogesterone acetate was the most effective from the point of view of side effects and overall symptomatic improvement. Usually, this medication is not used because of significant delays in return of ovarian function (7–9 months) and fertility (approximately 13 months), but it may be appropriate for adolescents in whom delayed childbearing is desired.

Conservative surgery during or following postoperative medical therapy should be performed only for persistent pain associated with endometriosis, subsequent infertility, or endometriosis compromising other organ systems. The symptomatic results of conservative surgery are favorable and may exceed those of operative laparoscopy and medical therapy.

COMMENTS

Evaluation of pelvic pain in the adolescent requires a systematic approach. The patient with recurrent lower abdominal pain in a cyclical pattern who has a normal pelvic examination is best treated initially with nonsteroidal antiinflammatory agents, next by oral contraceptive therapy. If these measures fail to alleviate the symptoms, consideration should be given to diagnostic laparoscopy with intraoperative resection of the foci of endometriosis via either bipolar coagulation or laser vaporization. Depending on postoperative symptoms and reevaluation, ovulation suppression with any of several medical treatments is in order.

REFERENCES

1. EBERS, G. 1937. The papyrus ebers-1. Chap. 97, p. 112 Leipzig 1973; E. Bell, B. Lewin & E. Munksgaard, trans. Jnar Munksgaard. Copenhagen.
2. VON ROKITANSKY. 1960. Ueber Uterudausen-Newbildung in Uterus and Ovarial sarcomen. Ztschr. d.k.k. Gesell Schd. Aertte zu Wien **37:** 577.
3. RANNEY, B. 1980. Etiology, prevention, and inhibition of endometriosis. Clin. Obstet. Gynecol. **23:** 875.
4. MEIGS, J. 1948. Endometriosis. Ann. Surg. **127:** 795.
5. GOLDSTEIN, D., C. DECHOLNOKY & S. J. EMANS. 1980. Adolescent endometriosis. J. Adolesc. Health Care **1:** 37.
6. CHATMAN, D. 1976. Endometriosis in the black woman. Am. J. Obstet. Gynecol. **125:** 987.
7. HOUSTON, D. 1984. Evidence for the risk of pelvic endometriosis by age, race and economic status. Epidemiol. Rev. **6:** 167.
8. SCHIFRIN, B. 1973. Teen-age endometriosis. Am. J. Obstet. Gynecol. **116:** 973.
9. SANFILIPPO, J., N. WAKIM, K. SCHIKLER & M. YUSSMAN. 1986. Endometriosis in association with a uterine anomaly. Am. J. Obstet. Gynecol. **154:** 39.
10. FALLON, J. 1946. Endometriosis in youth. JAMA **131:** 1405.
11. DERRYBERRY, W. & W. BONNEY. 1968. Pelvic endometriosis in a 15-year-old. Obstet. Gynecol. **27:** 558.
12. BULLOCK, J., F. MASSEY & R. GAMBRELL. 1967. Symptomatic endometriosis in teenagers: A reappraisal. Obstet. Gynecol. **43:** 896.
13. HANTON, E., G. MALKASIAN, M. DOCKERTY, *et al.* 1967. Endometriosis in young women. Am. J. Obstet. Gynecol. **98:** 116.
14. HANTON, E., G. MALKASIAN, M. DOCKERTY, *et al.* 1966. Case report: Endometriosis associated with complete or partial obstruction of menstrual egress. Obstet. Gynecol. **28:** 626.
15. MOORE, J., B. SHIFRIN & S. EREZ. 1967. Ovarian tumors in infancy, childhood, and adolescence. Am. J. Obstet. Gynecol. **99:** 913.
16. BRUSER, N. 1955. The common occurrence of endometriosis in young women. Can. Med. Assoc. J. **72:** 190.
17. DEPP, O. & D. POPE. 1956. Early conservative surgery in endometriosis. South. Med. J. **49:** 1345.
18. TELINDE, R. 1961. Endometriosis. Clin. Obstet. Gynecol. **4:** 788.
19. SUTTON, L. 1941. The clinical features of endometriosis. N.Y. J. Med. **41:** 1343.
20. SUTTON, L. 1970. Etiologic factors in endometriosis with report of a case with reflux menstruation. N.C. Med. J. **31:** 45.
21. MCDONALD, R. 1943. Uterus didelphys with endometriosis. Am. J. Obstet. Gynecol. **45:** 1038.
22. KING, W. 1979. Metastatic endometriosis and abdominal scars. Can. J. Surg. **22:** 579.
23. MITTAL, G., T. CHOUDHURY & J. CORTEZ. 1981. Endometriosis of the appendix presenting as acute appendicitis. Am. J. Surg. **142:** 519.
24. CHATMAN, D. & A. WARD. 1982. Endometriosis in adolescents. J. Reprod. Med. **27:** 156.
25. WHITEHOUSE, H. 1925. Endometrioma invading the bladder removed from a patient who had never menstruated. Proc. R. Soc. Med. **19** (Obstet. Gynecol. Sec.): 15.
26. SEITZ, L. 1980. Uber genese, klinik und therapie der endometriosis (hetertopein der uterusschleimhaut). Arch. Gynaecol. **137:** 327.
27. SIMPSON, J., S. ELIAS, L. MALINAK & V. BUTTRAM. 1980. Heritable aspects of endometriosis. 1. Genetic studies. Am. J. Obstet. Gynecol. **137:** 327.
28. BASSLER, R., CH. THEELE & H. LABACH. 1982. Nodular and tumorlike gliomatosis peritonei with endometriosis caused by a mature ovarian teratoma. Pathol. Res. Pract. **175:** 392.

29. PUEBLITZ-PEREDO, S., E. LUEVANO-FLORES & R. RINCON-TARACENA. 1985. Uteruslike mass of the ovary: endometriosis or congenital malformation. Arch. Pathol. Lab. Med. **109:** 361.
30. ACOSTA, A., A. KAPLAN & R. KAUFMAN. 1972. Gynecologic cancer in children. Am. J. Obstet. Gynecol. **112:** 944.
31. BUSH, W., D. HALL & B. WARD. 1974. Adenomyosis of the gastric antrum in children. Pediatr. Radiol. **111:** 179.
32. HUFFMAN, J. 1981. Endometriosis in young teen-age girls. Pediatr. Ann. **10:** 44.
33. JONES, H. 1981. Reproductive impairment and the malformed uterus. Fertil. Steril. **36:** 137.
34. BARBIERI, R., J. CANICK, A. MAKRIS, R. TODD, I. DAVIES & K. RYAN. 1977. Danazol inhibits steroidogenesis. Fertil. Steril. **28:** 809.
35. LUCIANO, A., K. HAUSER, F. CHAPLER & R. WALLACE. 1983. Effects of danazol on plasma lipid and lipoprotein levels in healthy women and in women with endometriosis. Am. J. Obstet. Gynecol. **145:** 422.
36. BETZ, G., J. MILLER & D. HALES. 1981. Actions of danazol in vivo on cytochrome P-450 and steroidogenic enzymes in rat testis and liver microsomal preparations. Am. J. Obstet. Gynecol. **14:** 962.
37. SHAW, R. 1984. Female pseudohermaprhroditism associated with danazol exposure in utero case report. Br. J. Obstet. Gynecol. **91:** 386.
38. THURELL, J. & J. DYMLING. 1979. Effect of danazol on thyroid function in women. Postgrad. Med. J. **55**(Suppl 5): 33.
39. BUTTRAM, U., JR. 1979. Cyclic use of combination oral contraceptives and the severity of endometriosis. Fertil. Steril. **31:** 347.
40. CRAMER, D., E. WILSON, R. STILLMAN, M. BERGER, S. BELISLE, I. SCHIFF, B. ALBRECHT, M. GIBSON, B. STADEL & S. SCHOENBAUM. Association of endometriosis with oral contraceptive use. Presented at the American Fertility Society, Abstract 328, Toronto, 1986.
41. ORTIZ, A., M. HIROI, F. STANCZYK, U. GOEBELSMAN & D. MISHELL. 1977. Serum medroxyprogesterone acetate (MPA) concentrations and ovarian function following intramuscular injection of depo-MPA. J. Clin. Endocrinol. Metab. **44:** 32.

Modern Approach to Endometriosis

V. A. TZINGOUNIS AND E. CARDAMAKIS

Department of Obstetrics and Gynecology
University of Patras
Rion-Patron Street
265 00 Patras, Greece

MODERN DIAGNOSTIC APPROACH

Endometriosis is very common during the reproductive years. All investigators who are involved in the research of endometriosis recognize that it is still an enigmatic disease, and most of them agree that the diagnosis of endometriosis is frequently inaccurate. There are no reliable criteria for endometriosis and even the diagnosis by laparoscopy is unreliable. Although published data strongly suggest that during laparoscopy the accuracy of diagnosis improves with increasing experience of the surgeon, even the most experienced surgeon cannot visually identify microscopic disease, which probably represents the bulk of all present endometriosis; on the other hand, gross pathology does not confirm the diagnosis.

Global and Greek Issues of Endometriosis

Endometriosis, which is found in 10–15% of the women of reproductive age, is thought to be responsible for a high percentage (30–40%) of infertility.[1]

From 1980 to 1994, we performed laparoscopies in 1805 women (age 16–56 years, median 36 years) for primary or secondary sterility and acute or chronic pelvic pain. Of these, 1480 (81.99%) were diagnostic and 325 (18.01%) were operative. Findings were normal in 384 women (21.3%) and revealed pathology in 1421 (78.7%). The most frequent findings were adhesions (496, 27.5%) and endometriosis (244, 13.5%).[2]

Although the revised American Fertility Society classification system[3] has been a useful tool for many years of research into endometriosis, our present knowledge of the disease has shown the deficiency of the system.[4] In addition to the classic black or "powder burn" lesions of endometriosis, the disease may have a wide range of visual presentations,[5] including a white, opacified peritoneum, glandular excrescence on peritoneal surfaces, red flame-like lesions that are often raised above the peritoneal surface, otherwise unexplained adherence of the under surface of the ovary to the peritoneum of the ovarian fossa, peritoneal pockets or windows, and clear vesicles or yellow-brown patches of peritoneum. It has been postulated that any peritoneum that appears abnormal should be suspected of harboring endometriosis, and biopsies should be performed liberally in order to establish the diagnosis.[6]

Symptoms and Diagnosis: Ovarian Endometrioma and Subfertility

Sampson was unable to find a relationship between the extent of disease and severity of pain and compared this with the lack of correlation for adhesions in general.[7] Many subsequent studies have shown no correlation between symptoms such as pain, dysmenorrhea, and dyspareunia and the stage of endometriosis.[8–11] Others have suggested a similar lack of correlation between symptoms and absence or presence of various pathologic findings.[10,12–14]

The symptoms that endometriosis produces merge with those normally experienced during ovulatory menstrual cycles and include: (1) dysmenorrhea that increases rather than decreases with age, (2) acquired dyspareunia, (3) premenstrual spotting, and (4) infertility.

Premenstrual spotting, when it is present (about 50% of patients), has the greatest predictive power (over 80%). The differential diagnosis includes other putative abnormal pelvic sources of cytokines and prostaglandins as well as lesions of the endometrium that promote local endometrial instability. Empirical studies show that there is a significant (though loose) association between the degree of endometriosis and the duration of premenstrual spotting.

A large volume of epidemiological data supports the relationship between endometriosis and infertility. Mechanical reasons can explain infertility in mild and severe endometriosis when the disease involves the ovaries and causes adhesions that disturb or block the release or pick-up of the eggs from the ovaries. Such a condition is found in the presence of ovarian endometriomata, tuboovarian and peritubular adhesions, or obliterations of the ovarian fossa. On the other hand, in the minimal and mild forms of endometriosis there is no satisfactory answer to the question of how endometriosis causes sterility.

Recently, the CA-125 antigen of a membrane glycoprotein of the serous epithelium used as a marker to detect ovarian cancer has been found to be increased in the plasma of women with active endometriosis.[15]

Is cancer antigen CA-125 a useful tool in monitoring therapy and predicting recurrence of the endometriosis? We believe that CA-125 levels can predict active endometriosis in patients with advanced disease but cannot predict adhesions; these levels can also be useful in monitoring therapy and long-term follow-up in patients with advanced disease.

A preoperative evaluation of serum CA-125 levels must be made before endoscopic surgery in all women, especially in cases of large or multilocular endometriomas.

Abnormal Autoimmunity and Endometriosis

Much evidence suggests that endometriosis is associated with changes in the immune system. Startseva[16] was the first to report a change in the immune response in women with endometriosis and adenomyosis, with observation of increased B-cell and reduced T-cell activity, as well as changes in immunoglobulins.

Using immunofluorescence, immunodiffusion, and hemagglutination techniques, IgG and IgA autoantibodies to ovarian and endometrial tissue were identified in serum, cervical, and vaginal secretions in patients with endometriosis. When compared with fertile controls, although both have autoantibodies against some endometrial antigens, specific autoantibodies directed against antigens of 26 and 94 kDa were found in sera, peritoneal fluid, and endometrial tissue of patients with endometriosis. Also detected in patients with endometriosis are autoantibodies against subcellular elements or chemical substances integral to cell structure.[17] Gleicher *et al.*[18] noted that among 31 patients, 65% had IgG and 45% had IgM antibodies to at least 16 antigens tested, including phosphatidyl serine, histones, and nucleotides.

The peritoneal environment of women with endometriosis contains elevated levels of activated macrophages compared with fertile controls.[19,20] The presence of activated macrophages in the peritoneal cavity has been suggested to contribute to the cause and pathophysiologic mechanisms of endometriosis. Sharpe-Timms *et al.*[21] have demonstrated that granulocyte-macrophage colony-stimulating factor (GM-CSF) is localized in human endometrial and endometriotic epithelial cells. Thus, endometrial and endometriotic GM-CSF may play a role in macrophage chemotaxis, proliferation, and activation.

In contrast to other investigators, we do not believe that endometriosis is associated with a single immunological defect such as, for example, abnormal NK cell activity or abnormal peritoneal macrophage activation. Instead, we see endometriosis as only the visible tip of a much broader immunological abnormality that affects women and is characterized by decreased fecundity and increased pregnancy wastage. Because immunological abnormalities are basically identical in women with endometriosis and those with unexplained infertility, we believe that these two conditions may be largely identical in etiology and pathophysiology or reproductive failure. Moreover, considerable evidence suggests that this immunologically mediated condition is genetic in origin and may be the consequence of one or more endometriosis gene(s). Endometriosis could then, in its more severe expression, represent the homozygous occurrence of such endometriosis gene(s), whereas unexplained infertility may reflect a heterozygous expression.

The genetic aspects of endometriosis remain an interesting question. Simpson *et al.*[22] postulated a polygenic/multifactorial pattern of inheritance with a 69% concurrence in first-degree relatives. Sanfilippo *et al.*[23] reported three cases of endometriosis and a uterine anomaly, and they recommended consideration of endometriosis and/or a reproductive tract abnormality in the adolescent with persistent pelvic pain. Endometriosis may be present, especially in cases of hematometra and hematosalpinx.[24] In a series published by Creatsas *et al.*,[25] all cases with endometriosis (4/22) were associated with hematocolpos and hematometra.

No case report of primary hypogonadism and endometriosis has been published. Here, we present the case of a 33-year-old patient with primary amenorrhea and atypical endometriosis. During laparoscopy the uterus appeared hypoplastic; tubes with cystic changes and the ovaries were ribbon-like. Biopsy of the ovaries revealed cortical ovarian tissue without follicles. Near the broad ligament and under the ovarian fossa there was a focus of peritoneal endometriosis of the white opacification type. Biopsy revealed endometrial glands and stroma. Interestingly, when we examined her sister, we found that she also had primary hypogonadism and atypical endometriosis. We believe that these cases are of exceptional interest and will contribute to the discussion about the pathogenesis of endometriosis.

MODERN THERAPEUTIC APPROACH

The options for treatment include no treatment, medical treatment, and surgical treatment by laparoscopy or laparotomy. It has been difficult to determine the optimal treatment because prospective, randomized trials have rarely been performed. An array of studies have addressed these alternative treatments of endometriosis.[26–47] Many reports have significant limitations because they are retrospective or lack controls. Even prospective studies done with controls have limitations because of differences among the treatment groups, but they represent the best studies to date with respect to surgical treatment for endometriosis.

GnRH Analogues and Danazol in the Treatment of Endometriosis: Treatment of Atypical Endometriosis

During the last two decades, drugs such as danazol, gestrinone, and GnRH agonists[49,50] have been introduced as a therapeutic approach to endometriosis. Large, retrospective studies of the efficacy of danazol have reported crude pregnancy rates of 28% to 47%. Monthly fecundity rates (when reported) have ranged from 4% to 6%.[51–53] Pregnancy rates reported after treatment with GnRH agonists ranged from 24% to 62%.[54–56] The epidemiologic work of Vessey *et al.*[57] has revealed that by one year, approximately 82% of a normal female population will conceive; this translates into a monthly fecundity figure of approximately 12% among women who are not known to be infertile. Several studies of endometriosis-associated infertility have included a nontreatment, expectant-management arm; and monthly fecundity rates have ranges from approximately 2% to >10%.[58–61] These figures should be kept in mind when treating women with infertility caused by endometriosis.

In a study conducted in the University of Patras,[62] we analyzed the results of three pharmacological treatments, danazol, danazol plus clomiphene citrate, and triptorelin, administered to infertile women with endometriosis compared to a control group of women who did not receive any kind of treatment; moreover, we tried to assess the impact of atypical endometriosis on fertility as well as the effect of treatments in atypical endometriosis. A true comparison of the efficacy of these therapies in the treatment of endometriosis-associated infertility would have to ensure that the severity of disease is similar among treatment groups, the women are of similar ages, and the duration of infertility is comparable in all treatment groups.

Using these criteria, the overall crude pregnancy rate was 47.38% in the treatment groups and 20.93% in the expectant management group. Moreover, among the patients who received triptorelin, the pregnancy rate was 66.66%, and among those who received danazol plus clomiphene citrate the pregnancy rate was 41.33%. These rates are not statistically significantly different, but comparing the monthly fecundity rate (MFR) showed a higher rate with triptorelin than with danazol and clomiphene citrate (0.11 vs. 0.06, $p = 0.041$).

The question of whether or not to treat atypical endometriosis has to be clarified. In infertile patients, long-term medical therapy is inadvisable, because prospective placebo-controlled randomized studies have failed to show a beneficial effect on pregnancy rates. It is interesting to note, however, that pregnancy following medical treatment is most likely to occur within the first months after treatment, as was observed in our study using triptorelin and danazol plus clomiphene citrate groups; thus, a medical approach may yet have a role to play.

Interferon α-2a in the Treatment of Endometriosis

It has recently been observed that the increase in pelvic endometriosis correlates with an increase of factors that inhibit the immune system (such as smoking, alcohol abuse, psychological and professional stress). As a result of these considerations, we have treated endometriotic pelvic disease with an association of GnRH analogues and interferon α-2a (IFNα-2a). We have treated 30 patients, and our preliminary results indicate an increased pregnancy rate and a higher monthly fecundity rate in the group that received combined therapy compared with the group that received triptorelin alone or danazol alone.

Possible explanations for these encouraging preliminary results could include the following:

1. Interferon administration significantly increases plasma growth hormone (GH) and, consequently, insulin growth factor-I (IGF-I), resulting in amplification of gonadotropic action, specifically an increase of FSH effect on the granulosa cells and on signaling cascades in LH and hCG receptors.[63]
2. After IFNα treatment, estrogen (ER) and progesterone receptor (PR) levels were significantly increased in endometrial cells, with a simultaneous reduction of epidermal growth factor receptor (EGF-R) content (EGF is increased in women with polycystic ovaries).[64]
3. The human placenta has been demonstrated to be a site of IFNα production[65]; moreover, this cytokine has been shown to exert a protective effect on target cells from killing by NK cells (mechanism of abortion). Trophoblast cells are protected by IFNα from decidual LAK cells.[66]

Rationale for Surgery

The leading board members of the Third World Congress on Endometriosis were asked to evaluate the rationale for surgery in case of endometriosis and to find five major indications for surgery. Of the seven members of the Board, three concluded that peritoneal endometriosis should be treated surgically and two more agreed in the case of infertility. All seven Board members considered surgery appropriate in case of endometriotic cysts and peritoneal endometriotic adhesions related to infertility.[67] In conclusion, the major indications for surgery in endometriosis are:

1. Ovarian cysts, adhesions, and rectovaginal endometriosis are absolute indications;
2. Peritoneal endometriosis (mild or minimal) is considered by approximately half of the experts to be an indication;

3. Ureteral and/or digestive endometriosis are indications, if a ureteral or intestinal occlusion with deep wall involvement is diagnosed.

In our department a combination of medical and endoscopic surgical therapy has been proposed for the management of endometriosis. Presurgical treatment for 3 months with GnRH agonist has the following advantages:

1. Reduction of pelvic vascularity and inflammation,
2. Reduction in size and activity of endometriotic implants,
3. Reduction in ovarian cyst diameter,
4. A thinner cyst wall,
5. Absence of follicles or corpus luteum.

Hormone Replacement Therapy and Endometriosis

Several studies have documented a fall in bone mineral density in women with endometriosis treated with GnRH agonists.[68–75] For example, Johansen *et al.*[76] showed that after 6 months of therapy with nafarelin, vertebral mineral density declined by 6% and radial density fell by 2% (proximal radial) to 4% (distal radial). By 6 months after discontinuation of therapy, bone density had returned to levels not statistically different from baseline at all skeletal sites, suggesting that the decline in bone density was transient. Because of the risk of trabecular bone loss, treatment periods of longer than 6 months are not recommended at present. However, concurrent low-dose hormonal supplementation or other bone-sparing therapies may allow more extended treatment in the future.

CONCLUSIONS

1. Women with unexplained infertility should have studies of immune function to rule out subclinical forms of endometriosis.
2. Evaluation of infertility in women with endometriosis should include an assessment for presence of autoantibodies.
3. Efforts should be made to measure cytokine concentrations in the circulation of women, to test the potential utility of these as noninvasive markers of endometriosis.
4. Tissue studies have led to the conclusion that there is no uniform appearance that is always identifiable as endometriosis and no appearance that definitively rules out endometriosis.
5. Because staging of the disease by anatomic means does not correlate with any of the clinically important characteristics of endometriosis, it may be time to search for a functional classification of the disease; in this regard, autoimmune parameters present themselves as a promising first step.
6. A detection of the endometriosis gene(s) would allow for an accurate diagnosis of endometriosis (and of so-called unexplained infertility). The case re-

port of primary hypogonadism and atypical endometriosis enhance the gene theory.

7. Danazol followed by induction of ovulation with clomiphene citrate and triptorelin are equally effective in the treatment of endometriosis-related infertility.
8. Atypical endometriosis is distinct from active, inactive, and deep pelvic endometriosis.
9. Preliminary data indicate that the combination treatment of GnRH analogues and IFNα-2a increases pregnancy rate and monthly fecundity rate compared with GnRH analogues alone or danazol alone in women suffering from mild, moderate, or atypical endometriosis.
10. In most instances, GnRH agonist must be given before surgery and considered as chemotherapy before debulking surgery.
11. The conception of add-back hormonal replacement therapy (HRT) to prevent bone loss is promising because it may permit GnRH analogues to be used for longer treatment periods than the currently accepted limit of 6 months. This may enable repeated treatment courses in young women with recurrent endometriosis.
12. Endometriosis continues to baffle both scientists and clinicians. It is hoped that further insight into many areas of research will resolve the pathogenesis and the relationship between endometriosis and infertility.

REFERENCES

1. Kistner, R. W. 1979. Endometriosis and infertility. Clin. Obstet. Gynecol. **22:** 101.
2. Tzingounis, V. A., E. Cardamakis, G. P. Lioutas & A. P. Pappas. 1995. Diagnostic laparoscopy. J.A.A.G.L. **2**(Suppl.): S54.
3. American Fertility Society. 1985. Revised American Fertility Society classification of endometriosis. Fertil. Steril. **43:** 351–354.
4. Brosens, I. A. 1994. New principles in the management of endometriosis. Acta Obstet. Gynecol. Scand. **159**(Suppl.): 18–21.
5. Jansen, R. P. & P. Russell. 1986. Nonpigmented endometriosis: Clinical, laparoscopic and pathologic definition. Am. J. Obstet. Gynecol. **155:** 1154–1159.
6. Rock, J. A. & D. M. Moutos. 1992. Endometriosis: The present and the future. An overview of treatment options. Br. J. Obstet. Gynaecol. **92**(Suppl. 7): 1–4.
7. Sampson, J. A. 1921. Perforating hemorrhagic (chocolate) cysts of the ovary. Their importance and especially their relation to pelvic adenomas of the endometrial type ("adenomyoma" of the uterus, rectovaginal septum, sigmoid etc). Arch. Surg. **3:** 245–323.
8. Gray, L. A. 1958. The conservative operation for endometriosis: A report of its use in 200 cases. J. Ky. Med. Assoc. **56:** 1219.
9. Buttram, V. C. 1979. Conservative surgery for endometriosis in the infertile female: A study of 206 patients with implication for both medical and surgical therapy. Fertil. Steril. **31:** 117–123.
10. Cunanan, R. G., N. G. M. Courey & J. Lipper. 1983. Laparoscopic findings in patients with pelvic pain. Am. J. Obstet. Gynecol. **146:** 589–591.
11. Fedele, L., F. Parazzini, S. Bianchi, L. Arcaini & G. B. Candiani. 1990. Stage and localization of pelvic endometriosis and pain. Fertil. Steril. **53:** 155–158.

12. STOUT, A. L., J. E. STEEGE, W. C. DODSON & C. L. HUGHES. 1991. Relationship of laparoscopic findings to self-report of pelvic pain. Am. J. Obstet. Gynecol. **164:** 73–79.
13. FRANSEN, A. M. H. W., F. M. KAOER, D. R. CHADHA, J. A. ZIJSTRA & R. ROLLAND. 1989. Endometriosis: Treatment with gonadotropin-releasing hormone against buserelin. Fertil. Steril. **51:** 401–408.
14. KRESCH, A. 1984. Laparoscopy in 100 women with chronic pelvic pain. Obstet. Gynecol. **64:** 672.
15. PATTON, P. E., C. S. FIELD, R. W. HARMS & C. B. COULAN. 1986. CA-125 levels in endometriosis. Fertil. Steril. **45:** 770.
16. STARTSEVA, N. V. 1980. Clinico-immunological aspects of genital endometriosis. Akush. Ginekol. (Mosk.) **3:** 23.
17. MATHUR, S., *et al.* 1988. Endometrial antigens involved to the autoimmunity of endometriosis. Fertil. Steril. **50:** 860.
18. GLEICHER, N., *et al.* 1982. Abnormal autoantibodies in endometriosis. Is endometriosis an autoimmune disease? Obstet. Gynecol. **70:** 115.
19. HILL, J. A. & D. J. ANDERSON. 1989. Lymphocyte activity in the presence of peritoneal fluid from fertile women and infertile women with and without endometriosis. Am. J. Obstet. Gynecol. **161:** 861–864.
20. BRAUN, D. P., H. GEBEL, C. ROTMAN, N. RANA & W. P. DMOWSKI. 1992. The development of cytotoxicity in peritoneal macrophages from women with endometriosis. Fertil. Steril. **57:** 1203–1210.
21. SHARPE-TIMMS, K. L., P. L. BRUNO, L. K. PENNEY & J. T. BICKEL. 1994. Immunohistochemical localization of granulocyte-macrophage colony-stimulating factor in matched endometriosis and endometrial tissues. Am. J. Obstet. Gynecol. **171:** 740–745.
22. SIMPSON, T. L., S. ELIAS, I. R. MALINAK & V. C. BUTRAM, JR. 1980. Heritable aspects of endometriosis. I. Genetic studies. Am. J. Obstet. Gynecol. **137:** 327.
23. SANFILIPPO, J. S., N. G. WAKIN, K. N. SCHIKLER & M. A. YUSSMAN. 1986. Endometriosis in association with uterine anomaly. Am. J. Obstet. Gynecol. **154:** 39–43.
24. JONES, W. H. 1981. Reproductive impairment and malformed uterus. Fertil. Steril. **36:** 137.
25. CREATSAS, G., F. CARDAMAKIS, E. HASSAN, E. DELIGEOROGLOU, N. SALAKOS & D. ARAVANTINOS. 1994. Congenital uterine anomalies with obstructed cervix, hemivagina, or both during adolescence: Report of 22 cases. J. Gynecol. Surg. **10:** 159–167.
26. GARCIA, C. R. & S. S. DAVID. 1977. Pelvic endometriosis: Infertility and pelvic pain. Am. J. Obstet. Gynecol. **129:** 740–747.
27. ADAMSON, G. D., L. FRISON & E. J. LAMB. 1982. Endometriosis: Studies of a method for the design of a surgical staging system. Fertil. Steril. **38:** 659–666.
28. SCHENKEN, R. S. & L. R. MALINAK. 1982. Conservative surgery versus expectant management for the infertile patient with mild endometriosis. Fertil. Steril. **37:** 183–186.
29. GUZICK, D. S. & J. A. ROCK. 1983. A comparison of danazol and conservative surgery for the treatment of infertility due to mild or moderate endometriosis. Fertil. Steril. **40:** 580–584.
30. RONNBERG, L. & P. A. JARVINEN. 1984. Pregnancy rates following various therapy modes for endometriosis in infertile patients. Acta Obstet. Gynecol. Scand. **123**(Suppl.): 69–72.
31. BUTTRAM, V. C., JR., R. C. REITER & S. WARD. 1985. Treatment of endometriosis with danazol: Report of a 6-year prospective study. Fertil. Steril. **43:** 353–360.
32. OLIVE, D. L. & K. L. LEE. 1986. Analysis of sequential treatment protocols for endometriosis-associated infertility. Am. J. Obstet. **154:** 613–619.
33. SEILER, J. C., G. GIDWANI & L. BALLARD. 1986. Laparoscopic cauterization of endometriosis for fertility: A controlled study. Fertil. Steril. **46:** 1098–1100.
34. HULL, M. E., K. S. MOGHISSI, D. F. MAGYAR & M. F. HANES. 1987. Comparison of different treatment modalities of endometriosis in infertile women. Fertil. Steril. **97:** 40–44.

35. Nowroozi, K., J. S. Chase, J. H. Check & Ch. Wu. 1987. The importance of laparoscopic coagulation of mild endometriosis in infertile women. Int. J. Fertil. **32:** 442–444.
36. Pouly, J. L., H. Manhes, G. Mage, M. Canis & M. A. Bruhat. 1987. Laparoscopic treatment of endometriosis (laser excluded). Contrib. Gynecol. Obstet. **16:** 280–285.
37. Thomas, E. J. & I. D. Cooke. 1987. Successful treatment of asymptomatic endometriosis: Does it benefit infertile women? Br. Med. J. **294:** 1117–1119.
38. Badawy, S. Z. A., M. M. El Bakry, F. Samuel & M. Dizer. 1988. Cumulative pregnancy rates in infertile women with endometriosis. J. Reprod. Med. **33:** 757–760.
39. Bayer, S. R., M. M. Seibel, D. S. Saffan, M. J. Berger & M. L. Taymor. 1988. Efficacy of danazol treatment for minimal endometriosis in infertile women. J. Reprod. Med. **33:** 179–183.
40. Fayez, J. A., L. M. Collaro & C. Verno. 1988. Comparison of different modalities of treatment for minimal and mild endometriosis. Am. J. Obstet. Gynecol. **159:** 927–932.
41. Federici, D., E. Conti, W. Costantin, *et al.* 1988. Endometriosis and infertility: Our experience over five years. Hum. Reprod. **3:** 109–111.
42. Telimaa, S. 1988. Danazol and medroxyprogesterone acetate inefficatious in the treatment of infertility in endometriosis. Fertil. Steril. **50:** 872–875.
43. Levinson, C. J. 1989. Endometriosis therapy: Rationale for expectant or minimal therapy in minimal/mild cases (AFSI) [Abstract]. *In* Proceedings of the Second World Congress on Gynecologic Endoscopy, Clarmont-Ferraud, France, 1989.
44. Chong, A. P., M. E. Keene & N. L. Thorton. 1990. Comparison of three modes of treatment for infertility patients with minimal pelvic endometriosis. Fertil. Steril. **53:** 407–410.
45. Arumugam, K. & R. Urquhort. 1991. Efficacy of laparoscopic electrocoagulation in infertile patients with minimal or mild endometriosis. Acta Obstet. Gynecol. Scand. **70:** 125–127.
46. Paulson, J. D., P. Asmar & D. S. Saffan. 1991. Mild and moderate endometriosis: Comparison of treatment modalities for infertile couples. J. Reprod. Med. **36:** 151–155.
47. Adamson, G. D., S. J. Hurd, D. J. Pasta & B. D. Rodriguez. 1993. Laparoscopic endometriosis treatment: Is it better? Fertil. Steril. **59:** 36–44.
48. Coutinho, E. M. 1982. Treatment of endometriosis with Gestinoma (R23-23) a synthetic anti-estrogen, anti-progesterone. Am. J. Obstet. Gynecol. **144:** 895–898.
49. Lemay, A., R. Maheux, N. Faure, C. Jean & A. T. A. Fezekas. 1984. Reversible hypogonadism induced by a luteinizing hormone releasing hormone (LHRH) agonist (Buserelin) as a new therapeutic approach of endometriosis. Fertil. Steril. **41:** 863–871.
50. Donnez, J., M. Nisolle, F. Clerckx & F. Casanas-Roux. 1988. Combined (hormonal and microsurgical) therapy in endometriosis. Gynecol. Endocrinol. **2:** 84.
51. Dmowski, W. P. & M. R. Cohen. 1978. Antigonadotropic (danazol) in the treatment of endometriosis: Evaluation of posttreatment fertility and three-year follow-up data. Am. J. Obstet. Gynecol. **130:** 41–48.
52. Greenblatt, R. B. & V. Tzingounis. 1978. Danazol treatment of endometriosis long term follow-up. Fertil. Steril. **32:** 518–520.
53. Butler, L., E. Wilson, S. Belisle, *et al.* 1984. Collaborative study of pregnancy rates following danazol therapy of stage I endometriosis. Fertil. Steril. **41:** 373–376.
54. Fedele, L., F. Parazzini, E. Radici, *et al.* 1992. Buserelin acetate versus expectant management in the treatment of infertility associated with minimal or mild endometriosis: A randomized clinical trial. Am. J. Obstet. Gynecol. **166:** 1345–1350.
55. Henzl, M. R., C. L. Corson, K. Moghissi, V. A. Buttram, C. Berguist & J. Jacobson. 1988. Administration of nasal nafarelin as compared with oral danazol for endometriosis. N. Engl. J. Med. **318:** 485–489.

56. FEDELE, L., S. BIANCHI, L. ARCAINI, P. VERCELLINI & G. B. CANDIANI. 1989. Buserelin versus danazol in the treatment of endometriosis-associated infertility. Am. J. Obstet. Gynecol. **161:** 871–876.
57. VESSEY, M. P., N. H. WRIGHT, K. MCPHERSON, *et al.* 1978. Fertility after stopping different methods of contraception. Br. Med. J. **1:** 265–267.
58. SCHENKEN, R. J. & L. R. MALINAK. 1978. Reoperation after initial treatment of endometriosis with conservative surgery. Am. J. Obstet. Gynecol. **131:** 416–424.
59. SEIBEL, M. M., M. J. BERGER, F. G. WEISTEIN, *et al.* 1982. The effectiveness of danazol on subsequent fertility in minimal endometriosis. Fertil. Steril. **38:** 534–537.
60. PORTUONDO, J. A., A. D. ECHANOJANREGNI, C. HERRAN, *et al.* 1983. Early conception in patients with untreated mild endometriosis. Fertil. Steril. **39:** 22–25.
61. OLIVE, D. L., G. F. STOHS, D. A. METZGER, *et al.* 1985. Expectant management and hydrotubations in the treatment of endometriosis associated with infertility. Fertil. Steril. **44:** 35–41.
62. TZINGOUNIS, V. & E. CARDAMAKIS. 1994. The role of GnRH analogues and Danazol in the treatment of endometriosis. 4th World Congress of Endometriosis, Salvador-Bahia-Brazil, 25–28 May 1994, Abstract FC-10.
63. ANGIOLI, S., F. PETRAGLIA, F. IORI, S. SARDELLI, A. VOLPE & A. R. GENAZZANI. 1993. Acute β-interferon and thymopentin administration increases plasma GH and cortisol levels in children. Gyn. Endocrin. **7**(Suppl. 1): 148.
64. SCAMBIA, G., P. B. PANICI, F. BATTAGLIA, G. FERRANDINA, G. BAIOCECHI, A. GALLO, G. SICA & S. MANCUSO. 1991. Effect of recombinant human interferon alpha-2b on receptors for steroid hormones and epidermal growth factor in patients with endometrial cancer. Eur. J. Canccr **27:** 51–53.
65. TAO, Y.-X. & Y.-Q. CAO. 1993. Modulation of interferon secretion by concanavalin A and interleukin-2 in first trimester placental expants in vitro. J. Reprod. Immun. **24:** 201–212.
66. KINY, A. & Y. W. LOKE. 1993. Effect of IFN-γ and IFN-α on killing of human trophoblast by decidual LAK cells. J. Reprod. Immun. **23:** 51–62.
67. DONNEZ, J., M. NISOLLE & F. CASANAS-ROUX. 1994. Endometriosis. Rationale for surgery. *In* An Atlas of Laser Operative Laparoscopy and Hysteroscopy. J. Donnez & M. Nisolle, Eds.: 53–62. Parthenon Publishing Co. Carnforth, U.K.
68. BIANCHI, G., S. COSTANTINI, P. ANSERINI, *et al.* 1989. Effects of gonadotropin-releasing hormone agonist on uterine fibroids and bone density. Maturity **11:** 179–185.
69. RICO, H., F. ARNANZ, M. REVILLA, *et al.* 1993. Total and regional bone mineral content in women treated with GnRH agonists. Calcif. Tissue Int. **52:** 354–357.
70. SCHARLA, S. H., H. W. MINNE, S. WAIBEL-TREBER, *et al.* 1990. Bone mass reduction after estrogen deprivation by long-acting gonadotropin-releasing hormone agonists and its relation to pretreatment serum concentrations of 1,25-dihydroxyvitamin D_3. J. Clin. Endocrinol. Metab. **70:** 1055–1061.
71. WAIBEL-TREBER, S., H. W. MINNE, S. H. SCHARLA, T. BREMEN, R. ZEGLER & G. LEYENDECKER. 1989. Reversible bone loss in women treated with GnRH-agonists for endometriosis and uterine leiomyoma. Hum. Reprod. **4:** 384–388.
72. CANN, C. E., M. HENZL, K. BURRY, *et al.* 1987. Reversible bone loss in produced by the GnRH agonist nafarelin. *In* Calcium Regulation and Bone Metabolism: Basic and Clinical Aspects. D. V. Cohn, T. J. Martin & P. J. Mennier, Eds.: 123–127. Proceedings of the Ninth International Conference on Calcium Regulating Hormones and Bone Metabolism, Nice, France, 25 October–1 November 1986. Elsevier. Amsterdam.
73. MATTA, W. H., R. W. SHAR, R. HESP & R. EVANS. 1988. Reversible trabecular bone density loss following induced hypo-oestrogenism with the GnRH analogue buserelin in premenopausal women. Clin. Endocrinol. **29:** 45–51.

74. SCIALLI, A. R., K. J. JESTILE & J. A. SIMON. 1993. Leuprolide acetate and bone mineral density measured by quantitative digitized radiography. Fertil. Steril. **59:** 674–676.
75. SURREY, E. S., N. FOURNET, B. VOIGT & H. L. JUDD. 1993. Effects of sodium etidronate in combination with low dose norethindrone in patients administered a long-acting GnRH agonis: A preliminary report. Obstet. Gynecol. **81:** 581–586.
76. JOHANSEN, J. S., B. J. RIIS, C. HASSAGER, M. MOEN, J. JACOBSON & C. CHRISTIANSEN. 1988. The effect of a gonadotropin-releasing hormone agonist analog (nafarelin) on bone metabolism. J. Clin. Endocrinol. Metab. **67:** 701–706.

Female Genital Tract Malignancies during Puberty

Uterine and Cervical Malignancies

GERHARD TSCHERNE

Department of Obstetrics and Gynecology
University of Graz
Univ.-Frauenklinik
Auenbruggerplatz 14
A-8036 Graz, Austria

Malignancies in the female genital tract are rare during puberty and extremely rare in the uterine corpus. More frequent and of real importance are malignancies in the uterine cervix, especially in form of preclinical lesions. Problems like sexual behavior in adolescence, contraception, and human papilloma virus (HPV) infection are becoming more and more of interest. Early detection of any malignancy is vital in planning an individualized, optimal treatment regime. New diagnostic possibilities may improve our ability to detect these malignancies early. The primary intention of therapy must be curative; on the other hand, preservation of fertility is also a central issue in this age group.

An exact diagnosis and estimation of the degree of malignancy as the basis for an adapted treatment including an efficient follow-up is only possible in a specialized oncological center. Centralization of gynecological health services may be desirable in order to develop optimal procedures for young patients. The gynecological university clinic of Graz is such an oncological center with a great deal of diagnostic and treatment experience. An outpatient unit for children and adolescents was established in 1976. But even there the frequency of uterine malignancies is low (TABLE 1).

MALIGNANCIES OF THE UTERINE CORPUS

There are no extensive reports in the literature because of the small number of uterine malignancies in adolescence. Mixed mesodermal tumors may occur as well as mixed Müllerian tumors, malignant tumors as carcinosarcoma. Adenocarcinomas, usually of mesonephric origin, have been reported as well as leiomyosarcomas, gliomas, and neuroectodermal tumors.

Diagnostic and therapeutic procedures should be performed according to oncological principles with individually adapted treatment regimes, including surgery, irradiation, and cytostatic chemotherapy.

TABLE 1. Malignancies of the Uterus in Patients up to 19 Years of Age and Overall[a]

Site	Patients (up to 19 yr)	Total
Cervix		
CIN III conization	58	3967
Invasive cancer	2	1803
Corpus	0	

[a]Study done at University Clinic Graz, Department of Obstetrics and Gynecology, Graz, Austria in 1970–1990.

MALIGNANCIES OF THE UTERINE CERVIX

Clinical cancer of the cervix is rare in adolescence. Preclinical stages in the form of CIN III and microcarcinoma are more frequent, raising questions and problems concerning etiology, tumor spreading and progression, the possibility of prevention, and optimal adapted treatment that is as conservative as possible. A recently published FIGO-staging is presented in part in TABLE 2.

In the case of invasive clinical cancer, radical surgery has to be performed, usually in the form of the Wertheim operation with pelvic and, if necessary, additional para-aortal lymphonodectomy. The ovaries may be preserved to maintain hormonal function. A typical procedure performed at the Graz clinic is shown in FIGURE 1. Adjuvant treatment has to be performed individually, continuous follow-up is obligatory.

There may be a possibility of preserving the uterus even in the case of invasive carcinoma. Dargent[6] demonstrated a vaginal method for relatively radical surgery similar to the Schauta operation. It may be carried out in cervical carcinoma stages Ia, Ib, and IIa. More or less up to the full length of the cervix, is removed, together with the upper part of vagina and parts of the parametrial tissue. Lymphonodectomy, if necessary, may be done by laparoscopy. An os externum of the uterine cavity re-

TABLE 2. The New FIGO Classification of Cervical Cancer

Stage	Description
0	Carcinoma *in situ,* intraepithelial carcinoma
I	Carcinoma strictly confined to the cervix
Ia	Invasive carcinoma of the cervix, diagnosed only by microscopy. Macroscopically detectable lesions—even with superficial invasion—belong to stage Ib.
Ia1	Measured stromal invasion with a depth of not more than 3 mm and a horizontal spread not more than 7 mm
Ia2	Lesions detected microscopically with a measured depth of stromal invasion more than 3 mm and not more than 5 mm and a horizontal spread not more than 7 mm

[a]Shown in part; developed in Montreal in 1994.

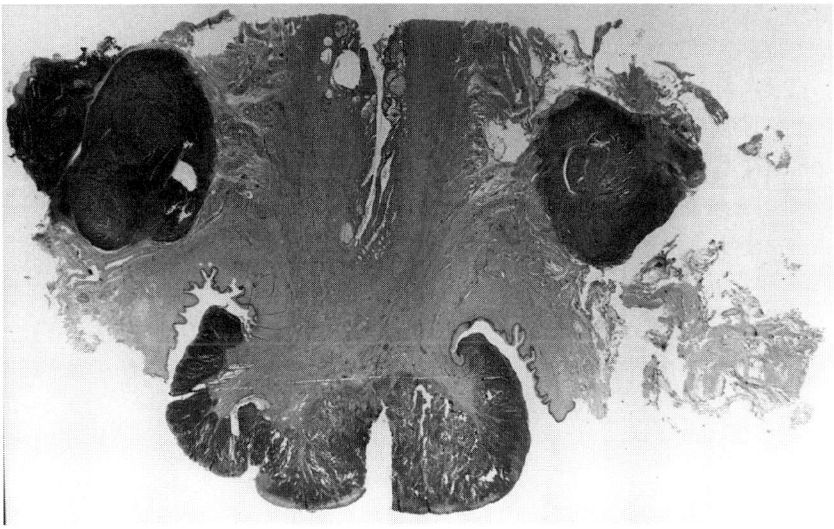

FIGURE 1. Frontal giant section through the cervix and the parametria, obtained at radical abdominal hysterectomy with pelvic and para-aortal lymphadenectomy because of clinical cancer stage IIb (Pat. P.U., 19 yrs; Op. 1994). Histologically, a neuroendocrine small cell carcinoma. Metastases in both parametria. (Provided by Dr. O. Reich, pathologist, University Clinic Graz, Department of Obstetrics and Gynecology, Graz, Austria.)

mains open. Dargent reported pregnancies and the birth of normal babies in six women.[6]

In the case of preclinical carcinomas of the cervix, an exact diagnosis is the basis for an optimal individualized treatment, and the spectrum of possibilities has been extended (TABLE 3).

Colposcopy and cytology are the first steps of diagnostic procedure. In the Graz clinic, it is standard to use both screening methods at every gynecological examination.[2] The first colposcopy should be done when an adolescent girl begins to have sexual intercourse. In adolescence, suspicious lesions are usually seen on the surface

TABLE 3. Diagnosis and Treatment of Preclinical Carcinomas of the Cervix Uteri: CIN III and Microinvasive Cancer

Diagnosis	Treatment
Colposcopy	Conization
Cytology	Loop Excision
Biopsy (directed)	
Histological examination	
Conization	Cryosurgery
Virology (HPV)	Electrocautery
DNA cytometry	Laserablation

of the cervix in connection with a transformation zone. In the case of colposcopic pictures like mosaicism, punctation, leukoplacia, or suspicious vessels, a biopsy has to be taken directly from the suspicious area viewed under the colposcope. The result of the histological examination determines the further steps. Only in case of a histologically confirmed diagnosis of CIN III (severe dysplasia or carcinoma *in situ*) is conization performed. In mild and moderate dysplasia, further observation by regular colposcopy and cytology is sufficient. A cytologically suspicious result also has to be confirmed by histological examination, that is, by biopsy or cervical curettage.

Conization is usually performed by cold knife excision[5] of a relatively flat cone, removing the whole transformation zone on the ectocervix, which is the typical form in adolescence. The cone is dissected in step-serial sections. In our own histological laboratory, it is possible to examine a series of 70 to 80 steps (FIG. 2). Thus, the two essential questions may be answered exactly: (1) Are there invasive formations anywhere? and (2) Is the CIN III removed totally?

If there is no invasion at all and the cone is removed *in sano,* the conization is to be seen as the treatment. An exact follow-up is the only necessary further procedure. If carcinoma *in situ* is not removed totally, the cone is not *in sano;* in adolescent girls observation by regular colposcopy and cytology is usually sufficient. Histological examination of specimens of a second conization has shown that in a great number of cases there are no more CIN III formations because of the coagulation of the margin on the occasion of the first conization. This method of coagulation of the defect after conization effects a re-formation of the cervix in an optimal form. Thus, fertility is preserved, following pregnancies and deliveries are nearly comparable to normal.[8] The frequency of cesarian section is insignificantly higher than in general.

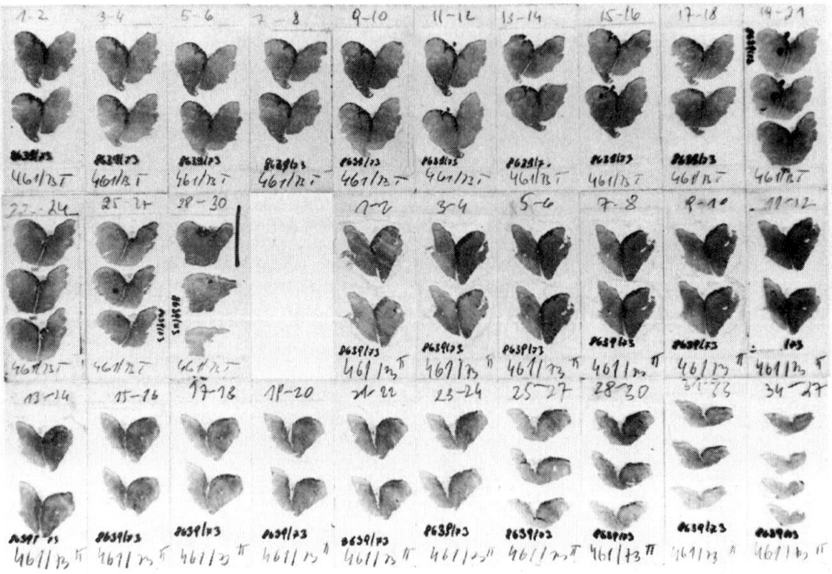

FIGURE 2. Step-serial sections of a conization specimen.

In case of microinvasive carcinoma (stages Ia1 and Ia2), conization is the treatment if the cone is removed *in sano.* If not, decisions about further procedures will depend on the situation, first of all on an exact histological diagnosis by a competent pathologist.[3]

Loop excision may be a method of treatment, at least in case of severe dysplasia. With large loops one may excise the whole transformation zone, but the histological examination is not as efficient as in a specimen of cold knife conization. Cryosurgery, electrocautery, and laser destruction are not suitable because of the lack of good surgical specimens for optimal histological examination.

Virology and DNA-Cytometry[1,7]: Human papilloma virus (HPV) should be considered to be a factor in the etiology of carcinoma of the cervix. Certain HPV types, such as 16 and 18, as well as 31 and 33, have oncogenic potency. They play a role in the occurrence of some intraepithelial lesions. Obviously, additional cofactors must become effective. Evidence of HPV DNA has become possible, so the DNA can be detected in carcinoma cells. HPV DNA analysis may become a prognostic factor or a factor for estimating the degree of malignancy.[9] The histological diagnosis may be complemented through the virological status. CIN can regress, persist, or proceed to invasive growth. We can carry out observation of mild and moderate dysplasia. Carcinoma *in situ* regresses rarely, if ever. Perhaps cytometric and virologic examination may help to establish the benign or malignant nature of the epithelial lesion and thus inform the decision about whether conization should be done or whether one can wait and see. Especially in adolescents, prevention of unnecessary surgical interventions is an obligation.

Another aspect of health care for adolescents is prevention. Perhaps we can, and should, identify those adolescent girls at risk of cervical carcinoma. Early sexual contact and multiple sexual partners play a role in tumor genesis in combination with HPV contamination. Additional factors like other infections (chlamydia?), hormones (pill), immunologic suppression, and environmental factors may play a role. Early colposcopic and cytologic examination and, in the future, HPV-DNA analysis and other diagnostic steps will establish a mosaic of data for the prognostic estimation. The best opportunity for starting this procedure is at the time of prescribing birth control pills, which should not be done without a gynecological examination.

Adenocarcinoma of the cervix is rarely found in adolescence, so that the *in situ* form of this malignancy hardly ever occurs.

Sarcoma botryoides is a standard tumor in the literature and is localized in the vagina in infants and children. In puberty or adolescence, it is localized in the cervix. Diagnosis will be made on the basis of clinical signs and examinations and on histological findings. The treatment is surgical removal, the extent of which depends on localization and volume. Again, the first issue is to cure the patient, but if it is possible, the uterus should be preserved. Such a case is presented in FIGURE 3.

SUMMARY

Malignancies of the uterine corpus are extremely rare. Diagnostic and therapeutic procedures should be performed according to oncological principles with individually adapted treatment regimes. Clinical cancer of the cervix is rare in adolescence; the

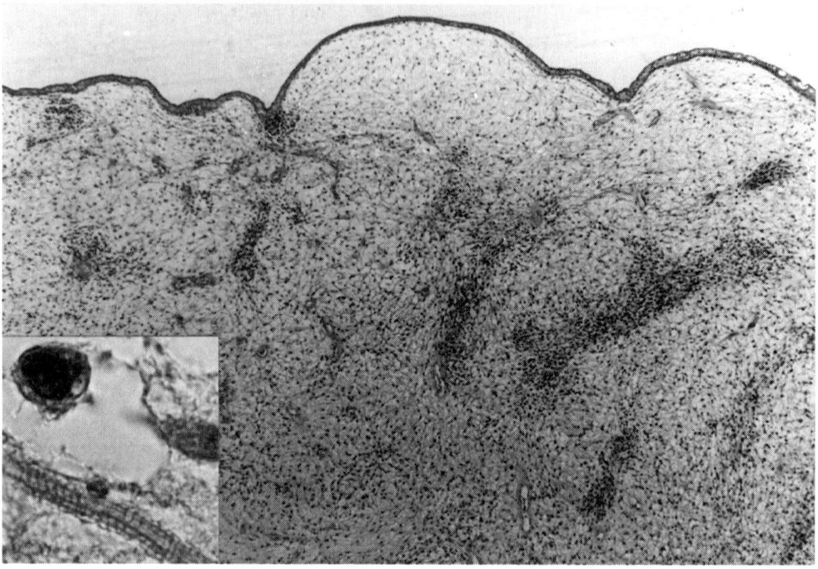

FIGURE 3. Embryonal rhabdomyosarcoma of the cervix, botryoide type. The inset shows the typical cross striations. The large exophytic tumor was removed together with a cone of the cervix, the uterus remained *in situ* (Pat. R.C., 19 yrs., Op. 1994). (Provided by Dr. O. Reich, as for FIG. 1.)

treatment is radical surgery. Preclinical stages, that is, CIN III (severe dysplasia, carcinoma *in situ*) and microinvasive cancer (stages Ia1, Ia2), are important, also because of their frequency. Diagnosis is based on colposcopy, cytology, direct biopsy, histological examination, and conization. In addition, virology (HPV) and DNA cytometry may become prognostic factors. Treatment consists of conization with an exact histological examination in serial sections as a basis for preserving the uterus. The sarcoma botryoides is localized in the cervix in adolescence, whereas it is in the vagina in infants and children.

REFERENCES

1. BÖCKING, A. 1993. Cervical cancer-DNA analysis. *In* Surgical Gynecologic Oncology. E. Burghardt, Ed.: 250. Georg Thieme Verlag. Stuttgart–New York.
2. BURGHARDT, E. 1991. Colposcopy–Cervical Pathology. Textbook and Atlas. 2nd edit. Georg Thieme Verlag. Stuttgart–New York.
3. BURGHARDT, E., F. GIRARDI, M. LAHOUSEN, H. PICKEL & K. TAMUSSINO. 1991. Microinvasive carcinoma of the uterine cervix (FIGO Stage Ia). Cancer **67:** 1037.
4. BURGHARDT, E., Ed. 1993. Surgical Gynecologic Oncology. Georg Thieme Verlag. Stuttgart–New York.
5. BURGHARDT, E. 1993. Cold-knife conization. *In* Surgical Gynecologic Oncology. E. Burghardt, Ed.: 269. Georg Thieme Verlag. Stuttgart–New York.

6. DARGENT, D. & F. LAFFARGUE. 1995. Fertility and pregnancies after genital tract surgery. Presented at Cervical Cancer: 15th World Congress on Fertility and Sterility, Sept. 17–22, Montpellier, France.
7. GIRARDI, F. & H. PFISTER. 1993. Cervical cancer-virology. *In* Surgical Gynecologic Oncology. E. Burghardt, Ed.: 252. Georg Thieme Verlag. Stuttgart–New York.
8. HOLZER, E. 1972. Fertilität, Schwangerschaft und Geburtsverlauf nach Konisation der Portio vaginalis uteri. Geburtshilfe Frauenheilk. **32:** 950.
9. JAKOBSEN, A. 1984. Prognostic impact of ploidy level in carcinoma of the cervix. Am. J. Clin. Onc. **7:** 475.

Ovarian Malignancies in Adolescence

S. K. FOTIOU

First Department of Gynecology
Hellenic Cancer Institute
St. Savas Hospital
Alexandras Ave 171
Athens 155 22, Greece

Malignant tumors arising in the ovaries of females younger than 20 years of age constitute a special group of neoplasms. This is mainly due to the histologic composition of these neoplasms, which defines their natural history, the peculiarities of the clinical course of the disease related to the immature (physically, hormonally, and immunologically) host, and the therapeutic implications of the patient's age. It is well understood that preservation of ovarian tissue in these patients is essential in order to ensure normal physical development and child-bearing potential. Nevertheless, it is even more important that the disease be properly eradicated.

Ovarian tumors are unusual in adolescents and account for less than 1–2% of all neoplasms in females younger than 16 years of age.[1] Nevertheless, they compose the most usual (60–70%) type of gynecologic neoplasms during childhood and adolescence.[1,2] Their incidence is difficult to define accurately, because nonneoplastic ovarian masses are often included in the reports. It is postulated that 5 to 10% of all ovarian tumors appear before the 20s[3,4] and one-fifth of them precede menarche.[5] The percentage of malignancies varies between 29 and 55% in the literature.[3,4,6,7]

CLASSIFICATION

Classification is based on histogenetic origin. There are three predominant classes: common epithelial tumors, germ cell tumors, and sex cord–stromal tumors. In the WHO classification, the remaining ovarian tumors are separated from these classes, because their histogenesis is undetermined, their histology is not specific, or they are of metastatic origin.[8] An understanding of histogenesis and biological behavior of these tumors is necessary for the proper evaluation and effective treatment of the patients.

The incidence of the different histogenetic classes depends mainly on the age period. In adults, common epithelial tumors account for 90% of ovarian cancers, and germ cell and sex cord–stromal tumors account for 5% each. During childhood and adolescence, the incidence of germ cell tumors far exceeds that of the epithelial ones. A compilation of the literature data from 12 reports (TABLE 1) reveals that in females younger than 20 years of age, germ cell tumors represent 61.5% and epithelial tumors only 20%.[7,9–19]

TABLE 1. Ovarian Tumors in Adolescence: Incidence and Histologic Categories[a]

Histogenetic Category	Cases	Percentage
Germ cell tumors	1134	61.5%
Common epithelial tumors	365	20%
Sex cord–stromal tumors	177	9.5%
Others	170	9%
Total	1846	100%

[a]Figures are compiled from 12 reports.[7,9–19] Patients were all younger than 20 years of age.

CLINICAL FEATURES

In young girls an ovarian mass can more easily be evident as an enlargement over the inguinal ligament or, higher up, at a supra-pelvic level. This is due to the shallow pelvis and the higher position of the ovary, which may simulate an abdominal rather than a pelvic organ.

The relative—in comparison with a mature woman—lack of space for tumor expansion in the pelvis of a young girl results more often in lower abdominal or pelvic pain, which seems to be the most common leading symptom, with abdominal enlargement being next in frequency.

Ovarian tumors in adolescence exhibit some special clinical characteristics that are summarized below. Acute symptoms due to torsion or necrosis of the tumor pedicle are relatively common in this age group. A germ cell tumor may, at times, present as acute appendicitis, leading to an emergency laparotomy. Dysgerminomas and mostly gonadoblastomas arise frequently in dysgenetic gonads, and they need to be excised.

Functional hormonal activity of these tumors is quite common and can result in precocious puberty, virilization, or dysfunctional bleeding, leading at times to the erroneous diagnosis of extra- or intrauterine pregnancy.

The preoperative diagnostic workup in young patients is similar to that used in elderly women, including blood tests and radiologic investigation of the urinary and gastrointestinal tract. Ultrasonography, CT scan, occasionally MRI of the abdomen and pelvis, and tumor markers estimation are also applied.

EPITHELIAL OVARIAN TUMORS

These tumors are exceedingly rare before menarche, increasing thereafter in frequency. If they occur in adolescence, they are usually benign.[20] Deprest *et al.*,[21] in a recent review of 2,225 cases of ovarian tumors in females younger than 20 years of age, estimated that 19.3% were of epithelial origin with a malignancy rate of 15.9%. Among the malignant tumors, 39.4% were of the mucinous type, compared to 12% in all age groups. It is possible that this subgroup represents monodermal teratomas originating from germ cells. An intestinal type of differentiation is present, in contrast to similar tumors in adults where a Müllerian-type epithelium is predominant.[22,23] The CA-125 levels in the sera of these patients are usually low. In certain cases, CEA and CA 19-9 levels are elevated, and measurement of these might be of value in clinical practice.[24,25]

The standard of treatment in epithelial ovarian cancer is well known. Conservative surgery, that is, unilateral salpingoophorectomy (USO), is justified only under strict criteria that include stage IA, well-differentiated tumors. Finally, some arguments in favor of conservatism in stage IB grade I and stage IA grade II or III have been expressed.[26]

Borderline tumors are of special interest in this age group, because of their high incidence (30.3% of ovarian tumors, instead of 6–10% in all ages). These neoplasms can at times be conservatively treated and have a high five-year survival of 93%.[27] Their potentially aggressive behavior, however, underlines the necessity to discriminate among them, in order to identify those that need to be more radically treated.

In accordance with our current knowledge, the following observations can be made:

- Successful management is mainly attributed to accurate staging and optimal cytoreduction (complete extirpation of the disease).
- In stage I patients, USO is considered adequate treatment. Wedge biopsy of the contralateral, normal-looking ovary is necessary in serous but not in mucinous tumors (minimizing the possibility of adhesion formation). These two distinct histologic types exhibit a different biologic behavior, which accounts for differences in treatment. Serous tumors are more aggressive, bilaterality is not uncommon (14–40%),[20,28–30] and relapses in the remaining ovary occur in about 15% of the cases if conservative treatment has been previously applied.[31] Mucinous tumors rarely develop in the remaining normal-looking ovary—especially if no peritoneal spread is present—and have a more favorable prognosis.[32]
- If the disease is disseminated in the peritoneal cavity, adequate cytoreduction is the treatment of choice. If cytoreduction is successful, removal of the uterus and the normal ovary does not seem to affect survival.[33] Should this not be the case, adjunctive chemotherapy is warranted.

GERM CELL TUMORS

Germ cell tumors originate from the primordial germ cells of the ovary. Germ cell tumors can arise even in extragonadal sites—most often retroperitoneal—deriving from arrested germ cells in the course of their embryonic migration from the yolk sac to the developing gonad.

They are the most common malignant ovarian neoplasms during the first two decades of life. The classification of germ cell tumors is presented in TABLE 2, along with the tumor markers produced by the different histologic subtypes. These markers can be very useful for diagnosis and for monitoring the disease after initial treatment.

Germ cell tumors are usually large and grow rapidly. Therefore, they often pro-

TABLE 2. Classification of Ovarian Germ Cell Tumors and Tumor Markers

Histologic Types	Tumor Markers
1. Dysgerminoma	LDH, PLAP
2. Teratoma: Immature	
Mature	
Monodermal specialized	—
3. Endodermal sinus tumor	AFP
4. Embryonal carcinoma	AFP-HCG
5. Polyembryoma	AFP-HCG
6. Choriocarcinoma	HCG
7. Mixed forms	AFP-HCG-LDH

duce pressure symptoms in the bladder and rectum and pelvic pain, related to hemorrhage or necrosis of the tumor. Hormonal disturbances in the form of precocious puberty or menstrual irregularities are usual. In preoperative evaluation, CT or MRI may disclose retroperitoneal lymphadenopathy or liver metastasis. A karyotype should be taken preoperatively on premenarcheal girls because of the propensity of these tumors to develop in dysgenetic gonads.[34,35]

Dysgerminoma

Dysgerminoma is the most common malignant germ cell neoplasm, representing 30 to 40% of all tumors in this group. In 5% of the cases, dysgerminoma arises in females with dysgenetic gonads and, in most of these cases, it coexists with gonadoblastoma. This is a benign, mixed tumor composed of germ and sex cord–stromal cells that if left *in situ* in patients with dysgenetic gonads will develop malignancy in more than 50% of the cases.[36,37]

Dysgerminoma is often diagnosed in stage I (75%), but it is the only germ cell tumor that involves the contralateral ovary at a significant (10–15%) rate. It is also distinguished from the other ovarian malignancies by its propensity to metastasize to the paraortic lymph nodes in the absence of peritoneal spread and to respond well to radiation treatment. The treatment is primarily surgical and consists of USO and proper staging. A thorough lymphadenectomy (pelvic and paraortic) and evaluation of the normal-looking ovary should be included.

In case of dysgenetic gonads, both ovaries should be removed, but the uterus may be left intact for possible future embryo transfer. In the case of extraovarian spread, cytoreductive surgery has to be carried out, but the contralateral ovary and the uterus may be retained in this highly chemosensitive disease. However, conservative surgical treatment even in stage IA is associated with a significant (17–35%) recurrence rate. For this reason, the adjuvant administration of three cycles of PVB, or VAC, or more recently PEB (platinum-etoposide-bleomycin) is the usual postoperative treatment today. In this way, five-year survival rates higher than 95% have been achieved, and the fertility of these patients is preserved.

Recurrences occur mostly within the first year after initial treatment. In this case other cytostatic combinations may be used, and consideration should also be given to high-dose chemotherapy. Sometimes, in spite of the disadvantage of loosing fertility, radiation therapy is required.[35–40]

Immature Teratoma

This is the second most frequent germ cell malignancy, and 50% of the cases affect girls between 10 and 20 years of age. Immature teratoma is classified in grades 1–3, according to the differentiation of the neural elements of the tumor, which is the main prognostic factor. Tumor markers are negative in pure tumors.

This neoplasm is usually diagnosed in stage IA. In adolescents, USO and surgical staging should be performed. Involvement of the contralateral ovary is rare, and wedge biopsy is not necessary.

Postoperative treatment in stage IA grade I lesions is not considered useful, and prognosis is excellent. In patients with tumors of stage IA but grades II or III, adjuvant chemotherapy should be given. Regardless of the tumor grade, chemotherapy should be administered if ascites was present. In the past the VAC regimen was most frequently administered, but recently, a prompt switch to the BEP combination has occurred, because of its better therapeutic index and lower toxicity.[36,40,41]

Endodermal Sinus Tumor

Endodermal sinus tumor (EST) is the third most common malignant germ cell tumor. The median age of patients is 18 years. ESTs have also been referred to as yolk sac tumors, and they secrete α-fetoprotein (AFP). The serum levels of AFP relate to the extent of the malignancy and are useful in monitoring the course of the disease. At laparotomy, the tumor is usually large and solid, and the contralateral ovary is rarely affected in the absence of extraovarian spread. Surgical treatment consists of USO and abdominal exploration, even though postoperative chemotherapy is indicated in all stages. In case of extraovarian spread, cytoreductive surgery should be performed. Removal of the uterus and the contralateral ovary does not affect survival.

Chemotherapy, adjuvant or therapeutic, is applied using platinum combinations (preferably PEB or POMB-ACE). The optimal number of treatment cycles has not yet been established and varies between three and six.[36,37,40,42]

Embryonal carcinoma, choriocarcinoma, and polyembryoma are extremely rare germ cell tumors. They usually affect young girls. Tumor markers (see TABLE 2) are positive and can be used to monitor the response to treatment and follow the course of the disease. During laparotomy, every effort should be made to preserve fertility, and postoperative chemotherapy is based on platinum combination regimens.

SEX CORD–STROMAL TUMORS

Sex cord–stromal tumors (SCST) represent 5–7% of malignant ovarian tumors. They derive from the sex cords—downgrowths of the celomic epithelium—and the mesenchyme of the embryonic gonad. These elements can be present in any possible combination or percentage and in any degree of differentiation. SCST are divided into four major categories: (a) Female cell type, in which granulosa- and theca-cell tumors are included; (b) male cell type, including Sertoli cell tumors, Leydig cell tumors, and Sertoli–Leydig cell tumors; (c) male and female cell type, including gynandroblastoma; and (d) unclassified SCST in which SCSTs with annular tubules (SCSTAT) and sclerosing stromal tumors are included.

Granulosa Cell Tumors

This is the most frequent (70%) representative of SCST. In 75% of the cases they are hormone—most often estrogen—secreting. Therefore, these tumors are associated with sexual pseudoprecosity in prepubertal girls. In the reproductive age group, most patients have menstrual irregularities or secondary amenorrhea and cystic hyperplasia of the endometrium. At times an endometrial cancer can even be developed.[36,37]

Scully's group described a variety of granulosa cell tumors with distinct histopathologic features that tends to occur in young women,[43] and therefore was called juvenile granulosa cell tumor (JGCT). The clinical features of this tumor seem to be similar to the adult type. Diagnosis of JGCT is usually made early in stage IA, and prognosis is very good (92%, 5-year survival in Scully's series).

Granulosa cell tumors are mostly slow-growing neoplasms, and recurrences may develop late (after 10–20 years). Therefore, they are considered of low malignant potential, and unilateral salpingoophorectomy is the treatment of choice if unilateral involvement is present. Accurate histologic diagnosis on frozen section is difficult. When it becomes possible, however, biopsy of the normal-looking contralateral ovary may be omitted. Provided that histologic diagnosis and staging are correct, adjuvant chcmo- or radiotherapy are not of substantial value.[37,44] In advanced-stage disease, VAC chemotherapy has accomplished quite good results.[45]

Male Cell Type

Pure Sertoli tumors are rare tumors, composed entirely of Sertoli cells, and are primarily estrogenic. The reported cases belonged to stage IA. In young women the management consists of USO.[46] Pure Leydig tumors are also rare virilizing tumors and affect women around the climacterium.

Sertoli–Leydig cell tumors, even though they account for fewer than 0.2% of ovarian cancers, represent the most usual subtype of this group of tumors. They occur most frequently in young women as low-grade malignancies, although occasionally they can be poorly differentiated and behave more aggressively.

They represent the most common virilizing ovarian tumors (70–85% of cases), even though, rarely, they can be estrogen producing. For this reason the term arrhenoblastoma or androblastoma, which was originally used, has been replaced by Sertoli-Leydig tumor.

These low-grade lesions are only rarely (<1%) bilateral, and therefore USO is the usual treatment in young women. The five-year survival rate is 70–90%. The value of chemo- or radiotherapy has not yet been well documented.[37,47]

Gynandroblastoma and SCSTAT tumors are rare neoplasms with a malignant potential similar to that of granulosa cell tumors. Gynandroblastoma contains granulosa and Sertoli or Leydig cells. Sclerosing stromal tumors with annular tubules were described by Scully.[48] They affect young women and are often associated with Peutz-Jeghers syndrome, in which case they behave in a more aggressive way. They are bilateral in two-thirds of the cases. Proper staging is considered necessary, and conservative surgery is acceptable in stage IA.

SUMMARY

Ovarian malignancies, although rare during adolescence, constitute the most common genital neoplasms in this age group. Germ cell tumors account for the majority of cases (61.5%), whereas 20% belong to the common epithelial group and 9.5% derive from sex cords and ovarian stroma.

Dysgerminomas are the most frequent germ cell tumors. They are usually large and often secrete hormones and tumor markers that can be useful in monitoring the course of the disease. Diagnosis is often made in stage IA, and conservative surgery is the treatment of choice.

In the epithelial neoplasm group, mucinous tumors are more common than usual (39.4% instead of 12%). The incidence of borderline tumors is also higher (30.3% versus 6–10%). Adnexectomy and, if needed, extirpation of peritoneal implants is considered adequate treatment.

Sex cord–stromal tumors consist of epithelial (granulosa-Sertoli cells) and mesenchymal elements in a variety of combinations. Granulosa cell tumor is the most common subtype, presenting as the juvenile form in young females. It is of low malignant potential and is adequately treated with adnexectomy only.

REFERENCES

1. Piver, M. S. & T. Patton. 1986. Ovarian cancer in children. Sem. Surg. Oncol. **2:** 163–169.
2. Barber, H. R. K. & E. A. Graber. 1973. Gynecological tumors in childhood and adolescence. Obstet. Gynecol. Surv. **28**(Suppl.): 357.
3. Abell, M. R., V. J. Johnson & F. Holtz. 1965. Ovarian neoplasms in childhood and adolescence. Tumors of germ cell origin. Am. J. Obstet. Gynecol. **92:** 1059.
4. Norris, H. J. & R. D. Jensen. 1972. Relative frequency of ovarian neoplasms in children and adolescents. Cancer **30:** 713.
5. Abell, M. R. 1977. Ovarian neoplasms of childhood and adolescence. *In* Pathology of the Female Genital Tract. A. Blaustein, Ed. Vol. 1: 586–626. Springer-Verlag. New York.
6. ACOG Technical Bulletin. 1991. Cancer of the ovary. Int. J. Gynecol. Obstet. **35:** 359–366.
7. Diamond, M. P., J. W. Baxter, C. G. Peerman & L. S. Burnett. 1988. Occurrence of ovarian malignancy in childhood and adolescence: A community-wide evaluation. Obstet. Gynecol. **71:** 858–860.
8. Serov, S. F., R. E. Scully & L. H. Sobin. 1975. Histological typing of ovarian tumors. International classification of tumors. World Health Organization. Geneva.

9. BREEN, J. L. & W. S. MAXSON. 1977. Ovarian tumors in children and adolescents. Clin. Obstet. Gynecol. **20:** 607–623.
10. LINDFORS, O. 1976. Primary ovarian neoplasms in infants and children. A study of 81 cases diagnosed in Finland and Sweden. Ann. Chir. Gynecol. **60:** 1–60.
11. LUCRAFT, H., J. R. MANN & V. PEARSON. 1980. Malignant ovarian tumors in children. Adv. Biopsy **26:** 97–114.
12. JUNAID, T. A. 1981. Ovarian neoplasms in children and adolescents in Ibadan, Nigeria. Cancer **47:** 610–614.
13. YAKUSHI, M., T. MATSUKUMA, M. ABE, T. MINISHIDA, H. NISHIMURA, A. TSUNAWAKI & T. KATO. 1981. Ovarian tumors in adolescents less than 20 years of age. Acta Obstet. Gynecol. Jpn. **33:** 833–838.
14. EHREM, I. M., G. H. MAHOUR & H. ISAACS. 1984. Benign and malignant ovarian tumors in children and adolescents. Am. J. Surg. **147:** 339–344.
15. SEGUPTA, S. K. & V. J. EVERETT. 1987. Ovarian neoplasms in children and adolescents in Papua New Guinea. Aust. N. Z. Obstet. Gynecol. **27:** 3235–3238.
16. SHAWIS, R. N., E. L. GOHARY & R. C. COOK. 1985. Ovarian cysts and tumors in infancy and childhood. Ann. R. Cool. Surg. **67:** 17–19.
17. CRONEN, R. W. & H. S. NAGARAJ. 1988. Ovarian tumors in children. South. Med. J. **81:** 464–468.
18. SCHWOBEL, M. G. & U. G. STAUFFER. 1991. Surgical treatment of ovarian tumors in childhood. Progr. Ped. Surg. **26:** 112–123.
19. GRIBBON, M., S. H. EIN & K. MANCER. 1992. Pediatric malignant ovarian tumors: A 43-year review. J. Ped. Surg. **27:** 480–484.
20. HART, W. R. 1992. Pathology of malignant and borderline epithelial tumors of ovary. *In* Gynecologic Oncology. M. Copplesson, Ed. Vol. 2: 863–887. Churchill Livingstone. Melbourne.
21. DEPREST, J., P. MOERMAN, P. CORNELLIE & P. IDE. 1992. Case report. Ovarian borderline mucinous tumor in a premenarchial girl. Review of ovarian epithelial cancer in young girls. Gynecol. Oncol. **45:** 219–224.
22. MORRIS, H. B., C. VECCHIA & G. L. DRAPER. 1984. Malignant epithelial tumors of the ovary in childhood. A clinicopathological study of 13 cases in Great Britain. Gynecol. Oncol. **19:** 290–297.
23. SCULLY, R. E., P. AGUIRRE & R. A. DE LELLIS. 1984. Argyrophilia serotonin and peptide hormones in the female genital tract and its tumors. Int. J. Gynecol. Pathol. **3:** 51–70.
24. VAN NAGEL, J. R., E. S. DONALDSON, E. C. GAY, R. M. C. SHARKEY, P. RAYBURN & D. M. GOLDENBERG. 1978. Carcinoembryonic antigen in ovarian epithelial cystadenocarcinomas: The prognostic value of tumor and serial plasma determinations. Cancer **41:** 2335.
25. CHARPIN, C., A. K. BHAN, U. R. ZURAWSKI & R. E. SCULLY. 1982. Carcinoembryonic antigen (CEA) and carbohydrate determinant 19-9 (Ca 19-9) localization in 121 primary and metastatic ovarian tumors. An immunohistochemical study with the use of monoclonal antibodies. Int. J. Gynecol. Pathol. **1:** 231.
26. MAGGINO, T., E. SARTORI, F. LANDONI, *et al.* 1995. Reduction in radicality in early stages ovarian carcinoma, with the possibility of preserving fertility. 5th Meeting of the IGCS. Int. J. Gyn. Cancer **5:** 25. (Abstr.).
27. PETTERSON, F. 1994. Annual report on the results of treatment in gynecological cancer. International Federation of Gynecology and Obstetrics. Vol. 22. Stockholm.
28. JULLIAN, C. G. & J. D. WOODRUFF. 1973. The biologic behavior of low grade papillary serous carcinoma of the ovary. Obstet. Gynecol. **40:** 860.
29. KATZENSTEIN, A. A., M. T. MAZUR, T. E. MORGAN & M. KAO. 1978. Proliferative serous tumors of the ovary. Histologic features and prognosis. Am. J. Surg. Pathol. **2:** 339.
30. RUSSELL, P. 1979. The pathological assessment of ovarian neoplasms. I. Introduction to the common epithelial tumors and analysis of "benign" epithelial tumors. Pathology **11:** 5.

31. Bostwick, D. G., H. D. Tazelaar, S. C. Ballin, M. R. Hendrickson & R. L. Kempson. 1986. Ovarian epithelial tumors of borderline malignancy: A clinical and pathologic study of 109 cases. Cancer **58:** 2052.
32. Hart, W. R. & H. J. Norris. 1973. Borderline and malignant mucinous tumors of the ovary: Histologic criteria and clinical behavior. Cancer **31:** 1031.
33. Koern, J., C. G. Trope & V. M. Abeler. 1993. A retrospective study of 370 borderline tumors of the ovary treated at the Norwegian Radium Hospital from 1970 to 1982. Cancer **71:** 1810–1820.
34. Norris, H. J. & R. D. Jensen. 1972. Relative frequency of ovarian neoplasms in children and adolescents. Cancer **30:** 713.
35. Gershenson, D. M. 1992. Malignant germ cell tumors of the ovary: Clinical features and management. *In* Gynecologic Oncology. M. Coppleson, Ed. Vol. 2: 935–945. Churchill Livingstone. Melbourne.
36. Berek, J. S. & N. F. Hacker. 1994. Nonepithelial ovarian and fallopian tube cancers. *In* Practical Gynecologic Oncology. J. S. Berek & N. F. Hacker, Eds. Vol. 1: 377. Williams and Wilkins. London.
37. Piver, S., J. Fanning & K. A. Craig. 1993. Ovarian cancer. *In* Gynecologic Oncology. R. C. Knapp & R. S. Berkowitz, Eds. Vol. 1: 250. McGraw-Hill. New York.
38. Kurman, R. J. & H. J. Norris. 1977. Malignant germ cell tumors of the ovary. Hum. Pathol. **8:** 551.
39. Slayton, R. E., R. C. Park, S. G. Silverberg, H. Shingleton, W. T. Creasman & J. A. Blessing. 1985. Vincristine, dacktinomycin and cyclophosphamide in the treatment of malignant germ cell tumors of the ovary. A Gynecologic Oncology Group Study (a final report). Cancer **56:** 243.
40. Gershenson, D. M., M. Morris, A. Cangir, J. Kavanagh, C. A. Stringer, C. L. Edwards, E. G. Silva & J. T. Wharton. 1990. Treatment of malignant germ cell tumors of the ovary with Bleomycin, Etoposide and Cisplatin. J. Clin. Oncol. **8:** 715–720.
41. Norris, H. J., H. J. Zirkin & W. L. Benson. 1976. Immature (malignant) teratoma of the ovary. A clinical and pathologic study of 58 cases. Cancer **37:** 2359.
42. Mangioni, C., C. Bonazzi, F. Peccatori, A. Pelegrino, S. Chiari & M. R. Pittelli. 1993. Nongerminomatous ovarian germ cell tumors: Conservative surgery and fertility. Int. J. Gynecol. Cancer **3:** 33. (Abstr.).
43. Scully, R. E. 1977. Ovarian tumors. Am. J. Pathol. **87:** 686.
44. Hoskins, W. J. & S. C. Rubin. 1992. Malignant gonadal stromal tumors of the ovary: Clinical features and management. *In* Gynecologic Oncology. M. Coppleson, Ed. Vol. 2: 961–970. Churchill Livingstone. Melbourne.
45. Colombo, N., C. Sessa, F. Landoni, E. Sartori, S. Pecorelli & E. Mangioni. 1986. Cisplatin, Vincristine and Bleomycin combination chemotherapy in metastatic granulosa cell tumor of the ovary. Obstet. Gynecol. **67:** 265.
46. Tavassoli, F. A. & H. J. Norris. 1980. Sertoli tumors of the ovary. A clinical study of 28 cases with ultra structural observations. Cancer **46:** 2281.
47. Zaloudek, C. & H. J. Norris. 1984. Sertoli–Leydig tumors of the ovary. A clinicopathologic study of 64 intermediate and poorly differentiated neoplasms. Am. J. Surg. Pathol. **8:** 409.
48. Scully, R. E. 1970. Sex cord tumors with annular tubules: A distinctive ovarian tumor of the Peutz-Jeghers syndrome. Cancer **25:** 1107.

Oncogenes and Onco-suppressor Genes in Female Genital Cancer

M. KOFFA AND D. A. SPANDIDOS[a]

Institute of Biological Research and Biotechnology
National Hellenic Research Foundation
Athens 11635, Greece
Laboratory of Virology
Medical School, University of Crete
Heraklion, Greece

INTRODUCTION

Oncogene or onco-suppressor gene activation in human cancer can result from increased gene copy number or structural changes, leading to increased expression of the gene product or production of an altered protein, respectively. Structural changes may take the form of point mutations or rearrangements, the latter usually resulting from chromosomal aberrations such as translocations and inversions. Changes resulting in increased gene expression include gene amplification, enhanced transcription or translation, and mRNA or protein stabilization.

Recently, another genetic alteration, microsatellite instability (MI), related to defects in the DNA repair system and manifested through the alteration of DNA repeat size, has been reported in some familial and sporadic tumors, including ovarian and endometrial tumors.[1,2]

Cervical cancer is widely regarded as a sexually transmitted disease, associated with human papilloma virus (HPV) infection, as well as with other sexually transmitted agents. Increased risk of developing this disease is associated with low socioeconomic status, early age at first coitus, multiple sexual partners, and multiple deliveries. Carcinoma of the uterine endometrium is the most frequent diagnosed gynecological malignancy in the Western world; nevertheless, it causes only 13% of all gynecological cancer deaths, owing to early diagnosis. On the basis of an analysis of the age-specific incidence of endometrial cancers, Renan[3] suggested that six genetic alterations are required for tumor formation. Ovarian carcinoma is the fourth commonest cancer in women and represents the most frequent cause of death from gynecological cancer.

Studies of these types of malignancies revealed involvement of several oncogenes and onco-suppressor genes (TABLE 1), some of them having prognostic significance (TABLE 2). In this review the involvement of such genes in cervical, endometrial, and ovarian carcinomas is considered.

[a]Address for correspondence: Institute of Biological Research and Biotechnology, National Hellenic Research Foundation, 48 Vas. Constantinou Ave., Athens 11635, Greece.

TABLE 1. Oncogenes and Onco-suppressor Genes Involved in Gynecological Cancer and Rate of Aberration

Genes	Cervical Cancer (%)	Ref. No.	Endometrial Cancer (%)	Ref. No.	Ovarian Cancer (%)	Ref. No.
Oncogenes						
ras	24.1	7	12-34	21, 22, 27	0–15.4	7,57
myc	38.7	12				
c-*erbB*-2			14	33	21.7	39
FGF-3/INT-2			14	33	10	38
akt-2					12.1	40
Onco-suppressor genes						
p53			32–73	34, 35	43–48	51, 58
DCC	30	54				
*BRCA*1					67	44

ONCOGENES AND ONCO-SUPPRESSOR GENES IN CERVICAL CANCER

Oncogenes

Activation of *ras* proto-oncogenes by point mutations has been detected in a number of tumors with a frequency that depends on the type of tumor[4]; most frequently, it is found in carcinomas of the pancreas (up to 90% of the tumors).[5] Mutations in the *ras* gene family have been reported less frequently in gynecological malignancies and mostly occur in codon 12 of the K-*ras* rather than 13 or 61 of K-*ras* or codons 12, 13,

TABLE 2. Genes with Prognostic Significance for Cervival, Endometrial, and Ovarian Cancer[a]

Gene Aberration Involved	Cervical Cancer	Endometrial Cancer	Ovarian Cancer
c-*erbB*-2 overexpression	Poor prognosis[12]	Advanced stage disease[29,30]	Shorter survival times[39]
c-*myc* amplification	Poor prognosis[9]	Advanced stage disease[31]	
ras mutations		Poor clinical outcome[23,24]	
c-*fms* overexpression		High-risk tumor[32]	
p53 overexpression, outcomemutations, LOH		Poor prognosis[34,35]	Poor prognosis[51]
FGF-3/INT-2		Advanced stage disease[33]	Aggressiveness of the disease[38]
akt-2 amplification			Poor prognosis[40]
*BRCA*1 mutations, LOH			Susceptibility[41,42]

[a]Superscript numbers refer to references.

and 61 of H-*ras* or N-*ras*, with the exception of squamous cell carcinomas of the cervix, in which mutations of H-*ras* have been reported in 11%.[6] Moreover, in our recent study focusing on the Greek population, mutations of the K-*ras* (28.1%), as well as H-*ras* (6.5%) and N-*ras* genes (6.9%), were detected. *ras* Gene mutations were also found in benign precursors (5.4%), suggesting a possible role in the initial stages of cervical carcinogenesis that contributes to their transition to more advanced lesions. The simultaneous presence of *ras* gene mutations and high-risk HPV DNA was also detected in 29% of the cases examined, suggesting a possible cooperation between *ras* activation and HPV infection in cervical cancer.[7] Although the role of HPV oncogenes E_6/E_7 is well established in cellular transformation, other viruses, such as CMV and HSV, are also implicated in cervical carcinogenesis, specifically in HPV-negative tumors.[8]

Overexpression of the c-*myc* oncogene, which codes for a DNA-binding protein and is believed to regulate cellular proliferation, has been associated with poor prognosis in patients with cervical cancer.[9] Alterations in *fos* expression, which appear to be an important facet of epidermal differentiation *in vivo*, could also contribute to the malignant progression of HPV-immortalized cells.[10]

The oncogene c-*erbB*-2 is located on chromosome 17 and encodes a membrane phosphoglycoprotein of 185 kDa.[11] Although the function of this protein is unknown, it has tyrosine-kinase activity and may act as a cell growth–regulating receptor. It has been suggested that overexpression of the c-*erbB*-2 protein could serve as a prognostic marker in cervical carcinomas and may help identify those patients for whom early adjuvant treatment might be beneficial.[12]

Amplification of MDM-2 has been reported in cervical cell lines as well as in carcinomas,[13] providing an alternative mechanism of p53 inactivation in HPV-negative primary cervical carcinoma. MDM-2 is a negative regulator of p53 protein activity, whereas p53 itself can stimulate MDM-2 expression, thus forming an MDM-2-p53 autoregulatory feedback loop.[14]

Onco-suppressor Genes

Mutations of the p53 tumor suppressor gene to date have been the most commonly found genetic alterations in human malignancies,[15] with the vast majority of the mutations occurring in the highly conserved exons 5–8.[16] Wild-type (wt) p53 protein can act as a positive and negative transcription factor, recognizing specific DNA sequences adjacent to p53-responsive genes[17,18] and inducing G1 growth arrest and apoptosis after DNA damage.[19]

p53 inactivation by mutations or deletions has been reported in cervical carcinomas,[13] whereas inactivation of the gene can also occur through HPV infection or amplification of MDM-2.[20]

ONCOGENES AND ONCO-SUPPRESSOR GENES IN ENDOMETRIAL CANCER

Oncogenes

The incidence of *ras* gene point mutations reported in endometrial carcinomas varies between 10 and 37%,[21,22] whereas its prognostic significance remains uncertain. It has been suggested that K-*ras* proto-oncogene activation plays an important role in determining the aggressiveness of endometrial carcinomas[23] and correlates with lymph node metastases,[24] whereas other investigators have reported the opposite.[25] Recently, *ras* oncogene activation has been found in endometrial hyperplasias, suggesting an involvement at the early stages of carcinogenesis.[26]

In a recent study of ours in endometrial carcinomas (unpublished data), point mutations at codon 12 of the K-*ras* (14.5%) as well as H-*ras* (7.3%) gene were detected, although activation of the H-*ras* gene has not been frequently reported. The *ras* gene activation occurs at a relatively lower frequency (21.8%) in endometrial carcinomas obtained from the Greek as compared to the Japanese population (30%),[27] probably due to different epidemiological and clinical characteristics.[25,28] Further work should demonstrate a correlation between geographic and ethnic differences, which may be of importance in epidemiological studies.

Other oncogenes that seem to be involved in endometrial carcinomas and have a prognostic significance are the c-*erbB*-2, *myc*, and *fms*. The overexpression of c-*erbB*-2 and *myc* oncogenes is often observed in patients with advanced stage disease and deep myometrial invasion.[29–31] Overexpression of the c-*fms* in endometrial cancer, a proto-oncogene that codes for the colony-stimulating factor-1 (CSF-1) receptor, may delineate a group of high-risk tumors.[32] Moreover, amplification of FGF-3/INT-2 detected in 14% of endometrial carcinomas was found to be associated with the advanced stages of disease in the endometrial tumorigenesis.[33]

Onco-suppressor Genes

p53 inactivation by mutations or deletions has been reported to serve as a prognostic indicator[34] in endometrial carcinomas. Overexpression of p53 is correlated with decreased survival in patients with uterine papillary serous carcinoma.[35] Mxi1, a tumor suppressor gene on 10q24-25, might also be involved in the development or progression of endometrial cancers. The gene encodes the MXI1 transcription factor, acting as a negative regulator of *myc* function.[36]

ONCOGENES AND ONCO-SUPPRESSOR GENES IN OVARIAN CARCINOMAS

It has been suggested that, although *ras* gene appears to play a minor role in the pathogenesis of invasive ovarian carcinomas, it might be more important in borderline ovarian tumors that exhibit low malignant potential.[37] In our study we found codon 12 point mutations in only 13% of invasive ovarian carcinomas.[7] INT-2 amplification in 10% of the ovarian carcinomas has been found to correlate with the aggressiveness of the disease.[38]

Patients with c-*erbB*-2 overexpression have a more advanced stage of disease, worse response to chemotherapy, and shorter survival time.[39] Moreover, ovarian cancer patients with *akt*-2 alterations appear to have a poor prognosis. It has been reported that amplification of *akt*-2 was especially frequent in undifferentiated tumors, suggesting that *akt*-2 alterations may be associated with tumor aggressiveness.[40] *akt*-

2 oncogene maps to 19q13.1-q13.2, encodes a serine–threonine protein kinase related to protein kinase C, and is one of the human cellular homologues of v-*akt*, the transduced oncogene of the AKT8 retrovirus, which induces lymphomas in mice.

Onco-suppressor Genes

In familial breast and ovarian cancers, a linkage has been demonstrated with the putative tumor suppressor gene *BRCA1* mapped on 17q12-q23. Women who carry mutations in the *BRCA1* gene have a 60% risk of ovarian cancer. Five to ten percent of ovarian carcinomas are reported to result from hereditary predisposition, with the germline inheritence of a mutation conferring autosomal dominant susceptibility.[41,42] However, detailed mapping studies[43] seem to indicate that the deleted 17q portion in sporadic ovarian cancers is associated with a distinct tumor suppressor gene.[44] *nm23*-H1 is located on the long arm of chromosome 17 and has been proposed as a metastasis suppressor gene.[45] The *nm23*-H1 and *nm23*-H2 gene products correspond to the human nucleoside diphosphate kinase A and B subunits, respectively. Although the exact mechanism underlying the supposed *nm23*-related metastatic suppression remains unknown, several distinct intracellular functions of *nm23*-nucleoside diphosphate kinase could influence the metastatic process: microtubule assembly, signal transduction, transcription regulation, and cellular adhesion.[46] It has been suggested that *nm23*-H1 gene product may exert an inhibitory effect on the lymphatic dissemination of human ovarian tumors. However, several other factors, biological as well as time and patient dependent, influence the complex metastatic progression of ovarian tumors and may cooperate with *nm23*-H1 in the promotion or inhibition of this process.[47]

It was recently reported that an inhibitor (p16/CDKN2) of cyclin D/cyclin-dependent kinase 4 complexes maps to 9p21 and is homozygously deleted in nearly 30% of ovarian cancer cell lines.[48] Other studies report infrequent observation of alterations in gene dosage, however, casting doubt on the involvement of CDKN2 in the pathogenesis of ovarian cancer.[49]

p53 abnormalities seem to be early events in epithelial carcinomas,[50] and they can serve as a marker of poor prognosis in a subset of patients with ovarian cancer,[51] although p53 mutations have also been found in borderline ovarian tumors.[52] However, alterations of the p53 gene may not be associated with the pathogenesis of ovarian germ cell tumors.[53] Relatively little is known of the molecular events that are associated with the development of such tumors, because most of the studies on ovarian cancer are focused on the epithelial carcinomas.

CHROMOSOME ABNORMALITIES

The presence of consistent chromosomal losses or deletions has suggested the involvement of known or candidate tumor suppressor genes at these locations. The detection of frequent loss of sequences from the long arm of chromosome 10 suggests the presence of a tumor suppressor gene important in endometrial tumorigenesis.[2] DCC allelic loss on chromosome 18q has been found in 30% of endometrial carcinomas.[54] Moreover, an additional genetic defect between chromosome 17p13.1 and 17p13.3, a telomeric region near the p53 gene, may have clinical implications, and other rogue genes in this region might be a topic of interest for future studies into the origin of human endometrial carcinoma.[34]

Studies on loss of heterozygosity have demonstrated a high incidence of chromosome 17q loss, indicating that one or more putative tumor suppressor genes, possibly implicated in ovarian carcinogenesis, might be located on this chromosomal arm. Loss of function of 17q located genes may be responsible for the frequent, rapid progression of ovarian carcinomas to an advanced stage.[43,55] Moreover, studies on chromosome 6q revealed a sharp contrast in the pattern of LOH between invasive and borderline ovarian tumors.[56]

CONCLUDING REMARKS

Further detailed studies are required to probe the relationships between mutations and factors such as genetic predisposition, prognosis, and diagnosis. Moreover, the most plausible strategy for cancer therapy is to learn how to induce such cells to commit suicide or how to eliminate them, preferentially by chemical or immunologic means. The need to apply our basic knowledge of oncogenes and onco-suppressor genes to more creative clinical applications, particularly in risk assessment and evaluation of new and existing drug therapies is stressed.

SUMMARY

Cancer is a multistep process resulting in the accumulation of genetic lesions in proto-oncogenes or tumor suppressor genes. In recent years, many biological studies have focused on the analysis of the genetic and molecular events occurring in genital tumors in order to identify genes involved in their initiation and progression. Understanding the genetic events that lead to initiation and progression of a disease remains an important challenge in gynecological research and ultimately may enable the development of better approaches for earlier diagnosis, in cases where current therapeutic strategies have a high cure rate.

REFERENCES

1. Risinger, J. I., A. Berchuck, M. F. Kohler, P. Watson, H. T. Lynch & J. Boyd. 1993. Genetic instability of microsatellites in endometrial carcinoma. Cancer Res. **53:** 5100–5103.
2. Peiffer, S. L., T. J. Herzog, D. J. Tribune, D. G. Mutch, D. J. Gersell & P. J. Goodfellow. 1995. Allelic loss of sequences from the long arm of chromosome 10 and replication errors in endometrial cancers. Cancer Res. **55:** 1922–1926.
3. Renan, M. J. 1993. How many mutations are required for tumorigenesis? Implications from the human cancer data. Mol. Carcinog. **7:** 139–146.
4. Spandidos, D. A., Ed. 1991. The superfamily of *ras* related genes. Plenum Press. New York and London. pp. 1–338.

5. CALDAS, C., S. A. HAHN, R. H. HRUBAN, M. S. REDSTON, C. J. YEO & S. E. KERN. 1994. Detection of K-*ras* mutations in the stools of patients with pancreatic adenocarcinoma and pancreatic ductal hyperplasia. Cancer Res. **54:** 3568–3573.
6. RIOU, G., M. BARROIS, Z.-M. SHENZ, P. DUVILLARD & C. LHOMME. 1988. Somatic deletions and mutations of c-Ha-*ras* gene in human cervical cancers. Oncogene **3:** 329–333.
7. KOFFA, M., E. KOUMANTAKIS, M. ERGAZAKI, V. MALAMOU-MITSI & D. A. SPANDIDOS. 1994. Detection of *ras* gene mutations and HPV in lesions of the human female reproductive tract. Int. J. Oncol. **5:** 189–195.
8. KOFFA, M., E. KOUMANTAKIS, M. ERGAZAKI, C. TSATSANIS & D. A. SPANDIDOS. 1995. Association of herpesvirus infection with the development of genital cancer. Int. J. Cancer **63:** 58–62.
9. RIOU, G., M. G. LÊ, M. FAVRE, D. JEANNEL, J. BOURHIS & G. ORTH. 1992. Human papillomavirus-negative status and c-*myc* gene overexpression: Independent prognostic indicators of distant metastasis for early-stage invasive cervical cancers. J. Natl. Cancer Inst. **84:** 1525–1526.
10. PEI, X. F., J. M. MECK, D. GREENHALGH & R. SCHLEGEL. 1993. Co-transfection of HPV-18 and v-*fos* DAN induces tumorigenicity of primary human keratinocytes. Virology **196:** 855–860.
11. PADHY, L. C., C. SHIH, D. COWING, R. FINKELSTIEN & R. A. WEINBERG. 1982. Identification of a phosphoprotein specifically induced by the transforming DNA of rat neuroblastomas. Cell **28:** 865–871.
12. HALE, R. J., C. H. BUCKLEY, H. FOX & J. WILLIAMS. 1992. Prognostic value of c-*erbB*-2 expression in uterine cervical carcinoma. J. Clin. Pathol. **45:** 594–596.
13. IKENBERG, H., K. MATTHAY, B. SCHMITT, T. BAUKNECHT, M. KIECHLE-SCHWARZ, A. GÖPPINGER & A. PFLEIDERER. 1995. P53 mutations and MDM-2 amplification are rare events in human papillomavirus-negative cervical carcinomas. Cancer **76:** 57–66.
14. BARAK, Y., T. JUVEN, R. HAFFNER & M. OREN. 1993. mdm-2 Expression is induced by wild-type p53 activity. EMBO J. **12:** 461–468.
15. HOLLSTEIN, M., D. SIDRANSKY, B. VOGELSTEIN & C. C. HARRIS. 1991. p53 Mutations in human cancers. Science **253:** 49–53.
16. HARRIS, C. & M. HOLLSTEIN. 1993. Clinical implications of the p53 tumor-suppressor gene. **329:** 1318–1327.
17. VOGELSTEIN, B. & K. KINZLER. 1992. p53 Function and dysfunction. Cell **70:** 523–526.
18. MACK, D., J. VARTIKAR, J. PIPAS & L. LAIMINS. 1993. Specific repression of TATA-mediated but not initiator-mediated transcription by wild-type p53. Nature **363:** 281–283.
19. CLARKE, A., C. PURDIE, D. HARRISON, *et al.* 1993. Thymocyte apoptosis induced by p53-dependent and independent pathways. Nature **362:** 849–852.
20. SCHEFFNER, M., B. WERNESS, J. HUIBREGTSE, A. LEVINE & P. HOWLEY. 1990. The E6 oncoprotein encoded by human papillomavirus types 16 and 18 promotes the degradation of p53. Cell **63:** 1129–1136.
21. CADUFF, R. F., C. M. JOHNSTON & T. S. FRANK. 1995. Mutations of the Ki-*ras* oncogene in carcinoma of the endometrium. Am. J. Pathol. **146:** 182–188.
22. IGNAR-TROWBRIDGE, D., J. I. RISINGER, G. A. DENT, M. KOHLER, A. BERCHUCK, J. A. MCLACHLAN & J. BOYD. 1992. Mutations of the Ki-*ras* oncogene in endometrial carcinoma. Am. J. Obstet. Gynecol. **167:** 227–232.
23. MIZUUCHI, H., S. NASIM, R. KUDO, S. G. SILVERBERG, S. GREENHOUSE & C. T. GARRETT. 1992. Clinical implications of K-*ras* mutations in maligmant epithelial tumors of the endometrium. Cancer Res. **52:** 2777–2781.
24. FUJIMOTO, I., Y. SHIMIZU, Y. HIRAI, J. T. CHEN, H. TESHIMA, K. HASUMI, K. MASUBUCHI & M. TAKAHASHI. 1993. Studies on *Ras* oncogene activation in endometrial carcinoma. Gynecol. Oncol. **48:** 196–202.
25. SASAKI, H., H. NISHII, H. TAKAHASHI, A. TADA, M. FURUSATO, Y. TERASHIMA, G. P. SIEGAL,

S. L. PARKER, M. F. KOHLER, A. BERCHUCK & J. BOYD. 1993. Mutation of the Ki-*ras* protooncogene in human endometrial hyperplasia and carcinoma. Cancer Res. **53:** 1906–1910.

26. DUGGAN, B. D., J. C. FELIX, L. I. MUDERSPACH, J. L. TSAO & D. K. SHIBATA. 1994. Early mutational activation of the c-Ki-*ras* oncogene in endometrial carcinoma. Cancer Res. **54:** 1604–1607.
27. ENOMOTO, T., M. INOUE, A. O. PERANTONI, G. S. BUZARD, H. MIKI, O. TANIZAWA & J. M. RICE. 1991. K-*ras* activation in premalignant and malignant epithelial lesions of the human uterus. Cancer Res. **51:** 5308–5314.
28. ENOMOTO, T., M. FUJITA, M. INOUE, T. NOMURA & K. R. SHROYER. 1995. Alteration of the p53 tumor suppressor gene and activation of c-K-*ras*-2 protooncogene in endometrial adenocarcinoma from Colorado. Am. J. Clin. Pathol. **103:** 224–230.
29. KHALIFA, M. A., R. S. MANNEL, S. D. HARAWAY, J. WALKER & K.-W. MIN. 1994. Expression of EGFR, HER-2 /neu, P53, and PCNA in endometrioid serous papillary, and clear cell endometrial adenocarcinomas. Gynecol. Oncol. **53:** 84–92.
30. BERCHUCK, A., G. RODRIGUEZ, R. B. KINNEY, J. T. SOPER, R. K. DODGE, D. L. CLARKE-PEARSON & R. C. BAST. 1991. Overexpression of HER-2/*neu* in endometrial cancer is associated with advanced stage disease. Am. J. Obstet. Gynecol. **164:** 15–21.
31. BORST, M. P., V. V. BAKER, D. DIXON, K. D. HATCH, H. M. SHINGLETON & D. M. MILLER. 1990. Oncogene alteration in endometrial carcinoma. Gynecol. Oncol. **38:** 364–366.
32. LEISEROWITZ, G. S., S. A. HARRIS, M. SUBRAMANIAM, G. L. KEENEY, K. C. PODRATZ & T. C. SPELSBERG. 1993. The proto-oncogene *c-fms* is overexpressed in endometrial cancer. Gynecol. Oncol. **49:** 190–196.
33. ESTELLER M., A. GARCIA, J. M. MARTINEZ, I. PALONES, A. CABERO & J. REVENTOS. 1995. Detection of c-*erbB*-2/neu and fibroblast growth factor -3/INT-2 but not epidermal growth factor receptor gene amplification in endometrial cancer by differential polymerase chain reaction. Cancer **75:** 2139–2146.
34. KIHANA, T., K. HAMADA, Y. INOUE, N. YANO, H. IKETANI, S.-I MURZO, M. UKITA & S. MATSUURA. 1995. Mutation and allelic loss of the p53 gene in endometrial carcinoma. Cancer **76:** 72–78.
35. KING, S. A., A. A. ADAS, V. A. LIVOLSI, H. TAKAHASHI, K. BEHBAKHT, P. MCGOVERN, I. BENJAMIN, S. C. RUBIN & J. BOYD. 1995. Expression and mutation analysis of the p53 gene in uterine papillary serous carcinoma. Cancer **75:** 2700–2705.
36. ZERVOS, A., J. GYURIS & R. BRENT. 1993. Mxi1, a protein that specifically interacts with Max to bind Myc-Max recognition sites. Cell **71:** 223–232.
37. MOK, S. C., D. A. BELL, R. C. KNAPP, P. M. FISHBAUGH, W. R. WELCH, M. G. MUTO, R. S. BERKOWITZ & S. W. TSAO. 1993. Mutation of K-*ras* proto-oncogene in human ovarian epithelial tumors of borderline malignancy. Cancer Res. **53:** 1489–1492.
38. ROSEN, A., P. SEVELDA, M. KLEIN, K. DOBIANER, C. HRUZA, K. CZERWENKA, *et al.* 1993. First experience with FGF-3 (INT-2) amplification in women with epithelial ovarian cancer. Br. J. Cancer **67:** 1122–1125.
39. FELIP, E., J. M. DEL CAMPO, D. RUBIO, M. T. VIDAL, R. COLOMER & B. BERMEJO. 1995. Overexpression of c-*erbB*-2 in epithelial ovarian cancer. Cancer **75:** 2147–2152.
40. BELLACOSA, A., D. DEFEO, A. K. GODWIN, D. W. BELL, J. Q. CHENG, D. A. ALTOMARE, M. WAN, L. DUBEAU, G. SCAMBIA, V. MASCIULLO, G. FERRANDINA, P. BENEDETTI PANICI, S. MANCUSO, G. NERI & J. R. TESTA. 1995. Molecular alterations of the *akt*-2 oncogene in ovarian and breast carcinomas. Int. J. Cancer (Pred. Oncol.) **64:** 280–285.
41. HALL, J. M., M. K. LEE, B. NEWMAN, J. E. MORROW, L. A. ANDERSON, B. HUEY & M.-C. KING. 1990. Linkage of early onset familial breast cancer to chromosome 17q21. Science **250:** 1684–1689.
42. FUTREAL, P. A., Q. LIU, D. SHATTUCK-EIDENS, *et al.* 1994. *BRCA*1 mutations in primary breast and ovarian carcinomas. Science **266:** 120–122.

43. YANG FENG, T. L., H. HAN, K. C. CHEN, S. B. LI, E. B. CLAUS, M. L. CARCANGIU, S. K. CHAMBERS, J. T. CHAMBERS & P. E. SCHWARTZ. 1993. Allelic loss in ovarian cancer. Int. J. Cancer **54:** 546–551.
44. TAKAHASHI, H., K. BEHBAKHT, P. E. MCGOVERN, *et al.* 1995. Mutation analysis of the *BRCA*1 gene in ovarian cancers. Cancer Res. **55:** 2998–3002.
45. STEEG, P. S., G. BEVILACQUA, L. KOPPER, U. P. THORGEIRSSON, J. E. TALMADGE, L. A. LIOTTA & M. E. SOBEL. 1988. Evidence for a novel gene associated with low tumor metastatic potential. J. Natl. Cancer Inst. **80:** 200–204.
46. POSTEL, E. H., S. J. BERBERICH, S. J. FLINT & C. A. FERRONE. 1993. Human c-*myc* transcription factor PuF identified as nm23-H2 nucleoside diphosphate kinase, a candidate suppressor of tumor metastasis [see comments]. Science **261:** 478–480.
47. VIEL, L., L. DALL' AGNESE, V. CANZONIERI, F. SOPRACORDEVOLE, E. CAPOZZI, A. CARBONE, M. C. VISENTIN & M. BOIOCCHI. 1995. Suppressive role of the metastasis related *nm23*-H1 gene in human ovarian carcinomas: Association of high messenger RNA expression with lack of lymph node metastasis. Cancer Res. **55:** 2645–2650.
48. KAMB, A., N. A. GRUIS, J. WEAVER-FELDHAUS, Q. LIU, K. HARSHMAN, S. V. TAVTIGIAN, E. STOCKERT, R. S. DAY, B. E. JOHNSON & M. H. SKOLNICK. 1994. A cell cycle regulator potentially involved in genesis of many tumor types. Science **264:** 434–440.
49. SCHULTZ, D. C., L. VANDERVEER, K. H. BUETOW, M. P. BOENTE, R. F. OZOLS, T. C. HAMLTON & A. K. GODWIN. 1995. Characterization of chromosome 9 in human ovarian neoplasia identifies frequent genetic imbalance on 9q and rare alterations involving 9p, including CDKN2. Cancer Res. **55:** 2150–2157.
50. KUPRYJANCZYK, J., D. A. BELL, D. W. YANDELL, R. E. SCULLY & A. D. THOR. 1994. p53 Expression in ovarian borderline tumors and stage I carcinomas. Am. J. Clin. Pathol. **102:** 671–676.
51. LEVESQUE, M. A., D. KATSAROS, H. YU, P. ZOLA, P. SISMONDI, G. GIARDINA & E. P. DIAMANDIS. 1995. Mutant p53 protein overexpression is associated with poor outcome in patients with well or moderately differentiated ovarian carcinoma. Cancer **75:** 1327–1338.
52. WERTHEIM, I., M. MUTO, W. R. WELCH, D. A. BELL, R. S. BERKOWITZ & S. C. MOK. 1994. p53 Gene mutation in human borderline epithelial ovarian tumors. J. Natl. Cancer Inst. **86:** 1549–1551.
53. LIU, F.-S., E. S.-C. HO, J.-T. CHEN, R. T.-P. SHIH, C.-H. YANG & A. SHIH. 1995. Overexpression or mutation of the p53 tumor suppressor gene does not occur in malignant ovarian germ cell tumors. Cancer **76:** 291–295.
54. GIMA, T., H. KATO, T. HONDA, T. IMAMURA, T. SASAZUKI & N. WAKE. 1994. DCC gene alteration in human endometrial carcinomas. Int. J. Cancer **57:** 480–485.
55. SHENSON, D. L., H. H. GALLION, D. E. POWELL & M. PIERETTI. 1995. Loss of heterozygosity and genomic instability in synchronous endometrioid tumors of the ovary and endometrium. Cancer **76:** 650–657.
56. RODABAUGH, K. J., G. BLANCHARD, W. R. WELCH, D. A. BELL, R. S. BERKOWITZ & S. C. MOK. 1995. Detailed deletion mapping of chromosome 6q in borderline epithelial ovarian tumors. Cancer Res. **55:** 2169–2172.
57. ENOMOTO, T., M. INOUE, A. O. PERANTONI, N. TERAKAWA, O. TANIZAWA & J. M. RICE. 1990. K-*ras* activation in neoplasms of human female reproductive tract. Cancer Res. **50:** 6139–6145.
58. TENERIELLO, M. G., M. EBINA, R. I. LINNOILA, M. HENRY, J. D. NASH, R. C. PARK & M. J. BIRRER. 1993. p53 and Ki-*ras* gene mutations in epithelial ovarian neoplasms. Cancer Res. **53:** 3103–3108.

Oncogenic Role of the Y Chromosome

PAUL G. McDONOUGH

Department of Obstetrics and Gynecology
Medical College of Georgia
Augusta, Georgia 30912

The purpose of this presentation is to summarize our current knowledge concerning the molecular biology of cancer and reexamine the oncogenic potential of the Y chromosome in the light of this current information. The latter is an important question because it appears that the presence of any portion of the Y chromosome predisposes dysgenetic gonads to tumor formation. The two principal tumors that occur in persons with dysgenetic gonads are gonadoblastomas and dysgerminomas. These tumors occur in persons with 46,XY gonadal dysgenesis (Swyer's syndrome) and in persons with mosaic 45,X,46,XY karyotypes. The Y chromosome in mosaic individuals may be morphologically normal or morphologically abnormal. In some instances, it is not possible to identify the Y chromosome on the basis of morphology alone, and DNA analysis with Y-specific probes by Southern blotting and/or fluorescent *in situ* hybridization (FISH) are necessary. The association of Y DNA with these tumors in dysgenetic individuals has been a source of considerable discussion over the past decade. It is difficult to know if this association is related as causality or is simply a manifestation of a disordered pituitary gonadal axis in a person with a primitive, disorganized, dysgenetic gonad.

It is only in the last two years that a coherent theory of the etiology of human cancer has developed. Information gleaned through nucleic acid technology has enabled us to make dramatic improvements in our understanding of genetic predisposition to cancer.[1] Although an inherited component to human cancer has been recognized for many decades, the evidence for predisposition to cancer has historically been based on anecdotal reports of families with unusually high numbers of cancer cases apparently consistent with Mendelian inheritance. Over the past decade, the genes for many of the clearly inherited cancer syndromes have been localized to chromosomal regions, usually by genetic linkage study, and more significantly a number of genes have been localized that are responsible for familial clustering of the more common cancers such as breast, ovarian, and colon cancer, for which the evidence of an inherited component was previously more equivocal.[2] As a result of these studies, it has become apparent that there are three fundamental mechanisms that give a cell a specific growth advantage and lead to uncontrolled cell growth and cancer.[3] These three mechanisms may be briefly categorized as (1) activation of proto-oncogenes, (2) inactivation of tumor suppressor genes, and (3) inactivation of mismatch repair genes.

PROTO-ONCOGENES

It has been apparent for at least two decades that there are many genes within the human genome that are involved in cell-signaling systems. These genes encode cell receptors, G-proteins, and other downstream proteins in the cell-signaling pathway. It has also become apparent that when such genes are constitutively active, they give a cell a significant growth advantage that can lead to malignancy.[4,5] A prototype for a proto-oncogene that is expressed in a time- and tissue-specific manner in man and, when constitutively active, causes cell transformation is the RET proto-oncogene. The RET proto-oncogene is a gene that maps to the long arm of the number 10 chromosome in man. The gene, when performing its normal function as a tyrosine kinase receptor, is activated only during early embryonic development. It appears that the protein encoded by this gene plays some role in the migration of neural crest cells into the thyroid gland and the migration of neural crest cells into sympathetic and enteric ganglion. Once the RET proto-oncogene has performed this function, it is turned off, and it is usually not expressed again throughout the person's life. The only exception to this is when mutations, particular missense mutations, occur within the RET proto-oncogenes that reactivate the gene, at which time it is expressed in a continuous fashion. This activation at the cellular level requires only a mutation in one allele of the RET gene. Consequently, the mutation is dominant in nature and activating in function because it confers upon the gene a continuous activation that gives to the cells in the thyroid gland a distinct growth advantage, leading to medullary thyroid carcinoma. Over 20% of the cases of medullary thyroid carcinoma are familial and due to dominant, activating mutations in the RET proto-oncogene that are transmitted through the germline of individuals. The majority of the activating mutations in the RET proto-oncogene occur within a single domain of this gene and are relatively easy to detect.[6] Consistent with the concept of a single hit necessary for tumor formation, individuals who do not inherit RET proto-oncogene mutations through the germline but acquire medullary thyroid carcinoma through a single somatic mutation in a cell in the thyroid gland have a similar type of mutation in the gene. As a result of these findings, it is possible to identify individuals at risk for medullary thyroid carcinoma by simply analyzing the RET proto-oncogene in lymphocytes of peripheral blood. All germline mutations can be identified in this fashion, whereas somatic mutations require the analysis of the medullary thyroid carcinomas for specific identification of the RET proto-oncogene mutation. In summary, the RET proto-oncogene mutation is a prototype for a dominant activating mutation that requires only a single allele to be mutated and maybe transmitted through the germline. In addition, the sporadic cases of medullary thyroid carcinoma have exactly the same type of mutations in the RET proto-oncogene. RET mutants provide a prototype for preclinical diagnosis and the identification of at-risk individuals early in life and prophylactically removing their thyroid glands.[7,8] This has now been done in over 30 families with familial medullary thyroid carcinoma.

TUMOR SUPPRESSOR GENES

The second mechanism whereby a cell can gain a growth advantage is the inactivation of a tumor suppressor gene. Perhaps the prototype gene for a tumor suppressor gene is the gene BRCA1 that is involved in familial breast–ovarian cancer syndromes.[9] Tumor suppressor genes function normally to limit or put a break on the normal cell cycle. It appears that they limit the transition of the cell from G-0 to G-1 under normal physiologic conditions. BRCA1 is a tumor suppressor gene that is involved in familial breast–ovarian cancer and maps to the proximal long arm of the number 17 chromosome in man.[10] Unlike the RET proto-oncogene, a single mutation in one allele of BRCA1 is not sufficient at the cellular level to provide a growth advantage for the cell. A growth advantage only occurs when the second allele at the same locus is lost or similarly mutated. Consequently, at the cellular level it does require two genetic hits for cancer to develop. Women with breast–ovarian cancer may inherit the first mutation through the germline and then acquire the second mutation or hit at the cellular level at some point during the life of the at-risk subject.[10,11] Viewed from this perspective, it is apparent that the mutations in BRCA1 are inactivating mutations, and mechanistically two distinct hits at the cellular level are necessary for tumor formation. For example, 5 to 8% of breast–ovarian cancers are familial in nature and occur as the result of a germline transmission of the first mutation in the BRCA1 proto-oncogene. Obviously, other persons with nonfamilial types of breast–ovarian cancer may acquire the first and the second hit as somatic mutations at some point in their lives. The BRCA1 gene has been isolated, and it is a large gene with apparently many mutations (up to 30) within the gene. At this juncture it is difficult to determine whether screening by analyzing peripheral or lymphocyte DNA will be a feasible method to determine at-risk individuals. It is possible that the gene is too large, and there are too many mutations to perform any type of analysis other than complete sequencing of the gene in each at-risk person. The latter may be cost prohibitive, and an alternative approach would involve protein analysis. It is apparent from most of the mutations that have been analyzed to date that they shorten or truncate the length of the protein product of BRCA1. It might be possible, therefore, to analyze the protein for this shortening or truncation rather than analyzing the gene itself. Time will tell whether this will be an effective method of screening for familial breast–ovarian cancer. Nevertheless, it does stand as a prototype for a tumor suppressor gene, and the mode of inheritance is recessive in the Mendelian sense.

MISMATCH REPAIR GENES (SPELL-CHECKER GENES)

The third mechanism for the development of cancer is unique in that it involves genes (MSH2, MLH1, PMS1, PMS2) that are involved in correcting DNA replication errors in the genome. The identification of these so-called mutator or spell-checker genes came about through an analysis of cancer cells in subjects with familial nonpolyposis colon cancer. It was apparent from the analysis of the DNA of these tumor cells that short, base-pair repeats (dinucleotide or trinucleotide repeats) had multiple mismatch errors and deletions of short runs of these microsatellite DNA strands. It was apparent that the gene or genes responsible for correcting these replication errors were not doing their job. Careful study of persons with familial nonpolyposis coli revealed a marker on the short arm of chromosome 2 and another marker on the short arm of chromosome 3 that appeared to segregate with this type of colon cancer. When the genes on each of these chromosomes were isolated and sequenced, it was apparent that they were homologous to repair genes that are present in bacteria and yeast. One of these genes (MSH2) had a base sequence that was almost identical to a well-known and well-characterized "spell-checker gene" in yeast.

It became apparent that individuals with colon cancer, because of inactivating mutations in these spell-checker genes, were unable to correct these replication errors. Consequently, over time the replication mistakes that were present in the DNA of colon cells reached a threshold that led to malignancy. Analysis of two of the four spell-checker genes to date reveals multiple different mutations in MSH2 and MLH1.[12] Nevertheless, people are working hard to develop a screening test that involves analysis of these spell-checker genes in order to identify persons at risk for familial colon cancer. At present, approximately 5 to 8% of colon cancers are familial in nature. It is also anticipated that perhaps more spell-checker genes will be found within the genome.[13]

It is clear that the identification of genes that predispose to cancer and the ability to test for them in at-risk individuals has posed a number of ethical problems. Unlike many genetic diseases, there is incomplete penetrance, and the carrying of the gene does not mean that the person has a 100% chance of developing cancer. It is hoped in the future that our ability to detect and predict cancer in a more accurate fashion at the genetic level will evolve. It is possible that other mechanisms may be identified that lead to cancer, but currently the roles of the proto-oncogenes, tumor suppressor genes, and mismatch repair genes are pivotal to our understanding of the molecular biology of the malignant process.

RELATIONSHIP OF CURRENT KNOWLEDGE TO THE ONCOGENIC POTENTIAL OF Y DNA

In trying to understand the oncogenic potential of the Y chromosome, it is important to point out the notable exceptions to this association. Approximately 90% of 46,XX sex-reversed males have Y DNA integrated into one of their X chromosomes. This integration occurs during paternal meiosis when a portion of the paternal Y, usually the region corresponding to the sex-determining gene (SRY), is translocated onto the paternal X chromosome.[14,15] If the translocated segment contains SRY and the sperm receiving the derivative X with YDNA participates in fertilization, then a 46,XX sex-reversed male is the outcome. In general, $46,XX^{+SRY}$ males do not develop any type of tumor in their hypoplastic, poorly developed testes. These males have testicular failure and azoospermia but do not develop testicular tumors. The second notable exception to the association between YDNA and tumor is normal individuals who carry a portion of the heterochromatic region of the long arm of the Y chromosome, which has been integrated into the short arm of one of the acrocentric chromosomes. The two most frequently involved autosomes are chromosome 15 and chromosome 22. It appears that these chromosomes have received this repetitive copy YDNA sometime during paternal meiosis. The Y chromosome in these persons is morphologically normal without any loss of the heterochromatic segment. This derivative autosome, which has additional Yq material, segregates in a normal way during meiosis and may be carried by females (46,XX) or males (46,XY). This additional Yq material does not have any adverse effect, and individuals carrying this additional material are not prone to dysgenetic tumors. The overall incidence of familial 15:Yq or 22:Yq derivative chromosomes segregating in a family is approximately one in 5,000 families. The 46,XX male and the familial transmission of Y heterochromatin are two exceptions to the association between YDNA and dysgenetic tumor. Alternatively, the absence of YDNA and the presence of dysgenetic tumor occurs rarely in 46,XX true hermaphrodites.[16] In these individuals, which are few in number, it appears that a type of degeneration resembling gonadoblastoma may occur within the ovotestes or ipsilateral testes of the 46,XX true hermaphrodite. The majority of true hermaphrodites studied to date do not have YDNA in their genome.

In those individuals such as 46,XY sex-reversed females (Swyers syndrome) and 45,X/46,XY individuals with a predisposition to tumor, it appears that the Yq11 region of the Y chromosome is the predisposing region.[17] Investigators suspect that a gene that has oncogenic potential resides within this region. There is no clear, unequivocal evidence at this time to confirm this hypothesis. Several investigators using probes for this region have attempted to hybridize these probes with the mRNAs of gonadoblastomas and dysgerminomas. The results remain uncertain and controversial. Studies done in our laboratory suggest that the SRY region is present in the majority of persons who develop dysgenetic tumors, but there are still exceptions to this finding.[17] It would appear that a specific portion of the Y chromosome cannot be clearly implicated at this time. Similarly, no proto-oncogenes, anti-proto-oncogenes, or mutator genes have been localized to the Y chromosome. It is possible that the association between YDNA and oncogenesis may have an underlying endocrine basis rather than relying entirely on the presence or absence of YDNA. It is conceivable that primitive germ cell elements migrate partially into these undifferentiated gonads, which are then subject to continuous gonadotropin stimulation. This combination during early childhood may set in place conditions that predispose an individual to cellular perforation and/or degeneration within these dysgenetic gonads. It is conceivable that now, with the current tools of molecular biology, the answer to this perplexing question of YDNA and tumor formation in dysgenetic individuals may be answered.

SUMMARY

The mechanism to explain the oncogenic role of genomic YDNA in dysgenetic individuals remains uncertain. At this time, it is a statistically significant association, but without a biological explanation.

REFERENCES

1. WEINBERG, R. A. 1991. Tumor suppressor genes. Science **254:** 1138–1146.
2. KNUDSON, A. G. 1993. All in the (cancer) family. Nature Genet. **5:** 103–104.
3. PETERS, J. A. 1994. Familial cancer risk (Part I: Impact on today's oncology practice). J. Oncol. Manage. **20:** 8–15.
4. COOPER, G. M. 1992. Oncogenes as markers for early detection of cancer. J. Cell. Biochem. **16G:** 131–136.
5. PONDER, B. A. J. 1990. Inherited predisposition to cancer. **6:** 213–218.
6. DELELLIS, R. A. 1995. Biology of disease: Multiple endocrine neoplasia syndromes revisited. **72:** 494–505.

7. Marsh, D. J., B. G. Robinson, S. Andrew, A.-L. Richardson, R. Pojer, M. Schnitzler, L. M. Mulligan & V. J. Hyland. 1994. A rapid screening method for the detection of mutations in the RET proto-oncogene in multiple endocrine neoplasia Type 2A and familial medullary thyroid carcinoma families. Genomics **23:** 477–479.
8. Goodfellow, P. J. 1994. Inherited cancers associated with the RET proto-oncogene. Curr. Opin. Genet. Dev. **4:** 446–452.
9. Karlan, B. Y. & D. Krakow. 1994. Genetic aspects of ovarian cancer. Curr. Opin. Obstet. Gynecol. **6:** 105–110.
10. Smith, S. A. & B. J. Ponder. 1993. Predisposing genes in breast and ovarian cancer: An overview. Tumori **19:** 291–296.
11. Eeles, R. A., M. R. Stratton, D. E. Goldgar & D. F. Easton. 1990. The genetics of familial breast cancer and their practical implications. Eur. J. Cancer **30A**(9): 1383–1390.
12. Nyström-Lahti, M., R. Parsons, P. Sistonen, L. Pylkkänen, L. A. Aaltonen, F. S. Leach, S. R. Hamilton, P. Watson, E. Bronson, R. Fusaro, J. Cavalieri, J. Lynch, S. Lanspa, T. Smyrk, P. Lynch, T. Drouhard, K. W. Kinzler, B. Vogelstein, H. T. Lynch, A. Dela Chapelle & P. Peltomäki. 1994. Mismatch repair genes on chromosomes 2p and 3p account for a major share of hereditary nonpolyposis colorectal cancer families evaluable by linkage. Am. J. Hum. Genet. **55:** 659–665.
13. Fishel, R. & R. D. Kolodner. 1995. Identification of mismatch repair genes and their role in the development of cancer. Curr. Opin. Genet. Dev. **5:** 382–395.
14. Tho, S. P. T. & P. G. McDonough. 1987. Use of Y DNA probes to identify children at risk for dysgenetic gonadal tumors. Clin. Obstet. Gynecol. **30**(3): 671–681.
15. Tho, P. T. & A. Behzadian. 1991. Detection and amplification of Y sequences. Sem. Reprod. Endocrinol. **9:** 46–55.
16. Tho, S. P. T., L. C. Layman, R. D. Lanclos, L. Plouffe, Jr., J. R. Byrd & P. G. McDonough. 1992. Absence of the testicular determining factor gene SRY in XX true hermaphrodites and presence of this locus in most subjects with gonadal dysgenesis caused by Y aneuploidy. Am. J. Obstet. Gynecol. **167:** 1794–1802.
17. Tho, S. P. T., A. Behzadian, J. R. Byrd & P. G. McDonough. 1990. Correlation of the testicular determinant factor sequence zinc finger Y with varying gonadal phenotypes in a series of 13 subjects with gonadal dysgenesis due to Y aneuploidy. Am. J. Obstet. Gynecol. **163:** 1968–1975.

Malignant Ovarian Neoplasms

The Place of Conservative Surgery

ALIKI J. TSERKEZOGLOU

First Department of Gynecology
Hellenic Cancer Institute
"St. Savas" Hospital
171 Alexandras Ave
115 22 Athens, Greece

INTRODUCTION

The standard of care in the management of malignant ovarian neoplasms (MON) is the radical procedure that involves total abdominal hysterectomy/bilateral salpingo-oophorectomy (TAH, BSO); omentectomy; staging and cytoreduction; followed, when appropriate, by systemic treatment.

Conservative management, however, may at times be considered in young patients wishing to preserve fertility, provided certain well-defined criteria are met, and survival is not jeopardized.

The idea of minimal surgical intervention in MON has long been discussed. As early as 1908 and more recently in 1969, reports in the literature have suggested that radical and minor operations can in some cases result in a similar survival benefit.[1]

This, however, was the era before the recognition of the different histopathological types of ovarian tumors, extensive surgicopathological staging, and laborious cytoreductive surgery. All these procedures reveal prognostic factors that help identify a subset of patients that can rather safely benefit from conservative treatment. It is therefore of clinical importance to study the different subgroups of MON separately.

Nevertheless, before the identification of the individual tumor characteristics that allow minimal surgery, certain general requirements should be mentioned. Candidates must be young, of low parity and desirous of childbearing, with an otherwise normal pelvis, and willing to undergo a strict follow-up program.[2]

BORDERLINE TUMORS OF THE OVARY

Borderline tumors of the ovary (BT) form a distinct subgroup of ovarian neoplasms that is common in young women, and they usually appear at an early stage (stage I = 75%). These tumors have a good prognosis (5-years survival for stage I >90%).[2]

The extensive and careful histologic evaluation of the primary tumor is important in order to establish the diagnosis of borderline malignancy. If the low malignant or frankly invasive nature of a tumor cannot be determined on frozen section, a conservative approach is recommended until final diagnosis is reached, especially in young patients.[3]

Regardless of the conservative or radical surgical management of the primary tumor, careful staging, as performed in invasive ovarian cancer, is always mandatory. Careful visualization and palpation of the abdominal cavity is followed by retrieval of peritoneal washings for cytology. Random biopsies from suspicious areas and tumor adhesions are collected. Omentectomy and retroperitoneal node sampling are also performed for staging purposes.[2]

When disease is confined to one ovary (stage Ia) unilateral salpingo-oophorectomy (USO) is considered adequate.[2,3]

The therapeutic efficacy and recommendations for simple cystectomy have been investigated by Lim Tan *et al.*[4] Based on 35 cases, recurrence or persistence of tumor was found in 12% (8% ipsilateral). Multilocality of tumor and positive resection margins were considered by the authors as contraindications to cystectomy.[4]

The need for wedge biopsy of the contralateral normal-appearing ovary has been debated for years. Lately, it has been recognized that the risk of occult metastases (5–7%) is lower than the possibility of subsequent infertility (14%), thus suggesting that its routine use should be avoided.[3,5,6]

If both ovaries are involved (stage Ib), USO combined with contralateral cystectomy or BSO can be practiced. The preservation of the uterus, even if no ovarian tissue remains, is recommended in some cases when childbearing, even with oocyte donation, is desired.[2,3,7]

In the rare cases of advanced-stage BT, meticulous cytoreduction of as many extraovarian foci of disease as possible is necessary.[8–10] Preservation in whole or in part of one ovary can be considered even in these cases, provided it does not interfere with tumor debulking.

Survival in advanced disease seems to depend mostly on the invasive (0–50%) or noninvasive (67–94%) nature of the implants and on cytoreduction.[7]

In case a proper staging had not been done, initially restaging is considered, and it sometimes reveals more extensive disease than originally thought. Combining three series, Trimbos *et al.* found that 17 of 71 patients (24%) were upstaged during this procedure. Because the survival benefit is unclear, however, the decision to restage should be based on the adequacy of the previous exploration, tumor subtype, and mainly on recommendations for further therapy.[7]

Recurrence rates after conservative management in BT are in the range of 6.8%.[7] It is interesting to notice that in many cases a recurrence was documented at the time of definite treatment and not because of progressive symptomatic disease.[7] Mucinous borderline tumors are thought to be at high risk of recurrence and are sometimes complicated with pseudomyxoma peritonei. Appendectomy is often recommended.[3]

A number of studies have investigated the role of adjuvant chemo- or radiotherapy in stage I BT.[2] There is no data so far to support that disease-free and overall survival are improved. On the contrary, many treatment-related deaths have been reported, thus suggesting systemic treatment should not be used.[7] If, however, invasive implants are found at laparotomy, adjunctive therapy is given, even though its effectiveness remains speculative.[9,10]

After childbearing is completed, removal of the remaining ovary and uterus are recommended because of the higher risk of developing an ovarian malignancy than in the general population.[3]

EPITHELIAL OVARIAN CANCER

Epithelial ovarian cancer is rarely confined to one ovary only (stage I = 25%), and even in these cases the role of conservative therapy is controversial and needs to be clearly defined.[11,12] The young patient who desires preservation of fertility should be informed of the risks involved and the probability of definite treatment in case disseminated disease is confirmed at laparotomy.[2] Needless to say, if fertility is not an issue radical surgery should be performed even in early disease. Careful staging, similar to the procedure described for BT, is mandatory in this category of tumors as in all others. Occult metastases have been reported in inadequately explored "stage I" patients in 31% of the cases.[11] The diaphragm (7.6%), omentum (7.1%), peritoneum (9.8%), abdominal cavity (cytology 18.8%), or retroperitoneal nodes (8%) can be involved even when disease seems restricted to the ovaries.[11]

USO is accepted as adequate treatment in stage Ia, grade I tumors.[2] Some authors have suggested that BSO can be applied in stage Ib, grade I tumors; and in these cases, preservation of the uterus can also be considered.[1,13]

The need for wedge biopsy of the normal-looking ovary is controversial. Occult micrometastases are reported to be present in 12–17.5% of the cases, being more frequent in serous tumors. It could therefore be suggested that routine biopsy is performed in neoplasms of serous histopathology and spared in the endometioid and mucinous variety.[2] Soon after childbearing is completed, removal of the genital organs is recommended.[2,11]

The role of adjuvant systemic treatment in stage I epithelial ovarian cancer has been investigated regardless of the extent of the primary surgical operation. A number of risk factors, that is, poor differentiation, ascites, positive peritoneal cytology, ruptured capsule, and the presence of lesions on the external tumor surface, increase the risk of relapse. A wide variety of local, regional (i.p. 32P, pelvic RT), and systemic (chemotherapy, abdominal–pelvic RT) treatments have been investigated in a retrospective and prospective fashion.[2,11] Even though they are currently recommended in high-risk cases, none of them has been shown to offer considerable survival benefit that is of statistical significance.[2,13]

Second-look laparotomy is not routinely performed in stage I cases that are without evidence of disease after comprehensive staging surgery and primary chemotherapy, since the positive yield is very low (5.5%).[11] Inaccurate staging might have been the reason for a higher percentage of positive results (20%) in earlier series.[11]

In summary, the requirements for conservative management in stage I patients with epithelial ovarian cancer are clearly illustrated in the textbook *Gynecologic Oncology* by Di Saia (TABLE 1).[2] These recommendations have been somewhat extended in the recent publication of the NIH Consensus Development Program on ovarian cancer that also includes guidelines for adjuvant chemotherapy (TABLE 2).

OVARIAN GERM CELL TUMORS

Ovarian germ cell tumors (OGCT)[14,15] are rare malignant ovarian neoplasms (5%) that are more common in young women. Before the development of effective chemotherapy that improved survival (5 years survival stage I = 95%, stage II–III =

TABLE 1. Requirements for Conservative Management in Epithelial Ovarian Cancer

1. Stage I_a
2. Well differentiated
3. Young woman of low parity
4. Otherwise normal pelvis
5. Encapsulated and free of adhesions
6. No invasion of capsule, lymphatics, or mesovarium
7. Peritoneal washings negative
8. Adequate evaluation of opposite ovary and omental biopsy negative
9. Close follow-up probable
10. Excision of residual ovary after completion of childbearing

75%), prognosis was dismal (5 years survival 10–15%). Most of these tumors (60–70%) present in stage I; whereas in advanced disease, it is believed that they metastasize more often to the lymph nodes and lung parenchyma. Both issues are important in considering conservative treatment.

Definitive therapy in this group also consists of radical surgery. Because many patients are young, however, and most studies suggest that survival is similar regardless of the extent of the primary surgical excision (TAH/BSO or USO), conservative treatment can be applied, provided appropriate chemotherapy is given.

Conservative surgery (USO) is the treatment of choice in early-stage disease. Careful staging is necessary as in all other groups of malignant ovarian neoplasms. If bilateral involvement is present, cystectomy of the less-affected ovary might be considered. It is of importance to remember that mature teratomas at times coexist with OGCT. A frozen section will confirm the benign nature of the mass and justify cystectomy only. Mixed tumors and gonadoblastomas often arise in dysgenetic gonads. Due to the high probability of bilateral involvement, BSO is the appropriate management.

Wedge biopsy of the contralateral, normal-looking ovary is not necessary in OGCT, except in dysgerminomas and mixed tumors with dysgenetic elements in which bilateral involvement is not uncommon (20%). Recurrence rates after conserv-

TABLE 2. Adjuvant Therapy in Subgroups of Stage I Epithelial Ovarian Cancer[a]

Therapy	Subgroups
No therapy	Stage I_a, grade I, most stage I_b, grade I
Therapy needed	All grade III tumors
	All clear cell tumors
	Most stage I_c
Therapy controversial	All other subgroups of stage I

[a]NIH, 1994 Consensus Development Program on Ovarian Cancer. (Reported in Gynecol. Oncol. **55:** S4–S14, 1994.)

ative treatment can be high (17–53% for dysgerminomas), but since salvage therapy is effective this does not prohibit its practice.

Recent reports suggest that conservative surgery (USO) might also be applied even in advanced disease, provided that cytoreduction is feasible. Controversy exists in the literature as to the appropriate extent of cytoreduction, especially when morbidity is expected. In the case of dysgerminomas, which are highly chemo- and radiosensitive tumors, it has been mentioned that cytoreduction can be less aggressive if major organs are involved and the risks of surgery are considerable. Adjuvant chemotherapy in OGCT is of primary importance. All patients, except for those with stage Ia, grade I, immature teratomas are submitted to postoperative chemotherapy.

A number of combination regimens have been used in the past with good results. VAC and PVB schemas have been replaced lately by the less toxic and more effective PEB regimen (platinum, etoposite, bleomycin) in many centers. The ideal number of treatment cycles remains to be established. Some authors favor three to four cycles for early disease and five to six for advanced cases.

Second-look surgery is rarely used in OGCT if residual disease was present at the initial operation. Tumor marker levels (AFP, CEA, BHCG, etc.) in the serum, if positive, allow for a satisfactory assessment of disease status on follow-up.

The desirable endpoint of conservative management of malignant ovarian tumors is the delivery of a healthy baby. Surgical treatment does not seem to adversely affect conception, at least not considerably. The role of chemotherapy as a potential teratogen has always been an issue of concern. However the limited data in the literature does not support this hypothesis.[14] In an MDA hospital study, 12 out of 16 patients with OGCT who attempted pregnancy succeeded. In an Italian study, 16 healthy babies were born among 17 women treated for epithelial ovarian cancer.[13]

SEX CORD–STROMAL TUMORS

Most sex cord–stromal tumors[15,16] (granulosa, thecomas, etc.) should be considered low-grade malignancies and treated as such except for a rare subgroup of Sertoli-Leydig cell tumors. In addition, in 95% of the cases they are unilateral, further supporting the recommendation that USO and staging are adequate treatment in most cases when fertility is desired.

Because some of these neoplasms are functional (i.e., granulosa cell: estrogen production), diagnostic curettage is essential if conservative treatment is applied. Although the incidence of bilaterality is low, most physicians would perform a wedge biopsy of the contralateral ovary.

If disseminated disease is present, radical surgery would be advised by most authors. The number of cases reported in the literature and the effectiveness of postoperative systemic treatment are inadequate to allow any firm conclusions on the outcome of conservative management in advanced disease.

Adjuvant treatment, mostly chemotherapy, is advised in any type of metastatic tumor spread and in some stage I Sertoli-Leydig subcategories (grade III, heterologous elements). The regimens usually used are PVB or PEB, as in OGCT, or PAC, as in epithelial ovarian cancers.

SUMMARY

Even though radical surgery is the treatment of choice in malignant neoplasms, a conservative approach may be considered in young patients who wish to preserve fertility, provided well-defined criteria are met and survival is not jeopardized. Unilateral, stage I, borderline (BT), germ cell (OGCT), sex cord stromal tumors, and grade I epithelial cancer can be treated with unilateral salpingoophorectomy (USO). If bilateral ovarian involvement is present, bilateral salpingoophorectomy (BSO) and preservation of the uterus can be considered. Cystectomy is rarely practiced, because of published contraindications,[4] in borderline tumors. Complete surgical staging is mandatory in all cases regardless of the type of surgery (USO or BSO). Conservative management of more advanced disease is considered in a few BT and OGCT cases, provided it can be combined with successful cytoreduction. Adjuvant chemotherapy is necessary in almost all OGCT and epithelial cancers, although its role in BT and sex cord tumors is unspecified yet. Current knowledge suggests that conception is possible after conservative management for malignant ovarian neoplasms and chemotherapy does not cause obvious genetic malformations in the newborn.

REFERENCES

1. Munnel, E. Q. 1969. Is conservative therapy ever justified in stage I (Ia) cancer of the ovary? Am. J. Obstet. Gynecol. **1:** 641–653.
2. Di Saia, P. & W. Creasman. 1993. The adnexal mass and early ovarian cancer. Epithelial ovarian cancer. *In* Clinical Gynecologic Oncology. S. Manning, Ed. Chapt. 10 and 11: 324–358. Mosby Year Book Inc. St. Louis, MO.
3. Morrow, P. 1992. Malignant and borderline epithelial tumors of the ovary: Clinical features, staging, diagnosis, intraoperative assessment and review of management. *In* Gynecologic Oncology. M. Coppleson, Ed. Vol. 2: 889 915. Churchill. Livingston. Hong Kong.
4. Lim-Tan, K. S., H. E. Cajigas & R. E. Scully. 1988. Ovarian cystectomy for serous borderline tumors. A follow-up study of 35 cases. Obstet. Gynecol. **72:** 775–780.
5. Bostwick, D. G., H. D. Tazelaar, S. C. Ballon, M. R. Hendrickson & R. L. Kempson. 1986. Ovarian epithelial tumors of borderline malignancy. Cancer **58:** 2052–2065.
6. Tazelaar, H. D., D. G. Bostwick, S. C. Ballon, M. R. Hendrickson & R. L. Kempson. 1985. Conservative treatment of borderline ovarian tumors. Obstet. Gynecol. **66:** 417–422.
7. Trimbos, C. L. & E. L. Trimble. 1994. Management of epithelial ovarian tumors of low malignant potential. Gynecol. Oncol. **55:** S52–61.
8. Kaern, J., C. Trope & V. M. Abeler. 1993. A retrospective study of 370 borderline tumors of the ovary treated at the Norwegian Radium Hospital from 1970 to 1982. Cancer **71:** 1810–1820.
9. Gershenson, D. M. & E. G. Silva. 1990. Serous ovarian tumors of low malignant potential with peritoneal implants. Cancer **65:** 578–585.
10. Sutton, G. P., B. N. Bundy, G. A. Omura, E. L. Yordan, J. B. Beecham & T. Bonfiglio. 1991. Stage III ovarian tumors of low malignant potential treated with cisplatin combination therapy. (A *Gynecologic Oncology* group study). Gynecol. Oncol. **41:** 230–233.
11. Benjamin, J. & S. C. Rubin. 1994. Management of early stage epithelial ovarian cancer. Obstet. Gynecol. Clin. N. Am. **21:** 107–120.

12. TRIMBLE, E. L. 1994. National Institutes of Health Consensus Development Conference Statement. Ovarian Cancer: Screening, Treatment and Follow Up. Gynecol. Oncol. **55:** S1–14.
13. COLOMBO, N., S. A. CHIARI, N. MAGGIONI, *et al.* 1994. Controversial issues in the management of early epithelial ovarian cancer: Conservative surgery and role of adjuvant therapy. Gynecol. Oncol. **55:** 547–551.
14. GERSHENSON, D. M. 1992. Malignant germ cell tumors of the ovary: Clinical features and management. *In* Gynecologic Oncology. M. Coppleson, Ed. Vol. 2: 935–945. Churchill. Livingston. Hong Kong.
15. GERSHENSON, D. M. 1994. Management of early ovarian cancer: Germ cell and sex cord–stromal tumors. Gynecol. Oncol. **55:** S62–72.
16. HOSKINS, W. L. & S. C. RUBIN. 1992. Malignant gonadal stromal tumors of the ovary: Clinical features and management. *In* Gynecologic Oncology. M. Coppleson, Ed. Vol. 2: 961–970. Churchill. Livingston. Hong Kong.

Acquired Clitoral Enlargement

Diagnosis and Treatment

JAN HOŘEJŠÍ[a]

Department of Obstetrics and
Adult and Pediatric Gynecology
Second Medical Faculty
Charles University Prague
Prague, Czech Republic

Clitoral hypertrophy is usually seen in congenital malformations, mainly in intersexual stages. Prader classified it under congenital adrenal hyperplasia syndrome, which is most often divided into five degrees.[1]

Acquired clitoral hypertrophy is a relatively rare condition, and literature data concerning this problem are very poor, consisting usually of case reports only.

Among the contributing factors in the etiology of acquired clitoral hypertrophy, hyperandrogenism was the one most often mentioned. The resource of higher levels of androgen can be demonstrated in some endocrinopathies: Ishizuka *et al.*[2] demonstrated clitoromegaly in nonneoplastic and nonpolycystic ovarian hypertestosteronism. Clitoral hypertrophy due to hyperandrogenism may be caused by polycystic ovary (PCO) syndrome[3–5] or by late onset of the 21-hydroxylase deficit.[6] In those cases, clitoral enlargement is not very apparent.

The more pronounced clitoral enlargement or hypertrophy is obvious in hormonally active, masculinizing tumors: Such tumors are most often ovarian virilizing tumors, as Leydig-cell tumor,[7] lipid-cell tumor,[8] or arrhenoblastoma.[9,10] Virilizing cortical carcinoma[11,12] or adenoma[13] of adrenals can also develop clitoromegaly. There are references that also demonstrate androgenic activity of gonadoblastoma that results in clitoromegaly.[14,15] Howe *et al.*[16] demonstrated clitoral hypertrophy in women after self injection of long-acting synthetic androgens.

Nonhormonal causes of acquired clitoral enlargement is even rarer than the hormonal causes mentioned above. There are reports in the literature concerning clitoral enlargement caused by neurofibromatosis. Neurofibromatosis affects either the clitoris itself[17,18] or the clitoral prepuce only, creating clitoral pseudohypertrophy.[19]

Another type or pseudohypertrophy of the clitoris is often seen in small girls due to masturbation: Manipulations with skin of prepuce represents repeating mechanical insult, which enlarges prepuce and labia minora, thus imitating true clitoral enlargement.

[a]Address for correspondence: Professor Jan Hořejší, M.D., Dr. Sc., Dept. Ob/Gyn, 84, Vúralu, CZ 150 06 Praha 5, Czech Republic.

DIAGNOSIS

Diagnosis of acquired clitoral enlargement must take into consideration all the above-mentioned etiological factors. Careful clinical examination is the first step for proper diagnosis: It helps us first to differentiate between true clitoral enlargement and pseudohypertrophy produced by hypertrophy of prepuce and labia minora. If clitoral enlargement also involves corpora cavernosa, then the shape of other components of external genitalia plays an important role in the diagnosis: In congenital clitoromegaly, we often see malformations of the external orifice of urethra and vagina. We usually can see only the opening of the urogenital sinus, and endoscopic examination helps us determine the degree of malformation according to Prader's classification.[1] In isolated clitoral hypertrophy, we have to observe whether it is symmetrical, homogenous, and smooth or not. Cases of clitoral neurofibromatosis tend to be irregular in shape, often nonsymmetrical and rough.

Endocrinologic examination is essential, of course. The whole spectrum of androgen tests is necessary. Native 17-hydroxyprogesterone levels and levels after stimulation with adrenocorticotrophic hormone (Synacten), levels of FSH and LH and the FSH:LH ratio, estrogen, and progesterone levels are obligatory. We have to think about exogenous androgen intake in top-level sportswomen! In cases in which masturbation is suspected, psychological or even psychiatric examination of child may be necessary.

TREATMENT

The first steps in correcting and curing acquired clitoral enlargement have to focus on determining and blocking the hypertrophy-evoking cause: This could mean suppressing ovarian or adrenal hyperproduction of androgens, removing a hormonally active virilizing tumor, stopping exogenous androgen intake, or influencing a child's masturbating activities. Then a period of waiting and observing is indicated. If clitoral enlargement does not display any regression or does not disappear, surgical correction becomes necessary.

In refractory simple clitoral hypertrophy, reductive clitoroplasty is performed.[20] Surgical technique involves preserving the glans clitoridis with its innervation, which is necessary for future sexual function.

In more serious cases, such as those involving congenital adrenal hypertrophy, Hořejší and Fára[21,22] recommend clitoridectomy with neoplastic reformation of labia minora including opening and enlargement of stenotic vagina or persistent urogenital sinus.[22,23]

Neurofibromatosis of the clitoris or of its prepuce requires surgery performed by a skilled gynecologic or plastic surgeon or urologist.[19]

SUMMARY

Clitoral hypertrophy is usually seen in congenital malformations, specifically in intersexual stages of hormonal expression. Acquired clitoral hypertrophy is a relatively rare condition, and data in the literature concerning this problem are sparse. Articles usually consist only of case reports.

Among the contributing factors in the etiology of acquired clitoral hypertrophy, the following three are the most frequent: (1) endocrinopathies including virilizing tumors of the ovaries or adrenals, (2) neurofibromatosis (of both clitoral subcutis and corpora cavernosa), and (3) pseudohypertrophy of the clitoris.

The first step in correcting acquired clitoral enlargement must be to determine and stop the cause of the hypertrophy, followed by a period of simple observation. If clitoral enlargement does not disappear over time, surgical correction is necessary.

REFERENCES

1. Prader, A. 1954. Der Genitalbefund beim Pseudohermaphroditismus femininus des kongenitalen adrenogenitalen Syndroms. Helv. Paed. Acta **9:** 231–240.
2. Ishizuka, B., Y. Kuribayashi, K. Watanabe, *et al.* 1992. A case of significant, non-neoplastic, ovarian hypertestosteronism. Nippon Naibunpi Gakkai Zasshi **68**(1): 19–29.
3. Derman, R. J. 1995. Effects of sex steroids on women's health: Implications for practitioners. Am. J. Medic. **98**(1): 137–143.
4. Muritano, M., M. Zachmann, B. Manella, *et al.* 1988. Transient ovarian testosterone and androstendione hypersecretion: A cause of virilization or premature pubarche in prepubertal girls. Horm. Res. **28**(1): 37–41.
5. Creatsas, G. 1987. Neonatal, Pediatric and Adolescent Gynecology with endocrinology appendix (in Greek). Entopia. Athens: 294 p.
6. Emans, S. J. H. & D. P. Goldstein. 1990. Pediatric and Adolescent Gynecology. Little, Brown. Boston/Toronto/London. pp. 243–272.
7. Ichinohasama, R., S. Teshima, K. Kishi, *et al.* 1989. Leydig cell tumor of the ovary associated with endometrial carcinoma and containing 17-beta-hydroxysteroid dehydrogenase. Int. J. Gynecol. Pathol. **8**(1): 64–71.
8. De Freitas, E. A., M. R. Dudzinski, J. C. La Rocque & C. C. Coddington. 1991. Ovarian vein sampling in rapidly progressing virilization. A case report. J. Reprod. Med. **36**(7): 546–548.
9. Hořejší, J. 1990. Dětská gynekologie (Pediatric Gynecology—in Czech). Avicenum. Praha. 284 pp.
10. Heinz, M. 1989. Gynäkologie im Kindes- und Jugendalter. Georg Thieme. Leipzig. pp. 67–88.
11. Tsujimura, A., T. Imazu, K. Nishimura, *et al.* 1993. A case of virilizing adrenocortical carcinoma in adult. Hinyokika Kiyo **39**(4): 345–348.
12. Pardo, J. M. 1986. Virilization of a female infant due to an adrenal tumor. Clin. Pediatr. Hygerstown **25**(9): 456–458.
13. Nakagawa, Y., Y. Hirao, S. Tsujimoto, *et al.* 1989. A case of infantile virilizing adrenocortical tumor. Hinyokika Kiyo **35**(10): 1731–1736.
14. Yakizane, S., R. Yamakawa, T. Murakami, *et al.* 1994. A 15-year-old girl with pubertal masculinization due to bilateral gonadoblastoma and 45,X/46,X,+mar. karyotype. Kurume Med. J. **41**(3): 155–159.
15. Dumic, M., S. Jukic, S. Batinica, *et al.* 1993. Bilateral gonadoblastoma in a 9-month-old infant with 46,XY gonadal dysgenesis. J. Endocrinol. Invest. **16**(4): 291–293.
16. Howe, R. S., R. P. Chow & C. L. Stevens. 1994. Use of flutamide for self-induced androgen excess. A case report. J. Reprod. Med. **39**(10): 838–840.

17. Nishimura, K., H. Sugao, K. Sato, *et al.* 1991. Neurofibroma of the clitoris. A case report. Urol. Int. **46**(1): 109–111.
18. Sutphen, R., E. Galan-Gomez & B. G. Kousseff. 1995. Clitoromegaly in neurofibromatosis. Am. J. Med. Genet. **55**(3): 325–330.
19. Griebel, M. L., J. F. Redman, S. F. Kemp, *et al.* 1991. Hypertrophy of clitoral hood: Presenting sign of neurofibromatosis in female child. Urology **37**(4): 337–339.
20. Shaw, A. 1977. Subcutaneous reduction clitoroplasty. J. Pediat. Surg. **12:** 331–336.
21. Hořejší, J. 1981. Clitoridectomia cum neoplastica labiorum minorum et plastica vestibuli vaginae. Acta Chir. Plast. **23**(1): 18–26.
22. Hořejší, J. 1991. Reconstruction of ambiguous genitalia. *In* Advances in Pediatric and Adolescent Gynecology. G. Creatsas & E. Deligeoroglou, Eds.: 71–76. Hellenic Society of Pediatric and Adolescent Gynecology. Athens.
23. Hořejší, J. 1987. Plastic reconstruction of the vaginal vestibule in women with masculinized external genitalia. Acta Chir. Plast. **29**(4): 229–241.

Karyotype–Phenotype Correlation in Females with X Chromosome Abnormalities

ZOE KOSMAIDOU-ARAVIDOU

Department of Genetics
Alexandra University Hospital
80, Vassilissis Sofias Avenue
11528 Athens, Greece

In mammals, females have a pair of X chromosomes, whereas males have one X chromosome and one Y chromosome. The normal X chromosome accounts for about 6% of the human genome, whereas the Y chromosome accounts for only about 1% of the human genome and is smaller than any other autosome. One of the pair of X chromosomes is inactivated in females. The inactivated X chromosome is late replicating, heterochromatic, and genetically unexpressed.

Consequently, dosage equivalence between males and females is achieved.[14] An X inactivation center (XIC) located at a proximal region on Xq is thought to control inactivation of an X chromosome as a whole in *cis*-limited fashion.[24] The recently discovered XIST gene[2] may be involved in the initiation process, and methylation seems to maintain the inactive status.[1,20] However, not all X chromosomal genes undergo inactivation. Genes that are located in the pseudoautosomal region (PAR), a region at the tip of the short arm of the X (band Xp 22.3) and sharing homology with the Y chromosome (band Yp 11.32), are exempt from X inactivation.[10,19]

The X and Y chromosomes evolved from a homologous ancestral chromosome pair, accompanied by rearrangements that resulted in a gradual differentiation of the sex chromosomes.[18]

Short stature and gonadal dysgenesis are the main manifestations of Ullrich-Turner syndrome, which occurs with X monosomy as well as with structurally aberrant X chromosomes.

For short stature, two types of major growth genes have been postulated on the sex chromosomes, a pseudoautosomal growth gene located in the distal part of the pseudoautosomal region and a Y-specific growth gene located at the proximal part of the Yq. An X-specific growth gene escaping inactivation is unlikely to exist, although the possibility that such a gene might be present in the proximal part of Xp has not been excluded formally.[17]

The fully Turner phenotype is most frequently manifested by patients with a 45,X karyotype. The fully or partial Turner phenotype is also exhibited by apparently nonupsaic patients with various sex chromosome rearrangements.

All 45,X women and 88% of the carriers of a terminally deleted Xp are short; 43% of the Xq-carriers also show short stature. The growth pattern in 45,X syndrome is characterized by intrauterine growth retardation, progressive decline in growth velocity in childhood, lack of pubertal growth spurt, and delayed growth cessation.

The severe short stature in 45,X, 46,X,del(X)(p11) and 46,X,i(Xq) are due to the total effects of the loss of P-growth gene(s) and the growth disadvantage caused by alteration of the amount of noninactivated region. Height comparisons between 45,X; 46,X del(X)(p22:32); 46,X,del(X)(p11); and 46,X,i(Xq), in which the P-growth gene(s) is present in a single copy, suggest that the degree of growth disadvantage correlates with the degree of chromosome imbalance.

The height decrease in 46,X,delX(q13-21) appears to be inexplicable without assuming the growth disadvantage caused by the loss of noninactivated region.

A large number of factors has been discussed that might influence the absence or presence of the different symptoms of these patients.[17,25] Two factors are (1) mosaicism (undetected 46,XX line) as well as UTS (undetected 45,X line) and (2) the hormonal status (as indicated by absence or presence of menarche). Treatment of UTS patients with hormones only leads to minor effects on height with a gain of 4 to 5 cm.

Gonadal dysgenesis in female sex chromosome aberrations would primarily be attributable to chromosome-pairing failure during mitotic prophase.

The Xq13-q26 region is the critical region for ovarian development, and the integrity of the region is required for normal ovarian development.[15,25]

However, the hypothesis would not explain adequately why gonadal dysfunction is so mild in patients with 46,X, i(Xq) accompanied by chromosomal breakage on the critical region. Of the 45,X Turner patients, 91% have streak gonads. Gonadal dysfunction varied in severity among different karyotypes, 45,X,46X,i(Xq); 46,X,idic(Xq); and 46,X,idic(Xp) were associated with severe gonadal dysfunction. In terminal X deletions, the degree of gonadal dysfunction was roughly correlated with the deletional site.

Xq carriers suffer from gonadal abnormalities more often than do carriers of Xp chromosomes. In the Xq carriers, ovarian dysgenesis seems to be caused by breaks in Xq 13-q24. Gonadal dysfunction appears to be mild in interstitial X deletions and in X inversions. The phenotype of a female with a balanced X-autosome translocation depends predominantly on two factors: (1) the position of the break points and (2) the functional status of the Xt. The combined effect of these factors results in a variety of clinical conditions that can be subdivided into distinct categories:

1. Xt is active in all cells and the break points do not disrupt any functional gene. Individuals from this group are either asymptomatic (30–50% of cases) or have gonadal dysgenesis. The two phenotypes are clearly delineated by the position of the X break point, which falls within the region Xq13-q26 in the patients with reproductive malfunctions.[4,13,21,27]

2. Xt is active in all cells, yet one or both of the break points disrupt coding sequences. This category of patients differs from the previous group in that the clinical picture is usually dominated by a single gene disorder.

3. Xt is subject to inactivation in a proportion of cells. This situation, occurring in about 23% of balanced X autosome translocations, creates a variety of abnormal phenotypes often puzzling for clinical interpretations. Typically, the symptoms represent an aneuploidy effect with multiple congenital anomalies and mental retardation, sometimes accompanied by contiguous gene syndromes and/or single gene disorders.

Among individuals with Turner syndrome, 6 to 11% possess a cell line containing one or more small markers,[5,7,22] of which a majority are X-chromosome derived, as determined by *in situ* hybridization.[3,6,13,23]

Individuals with a cell line containing a small mark (X) chromosome often have mental retardation and dysmorphic features not typical of the phenotype associated with Turner syndrome.[8,11,12,13,26]

Karyotype studies of these females show that the XIST locus on their small markers X chromosomes is either not present or not expressed. Because XIST transcription is well correlated with inactivation of the X chromosome in female somatic cells and spermatogonia, monoexpression of the locus even when it is present suggests that the chromosomes are transcriptionally active. The severe phenotype and mental retardation are due to functional disomy resulting from lack of dosage compensation for genes present within the mark (X) chromosome.

Turner syndrome is associated with various somatic stigmata such as (1) anomalies to lymphatic obstruction, (2) skeletal anomalies, (3) cardiovascular and renal anomalies, and (4) miscellaneous anomalies, such as multiple pigmented nevi. Somatic stigmata were frequently found in 45,X; 46,X,i(Xq); 46,X,del(X)(p11); and 46,X,Yp.[17]

The characteristic stigmata of Turner syndrome would primarily be ascribed to haploinsufficiency of the Xp-Yp homologous lymphogenic gene(s). Loss of the Xp-Yp homologous lymphogenic gene(s) constitutes the underlying factor of characteristic somatic stigmata and prenatal lethality.

The clinical presentation of characteristic stigmata appears to change with age. Lymphatic obstruction stigmata (e.g., puffy hands and feet) are conspicuous during infancy but tend to resolve with age, whereas skeletal anomalies (e.g., short metacarpals and cubitus valgus) usually become obvious after infancy. Lymphatic stigmata is compatible with that of cystic hygroma in fetal life, implying an amelioration of lymphatic flow with age. Development of skeletal anomalies at a later age is related to the timing of appearance of ossification centers.

The chromosome imbalance (quantitative alteration of a euchromatic or noninactivated region), dose effect of the P and the Y growth genes and of the Xp-Yp homologous lymphogenic gene, chromosome pairing failure, and other factors are likely to be the underlying mechanisms for the development of Turner features.

SUMMARY

In mammals, females have a pair of X chromosomes, whereas males have one X chromosome and one Y chromosome, which is much smaller and contains fewer genes than a X chromosome. One of the pair of X chromosomes is inactivated in females. The inactivated X chromosome is late-replicating, heterochromatic, and genetically unexpressed. An X inactivation center (XIC) located at a proximal region on Xq is thought to control inactivation of an X chromosome.

There has been increasing scientific interest in the relationship between chromosomal and clinical findings in different chromosomal aberrations, whether affecting the sex chromosomes or the autosomes. The genetic and molecular implications of the karyotype/phenotype controversy have recently been considered with the aim of better understanding the interplay of specific genes carried on different chromosomes in organ development and differentiation.

Karyotype/phenotype correlation showed the gradation of severity of clinical phenotype to be related to the number of X chromosomes.

REFERENCES

1. Ballabion, A. & H. F. Willard. 1992. Mammalian X-chromosome inactivation and the XIST gene. Curr. Opin. Genet. Dev. **2:** 439–447.
2. Brown, G. J., A. Ballabion, J. L. Rupert, R. G. Lafreniere, M. Grompe, R. Tonlorenzi & H. F. Willard. 1991. A gene from the region of the human X inactivation centre is expressed exclusively from the inactive X chromosome. Nature **349:** 38–44.
3. Callen, D. F., H. J. Eyre, M. I. Ringenbergs, G. J. Freemantle, C. P. Woodroffe & E. P. Ilaan. 1991. Chromosomal origin of small ring marker chromosomes in man: Characterization by molecular genetics. Am. J. Hum. Genet. **48:** 769–782.
4. Carpenter, N. J. 1983. Balanced X-autosome translocations and gonadal dysfunction in female and males. *In* Cytogenetics of the Mammalian X Chromosome, Part B. A. A. Sandberg, Ed.: 211–227. Alan R. Liss. New York.
5. Coco, R. & C. Bergada. 1977. Cytogenetic findings in 125 patients with Turner's syndrome and abnormal karyotypes. J. Genet. Hum. **25:** 95–104.
6. Crolla, J. A. & J. C. Llerena. 1988. A mosaic 45,X/46,X,r(?) karyotype investigated with X and Y centromere-specific probes using a uon radiographic *in situ* hybridization technique. Hum. Genet. **81:** 81–84.
7. de Almeida, J. C. C., J. C. Llerena, Jr., M. D. Gomes, R. R. Martins, M. Jung, D. F. Reis & A. G. Gund. 1985. G-11 staining in Turner's syndrome with mos 45,X/46,X,r(X). Ann. Genet. **28:** 37–41.
8. Dennis, N. R., A. L. Collins, J. A. Crolla, A. E. Cockwell, A. M. Fisher & P. A. Jacobs. 1993. Three patients with ring (X) chromosomes and a severe phenotype. J. Med. Genet. **30:** 482–486.
9. Elejalde, B. R. & M. M. de Elejalde. 1983. Phenotypic manifestations of X-autosome translocations. *In* Cytogenetica of the Mammalian X Chromosome. Part B. A. A. Sanderberg, Ed.: 225–244. Alan R. Liss. New York.
10. Ellis, N. & P. N. Goodfellow. 1989. The mammalian pseudoautosomal region. Trends Genet. **5:** 406–410.
11. Grompe, M., N. Rao, F. F. B. Elder, C. T. Caskey & F. Greenberg. 1992. 45,X/46,X,tr(X) can have a distinct phenotype different from Ullrich-Turner syndrome. Am. J. Med. Genet. **42:** 39–43.
12. Kushnick, T., T. G. Irons, J. E. Wiley, E. A. Gettig, K. W. Rao & S. Bower. 1987. 45X/46,X,r(X) with syndactyly and severe mental retardation. Am. J. Med. Genet. **28:** 567–574.
13. Lindgren, V., C. Chen, C. R. Bryke, P. Lichter, D. C. Page & T. Yang-Feng. 1992. Cytogenetic karyotypes. Hum. Genet. **88:** 393–398.
14. Lyon, M. F. 1962. Sex chromatin and gene action in mammalian X-chromosome. Am. J. Hum. Genet. **14:** 135–148.
15. Madan, K. 1983. Balanced structural changes involving the human X: Effect on sexual phenotype. Hum. Genet. **63:** 216–221.
16. Ogata, T. & N. Matsuo. 1993. Sex chromosome aberration, and stature deduction of the principal factors involved in the determination of adult height. Hum. Genet. **91:** 551–562.
17. Ogata, T. & N. Matsuo. 1995. Turner syndrome and female sex chromosome aberrations deduction of the principal factors involved in the development of clinical features. Hum. Genet. **95:** 607–629.
18. Ohno, S. 1967. Sex chromosomes and sex-linked genes. Springer. Berlin, Heidelberg, New York.
19. Rappold, G. A. 1993. The pseudoautosomal regions of the human sex chromosomes. Hum. Genet. **92:** 315–324.
20. Riggs, A. P. & G. P. Pfeifer. 1992. X-chromosome inactivation and cell memory. Trends Genet. **8:** 169–174.

21. SPARTO, G. E., E. THERMAN & K. PATAU. 1973. X inactivation in man: A woman with t(Xq; 12p^{+}). Am. J. Hum. Genet. **25:** 262.
22. SCHMID, W., E. NAEF, G. MURSET & A. PRADOR. 1974. Gytogenetic findings in 89 cases of Turner's syndrome with abnormal karyotypes. Hum. Genet. **24:** 93–104.
23. SCHWARTZ, S., T. W. DEPINET, J. LEANA-COX, N. B. ISADA, E. M. KARSON, L. M. PASZTOR, L. C. SHEPPARD, *et al.* 1997. Characterization of sex chromosome markers using fluorescence *in situ* hybridization and review of the literature. Ann. J. Med. Genet. In press.
24. THERMAN, E., G. E. SARTO & K. PATAU. 1974. Center for barr body condensation on the proximal part of the human Xq: A hypothesis. Chromosoma. **44:** 361–366.
25. THERMAN, E. & B. SUSMAN. 1990. The similarity of phenotypic effects caused by Xp and Xq deletions in the human female: A hypothesis. Hum. Genet. **85:** 175–183.
26. VAN DYKE, D. L., A. WIKTOR, C. G. PALMER, D. A. MILLER, M. WITT, V. R. BADU, M. J. WORSHAM, *et al.* 1992. Ullrich-Turner syndrome with a small ring X chromosome and presence of mental retardation. Am. J. Med. Genet. **43:** 996–1005.
27. ZUFFARDI, O. 1983. Cytogenetics of human X/autosome translocations. *In* Cytogenetics of the Mammalian X Chromosome, Part B. A. A. Sandberg, Ed.: 193–209. Alan R. Liss. New York.

The Ethics of Somatic and Germline Gene Therapy

PAUL G. McDONOUGH

Department of Obstetrics and Gynecology
Medical College of Georgia
Augusta, Georgia 30912

Recent developments in the understanding of the molecular basis of inherited and acquired diseases have led to novel experimental approaches to treatment that attempt to replace the mutated gene. This form of therapy is appropriately referred to as gene therapy. Gene therapy is defined as the delivery of a functional gene for expression in somatic tissues with the intent to cure a disease. It is clear from the work of the last decade that a single method of gene transfer will not be applicable to all clinical situations. Different gene transfer strategies may be required to target different tissues. Somatic gene therapy is a conceptually new approach to treating human disease, but it is rapidly becoming accepted by all parts of the biomedical community. The current models for gene therapy of specific diseases are quite crude and will require extensive refining. Research into the practical development of gene therapy protocols is in a phase of rapid technological progress. At the present time, there are approximately 100 approved protocols for gene therapy in man. At this time, even though there is not convincing evidence of clinical success, it is evident that many kinds of human diseases will eventually be treated by introducing heterologous genetic information into defective or damaged tissues. Gene therapy at the somatic level is basically the correction of a disease phenotype at the level of the fundamental gene defect. The potential for somatic gene therapy began to emerge in the 1970s with the development of genetically marked mammalian cell lines and the early approaches toward the introduction of functional macromolecular DNA into cells. Next in 1970 came the demonstration that mammalian genomes are amenable to genetic modification by viruses. The appearance of recombinant DNA (rDNA) technology in 1972 combined with the earlier advances to suggest that viruses might be genetically engineered to permit deliberate and potentially therapeutic gene transfer into defective cells to correct genetic defects.[1] The first workshop on gene therapy was held in 1971, and recombinant DNA technology provided the first approaches for the transfer of disease-related genes (i.e., beta globin, hypoxanthine-guanine phosphoribosyltransferase (HPRT), Lesch-Nyhan syndrome). It became clear at that time that replication-defective viral vectors were practical and safe vehicles for gene transfer. The development of these vectors, which was based on research into the life cycle and cellular-transforming capabilities of these retroviruses, was a major achievement toward somatic gene therapy.[2,3] In 1988, the rDNA Advisory Committee of the National Institute of Health, Bethesda, Maryland (NIH) approved guidelines for human gene therapy trials. The early gene therapy studies evaluated the safety of gene transfer therapy in humans.[4,5] Efficacy was actually evaluated subsequently in a separate group of experiments. Over the last five years, many additional viral vectors and new chemical methods of gene delivery have been developed. These developments have occurred in order to address some of the specialized needs of gene therapy such as targeting actively dividing versus nondividing quiescent cells and organ-specific delivery.

In general, a series of milestones usually punctuate progress toward gene therapy of any specific genetic disorder. The first is the isolation of the diseased gene and demonstration of its authenticity by expression in cultured cells. Safe gene delivery vectors are then used for evaluation of efficacy and safety in cultured cells and animal models before embarking on human trials. In any discussion of the ethics surrounding somatic gene therapy, it is important to understand each of these steps along the way to the final human experiment. Once the gene and its vector are considered to be effective and safe, then one must turn one's attention to the promoters or enhancers that regulate the cell-specific expression of this gene. These regulatory promoters provide the means for control of the transfer gene in the desired cell type. The mouse transgenic model has been especially valuable in testing gene transfer strategies for human diseases and for creating mouse models of human diseases.

The first truly successful gene therapy demonstration has come not through the application of molecular biological RNA/DNA techniques but rather from the extension of the now-standard methods of tissue transplantation. Bone marrow transplantation has been generally used for the treatment of neoplastic disease, but it has now been shown that it is possible to achieve a permanent correction of thalassemia by repopulation of the marrow with normal hematopoietic stem cells. It was in 1981 and 1982 that techniques for the preparation of the first truly effective gene transfer vehicles, the retroviral vectors, were developed. A number of important conceptual and technical changes have occurred in gene therapy since its inception. Although retroviral vectors are very useful for many models, they are limited primarily by the requirement for replication of their target cells. A number of other kinds of viral and nonviral techniques have recently been developed that promise to allow gene transfer into nonreplicating cells such as neurons and hepatocytes. These techniques will also permit direct gene therapy to defective cells *in vivo*. These tools include vectors derived from adenoviruses, adeno-associated viruses, and herpes viruses, as well as nonviral gene transfer techniques of lipofection and electroporation. Several of these approaches have already been applied to human studies including, for instance, the delivery of the cystic fibrosis transmembrane conductance regulator (CFTR) cDDA to cells of the airways of patients with cystic fibrosis.

ETHICAL ISSUES

Ethical issues raised by the prospect of human gene transfer therapy have been actively addressed by ethical research policy conferences. A view of human gene therapy has been developed in the United States that is the product of prolonged, detailed analysis of all of the relevant issues. In response to the meeting at Asilomar in 1975, the NIH established an office of DNA activities and developed the NIH guidelines for research involving DNA molecules. The issue of human gene therapy became a focus of public discussion in the early 1980s. As a result of these public discussions, the NIH DNA Advisory Committee (RAC) established a working group on human gene therapy that carried out a thorough study of the science and ethics of this technology. The document, "Points to Consider in the Design and Submission of Protocols for the Transfer of DNA into the Genome of Human Subjects," was developed over the period from 1984 to 1986 and was adapted by the RAC in 1986.[6] Periodic revisions were included as the technology for gene therapy became defined more precisely. In 1989 the first human gene transfer protocol was approved, and in 1990 the first human gene therapy protocol using a marker gene was approved.[7–9] As of March 1995, approximately 100 protocols had been approved by the RAC committee of the NIH. In general, the policies emanating from these committees state that somatic gene therapy (gene transfer targeted to one or more tissues of the body) should be treated as a conventional medical therapy in determining risk/benefit ratios. On the other hand, gene transfer of human embryos (germline gene transfer) is not currently considered justifiable. The regulatory responsibilities to implement these decisions are performed by local institutional review boards, the NIH, the DNA Advisory Committee, and the Food and Drug Administration. In all of these decisions, there must be concern for the clinical benefit to the research subject, concern regarding the informed participation of research subjects, concern about fair subject selection, and the need for special biosafety precautions when there is genetic uncertainty. For example, certain types of vectors used to deliver genes pose a small risk of causing cancer. An assessment of the risk of the treatment versus the benefit to the patient, the scientific validity of the experiments, and the safety parameters that need to be addressed are of utmost importance. In the view of the RAC committee, there must be sufficient prior knowledge to conclude that the probable benefits of the therapy outweigh the possible risks to the patient and the known benefits of available alternative treatments. The toxicity of the gene product is a principal consideration, because overexpression or inappropriate expression could create a clinical emergency. *In vitro* assays to assess the functional aspects of the gene delivery system are essential. It is necessary to establish *in vitro* that the same target cells that will be transduced in the patient can be transduced and that sufficient levels of expression can be maintained for a sufficiently prolonged period to achieve a clinical effect. The prior use of animal models is exceedingly important, although it is recognized that a precise model such as the Watanabe rabbit for familial hypercholesterolemia is relatively rare.

GENE THERAPY—FEASIBILITY AND ETHICS

Ultimately, somatic gene therapy will be added to the choices appropriate to those persons at high risk for any serious disease. Every week there is another feature in the press or on television discussing gene therapy. Sometimes it is described in terms of its potential to treat genetic disorders in a new and more effective way. Rarely, its wider potential to deliver genes for multifactorial conditions such as cancer or heart disease is discussed. Invariably the ethical dilemmas, that phrase so beloved of subeditors, appears as a bold heading. Is all this new-found optimism justified or is it the "flavor of the month," a mixture of hype by the practitioners (who stand to win large research grants), the biotechnology companies (which might otherwise languish in the corporate stakes), the large number of ethicists now competing for a public platform in which to air their personal views, and the journalists whose favorite words seem to be cure and breakthrough?

In general, there is a reason to be optimistic. Deficiency of the gene for adenine deaminase (ADA deficiency) creates a form of severe combined immune deficiency (SCID). When the mutated gene for adenosine deaminase (ADA) is replaced with a normal one in the lymphocytes of several children affected by SCID, there has been a clear clinical improvement. Recent studies show that targeting normal genes to enter cells (from bone marrow, the lung and gut, liver and skin) may be easier than was first thought and that DNA will function more or less normally once it is introduced into the cell. Finally, there is a growing consensus that it is ethical to use gene therapy in a wide variety of somatic ways but not in gametes or embryos. In addition, gene therapy may provide a new, general, enabling technology for protein and drug delivery, as well as for gene therapy, through the introduction of normal genes.

One can anticipate that gene therapy is coming in the future for serious disease. It is already here for ADA deficiency. Other single gene disorders such as cystic fibrosis and hemophilia B should follow quickly. Hemophilia B has been corrected in the canine species through liver transfer of the appropriate gene. However, the true excitement will be in the novel use of the technology to treat the common multifactorial diseases, even those not due primarily to a genetic defect, by genetic means at the somatic level. The obvious examples are hypercholesterolemia, cancer of the colon, and autoimmune disease. The time to begin thinking of these approaches is now while the ethical issue concerns are real. None of these issues are novel in medicine or in technology and are worth confronting for the benefits that will come to patients.

It is important to point out that there are two independent systems for reviewing human gene therapy protocols in the United States, one at the NIH and one at the FDA. The NIH and its RAC function responded to the perceived need for public participation in genetic research policy.[9] As a result the RAC meetings are completely open to the public, the meetings are announced in advance with provision for public comments, and all the review materials are available to the public on request. Given the provisions of the NIH guidelines, only those investigators who receive NIH funding, or who work in institutions that receive NIH funding for rDNA research, are required to undergo review by the RAC. However, approval by the FDA is also required. Those investigators and institutions who do not receive NIH funding are exempt from RAC review but must undergo FDA review. Unlike the RAC, FDA review does not have to be conducted in a public forum; the precedent for this derives from the fact that the FDA has a responsibility for reviewing proprietary information. These methods of surveillance have increased the potential for flexibility and have been one of the principal virtues of the process as gene therapy has moved from its infancy to a form of treatment with demonstrated efficacy.

SUMMARY

Somatic gene therapy research in humans is still searching for appropriate vector systems and remains experimental. Germline therapy is a major technical challenge and can be considered only for the future.

REFERENCES

1. FRIEDMANN, T. & R. ROBLIN. 1972. Gene therapy for human genetic disease? Science **175:** 949–955.
2. FRIEDMANN, T., Ed. 1991. Therapy for Genetic Disease. Oxford University Press. Oxford, England.
3. FRIEDMANN, T. 1992. A brief history of gene therapy. Nature Genet. **2:** 93–98.
4. KANTOFF, P. W., S. W. FREEMAN & W. F. ANDERSON. 1988. Prospects for gene therapy for immunodeficiency diseases. Annu. Rev. Immunol. **6:** 581–594.
5. FRIEDMANN, T. 1989. Progress toward human gene therapy. Science **244:** 1275–1281.
6. *Splicing Life.* 1982. President's Commission for the Study of Ethical Problems in Medicine and Biomedical and Behavioral Research. Government Printing Office. Washington, DC. pp. 1–115.
7. ANONYMOUS. 1990. The revised "Points to Consider" document. Hum. Gene Ther. **1:** 93–103.
8. JUENGST, E. T. 1990. The NIH "Points to Consider" and the limits of human gene therapy. Hum. Gene Ther. **1:** 425–433.
9. ANONYMOUS. 1991. Draft of FDA's Points to Consider in Human Somatic Cell Therapy and Gene Therapy. Hum. Gene Ther. **2:** 251–256.

Genetic Screening for RET Mutations in Families with Multiple Endocrine Neoplasia 2 Syndromes

M. ALEVIZAKI, H. SARIKA, D. A. KOUTRAS,
AND A. SOUVATZOGLOU

Endocrine Section
Department of Medical Therapeutics
Alexandra University Hospital
80, Vassilissis Sofias Avenue
11528 Athens, Greece

INTRODUCTION

Recent advances in molecular genetics have shed new light on the pathogenesis of multiple endocrine neoplasia syndromes. These new advances have led to the development of genetic tests, which may now be used for the identification of carriers in childhood. Physicians belonging to several specialties, such as endocrinologists, pediatric endocrinologists, surgeons, and geneticists, treat these patients at the preclinical stage.

Multiple Endocrine Neoplasia Type 2 Syndrome

The multiple endocrine neoplasia (MEN) type 2 syndrome is an autosomal dominant cancer syndrome characterized by the development of medullary carcinoma of the thyroid (MTC) and other neoplasms. An interesting feature of MTC in MEN2 is that C-cell hyperplasia precedes tumor development; at this stage serum calcitonin, the normal secretory product of thyroid C cells, is a very useful marker that can be used for detection of the disease at its early stages. The MEN2 syndrome includes three distinct entities: (1) the MEN2A syndrome, in which, apart from medullary carcinoma of the thyroid, there is involvement of the adrenal medulla (pheochromocytomas) in about 50% of the cases and hyperparathyroidism in 15 to 40% of the cases; (2) the MEN2B syndrome, in which, apart from MTC (100%) and pheochromocytoma (50%), there is involvement of the enteric autonomic nervous plexes and various dysplastic features; (3) the familial MTC, in which only thyroid C cells are involved.[1–3]

The search for the MEN2 locus has gone through various stages. The original studies had failed to show a consistent pattern of allelic chromosomal loss from the tumor cells, as would be expected if the MEN2 "gene" was a suppressor gene, as is usually the case with inherited cancer syndromes.[4,5] The next step was linkage analysis using DNA markers. With such studies, the genetic locus of MEN2A was roughly localized on chromosome 10 at the pericentromeric region.[6] High "lod scores" were obtained with certain of the markers, and the RET proto-oncogene was recognized as a "candidate" gene, since it had previously been mapped to this region.[7] Recently, germline mutations in the coding region of the RET proto-oncogene were described in patients with the MEN2 syndromes, which are responsible for the transmittance of the disease, in all three subtypes of MEN2.[8–12] The mutation is present in all cells, in one allele.

The RET Proto-oncogene

The RET protooncogene is a tyrosine kinase receptor of the cell membrane belonging to the same family as the platelet-derived growth factor receptor.[11] RET may participate in the migration of the neural crest in embryogenesis. GDNF (glial-cell-line derived neurotrophic factor) has recently been recognized as a putative ligand for RET.[13] Somatic mutations of this gene (in tumor cells only) have also been described in sporadic medullary thyroid carcinoma (30–65% of cases),[11,12,14] as well as in papillary thyroid carcinoma. In the latter case, there is rearrangement of RET in 10 to 25% of the tumors.[15]

The oncogenic mechanism is dominant, since the presence of the normal allele is not enough to restrain the cell from undergoing malignant transformation.[8] The mutations in MEN2 syndromes are practically all clustered in the cysteine-rich region, which is located in the extracellular domain near the transmembrane part of the protein encoded by exons 10 and 11.[8,10,16,17] They affect roughly the same cysteine residues in both the MEN2A and familial MTC syndromes. In the MEN2B syndrome, the mutation affects one totally different part of the protein in the intracellular region, which has protein kinase activity. It always involves the same residue, a methionine in exon 16.[11,12,18] The MEN2 mutations have not been found in the normal population.[8] Recent work has shown the occasional presence of more unusual mutations in certain families.[2]

Recent *in vitro* studies by Santoro *et al.* showed that transfection of cell lines with the mutated RET gene (both mutations found in MEN2A and B) is accompanied by increased transforming efficiency.[19] The MEN2A mutation causes dimerization of the RET protein, activation of the protein kinase receptor, and increased transforming ability. The presence of the MEN2B mutation is not accompanied by dimerization of the molecule; it probably alters the substrate specificity, making the RET receptor respond to nonphysiological ligand(s).[19]

DISCUSSION

The recognition that the majority of MEN mutations lie in a specific region of the RET gene allowed the genetic tests to replace the calcitonin stimulation tests that were previously used for the identification of gene carriers. Such tests were both unpleasant and required frequent screening up to at least the age of 35 years. Furthermore, reevaluation of results obtained with the use of these tests revealed that they would give both false positive as well as false negative results.[3,16] The genetic test is simple to perform and has a 100% accuracy once the mutation has been characterized in a family.

Recently, several groups have reported the use of various genetic tests to screen individuals with MEN2 syndromes for RET mutations.[10,16,20,21] The tests, which are commonly used, include PCR amplification of the exons where the mutations usually occur. The PCR product is subsequently analyzed either by direct electrophoresis if the mutation has been included in the primer sequence, or after digestion with a restriction enzyme in cases where a recognition site is affected by the mutation. The PCR product may be sequenced directly, in which case all possible mutation sites may be checked at the same time.[2,3,21]

We have studied the RET mutations in Greek families with MEN2 syndromes and have started to use the genetic analysis in the screening of young persons belonging to such families.

We studied patients from 12 distinct families with MEN2 syndromes who had a positive family history. Six came from typical MEN2A families. Five patients came from families with familial MTC. One additional patient had a typical MEN2B syndrome but a negative family history. The DNA was extracted from peripheral lymphocytes for analysis. Exons 10, 11, and 16 of the RET gene, where mutations are found in the majority of cases, were amplified using the polymerase chain reaction (PCR). The PCR product was sequenced directly using cycle sequencing.[10] RFLP analysis of the PCR product was used in the case of exon 16 where the restriction site of the enzyme Fok1 is affected by the sole mutation found in this position.

The patient with MEN2B had a heterozygous mutation of the RET gene in exon 16 (Met918-Tyr). Two patients with familial MTC had heterozygous mutations in exon 10 (Cys620-Tyr and Cys620-Arg, respectively). One additional patient with familial MTC had a Cys618-Ser mutation, whereas one case with MEN2A carried a heterozygous Cys618-Arg mutation. Finally, five patients with MEN2A had heterozygous mutations in exon 11 (Cys634-Arg in three and Cys634-Tyr in two cases). The Cys634-Arg mutation in exon 11 appears to be the commonest mutation in all studies (FIG. 1).[17] The same MEN2 mutation was always present in the same family. It was found only in affected and never found in unaffected members in a family.[22] No mutations were identified in the positions studied in two of the families with familial MTC.

We used the results of our sequence analysis to screen offspring of affected patients in a few families. The test has a 100% accuracy in identifying carriers among at-risk individuals. So far, we have been able to use the test in nine offspring of MEN2 families aged 14 to 25 years. Three belonged to a MEN2B family. They were all negative (the index case probably represents a new mutation because the relatives do not carry the characteristic phenotype). Six were from families with MEN2A syndrome. The MEN2 mutation was detected in one. Prophylactic thyroidectomy was offered to this individual; C-cell hyperplasia and C-cell tumors were present. The molecular study is recommended to the offspring (and in fact to all the relatives) in a family where the mutation has been characterized in one affected individual. The recommended age for screening is 4 years.[2,21] The age at which prophylactic thyroidectomy should be performed has been recommended to be as early as 6 years.[21]

There is still a small percentage of families where it has not been possible to identify the mutation. In a recent publication of a large series, where 361 families were collected, the mutation was identified in 87% of the cases.[17] It is not possible at present to speculate about the type of mutation in the remaining families. The identifica-

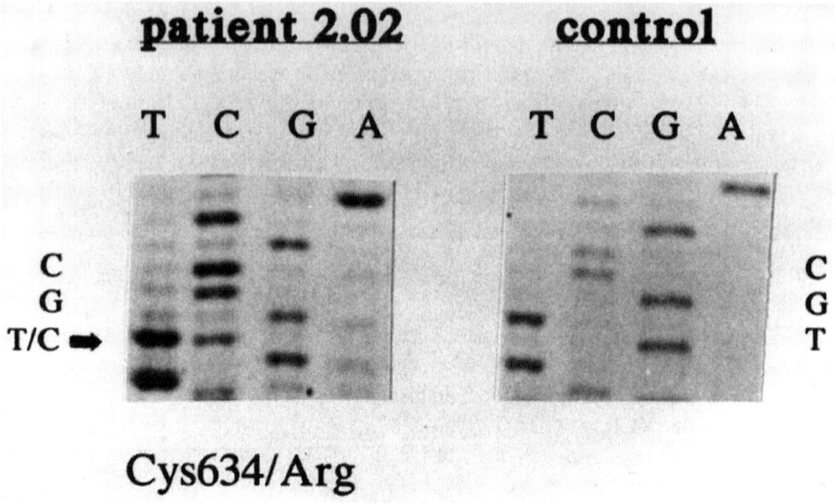

FIGURE 1. Sequence analysis of exon 11 of the RET proto-oncogene in patient 2.02 with MEN2A syndrome (MTC and bilateral pheochromocytomas). The heterozygous mutation is a T to C transition (*arrow*) and affects the first nucleotide in codon 634. The normal cysteine in this position is replaced by an arginine in one allele. This mutation was detected in germline DNA of all affected members in the family.

tion of these mutations too in the future will be very interesting, as it may reveal further pathogenetic mechanisms in this rare neoplasm and will also possibly clarify further the role of the RET oncogene in tumorigenesis in general.

Whether the RET mutation itself is sufficient for tumor development, or further genetic events are also required, is not known at present. Individuals who have had operations at a very young age based on genetic tests alone and before their calcitonin tests became positive had C-cell hyperplasia and on certain occasions small tumors as well.[21] A completely different mutation of the RET proto-oncogene involving rearrangement of genetic material, which is found in papillary thyroid carcinoma, induced the development of tumors in transgenic mice.[23] One may expect that in the near future the mechanisms involved in the pathogenesis of MEN syndromes will be clarified further.

SUMMARY

Mutations in the RET proto-oncogene have recently been recognized to be responsible for the inherited multiple endocrine neoplasia type 2 syndrome. As expected, Greek patients with MEN2 and FMTC carry RET mutations similar to those of other ethnic groups. In those regions of the gene that were analyzed, mutations were detected in six out of six families with classical MEN2A, three out of five of the families with familial MTC, and one case with MEN2B. Presymptomatic screening using DNA analysis has now replaced calcitonin stimulation tests in the offspring of families where the mutation has been characterized. The use of these methods will improve the prognosis in MEN2 patients and will also reduce the psychological burden of risk for a potentially lethal disease on family members.

REFERENCES

1. Eng, C., M. Stratton, B. Ponder, V. Murday, D. Easton, N. Sacks, M. Watson & R. Eeles. 1994. Familial cancer syndromes. Lancet **343:** 709–713.
2. Mulligan, L. M. & B. A. J. Ponder. 1995. Genetic basis of endocrine disease: Multiple endocrine neoplasia type 2. J. Clin. Endocrinol. Metab. **80:** 1989–1995.
3. Marsh, D. J., D. L. Learoyd & B. G. Robinson. 1995. Medullary thyroid carcinoma: Recent advances and management update. Thyroid **5:** 407–423.
4. Thakker, R. V. 1993. The molecular genetics of the multiple endocrine neoplasia syndromes. Clin. Endocrinol. **38:** 1–14.
5. Ponder, B. A. J., B. A. Smith, E. M. Marcus, Y. Nakamura, R. M. Landsvater, C. H. C. M. Buys & C. P. G. Mathew. 1989. Genetic events in tumorigenesis in multiple endocrine neoplasia type 2. Cancer Cells **7:** 219–221.
6. Matthew, C. G., K. S. Chin, D. F. Easton, K. Thorpe, C. Carter, G. I. Liou, S. L. Fong, C. D. Brodges, K. Haak, *et al.* 1987. A linked genetic marker for multiple endocrine neoplasia type 2A on chromosome 10. Nature **328:** 527–528.
7. Lairmore, T. C., S. Dou, J. R. Howe, D. Chi, K. Carlson, R. Veile, S. K. Mishra, S. A. Wells & H. Donis Keller. 1993. A 1.5-megabase yeast artificial chromosome contig from human chromosome 10q11.2 connecting three genetic loci (RET, D10S94, and D10S102) closely linked to the MEN2A locus. Proc. Natl. Acad. Sci. USA **90:** 492–496.
8. Mulligan, L. M., J. B. Kwok, C. S. Healey, M. J. Elsdon, C. Eng, E. Gardner, D. R. Love, S. E. Mole, J. K. Moore, L. Papi, M. A. Ponder, H. Telenius, A. Tunnacliffe & B. A. J. Ponder. 1993. Germ-line mutations of the RET proto-oncogene in multiple endocrine neoplasia type 2A. Nature **363:** 458–460.
9. Donis-Keller, H., S. Dou, D. Chi, *et al.* 1993. Mutations in the RET protooncogene are associated with MEN2A and FMTC. Hum. Molec. Genet. **2:** 851–856.
10. Mulligan, L. M., C. Eng, C. S. Healey, D. Clayton, J. B. J. Kwok, E. Gardner, M. A. Ponder, A. Frilling, C. E. Jackson, H. Lehnert, H. P. H. Neumann, S. N. Thibodeau & B. A. J. Ponder. 1994. Specific mutations of the RET proto-oncogene are related to disease phenotype in MEN2A and FMTC. Nature Genet. **6:** 70 74.
11. Hofstra, R. M. W., R. M. Landsvater, I. Caccherini, R. P. Stulp, T. Stelwagen, Y. Luo, B. Pasini, J. W. M. Hoppener, H. K. P. Vanamstel, G. Romeo, C. J. M. Lips & C. H. C. M. Buys. 1994. A mutation in the RET protooncogene associated with multiple endocrine neoplasia type 2B and sporadic medullary thyroid carcinoma. Nature **367:** 375–378.
12. Eng, C., D. P. Smith, L. M. Mulligan, M. A. Nagai, C. S. Healey, M. A. Ponder, E. Gardner, G. F. W. Scheumann, C. E. Jackson, A. Tunnacliffe & B. A. J. Ponder. 1994. Point mutation within the tyrosine kinase domain of the RET proto-oncogene in multiple endocrine neoplasia type 2B and related sporadic tumors. Hum. Mol. Genet. **3:** 237–241.
13. Durbec, P., C. V. Marcos Gutierrez, C. Kilkenny, M. Grigoriou, K. Wartiowaara, P. Suvanto, D. Smith, B. Ponder, F. Costantini, M. Saarma, H. Sariola & V. Pachnis. 1996. GDNF signalling through the Ret receptor tyrosine kinase. Nature **381:** 789–793.
14. Zedenius, J., C. Larsson, U. Bergholm, J. Bovee, A. Svensson, B. Hallengren, L.

GRIMELIUS, M. BACKDAHL, G. WEBER & G. WALLIN. 1995. Mutations in the RET proto-oncogene correlate to poor prognosis in sporadic medullary thyroid carcinoma. J. Clin. Endocrinol. Metab. **80:** 3088–3090.

15. GRIECO, M., M. SANTORO, M. T. BERLINGIERI, *et al.* 1990. PTC is a novel rearranged form of the RET proto-oncogene and is frequently detected *in vivo* in human thyroid papillary carcinoma. Cell **60:** 557–563.
16. LIPS, C. J. M., R. M. LANDSVATER, J. W. M. HOPPENER, R. A. GEERDINK, G. BLIJHAM, J. M. JANSEN-SCHILLHORN VAN HEEN, *et al.* 1994. Clinical screening as compared with DNA analysis in families with multiple endocrine neoplasia type 2A. N. Engl. J. Med. **331:** 828–835.
17. MULLIGAN, L. M., D. J. MARSH, D. G. ROBINSON, I. SCHUFFENECKER, J. ZEDENIUS, C. J. M. LIPS, *et al.* 1995. Genotype–phenotype correlation in MEN2: Report of the international RET mutation registry. J. Intern. Med. **238:** 343–346.
18. CARLSON, K. M., S. DOU, D. CHI, N. SCAVARDA, K. TOSHIMA, C. E. JACKSON, S. A. WELLS, P. J. GOODFELLOW & H. DONIS-KELLER. 1994. Single missense mutation in the tyrosine kinase catalytic domain of the RET proto-oncogene is associated with multiple endocrine neoplasia type 2B. Proc. Natl. Acad. Sci. **91:** 1579–1583.
19. SANTORO, M., F. CARLOMAGNO, A. ROMANO, D. P. BOTTATO, N. A. DATHAN, M. GRIECO, A. FUSCO, *et al.* 1995. Activation of RET as a dominant transforming gene by germline mutations of MEN2A and MEN2B. Science **267:** 381–383.
20. QUADRO, L., L. PANARIELLO, D. SALVATORE, F. CARLOMAGNO, M. DEL PRETE, V. NUNZIATA, V. COLABTUONI, G. DI GIOVANNI, L. M. BRANDI, M. MANELLI, M. GRIECO & M. SANTORO. 1994. Frequent RET protooncogene mutations in multiple endocrine neoplasia type 2A. J. Clin. Endocrinol. Metab. **79:** 590–594.
21. WELLS, S. A., D. D. CHI, K. TOSHIMA, L. P. DEHNER, C. M. COFFIN, B. DOWTON, *et al.* 1994. Predictive DNA testing and prophylactic thyroidectomy in patients at risk for multiple endocrine neoplasia type 2A. Ann. Surg. **220:** 237–250.
22. ALEVIZAKI, M., L. SARIKA, G. PHILIPPOU, S. I. GRIGORAKIS, P. PAPAPETROU, A. SOUVATZOGLOU & D. A. KOUTRAS. 1995. Study of the MEN2A "gene" in Greek patients with familial medullary thyroid carcinoma (MTC) and related syndromes. 8th Balkan Congress of Endocrinology, Abstract Book p. 242. Bursa. May 1995.
23. JHIANG, S. M., J. E. SAGARTZ, Q. TONG, J. PARKER-THORNBURG, C. C. CAPEN, J. Y. CHO, S. XING & C. LEDENT. 1996. Targeted expression of the ret/PTC1 oncogene induces papillary thyroid carcinomas. Endocrinology **137:** 375–378.

Gonadal Dysgenesis: Fertility Options

D. LOUTRADIS AND P. DRAKAKIS[a]

IVF Unit, Alexandra Maternity Hospital
First Department of Obstetrics and Gynecology
Athens University Medical School
Athens, Greece

INTRODUCTION

Gonadal dysgenesis is the most common cause of primary amenorrhea.[1] Patients with Turner's syndrome have a 45,XO karyotype, but mosaicism is common among them and may include 45,XO; 46,XX; and ringed X chromosomes. These patients present with short stature, cardiovascular abnormalities, developmental abnormalities of the genitourinary tract, high arched palate, increased freckling, and a shield chest.[1]

Although these patients have a high number of primordial follicles *in utero,*[2,3] the latter become atretic at a high rate and are exhausted before menarche.[3] Therefore, Turner's syndrome is associated with primary amenorrhea, high gonadotropin, and low estradiol serum values.[1] If the rate of atresia is slower, these patients may have secondary amenorrhea, but infertility is still the endpoint, although some women have conceived naturally and have even delivered healthy babies,[3–7] although this is not the rule. But even for these patients, fetal wastage and chromosomal errors in the offspring are significantly increased.[5,6,8] As a consequence, conception after *in vitro* fertilization of donor oocytes provides these patients with a chance to conceive and, furthermore, to deliver normal children at full term.

Oocyte donation,[9–10] a treatment similar to artificial insemination by donor for male infertility, has extended the indications of assisted reproduction for infertile couples.[11,12] One of these indications is ovarian failure.[13–15] Advanced age is another one, because patients over 40 years old undergoing IVF-ET[16] have pregnancy rates considerably lower when compared to those with ovum donation.[11] Multiple previous failures for conception in an *in vitro* fertilization and embryo transfer (IVF-ET) program, due mainly to poor ovarian stimulation or poor quality oocytes, is another common indication for oocyte donation.

Genetic disorders related to the X chromosome are also a major indication for entering such a program,[8,17–20] because this method provides an option for patients that lack their own oocytes, but also for those that have experienced or would like to avoid increased pregnancy complications or increased risk for offspring abnormalities.

The purpose of this study was to investigate whether oocyte donation is a viable option for conception for patients with Turner's syndrome and whether the outcome of this procedure is different for these patients and for those with other causes for ovum donation.

[a]Address for correspondence: Assistant Prof. D. Loutradis, Sirinon 62, P. Faliron 17561, Athens, Greece.

MATERIALS AND METHODS

One hundred and twenty-four women that have entered the oocyte donation program in our center were included in this study (from 1992 till 1994). Among these patients, seven had gonadal dysgenesis. For the rest, the indications for entering the program were either elevated serum FSH values (FSH $\geq$ 14 mIU/ml) or advanced age ($\geq$39 years old) with normal serum FSH levels or multiple failures to conceive (>3) in previous IVF-ET programs. Their mean age was 39.2 years (range: 25–48 years). The mean age of the patients with gonadal dysgenesis was 26.0 years (range: 23 to 29 years).

All recipients were subjected to a careful precycle medical screening in order to prevent the inclusion of patients with known preexisting diseases (especially cardiovascular and diabetic)[21] (TABLE 1). For the patients with Turner's syndrome, a special cardiopulmonary work-up was performed. The possible adverse effects on the already compromised cardiovascular system were taken into consideration. In addition, any associated congenital abnormalities that would adversely affect the pregnancy were screened for.

In our program, we use excess oocytes of IVF-ET cycles that are voluntarily donated by the patients after informed consent. The anonymity of recipients and donors is strictly maintained. All donors are less than 34 years old and are screened for hepatitis B and C, HIV-I and II, syphilis, chlamydia, and for vaginal infections. A detailed history is obtained in order to exclude potential carriers of genetic disease.

Superovulation in the donors was induced by GnRH analogues and gonadotropins.[22] Briefly, buserelin intranasal spray (Suprefact, Hoechst, Frankfurt, Germany) administration commenced on day 21 of the previous cycle at a dose of 100 μg 5 times daily (every 4 hours, omitting the 3 A.M. dose). When serum E_2 levels fell below 40 pg/ml and menses had started, hMG (Pergonal, Serono, Rome, Italy) administration commenced with 3 ampoules daily i.m. and was adjusted according to the patient's response. When the mean diameter of the leading follicle was $\geq$ 18 mm with 2–3 others $\geq$ 16 mm. Buserelin and hMG administration was then discontinued

TABLE 1. Medical Screening for the Recipients of Our Study before Entering the Oocyte Donation Program

- Electrocardiogram
- Mammography
- Chest X-ray
- Glucose tolerance test
- Blood urea
- Liver function assays
- Coagulation profile
- Full blood count
- Papanicolaou smear
- HIV I-II antibodies
- Hepatitis B and C screening
- Syphilis screening

and, within 24 hours, 10,000 IU of hCG (Profasi, Serono, Rome, Italy) were given i.m.

Follicular aspiration and oocyte retrieval was performed by transvaginal ultrasonographically guided puncture 34 to 36 hours after hCG administration. The oocytes were cultured in Ham's F-10 without hypoxanthine with 4% bovine serum albumin as previously described.[23] Because the potential donors were IVF patients themselves, only those that produced more than six oocytes were considered as donors. Their excess oocytes were then donated to the matched recipients.

Recipients were given 2 mg of estradiol valerate *per os* (Cyclacur, Shering, Berlin, Germany) 4 times daily followed by the daily addition of 100 mg of progesterone in oil (Lutorm, Chropi, Athens, Greece) i.m.[24] Patients were prospectively followed using a protocol that allowed for estradiol administration between 6 and 17 days before the addition of progesterone.[25] Menstruating patients started receiving estradiol on the second day of their cycle. In amenorrheic patients, estradiol was started arbitrarily.

Recipients were synchronized with donors so that the day before oocyte retrieval the recipient started progesterone. The first day of progesterone administration was considered "day 15" of the artificial cycle irrespective of the days of estradiol administration. Concepti were then transferred to the recipients the third (day 17), fourth (day 18), or fifth (day 19) day after progesterone administration depending on the availability of good-quality oocytes (from consecutive donors) and, eventually, good-quality embryos. In the majority of the cycles (140 cycles), embryo transfer was performed on the fourth day after progesterone administration, in 24 cycles on the third day, and in eight on the fifth day.

All embryos transferred were day 2 embryos. In the majority of cases, three or four embryos were transferred into the uterus of the recipient, although two, five, or six embryos were also transferred in some cases. All embryos were fresh; there was no transfer of frozen–thawed embryos.

The luteal phase of the recipients was supported by estradiol valerate *per os* and progesterone i.m. (same scheme as before transfer) and, if a pregnancy occurred, hormonal administration was continued until the 14th week of pregnancy.

RESULTS

Group A consisted of 165 cycles from 117 women with various reasons for oocyte donation as analyzed below and Group B consisted of 7 cycles from 7 women with Turner's syndrome.

Seventy-four cycles were from patients with serum FSH $\geq$ 14 mIU/ml (mean serum FSH value: 25.5 mIU/ml; mean age of patients: 39.3 yrs).

Fifty-five cycles were from women of advanced age (mean age: 41.2 yrs; range: 39–48 years). Their serum FSH value was $\leq$14 mIU/ml.

Thirty-six cycles were from patients that had already had at least three previous failures for conception in an IVF-ET program (mean age: 36.0 years; serum FSH value $\leq$14 mIU/ml).

The results of ovum donation for the patients of our study are shown in TABLE 2.

In Group A, a total of 581 embryos were transferred, resulting in 101 viable gesta-

TABLE 2. Results of Ovum Donation for the Patients—Except Those with Turner's Syndrome—of Our Unit (Group A) and for the Recipients with Turner's Syndrome (Group B)

	Group A	Group B
No. of women	117	7
No. of cycles	165	7
No. of embryos transferred	581	26
Gestational sacs with fetal heart beat by ultrasound	101	4
Implantation rate[a]	17.4%[b]	15.4%[b]
Clinical pregnancies	57	4
Clinical pregnancy rate per cycle	34.5%[b]	57.1%[b]
Deliveries	43	4
Live birth rate per cycle	26.1%[b]	57.1%[b]
Multiple pregnancies (twins)	10	0
Multiple pregnancy rate	17.5%	0%
Total No. of babies born	53	4
Abortion rate	24.5%	0%

[a]Number of gestational sacs with fetal heart beat by ultrasound divided by the number of embryos transferred (×100).

[b]$p > 0.05$; results not statistically different; χ^2 test.

tional sacs (with fetal heart beat by ultrasound). Implantation rate was 17.4%. There were 57 clinical pregnancies giving a pregnancy rate of 34.5% per cycle.

Forty-three patients delivered (live birth rate per cycle: 26.1%), and 10 of those gave birth to twins (17.5%). The total number of babies born was 53. Abortion rate was 24.5%.

In Group B, a total of 26 embryos was transferred, resulting in four viable gestational sacs (with fetal heart beat by ultrasound). Implantation rate was 15.4%. There were four clinical pregnancies, giving a pregnancy rate of 57.1% per cycle.

Four patients delivered (live birth rate per cycle: 57.1%). There were no multiple pregnancies: The total number of babies born was four, and there were no miscarriages.

There were no statistical differences between the two groups, although the number of cases in Group B was too small to draw any definite conclusions.

DISCUSSION

The data presented above show that *in vitro* fertilization of donor oocytes is a successful fertility option for patients with gonadal dysgenesis who had to be considered sterile a decade ago.

Although spontaneous conception does occur in patients with mosaic or nonmosaic Turner's syndrome,[3–7] the rate of miscarriage and the percentage of fetal malformations is greatly increased.[5,6,8,26] A specialized obstetrical department is needed to follow up these pregnancies, and there are always ethical problems to be considered surrounding the conception and birth of the offspring. Oocyte donation from young, healthy female volunteers is, thus, a very promising option for these patients.

This method has been used on many occasions in recent years. It has been suggested by some that the outcome of oocyte donation in Turner's syndrome patients is poorer than in other groups.[27–29] Others, though, including the authors, have found that the outcome is comparable.[20]

Because the endometrial response to hormonal replacement therapy was found to be suboptimal in cases of poorer outcome compared to other groups,[28] but endometrial response was comparable to the other groups when the outcome was also comparable,[20] it seems that the right preparation of the endometrium with the hormone replacement therapy is a very important factor of increased pregnancy rates for these patients.

In our data, the regimen used[25] seems to prepare the endometrium suitably for implantation since implantation and pregnancy rates were high. Of the seven patients that entered the study, four had been using hormonal therapy for a long time (three of them became pregnant), and three had not used any replacement therapy (one of them became pregnant). The latter were administered the same hormonal replacement therapy used for the donation cycles for 3 months before entering the program.

Previous treatment of the endometrium seems to be essential for high conception rates, and these patients should be given hormonal therapy for a period of time before entering the program. In addition, hormone treatment helps to avoid hypoplasia and hypovascularization of the uterus. In the absence of it, the risk for premature labor and pre-eclampsia is increased.[8]

In conclusion, oocyte donation is a successful conception option for patients with Turner's syndrome with results comparable to those of the other patients that undergo ovum donation. The preparation of the endometrium is a very important factor for the success of this treatment, something that also holds true for non-Turner's syndrome patients. The above-presented protocol gives equally good results for all candidates for ovum donation. A further investigation of the proper time for implantation ("implantation window") by sampling the endometrium for appearance and disappearance of pinopodes[24] would provide these—otherwise mainly sterile patients—with even higher conception rates.

REFERENCES

1. VAITUKAITIS, J. L. 1990. Anovulation and amenorrhea. *In* Infertility. A Comprehensive Test. M. Seibel, Ed.: 51–59. Appleton & Lange. Norwalk, CT.
2. NIELSEN, J., I. SILLESEN & K. B. HANSEN. 1979. Br. J. Obstet. Gynaecol. **86:** 833–839.
3. SINGH, R. P. & D. H. CARR. 1966. Anat. Rec. **155:** 369–372.
4. BAUDIER, S. M. M., H. J. CHIHAL & R. P. DICKEY. 1985. Obstet. Gynecol. **65**(3 Suppl.): 60S–64S.
5. MEYER, L., M. BIRKHAUSER, E. BUHLER & N. PAVIC. 1989. Geburtshilfe Frauenheilkd. **49**(9): 825–829.
6. KANEKO, N., S. KAWAGOE & M. HIROI. 1990. Gynecol. Obstet. Invest. **29**(2): 81–87.
7. BALEN, A. H. & M. G. PRENTICE. J. Obstet. Gynecol. **14**(2): 117–118.
8. LECLERCQ, G., M. BUVAT-HERBAUT, J. C. MONNIER, D. VIVATIER & P. DUFOUR. 1992. J. Gynecol. Obstet. Biol. Reprod. **21**(6): 635–640.

9. LUTJEN, P., A. TROUNSON, J. LEETON, J. FINDLAY, C. WOOD & P. RENOU. 1984. Nature **307:** 174–175.
10. BUSTILLO, M., J. E. BUSTER, S. W. COHEN, I. H. THORNEYCROFT, J. A. SIMON, S. P. BOYERS, J. R. MARSHALL, R. W. SEED, J. A. LOUW & R. G. SEED. 1984. JAMA **251:** 1171–1173.
11. SAUER, M. V. & R. J. PAULSON. 1992. Fertil. Steril. **58:** 16–18.
12. BENSHUSHAN, A. & J. G. SCHENKER. 1993. J. Assist. Reprod. Genet. **10:** 105–111.
13. EDWARDS, R. G., S. MARCOS, M. MACNAMEE, J. P. BALMACEDA, D. E. WALTERS & R. ASCH. 1991. Lancet **338:** 292–294.
14. COHEN, I. & L. SPEROFF. 1991. Obstet. Gynecol. Surv. **46:** 156–161.
15. COULAM, C. B., S. C. ANDERSON & J. F. ANNEGERS. 1986. Obstet. Gynecol. **67:** 604–606.
16. EDWARDS, R. G., S. B. FISHEL & J. COHEN. 1984. J. In Vitro Fertil. Embryo Trans. **1:** 3–23.
17. ABDALLA, H. I., R. J. BABER, A. KIRKLAND, T. LEONARD & J. W. W. STUDD. 1989. Br. J. Obstet. Gynaecol. **96**(9): 1071–1075.
18. CRITCHLEY, H. O. D., T. CHARD, B. A. LIEBERMAN, C. H. BUCKLEY & D. C. ANDERSON. 1990. Hum. Reprod. **5**(3): 250–254.
19. BARRI, P. N., B. COROLA, F. MARTINEZ, N. PARERA, A. VEIGA & G. CALDERON. 1992. Hum. Reprod. **7:** 85–88.
20. PRESS, F., H. M. SHAPIRO, C. A. COWELL & G. A. OLIVER. 1995. Fertil. Steril. **64**(5): 995–998.
21. BECKETT, V. & P. SEHRAL. 1994. Hum. Reprod. **9:** 2444–2445.
22. MICHALAS, S., D. LOUTRADIS, K. KALLIANIDIS, P. DRAKAKIS & D. ARAVANTINOS. 1994. ARTA **5:** 47–52.
23. KIESSLING, A. A., D. LOUTRADIS, P. MCSHANE & K. JACKSON. 1988. Ann. N.Y. Acad. Sci. **541:** 614–620.
24. NIKAS, G., P. DRAKAKIS, D. LOUTRADIS, C. MARA-SKOUFARI, E. KOUMANTAKIS, S. MICHALAS & A. PSYCHOYOS. 1995. Hum. Reprod. **10:** 1208–1213.
25. MICHALAS, S., D. LOUTRADIS, P. DRAKAKIS, K. KALLIANIDIS, S. MILINGOS, G. DELIGEOROGLOU & D. ARAVANTINOS. 1996. Hum. Reprod. In press.
26. PASQUALINI, A. J. 1988. Rev. Fr. Gynecol. Obstet. **83**(11): 717–721.
27. CHAN, C. L. K., I. T. CAMERON, J. K. FINDLAY, D. HEALY, J. F. LEETON & P. J. LUFJEN. 1987. Obstet. Gynecol. Surv. **42:** 350–353.
28. LI, T. C., P. DOCKERY, S. S. RAMSEWAK, L. KLENTZERIS, E. A. LENTON & I. D. COOKE. 1991. Br. J. Obstet. Gynaecol. **98:** 656–661.
29. HEINZE, H. J. 1994. Adol. Pediatr. Gynecol. **7:** 3–8.

Adolescent Sexuality

ALVIN F. GOLDFARB[a]

Department of Obstetrics and Gynecology
Jefferson Medical College of Thomas Jefferson University
and
North American Society for Pediatric and Adolescent Gynecology
Philadelphia, Pennsylvania 19107

We have always thought that problems referable to adolescent sexuality are uniquely problems of the 20th century. This is not so. One can date discussions concerning adolescent sexuality and the syndrome of "raging hormones" to the ancient Greeks and Egyptians and to modern Europeans. What is of major concern today, however, is the phenomenon of the unwed adolescent becoming pregnant. As the result of coital activity, with an absence of sex education, there is an increased risk for sexually transmitted disease and unwanted pregnancies. The adolescent who has an unintended pregnancy suffers from socioeconomic dysfunction characterized by failure to acquire an appropriate education for today's work force and is at risk to become dependent on the welfare system.

During the course of the past two decades, the rates of sexual activity in the United States have, in the adolescent population, increased almost by a geometric progression. In 1970, children 15 years of age represented only 5% of the population between the ages of 15 and 19 who were sexually active. Now 24% of 15-year-olds are sexually active. In 1970, 50% of the females did not become sexually active until they were nineteen years of age and in the 1990s over 50% were sexually active by the age of 17. This increase in the rate of sexual activity among adolescent women is illustrated in TABLE 1.

Whereas adults—particularly physicians—are all too cognizant of the risks involved in premature sexual intercourse, teenagers often do not comprehend that pregnancy and sexually transmitted disease may follow even the first episode of intercourse. Their unique psychology and unusual thinking make them immune to such worries but, unfortunately, not to the inevitable consequences of their sexual activity.

ADOLESCENT SEXUAL PRACTICES

With increased sexual activity among the teen population, it becomes important to understand teen sexual practices. As cognitive behavior has not completely matured, there is an attitudinal facet to their thinking that can best be stated by, "It can't happen to me." As health care providers, we are concerned about the increase in the incidence and the relative risk for the development of numerous sexually transmitted dis-

[a]Address for correspondence: Alvin F. Goldfarb, M.D., 1015 Chestnut St., Suite 1225, Philadelphia, PA 19107.

TABLE 1. Rates of Sexual Activity 1970 to 1990 in Adolescent Women[a]

Age	Year 1970	Year 1990
15	5%	24%
17	25%	50%
18	38%	68%
19	50%	>75%

[a]Note that 50% of all adolescent women were sexually active two years earlier in life in 1990.

eases in this age group, including hepatitis B and AIDS. In addition, the frequency of unwanted pregnancies increases in this age group.

The incidence of sexually transmitted diseases increases in this population in proportion to the number of new partners that an individual has. From a contraceptive standpoint the compliance rate is not quite as good as it should be. The majority of adolescents having their first coital experience do not use a contraceptive method. As a result of this, two outcomes may result: (1) they become poor compliers for contraception and (2) having more than one partner (which is not unusual in the adolescent) allows for an increase in unintended pregnancies as well as the acquisition and transmission of sexually transmitted diseases.

Once sexual intercourse is initiated, teens participate in the activity more persistently. Sexual initiation also appears to be related to other coming-of-age activities such as substance use, tobacco use, alcohol abuse, and delinquent behaviors. In addition, many adolescents are street persons, runaways, and prostitutes. These behaviors lead to increased sexual activity.

Experimentation with various forms of sexual practices have important implications for preventing the spread of AIDS. In a small study comparing affluent New York 12th grade students to inner city youth attending an adolescent clinic, it was noted that 27% of the latter group had anal intercourse versus 7% of the upper middle class students. More importantly, 70% of the teenagers reported never using condoms during such intercourse.

The number of gay and lesbian adolescents is difficult to estimate among this population. Two conflicting factors make estimating homosexual behavior among teenagers difficult: (1) Experimentation with the same sex is common during adolescence, but (2) same-sex orientation probably begins even before then.

The U.S. Department of Health and Human Services estimated in 1983 that throughout the United States between 730,000 and 1.3 million youths run away each year. Approximately 25% of these teenagers are considered "street kids" with no permanent support. A high number of homeless have a history of being abused or neglected by their families. In addition, many of these are homosexual or lesbian adolescents. The Youth Services Department of the Los Angeles Gay and Lesbian Community Service Center provides services to street youth with street outreach, drop-in assistance and referral, as well as comprehensive residential life stabilization. Approximately 65 to 70% of clients self-identify as being gay. They are usually 18 to 23 years of age, although 17% are 13–17 years of age. On the average, 89% are males.

Sexual orientation is probably under-reported because many teenagers do not feel comfortable in reporting their alternate sexual preference. Because much of the research has focused on gay men rather than lesbians, it is estimated that there are in fact more lesbians than reported by the various community services.

Runaway and street youth, in association with sex orientation, are related to the practice of survival sex (prostitution). A nationwide sample from the United States reported that approximately 12% of the runaway population (both males and females) engage in prostitution. The adolescent prostitute faces several risks. The major risk is acquiring an STD. The abortion rate is also increased among prostitutes: birth weights for children born to adolescent prostitutes are low. The appropriate emphasis, therefore, has not been given to the many psychological social and legal aspects of this population.

Suicide is another problem among adolescents presenting this kind of sexual behavior. In an adolescent care center in the United States, 25% of the visitors reported to have considered suicide seriously and one in six to have already attempted it. There are a number of studies cited by the Department of Health and Human Services showing the rate of suicide in gay teenagers to be three to six times more when compared with non-gay teenagers.

Age is the most important factor in determining whether a teenager is sexually experienced. Sex in the teenage years is becoming increasingly more common. Although the likelihood of having intercourse increases steadily with age, nearly 20% of adolescents do not have sex at all during their teenage years. For some young people, having sex is not a voluntary choice. The youngest teenagers are specially vulnerable to coercive sex. Some 75% of women who had intercourse before age 14 and 60% of those who have had sex before age 15 report having sex involuntarily. In addition, most of their experiences were with older men, meaning men that were five or more years older than the adolescent girls. It is not unusual for unmarried people, young and old alike, often to enter into, "serial monogamy." In other words, they remain faithful to their partner until the relationship breaks up, but then move into another relationship, thereby increasing their risk of acquiring an STD.

The latest statistics would suggest that perhaps sexual activity is leveling off in the adolescent population. Abstinence is being discussed in adolescent clinics and is influencing in a positive manner the lowering of the rate of adolescent coital activity. In addition, one can probably include in this data the statement that with the concern and risk for AIDS in promiscuous intercourse, even the adolescent is beginning to understand the relationship between promiscuity and disease.

SEXUALLY TRANSMITTED DISEASES

Every year 3,000,000 teenagers acquire an STD. Adolescents thus account for a quarter of the 12,000,000 new sexually transmitted infections that occur annually in the United States. Approximately 25% of all sexually experienced adolescents become infected each year. Roughly 13% of the young people between the ages of 13 and 19 contract an STD annually.

The following figures illustrate the incidents of chlamydia and gonorrhea seen in various population age groups. (FIGS. 1 and 2). It is quite apparent that the greatest incidence for chlamydia and gonorrhea is in the adolescent population. A wide variety of diseases can be transmitted through sexual intimacy. Chlamydia, trichomoniasis, gonorrhea, human papilloma virus (HPV), genital herpes, hepatitis B, syphilis, and HIV are among the most common STDs. Some of these diseases can be cured, including chlamydia, gonorrhea, trichomoniasis, and syphilis; that is, these diseases can be cured if they are detected early and treated vigorously. On the other hand, such viral diseases as genital herpes, HPV, and HIV cannot be cured and can be transmitted to sexual partners, years after initial infection. Hepatitis B is a viral illness that has as sequelae an increased risk factor for carcinoma of the liver and cirrhosis. This viral illness can be prevented with the use of hepatitis B vaccine.

It has been estimated that between 10 and 29% of the sexually experienced adolescent women tested for STDs have been found to have chlamydia. Up to 15% of sexually experienced teenage women are infected with HPV. Since 1980 the rate of reported cases of infectious syphilis among adolescent women has more than doubled. Sexually experienced men and women age 15 to 19 have higher rates of gonorrhea than any other 5-year age group between the ages of 20 and 44. Although the reported number of AIDS cases among teenagers is very small, about 20% of AIDS cases are diagnosed in people in their 20s. Most of them probably contracted HIV during adolescence. It is important to educate the adolescent about the fact that with increasing numbers of consorts, there is an increasing risk for the acquisition of an STD.

Both men and women can suffer serious health problems such as infertility, cancer, pelvic inflammatory disease, or HIV infection as a consequence of a sexually transmitted infection. Sexually transmitted diseases have a disproportionate impact on women, because these diseases are more easily transmitted to and more difficult to detect in women. As a result, complications of undiagnosed infections are far more

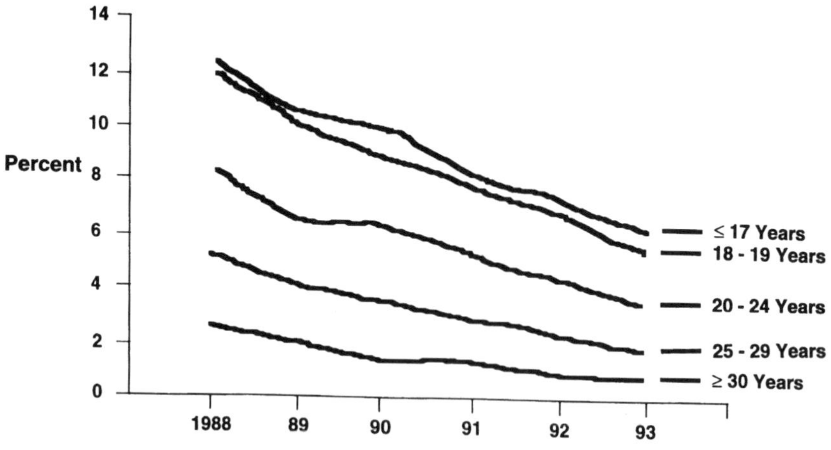

FIGURE 1. Chlamydia: Percent positivity among women tested in family-planning clinics by age group; region X, 1988–1993.

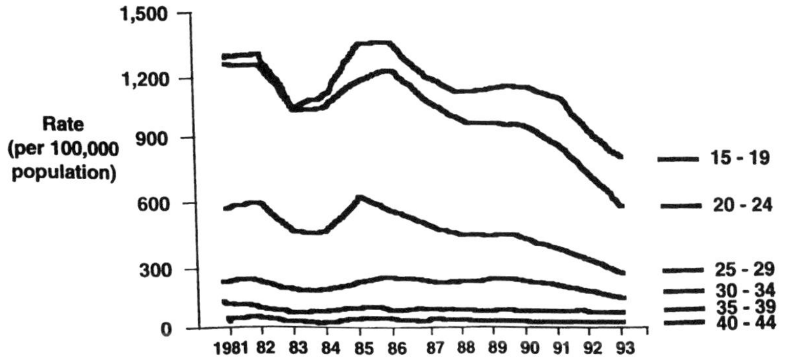

FIGURE 2. Gonorrhea: Age-specific rates among women 15 to 44 years of age; United States, 1981–1993.

common and severe in women. In addition, women can transmit an STD to her offspring during pregnancy or childbirth, sometimes with devastating consequences. A sexually experienced woman's risk of becoming infertile as a consequence of an upper genital tract infection (usually caused by untreated chlamydia or gonorrhea) or having an ectopic pregnancy (a possible result of an upper genital tract infection) is almost nonexistent if her risk of contracting an STD is low; that is to say, if she is in a mutually monogamous relationship with an uninfected partner. The risk of infection is substantially higher if the relationship is not mutually monogamous. Mutually monogamous relationships have a greater impact on reducing the risk of becoming infertile than does the choice of a contraceptive method.

Sexually experienced women and men age 15 to 19 have higher rates of gonorrhea than any 5-year age group between the ages of 20 and 44. Even women at high risk for acquiring an STD can avoid infection and reduced fertility if they choose the right contraceptive method, especially if they use it consistently. Barrier and spermadicidal methods, especially latex condoms, offer the maximum protection. Even when used imperfectly, condoms will reduce a woman's risk of infertility to an estimated 2%; used consistently, they provide still greater protection. The pill and other hormonal methods offer no protection against the risk of acquiring an STD; however, they probably lower a woman's risk of ultimately developing tubal infertility because they reduce the chances that lower genital tract infection will ascend into the upper genital tract where it could develop into PID and its sequelae, and they help prevent ectopic pregnancies, which can lead to infertility.

Early detection and treatment of STDs can reduce the chances that men and women will develop cancers associated with HPV and hepatitis B. STDs are extremely common among sexually experienced teenagers and can have serious, even life-threatening consequences. The surest means of preventing these problems is to be in a mutually monogamous relationship. Use of contraceptives, particularly latex condoms, can significantly reduce the likelihood of experiencing serious consequences, usually by lowering the risk of acquiring an STD. When infection does occur, timely treatment can be crucial to protecting one's health. STDs, of course, are not the only negative consequence of unprotected sex.

ADOLESCENT PREGNANCY

The United States has the highest rate of teenage pregnancy and abortion in the industrialized Western World, despite the fact that American teenagers are no more sexually active than their European counterparts. Overall, this amounts to more than one million teenage pregnancies in the United States, resulting annually in 400,000 abortions and 470,000 live births. One in ten female teenagers becomes pregnant each year in the United States, and, at present rates, four in ten will become pregnant while still in their teens. An estimated 12 million of the 29 million American young people age 13 to 19 have had sexual intercourse. The average age of first intercourse for American girls is 16 years. Of teens 15 years or younger, more than 30,000 become pregnant annually. Teenage girls have a disproportionately high number of abortions—26% of the total, although teens represent only 15% of the population.

Teen pregnancy costs American taxpayers an estimated $20 billion yearly in public funding support. Adolescent sexual intercourse is sporadic; that is, 75% of the teens reported engaging in intercourse either rarely (a few times per year or less) or occasionally (one to four times per month). At all ages, metropolitan teenagers are more likely to begin having intercourse earlier than their rural counterparts.

The out-of-wedlock births by age show a decrease in numbers as the adolescent grows into adulthood; women from age 15 to 20 account for approximately 81% of all out-of-wedlock births. As they approach 18 or 19, the proportion decreases to 59% and beyond the age of 20, only 27%. This correlates with the fact that the percentage of mothers using public assistance for delivery coverage decreases with age: 56% of all 15- to 19-year-olds need public assistance for delivery coverage; 20 to 24-year-old women, only 39%; as the women pass the age of 25, only 15% need public assistance. This would suggest that the women past 25 have some form of health insurance, or conversely, that the adolescent cannot obtain adequate health insurance.

Having a child below the age of 19 and not graduating from high school influences the individual's eventual annual income. Young women, or adolescents, who become mothers have an income in later life that is annualized at $17,600. Should they become mothers between the ages of 20 and 24, their annual income approximates $24,000. Should they not achieve motherhood voluntarily until they are past the age of 25, their annual income is approximately $36,400. Thus, associated with age, responsibility, and planning a pregnancy, is a higher annual income. This also reflects higher levels of education. There are many positive social and economic benefits that are associated with having a child later in life.

Among the problems that the adolescent obstetrical patient faces are some brought on by her own decisions. For example, the greatest number of adolescents who achieve a pregnancy do not get adequate prenatal care. They are not seen until well into the pregnancy for their prenatal care. In addition, these individuals usually have a weaker educational background. They are at greater risk for the development of toxemia. Many of these young adolescents are using drugs that may not only influence their own body but also may influence the growth and development of their young infant in utero.

Some of the problems that a fetus of an adolescent may face are low Apgar scores, low birth weight, and slow cognitive development. In addition, children of mothers who are adolescent and young are at approximately one-third more risk for health problems than women who are 25 and older. The baby is exposed and at risk for twice as many infections if the mother is younger when compared with women who are 25 or older. Just achieving a pregnancy as an adolescent is associated with greater risks to the mother and newborn.

Adolescence can be a time of great and satisfying personal growth, but not if it is marred by a premature pregnancy or acquiring an STD. The medical and social consequences of teen pregnancy are now well known: Pregnancy in teens younger than 15 is associated with a 60% higher risk of death, particularly in the younger than 15 age group; pregnancy carries with it increased risk for anemia, toxemia, hypertension, cephalopelvic disproportion, prematurity, and low-birth-weight babies. Fifty percent of teen mothers who marry the father of their children are divorced within five years. Without intensive school-based programs and efforts at secondary prevention, the drop-out rate for teenage mothers approaches 80%, and teen fathers are less likely to complete their high school education. Teen pregnancy takes a staggering socioeconomic toll including lowering levels of income, job success, and satisfaction. Society must also bear a major share of the impact.

THE ROLE OF THE HEALTH PROFESSIONAL

There are greater risks to the offspring of teenagers, including lower levels of school achievement, more emotional problems, and the possibility of increased abuse. Even if teenage pregnancy were not a factor, the risk of STDs alone, especially AIDS and hepatitis B, would well warrant the intervention of concerned health professionals. The roles of the health professionals in caring for the adolescent should be almost standardized. Confidentiality must be guaranteed. Confidentiality is the number one issue for teenagers seeking health care. Ensuring confidentiality may mean keeping separate files for those sensitive health visits that are required and not sending a bill home to parents. Alternatively, parents may agree, prospectively, to pay for visits without knowing why the visit was made. Physicians should be interested in seeing teenagers and should be skilled in the basics of adolescent medicine. Otherwise, the health visit becomes counterproductive for both the teenager and the professional.

There is no evidence that sex education increases, or for that matter decreases, levels of adolescent sexual activity. What it does accomplish is to make teenagers more knowledgeable about sexual matters and more tolerant of others. Teaching children about sex is no more likely to make them immediately become sexually involved than teaching them about geography is likely to make them drop out of school to join an expedition to Antarctica. One reason that sex education is not the panacea it was once believed to be is that a large number of teenagers are beginning sexual intercourse before they can be exposed to a sex education program. Nearly one-third of sex education teachers believe that their biggest obstacle to presenting information was pressure from parents and school administrators, particularly if teachers try to address issues of homosexuality, condoms, or abortion. Ideally, physicians should play a major role in the dissemination of sex education at home, in the office or clinic, and in school.

Counseling teenagers about sex can be difficult for both the health professional and a teenager. It requires skills best learned through practice. The style of the conversations is as important as the substance. Never be challenging in questioning. If you ask a teenager whether he or she has any questions about sex, the answer will invariably be no. If you ask, however, about their dating situation, they will give an honest answer, and this can gently lead to a discussion of other matters relating to human sexuality. Avoid discussion using the adolescent's jargon. Do not immediately assume that you are being understood. Avoid lectures, the teenager's parents do that. Give the patient credit for being intelligent, thoughtful, and responsible. Do not be afraid to offer your opinions and counsel in a straightforward manner. Teenagers will respond to this approach.

Information concerning sexuality really begins with talking about differences in human body parts. Not all women have the same size breast, not all males have the same size of penis. Sexual fantasies about an experience with members of the same sex do not necessarily mean a teenager is a homosexual. Sexual fantasies and masturbation are normal. The decision to begin having intercourse places the teen at risk for pregnancy and STDs. These risks can be lessened. There is nothing as safe as abstinence. Offering "no" as a form of contraception is perfectly acceptable. Taking oral contraceptives is a most efficient method for preventing pregnancy, but not for preventing STDs. Therefore, the "belt and garter approach" is in order; that is, the use of condoms to prevent STDs combined with oral contraceptives to prevent pregnancy is the most efficient manner for managing contraceptives in the adolescent.

The health professional who cares for the adolescent patient must be able to act as an educator and be comfortable reviewing, not only matters of sexuality, but also the information needed to prescribe good health: nutrition, exercise, and avoiding addictive behavior. In reality, the health professional treating adolescents must be an informed health educator who is nonjudgmental and gives information in a forthright manner.

SUMMARY

Sex education is almost mandated in the United States. The data reviewing sexual activity in the adolescent population indicates that large numbers of women under the age of 19 who have unintended pregnancies are at risk for an increased frequency of sexually transmitted diseases which will affect their future. It is essential that good educational programs and preventive service programs be developed and mandated for the adolescent population. Experience in Western Europe demonstrates that the adolescent who has a proper education concerning sexual activity, sexually transmitted disease, and contraception is at lower risk for the many problems that we see in the United States. There must be cross-cultural data that can be translated for use in the entire world. As the population of this world ages, we must protect those who are entering adulthood from being exposed to the STDs and undertaking the responsibility of parenting without having reached full maturity. The cost in dollars of the sequelae of adolescent pregnancies are great. These costs are not only financial, but also emotional and social, and they have a negative impact on the country in which the adolescent lives. We have a heavy responsibility as physicians and health care professionals to see that the adolescents of the world are given the knowledge and models to use to reduce the risk for pregnancy and the acquisition of a sexually transmitted disease.

REFERENCES

1. CREATSAS, G. K. 1994. Sexuality: Sexual activity and contraception during adolescence. Curr. Opin. Obstet. Gynecol. **5:** 774–783.
2. HENSHAW, S. K. & J. VANWORT. 1989. Teenage abortion, birth and pregnancy statistics: An update. Fam. Plan. Perspect. **21:** 85–88.
3. POKORNY, S. F. 1994. Reaching adolescents before they become sexually active. Female Patient **19:** 14–19. (Suppl. Apr.)
4. FUTTERMAN, D., K. HEIN, N. REUBEN, R. DELL & N. SHAFFER. 1993. Human immunodeficiency virus-infected adolescents: The first 50 patients in a New York City program. Pediatrics **91:** 730–735.
5. HILLARD, P. J. A. 1993. Family planning in the teen population. Curr. Opin. Obstet. Gynecol. **5:** 798–804.
6. Massachusetts Department of Education, Bureau of Student Development and Health. 1993.Massachusetts 1992, Youth Risk Behavior Survey Results. (January, 1993).
7. Pediatric and Adolescent Gynecology—A challenge for the 90s. Highlight of symposium presented by the North American Society for Pediatric and Adolescent Gynecology. Sponsored by Wyeth-Ayerst Laboratories, 1993.
8. Sex and American Teenagers. 1994. Alan Guttmacher Institute. Baltimore, MD.

Sexually Transmitted Diseases and Oral Contraceptive Use during Adolescence

G. CREATSAS[a]

First Department of Obstetrics and Gynecology
Division of Pediatric and Adolescent Gynecology
Medical School University of Athens
Athens, Greece

SEXUALLY TRANSMITTED DISEASES DURING ADOLESCENCE

Sexually transmitted disease (STD) during adolescence is a result of premature sexual life.[1] Infections involve the genital tract or may produce systemic disease (TABLE 1). Most of them, such as the human papilloma virus (HPV), involve the lower genital tract and cause cervicitis. An incidence of 32% HPV infection has been reported by Fisher *et al.*[2] among 107 teenagers. HPV anogenital infection has also occurred in 18.8% of the microbiological diagnoses in 32 teenaged girls attending a Dublin STD clinic.[3]

Chlamydia trachomatis (CT) and *Neisseria gonorrhoeae* (*N. gonorrhoeae*) may cause ascending infections involving the fallopian tubes.[4] These infections may also be found in asymptomatic sexually active adolescents. An incidence of 5.3% and 12.3% of *N. gonorrhoeae* and CT, respectively, has been reported among 19 asymptomatic adolescents.[5] Aerobic, anaerobic, or mixed pathogens may also be involved in ascending infections and cause pelvic inflammatory disease (PID) and pyeloperitonitis. Syphilis and other viral STD infections such as those of the human immunodeficiency virus (HIV), hepatitis B, herpes simplex and cytomegalovirus are also possible STDs during adolescence.[6] Finally, trichomoniasis, candidiasis, and bacterial vaginosis are common causes of cervicitis and vaginitis.[7]

A coincidence of various pathogens has been reported by Cox *et al.*[8] who found concomitantly the presence of *N. gonorrhoeae* in 22%, CT in 19%, *Trichomonas vaginalis* in 7%, and HIV in 7% of cases infected with syphilis. Street youth, runaways, homeless youth, prostitution, drug addiction, and sexual abuse in correlation with teenagers' incomplete knowledge on sexual matters are predisposing factors for STDs. In other words, premature sexual life in uneducated adolescents is a primary predisposing factor of STDs.

Consultation should include information on safe and efficient contraceptive methods (CM), simple in their use, to avoid discontinuation of the method. The condom, the "double Dutch method" (concomitant use of condom and oral contraceptives

[a]Address for correspondence: G. Creatsas, M.D., FACS, 9 Kanari str. 106 71 Athens, Greece.

TABLE 1. STDs and Related Infections during Adolescence[a]

Lower Genital Tract	Upper Genital Tract	Systemic Disease
HPV	*N. gonorrhoeae*	HIV
HSV	CT	Syphilis
CMV	CMV	Hepatitis
N. gonorrhoeae	Other pathogens	
CT		
Mycoplasma sp.		
Trichomonas vaginalis		
Candida albicans		
Vaginosis		

[a]ABBREVIATIONS: HPV, human papilloma virus; CT, *Chlamydia trachomatis*; HSV, Herpes simplex virus; HIV, human immunodeficiency virus; CMV, cytomegalovirus.

[OCs]) and other barrier methods such as vaginal sponges, which have both contraceptive and anti-STD properties, may be suggested as first-choice CMs.[9,10]

STDs AND ORAL CONTRACEPTIVE USE DURING ADOLESCENCE

OCs are popular during adolescence. Data available from a multinational survey on adolescent sexuality indicate that OCs are a favorite CM during adolescence. OCs are also suggested as a CM to adolescents presenting with menstrual irregularities, which is a common problem during the first two gynecological years. Low-dose OCs are preferable in most cases.[11,12]

Although OCs have been considered safe and effective during adolescence, their relationship with STDs remains unclear. It has been reported that OCs do not reduce the risk of gonococcal or CT infections of the lower genital tract. On the contrary, there is data indicating that the use of OCs is associated with higher rates of CT infection.[13,14] The findings of Kim *et al.*[15] have suggested that OC use may promote CT cervical infections or enhance the detection of the pathogen from the cervix in the population studied. They have also shown that the use of OCs for 6 months or longer was associated with higher prevalence of CT infection in comparison to less than 6 months' use. Other experimental studies on guinea pigs have shown that the use of sex steroids is more likely to result in development of salpingitis as compared with control animals when their lower genital tract was contaminated by CT.[15,16] Nevertheless, the above observation cannot be assumed to occur in a similar way for human beings. The effects of the OCs' use on the cervix include an eversion of the endocervical epithelium and enlargement of columnar villi resulting in cervical ectopy. Critchlow *et al.*[17] have shown that the prevalence of cervical ectopia is higher in OC users in women attending an STD clinic and a student health center. CT infects the columnar epithelium. It is also possible that the high CT prevalence seen in OC users is due to more efficient collection of cervical specimens from the increased area of the cervical ectopia accessible to specimen collection.[18]

Other studies report a 50% reduction in the risk of PID hospitalization rate for OC users in comparison to nonusers.[19] Today, the protection of OCs against PID has been reported as one of the well-established noncontraceptive OC benefits.[20] Among OC users, there is an apparent increased risk of CT cervical infection but a decreased risk of symptomatic PID[21] and no overall significant effects on tubal infertility.[22]

Westrom[23] has reported that OC users are associated with reduction in CT salpingitis and a lesser putative productive effect for gonococcal salpingitis. This association is supported by the findings of Cramer *et al.*,[22] who showed that primary tubal infertility is less common in former OC users. Among OC users CT tubal infections had less perihepatitis, perisplenitis, and pericolitis as well as lower geometric mean antibody levels against CT as compared to nonusers.[24] It has also been shown that at least a one-year use of OCs is necessary before protection occurs.[25] A relative study on the severity of PID in OC users indicates that OC users present a higher rate of mild PID infections instead of severe disease as compared to intrauterine device users.[20]

A similar effect is also expected with the use of long-acting progestogens. The injectable depot medroxyprogesterone acetate or norethindrone enanthate have a relative risk of acute PID of 0.5 as compared with controls.[26] Finally, in various laboratory studies progesterone depresses the growth of *N. gonorrhoeae,* whereas estrogens have little effect or slightly increase growth. *Trichononas vaginalis* and *Candida* sp. also express estrogen receptors.[21]

Several mechanisms have been suggested to explain the protective role of OCs against PID, such as thickening of cervical mucus produced by the progestogen component. This would lead to a reduced ascent of pathogens or enhanced immunological activities and decreased menstrual flow. Finally, a less favorable environment in bacterial growth has resulted.[27]

Bacterial vaginosis, trichomoniasis, and candidiasis have also been noted less frequently in women using OCs in comparison to IUDs and tubal ligation.[28] This finding is also confirmed by similar control and cohort studies.[29] There are also studies showing an increased risk of HPV infection associated with cervical intraepithelial neoplasia in OC users; however, these studies did not test for oncogenic HPV strains.[30,31]

Most data on OCs and HIV infection have been collected from Africa. A controlled Kenyan study reports that OC use is independently associated with HIV-1 seroconversion.[32] Although there are studies emphasizing that OC use is not associated with an increase risk of HIV infections, the increased ectopy with OC use and the increased risk of CT infection, which in turn increases the risk of HIV acquisition, are considered to be potential mechanisms for increased seroconversion.[33,34]

In the present study we have included sixty-nine sexually active adolescents (aged 16–18 years), divided into three groups according to the CM chosen. Young women were advised to use the same method for a 3-month period. Those with positive cervicovaginal cultures were properly treated before entering the study. Group A cases consisted of 22 adolescents who had chosen the condom as a CM and group B of 29 cases who preferred OCs. The same low-dose OC was used for the studied period. A third group (group C), who served as controls, consisted of 18 adolescents who did not agree to use prophylaxis although they were properly advised. As TABLE 2 shows, a higher prevalence of CT (27.8%) and *Mycoplasma* infections (11.1%) was found in

TABLE 2. Prevalence of STDs among 69 Adolescents Using the Same CM for a 3-Month Period

Group A STD	Group B Condom ($n = 22$)	Group C OC ($n = 29$)	NP ($n = 18$)
CT	0^b	3 (10.3%)	5 (27.8%)^b
Mycoplasma sp.	1 (4.5%)	2 (6.9%)	2 (11.1%)
Common pathogens	6 (27.3%)	14 (48.3%)	9 (50.0%)
HIV-1	0	0	0
HPV	2 (9.0%)	3 (10.3%)	2 (11.1%)
CMV	0	0	0
Syphilis	0	0	0
Hepatitis B (HepB sAg)	2 (9.0%)	2 (6.9%)	3 (16.7%)

[a]ABBREVIATIONS: NP, no prophylaxis; CT, *Chlamydia trachomatis*; HIV-1, human immunodeficiency virus; HPV, human papilloma virus; CMV, cytomegalovirus.

[b]$p < 0.05$.

group C cases when compared to condom and OC users. A statistically significant difference ($p<0.05$) was found in CT prevalence between group C and A cases. Common pathogens were also found at a higher incidence in group B (48%) and C cases (50%) when compared to condom users (27.3%). Nevertheless, no statistically significant difference was recorded. There were no cases of HIV-1 and syphilis. HepB sAg was detected in 16.7% of adolescents with no prophylaxis and in 9% and 6.9%, respectively, in condom and OC users. Finally there were no PIDs or pregnancies in any of the groups tested.

COMMENT

The control of STDs is one of the fundamental goals of reproductive health policy. It has been estimated that each year almost 250 million new STD cases appear, including genital CT, 30 million cases of HPV, 25 million of *N. gonorrhoeae,* and 20 million of genital herpes. In addition, WHO reports almost 3.5 million new cases of syphilis, 2.0 million cases of chancroid, and more than one million HIV infections. WHO predicts that for the next 8 years the cumulative number of both adults and children infected by HIV will be triple or quadruple the current number, so that by the end of the year 2000 it is expected to rise up 30 to 40 million cases.[36,37]

The best CM is that which provides safe and reliable contraception. Today, however, the increase of STDs indicate the use of CMs that at the same time provide anti-STD properties. OCs have many noncontraceptive benefits. Among these is protection from PID; CT is one of the common causes of PID. Although the effects of OCs on CT prevalence is not clear and several studies have indicated an increased incidence of CT cervical infection, it is clear today that PID is reduced in OC users. This is possibly due to the cervical mucus produced by the progestin, which results in a less favorable environment for bacterial growth. This beneficial effect becomes clearer after six months of OC use.

The above results have shown that the condom is the safest CM in terms of the prevention of STDs. However, OC users also had a lower incidence of CT, *Mycoplasma,* and infections from common pathogens when compared to group C cases.

Screening for CT and *Mycoplasma* infections is suggested for all sexually active adolescents, especially those presenting with a vaginal discharge. If an OC is chosen as a CM during adolescence, the use of condoms should also be advised. Otherwise, another barrier method, such as a sponge, should be prescribed as an alternative method.[10]

CONCLUSION

OCs play a protective role against PID by thickening the cervical mucus, thus reducing the ascent of pathogens into the endometrial cavity. They also enhance local immunological activities but increase cervical ectopia, which is a risk factor for HIV, CT, and gonococcal infections. Because data on the relationship between OCs and STDs are still not clear, we advise the use of a barrier method together with OCs.

SUMMARY

Sexually transmitted diseases (STD) cause lower genital tract infections (cervicitis, vaginitis) or ascending infections of the fallopian tubes and, possibly, pelvic inflammatory disease (PID). The syphilis bacterium, human immunodeficiency virus (HIV), and the hepatitis virus cause systematic disease. Although oral contraceptives (OCs) are the most reliable contraceptive method, they have limited anti-STD properties and their relationship with STDs remain unclear. Various mechanisms explain a protective role of OCs against STDs; however, in no way can OCs be considered a safe anti-STD contraceptive method, when compared to specific barrier methods, which provide both contraception and anti-STD protection. The above has been confirmed by a recent study performed in our institution where 10.3% and 6.9% of OC users presented a prevalence of *Chlamydia trachomatis* and *Mycoplasma,* respectively, when compared to 0% and 4.5% infection rates found among condom users. It is concluded that although OCs possess some anti-STD properties, mainly in the prevention of PID, they should be used in combination with a barrier method.

REFERENCES

1. Creatsas, G. 1995. Sequelae of premature sexual life. J. R. Soc. Med. **88:** 369–37.
2. Fisher, M., W. D. Rosenfeld & R. D. Burk. 1991. Cervicovaginal human papillomavirus infection in suburban adolescents and young adults. J. Pediatr. **119:** 821–825.
3. Fitzpatric, C., P. McKenna & R. Hone. 1992. Teenage girls attending a Dublin sexually transmitted disease clinic. A socio-sexual diagnostic profile. Ir. J. Med. Sci. **161:** 460–462.
4. Creatsas, G., M. Pavlatos, E. Koumantakis, I. Zolotas & D. Kaskarelis. 1982. Bacteriologic aspects of pelvic inflammatory disease. Gynecol. Obst. Inv. **13:** 1–8.

5. BRAVERMAN, P. K., F. M. BIRO, R. L. BRUNNER, M. GILCHRIST & H. J. L. RAY. 1990. Screening asymptomatic adolescent males for chlamydia. J. Adolesc. Health Care **11:** 141–144.
6. AIDS Policies on Youth Work Group. 1989. Recommendations. J. Adolesc. Health Care **10:** 45S–47S.
7. BARBONE, F., H. AUSTIN, W. C. LOUV & W. J. ALEXANDER. 1990. A follow-up study of methods of contraception, sexual activity, and rates of trichomoniasis candidiasis and bacterial vaginosis. Am. J. Obstet. Gynecol. **163:** 510–514.
8. COX, J. M., J. LAWRENCE & J. J. SILBER. 1992. Substance abuse and syphilis in urban adolescents: A new risk factor for an old disease. J. Adolesc. Health Care **13:** 483–486.
9. CREATSAS, G. 1993. Sexuality: Sexual activity and contraception during adolescence. Curr. Opin. Obstet. Gynecol. **5:** 774–783.
10. PSYCHOYOS, A., A. CREATSAS, E. HASSAN, V. GEORGOULIAS & A. GRAVANIS. 1993. Spermicidal and antiviral properties of cholic acid: Contraceptive efficacy of a new vaginal sponge (Protectaid®) containing sodium cholade. Hum. Reprod. **8:** 866–869.
11. CREATSAS, G., P. ADAMOPOULOS, N. ELEFTEHRIOU, E. DELIGEOROGLOU, N. AREFETZ, N. GOUMALATSOS & D. LOUTRADIS. 1991. Clinical and metabolic effects of the monophasic Gestodene/Ethinystradiol pill for contraception during adolescence. Adolesc. Pediatr. Gynecol. **4:** 76–79.
12. CREATSAS, G. 1991. Progestagens in reproductive endocrinology. Eur. J. Obstet. Gynecol. Reprod. **41:** 28.
13. WASHINGTON, A. E., S. GOVE, J. SCHACHTER, *et al.* 1985. Oral contraceptives, *Chlamydia trachomatis* infection and pelvic inflammatory disease: A word of caution about protection. JAMA **253:** 2246–2250.
14. HANDSFIELD, H. J., L. L. JASMAN, P. L. ROBERT, *et al.* 1986. Criteria for selective screening for *Chlamydia trachomatis* infection in women attending family planning clinics. JAMA **255:** 1730–1734.
15. KIM, O. H. M., R. A. FEINSTEIN, E. J. SOILEAU, *et al.* 1989. *Chlamydia trachomatis* cervical infection and oral contraceptive use among adolescent girls. J. Adolesc. Health Care **10:** 376–381.
16. BARRON, A. L., J. N. PASLEY, R. G. RANK, *et al.* 1988. Chlamydial salpingitis in female guinea pigs receiving oral contraceptives. Sex. Transm. Dis. **15:** 169–173.
17. CRITCHLOW, C. W., P W. HANSSEN, D. A. ESCTENBACH, *et al.* 1995. Determinants of cervical ectopia and of cervicitis: Age, oral contraception, specific cervical infection, smoking and douching. Am. J. Obstet. Gynecol. **173:** 534–543.
18. JORDAN, J. A. & A. SINGER. 1976. Effect of oral contraceptive steroids upon epithelium and mucus. *In* The Cervix. J. A. Jordan & A. Singer, Eds.: 192–209. WB Saunders Co. London.
19. WOLNER-HANSSEN, P., D. A. ESCHENBACH, J. PAAVONEN, *et al.* 1990. Decreased risk of symptomatic chlamydial pelvic inflammatory disease associated with oral contraceptive use. JAMA **263:** 54–59.
20. SVENSSON, L., L. WESTRO & P. A. MARDH. 1984. Contraceptives and acute salpingitis. JAMA **251:** 2553–2555.
21. MCGREGOR, J. & H. HAMMIL. 1993. Contraception and sexually transmitted diseases: Interactions and opportunities. Am. J. Obstet. Gynecol. **168:** 2033–2041.
22. CRAMER, D. W., M. D. GOLDMAN, I. SCHIFF, *et al.* 1987. The relationship of tubal infertility to barrier method and oral contraceptive use. JAMA **257:** 2446–2450.
23. WESTROM, L. 1980. Incidence, prevalence and trends of acute pelvic inflammatory disease and its consequences in industrialized countries. Am. J. Obstet. Gynecol. **138:** 880–892.
24. WOLNER-HANSSEN, P., L. SVENSSON, P. A. MARDH & C. WESTROM. 1988. Laparoscopic findings and contraceptive use in women with signs and symptoms suggestive of acute salpingitis. Obstet. Gynecol. **66:** 233–238.

25. Panser, L. A. & W. R. Phipps. 1991. Type of oral contraceptive in relation to acute, initial episodes of pelvic inflammatory disease. Contraception **43:** 91–99.
26. Gray, R. H. 1985. Reduced risk of pelvic inflammatory disease with injectable contraceptives. Lancet **1:** 1046.
27. Burkman, R. T., Jr. 1994. Noncontraceptive effects of hormonal contraceptives. Bonk mass, sexually transmitted disease and pelvic inflammatory disease, cardiovascular disease, menstrual function and future fertility. Am. J. Obstet. Gynecol. **170:** 1569–1575.
28. Barbone, F., H. Austin, W. C. Louv & W. J. Alexander. 1990. A follow-up study of methods of contraception, sexual activity and rates of trichomoniasis, candidiasis and bacterial vaginosis. Am. J. Obstet. Gynecol. **163:** 510–514.
29. Roy, S. 1991. Non-barrier contraceptives and vaginitis and vaginosis. Am. J. Obstet. Gynecol. **165:** 1240–1244.
30. Stendahl, U. & K. Rogo. 1990. Cervical cancer: Role for progesterone during pregnancy and contraception. Am. J. Obstet. Gynecol. **163:** 685–686.
31. Hicks, D. 1994. Sexually transmitted diseases and contraceptive methods. Fertil. Control Rev. **3:** 3–7.
32. Plummer, F. A., J. N. Simonsen, D. W. Cameron, *et al.* 1991. Co-factors in male–female sexual transmission of human immunodeficiency virus type 1. J. Infect. Dis. **163:** 233–239.
33. European Study Group. 1989. Risk factors for male to female transmission of HIV. Br. Med. J. **298:** 411–415.
34. Burkman, R. T. 1990. Modern trends in contraception. Obstet. Gynecol. Clin. N. Am. **17:** 759–774.
35. Creatsas, G. 1993. Consensus meeting for a European preventive programme for genital chlamydial infections and allied conditions in contraceptive centers. November 20, 1993. Unpublished data. Paris.
36. Crosignani, P. G., E. Disfalutzy, J. Newton & B. Rubin. 1992. Sexually transmitted diseases. Hum. Reprod. **7:** 1330–1334.
37. Fathalla, M. F. 1991. Reproductive health: A global overview. Ann. N.Y. Acad. Sci. **626:** 1–10.

Adolescent Sexuality: An Educational and Counseling Challenge

LEENA RUUSUVAARA

Adolescent Health Care Center
Department of Obstetrics and Gynaecology
Uppsala University Hospital
S-751 85 Uppsala, Sweden

Each society shapes the sexuality of its members according to accepted rules by controlling sexuality through different mechanisms, which may vary over time. Children and young people are thus made participants in the prevailing value system in which they are growing up. Adults have always been busy protecting young people and have had anxious concerns about adolescent sexual behavior.

Sex education of young people is also colored by society's reluctance to accept adolescent sexuality. The information given is limited to the dangers and negative consequences of sexual activity, for example, unwanted pregnancies, abortions, and sexually transmitted diseases (STDs). Many societies emphasize sexuality as a problem and would like adolescents to postpone sexual activity until they are "mature enough."[1] Sexuality itself and sexual feelings and desire are veiled in silence. Thus, young people are left to learn from their peers and the media what adults do not teach them about sex, and they tend to form their own social norms.

A review of family-planning literature reveals that researchers adopt narrow definitions of sexual behavior and focus almost exclusively on risks of pregnancy and diseases. Little concern is shown in these articles about promoting the idea of more communicative, pleasurable, and egalitarian sexual relations among teenagers because the focus is on avoiding behaviors that are defined as "high risk."[2]

The world-wide epidemics of chlamydia infection and other STDs are an indication that there is a need for even more extensive education related to contraception and safer sex. In the United States, however, there is little evidence that these contraceptive-based sex education programs have resulted in reduced sexual activity, diminished teenage-pregnancy rates, or increased effective contraceptive use.[3,4] In Canada the clinical evidence is that existing prevention strategies are not working.[3,4] In Sweden, where sex education has been mandatory for decades, the increasing rates of STDs and teenage pregnancies in the late 1980s worried authorities. The figures were brought down in the 1990s by extensive efforts both in schools and at publicly funded adolescent health clinics and family-planning units.[5,6] The use of condoms by adolescents increased, and one of the reasons reported for this was various campaigns at schools and the dissemination of information via adolescent health clinics.[5,6] Statistics from different European countries show that the unwanted consequences of adolescent sexual activity are a major problem.[7]

Sex education might be more successful in influencing behavior and creating positive health effects if more of the focus were directed at adolescent needs. Sex education programs should also take the psychology of childhood and adolescence, with their different developmental phases, into account. During early adolescence (10–13 or 14 years) the youngsters need concrete, straightforward information that is applicable in his/her actual life situation. During middle adolescence (14–16 or 17 years), adolescents usually are in the middle of the liberation process. They are testing new "adult" behaviors and are not easy to influence. At 17 to 20 years of age, during late adolescence, they are capable of abstract thought and are able to undertake preventive safety measures (which may be very difficult earlier).[8]

The correct timing of sex education is both difficult and important. If the information given comes too late, it might not be able to change the already established, risk-taking behavior. If it comes too early, it will not be understood and might be forgotten when it is time to use it.[9]

It has been shown in the follow-up of a prospective study that girls with good self-esteem and a sense of responsibility avoided pregnancies and STDs in follow-up. Girls with high degree of risk-prone behavior or attitudes and girls with a problematic life situation and without adequate family support were those who became accidentally pregnant and/or acquired an STD.[10] Adolescent girls apparently arrive at different solutions to problems during their developmental crises, and the author recommends extra social and psychosexual and behavioral counseling.

Countries where sex education has been accepted, combined with widely spread family-planning services and abortion on demand, have the lowest pregnancy and abortion rates in the world. But even they could do a better job of putting sex education in its proper place in society and in using both old and new methods. Sex education in schools is important but should be kept up to date. Teachers and counselors need continuous education in these matters, too. Midwives, nurses, and doctors should be aware of the trends and changes in the young society. With open minds they will get this information during their daily contact with teenagers. Drama and awareness-enhancing interactions and peer education, youth-to-youth information, are all valuable.

We have a responsibility to give a balanced and positive view of sexuality and to deal with matters like respect and responsibility both for males and females. Focusing solely on the technical information and the risks has been found to be insufficient in preventing the unwanted consequences of sexuality. Sex education programs may have very different approaches in different cultural and religious settings. Sexual enjoyment should be regarded as a natural and respectable topic. Both genders should have equal rights in fulfillment of this pleasure. Women, particularly, should understand that they have the right to determine what happens to their own bodies.

SUMMARY

A review of family-planning literature reveals that researchers adopt narrow definitions of sexual behavior and focus almost exclusively on risks of pregnancy and diseases. Little concern is shown in these articles about promoting the idea of more communicative, pleasurable, and egalitarian sexual relations among teenagers, because the focus is on avoiding behaviors that are defined as "high risk."

In the United States, there is little evidence that these contraceptive-based sex education programs have resulted in reduced sexual activity, diminished teenage-pregnancy rates, or increased effective contraceptive use. In Canada the clinical evidence is that existing prevention strategies are not working. In Sweden the increasing rates of STDs and teenage pregnancies in the late 1980s worried authorities. The figures were brought down in the 1990s by extensive efforts both in schools and at publicly funded adolescent health clinics and family-planning units.

It has been shown that girls with good self-esteem and a sense of responsibility avoided pregnancies and STDs in follow-up studies. Girls with a high degree of risk-prone behavior or attitudes and girls with a problematic life situation and without adequate family support were those who became unintentionally pregnant and/or acquired an STD.

Countries where sex education has been accepted, combined with widely spread family-planning services and abortion on demand, have the lowest pregnancy and abortion rates in the world. But even they could do better by putting sex education in its proper place in society and by using both old and new methods.

REFERENCES

1. Helmius, G. 1990. Mature enough for sex? The sexually restricting society and adolescent heterosexual joy. Ph.D. thesis, Dept. of Sociology, University of Uppsala, Uppsala, Sweden.
2. Dixon-Mueller, R. 1993. The sexuality connection in reproductive health. Stud. Fam. Plann. **24**(5): 269–282.
3. Genuis, J. S. & S. K. Genuis. 1995. Adolescent sexual involvement: Time for primary prevention. Lancet **345:** 240–241.
4. Stout, J. W. & F. P. Rivara. 1989. Schools and sex education: does it work? Pediatrics **83:** 375–379.
5. Persson, E. & G. Jarlbro. 1992. Sexual behavior among youth clinic visitors in Sweden: Knowledge and experiences in an HIV perspective. Genitourin Med. **168:** 26–31.
6. Klanger, B., T. Tydén & L. Ruusuvaara. 1993. Sexual behavior among adolescents in Uppsala, Sweden. J. Adolesc. Health **14:** 468–474.
7. Creatsas, G. K., *et al.* 1995. Adolescent sexuality in Europe: A multicentric study. Adolesc. Pediatr. Gynecol. **8:** 59–63.
8. Berg-Kelly, K. 1992. Tonåringar, Graviditet och Abort (Teenagers, Pregnancy and Abortion). Rädda Barnen. Stockholm. pp. 17–23. In Swedish.
9. Kristjánsdottir, J. Personal communication. 1995. Adolescent Health Care Center, Uppsala.
10. Cacciatore, R. 1995. Risk-prone behavior in adolescent girls. Abstract IX: 133 World Congress of Pediatric & Adolescent Gynaecology (Singapore): Feb 23–26.
11. Editorial. 1995. Sex education in schools: Peers to the rescue? Lancet **344**(8927): 899–900.

The Genital Examination in Suspected Child Sexual Abuse

A Diagnostic Dilemma

FRANCESCA NAVRATIL[a]

Pediatric and Adolescent Gynecology Outpatient Department
University of Zürich Children's Hospital
Zürich, Switzerland

There is an increasing awareness of the broad spectrum of the problems that are seen in connection with a sexual abuse situation; and, among other professionals, physicians may be involved in the detection, diagnosis, and management of sexual abuse cases. In our institution 2% of the patients seen at the pediatric and adolescent gynecological outpatient clinic in 1982 had problems related to a sexual abuse situation. In 1989 the number had increased to 10% and had reached 22% in 1994; of these 44% were younger than 7 years. The youngest was 8 months old.

DEFINITION

Sexual abuse is the involvement of children and adolescents in sexual activities they do not understand, to which they cannot give informed consent, or that violate social taboos. Sexual abuse can involve touching; fondling; oral contact with breasts or genitals; insertion of fingers or objects into vulva or anus; vaginal, anal, and oral intercourse; masturbation; prostitution; exhibitionism; and pornography. The abuse is an abuse of power and can be perpetrated by male or female adults and teenagers as well as older children.

In the majority of cases, the perpetrator is known or related to the victim. Victims include boys and girls of all ages, races, and socioeconomic groups. Some children and adolescents can be at increased risk for victimization: for example, preverbal children and children and adolescents with malformations, developmental disabilities, or chronic disease.

WHAT CAN CONTRIBUTE TO THE DIAGNOSIS?

- The history obtained from the victim is usually the most important evidence, although there are many problems associated with children's and adolescents' disclosures.

[a]Address for correspondence: Dr. Francesca Navratil, 63 Forsterstrasse, 8044 Zürich, Switzerland.

- Behavioral and psychological problems may be indicative of sexual abuse and may be useful diagnostically. They should alert caretakers and professionals, although most of them are not specific.
- Medical evidence can contribute to the diagnosis; but there can be many problems and difficulties in the differentiation of normal findings, normal variations, and low and high probability indicators; and unequivocal physical evidence is seldom encountered.

Sexual abuse does not necessarily implicate vaginal or anal penetration, which means that in a great number of victims no abnormalities are going to be found on physical examination. On the other hand, even after vaginal penetration has occurred, the majority of lesions heal without leaving specific changes; and the genitoanal examination, which in most cases occurs weeks or months after the abusive act, will fail to detect any abnormal or suspicious genital findings.

GENERAL ASPECTS

After having examined a child for suspicion of sexual abuse, it is often difficult to determine with certainty that the findings confirm it; and the consequences of nonidentification or erroneous diagnosis can be very damaging for the victim, the family, and the alleged perpetrator.

For this reason all physicians involved in the examination of children and adolescents with any kind of genitoanal complaints; with any suspicion of sexual abuse by history, medical, or behavioral indicators; or having disclosed abuse should be able to perform the appropriate, nontraumatizing medical examination. They have also to be familiar with the normal anatomy, the variations of normal appearance of the genitoanal area, and the differential diagnosis of suspicious, suggestive, or abnormal findings for the different age groups and the different examining positions and techniques.

MEDICAL EXAMINATION

All children alleged to be or to have been sexually abused should have a complete medical examination. The timing and the extent of the physical examination depend on the history and the presenting complaint.

If the last abuse episode has occurred within 72 hours, the examination and documentation should be immediate for detection and treatment of acute and/or chronic injuries and for collection of forensic specimens. Screening (cultures, serology) and/or treatment for sexually transmitted diseases (STD) might be considered, and emergency post-coital contraception offered to the adolescent victim.

If the last abuse episode has occurred days, weeks, or months before, the physical examination should be scheduled as soon as possible after the disclosure interview and psychosocial evaluation. Screening and treatment for STD and a pregnancy test might be necessary, depending on the history and the symptomatology.

The examination of the genitoanal area should only occur as part of a complete physical examination, which helps the victim to feel he or she is being treated as a whole person and the professional to decide if other medical conditions could be responsible for the physical findings.

As a general rule, the genital examination (and especially so that of the prepubertal child) is principally an external visualization facilitated by varying positions and techniques. Digital examination should not be done and instrumentation (vaginoscope, speculum) is rarely necessary, but must always be considered in the presence of trauma, injuries, genital hemorrhages, suspicion of the presence of a foreign body, or recurrent genital infection.

The genital inspection is carried out with the patient lying supine with the legs in the frogleg position or on stirrups. Small children can be examined sitting on a parent's lap. In the supine position, the labial separation and traction technique are used for better visualization of the genital area.

The examination in the prone knee–chest position can be embarrassing for the victim of abuse; nevertheless, it is extremely important especially for the interpretation of unclear hymenal findings in the supine position (attenuated hymen, redundant tissue, rolled edges in the dorsal quadrants of the hymen).

On medical examination the high probability indicators of sexual abuse are pregnancy in a young adolescent; the presence of sexually transmitted diseases; and the presence of sperm in the genitoanal area, on other parts of the body, or on the victim's clothes.

There are other indicators of possible ongoing or past sexual abuse that can be found on examination of the genitoanal area, but there is a fair amount of variability in the shape and other characteristics of the hymen, the hymenal orifice (transhymenal diameter), and the structures of the vestibulum of nonabused children, which change with age, showing a gradual increase. Variability also exists in the examination method (TABLE 1).

Independent of the examining position and technique, the vertical transhymenal diameter consistently shows the largest measurements. The width of the posterior rim is difficult to determine, but if it cannot be visualized in the supine position the examination in the knee–chest position will succeed in demonstrating its presence in the nonabused girl, which leads to the conclusion that a congenital absence of the hymen has never been documented in normal, nonabused children.

It is important to acknowledge that the examination in the prone knee–chest position can give additional information about the normality, normal variability, or abnormality of a vestibular finding; and physicians should not be reluctant to include it in their genital inspection (FIGS. 1 and 2).

MEDICAL FINDINGS

There are findings that are nonspecific or represent normal variations of genitoanal anatomy and can be found in nonabused children and adolescents: erythema, periurethral bands, perihymenal bands, labial adhesions, lymphoid follicles, urethral dilatation, and friability of the posterior fourchette. (With the labial traction technique, superficial tears of the fourchette may occur.) (See TABLE 2.)

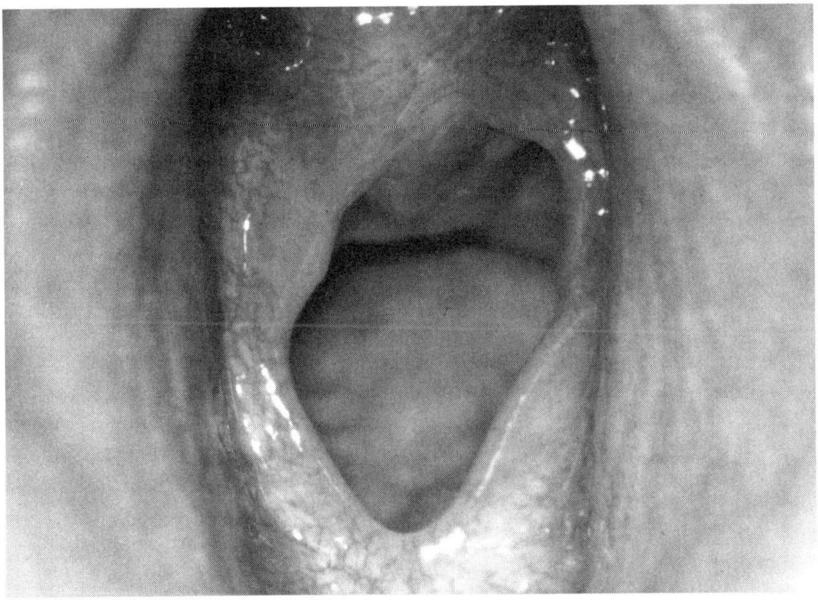

FIGURE 1. 5 2/12-year-old. Supine position, traction. Rolled, thickened hymenal edge.

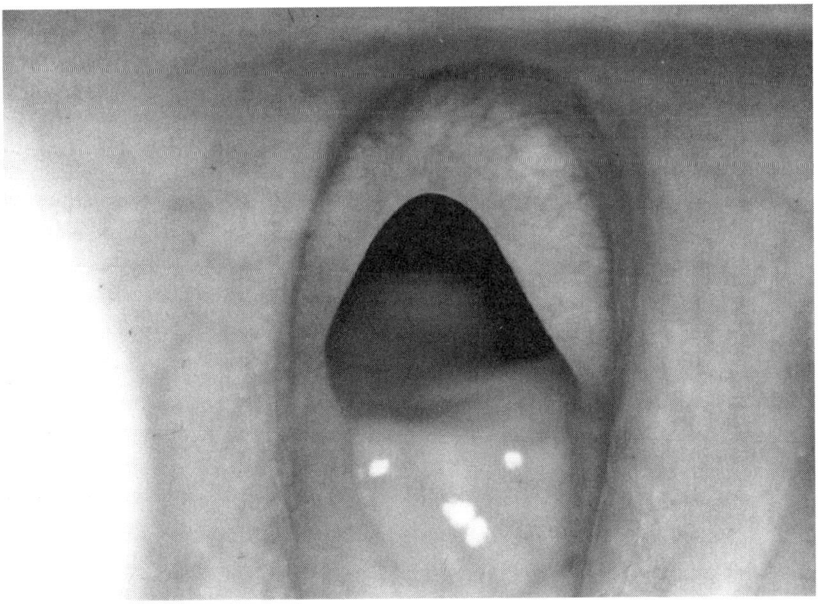

FIGURE 2. Same patient as in FIGURE 1. Prone knee-chest position. Hymen appears thinned out, normal width of hymenal rim.

TABLE 1. Frequency (%) of Hymenal Findings by Examination Method[a]

	Separ.	Tract.	Knee–Ch.
Absent	0	0	0
Hymenal edge			
Sharp	50.7	54.4	86.1
Thickened	51.3	53.8	26.3
Rolled	18.4	23.8	6.3
Mounds	23.7	33.8	17.9
Notches	4.1	6.6	2.2

[a]Patient ages ranged from 10 months to 10 years. Data from McCann and Wells.[1]

There are findings that may result from conditions other than sexual abuse: injuries, dermatological problems, non-sexually transmitted genital infections, urethral problems (urethral prolapse), and congenital anomalies.

There are findings associated with acute trauma and suggestive of sexual abuse: acute hematomas, abrasions, lacerations, and transections (vestibule, labia, hymen, posterior fourchette).

There are specific findings that can be associated with prior trauma and support suspicion of sexual abuse: vaginal orifice dilatation, hymenal narrowing (posterior hymenal rim), localized hymenal thickening, bumps (mounds, convexities), notches (U and V-shaped concavities, especially posteriorly), altered vascularity, scarring, adhesions (hymen-vagina/vestibular wall). An attenuation of the hymen posteriorly, bumps, notches, and any suspicious finding in the supine position should always be verified with the child in the prone knee-chest position (FIGS. 3 and 4).

In the majority of sexually abused children, no abnormalities or nonspecific genital findings are encountered, which means that a normal genital examination does not rule out the possibility of an ongoing or past sexual abuse situation. Even a history of vaginal penetration given by the victim or the perpetrator does not always have to correlate significantly with abnormal genital findings.

TABLE 2. Genital Findings in Nonabused Prepubertal Girls, Normal Variations[a]

Erythema	56%
Periurethral bands	50.6%
Labial adhesions	38.9%
Lymphoid follicles	33.7%
Perihymenal bands	16.0%
Urethral dilatation	15.3%
Friability post. fourchette	2.3%

[a]Results are given as percent of subjects. Patients ranged in age from 10 months to 10 years. Data from McCann and Wells.[1]

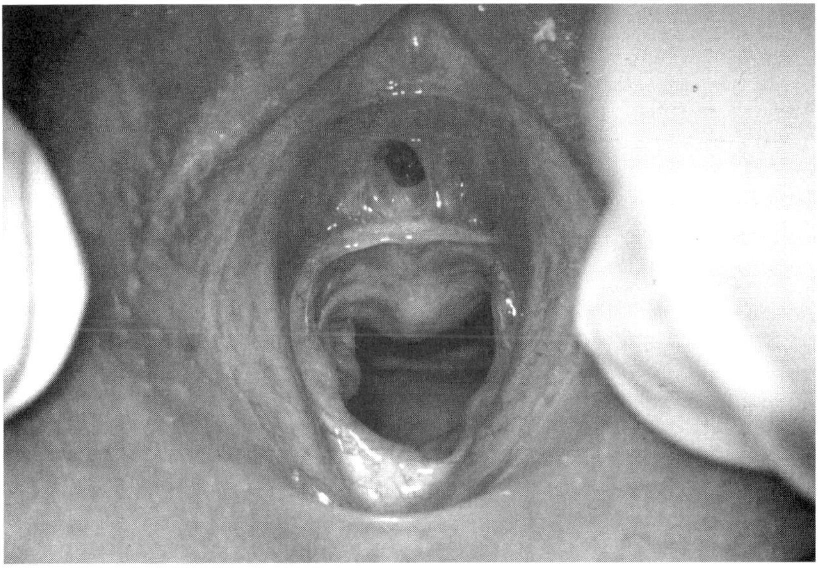

FIGURE 3. 5-year-old. Supine position, traction. Hymenal opening enlarged, asymmetrical, redundancy at the 6 to 8 o'clock position, concavity (?) at the 5 o'clock position. History of chronic abuse by mother's boyfriend.

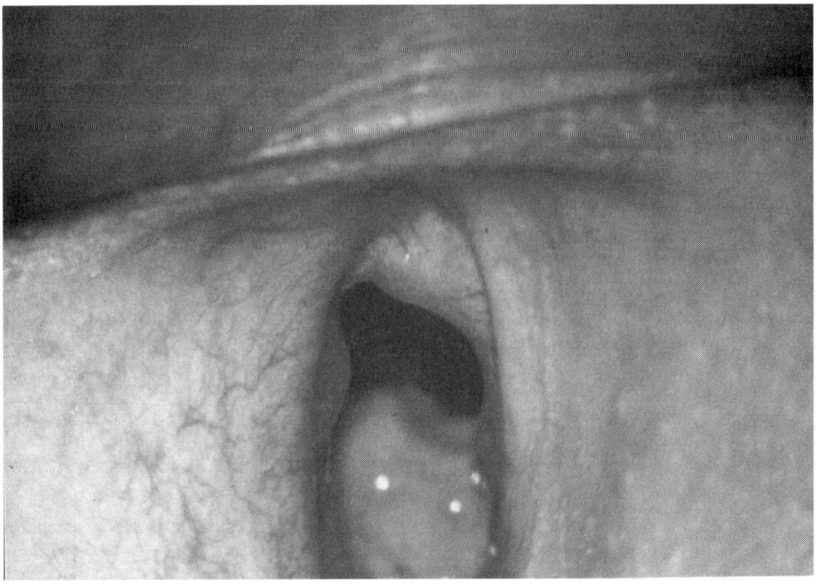

FIGURE 4. Same patient as in FIGURE 3. Prone knee-chest position. U-shaped concavity, healed interruption in the integrity of the hymen at the 11 o'clock position (5 o'clock supine).

TABLE 3. Genital Findings in Sexual Abuse

Normal	
Hymen appearance normal	50%
Ample posterior rim	48%
Estrogen changes	43%
Nonspecific	
Erythema	32%
Increased vascularity	25%
Labial adhesions	17%
Suspicious	
Posterior rim <1 mm	6%
Acute vestibule abrasions (Not involving hymen)	2%
Clear evidence	
Absence of hymenal tissue post.	4%
Hymenal Transection	5%

[a]Data from Adams.[2]

CONCLUSIONS

The first step in the recognition of child sexual abuse is to consider the possibility that an ongoing or past abuse might be a reality. There are physical and behavioral indicators of possible sexual abuse, but the history given by the victim is most important for the evaluation.

The medical examination should be carried out by experienced physicians, because the correct interpretation of the data can be difficult but is essential if mistakes are to be avoided and the victim not traumatized by multiple evaluations and hasty nonprofessional actions. Physicians should know that a normal genital examination does not rule out the possibility of sexual abuse and that the diagnosis of sexual abuse cannot be made on somatic findings alone. There is no simple test or procedure that can prove that sexual abuse has occurred.

If a sexual abuse situation is suspected, only a multidisciplinary team evaluation can result in an appropriate diagnostic, therapeutic, protective, and legal approach primarily contributing to the interruption of the vicious cycle from which there is otherwise no escape for the abused child.

REFERENCES

1. McCann, J., R. Wells, *et al.* 1990. Genital findings in prepubertal girls selected for nonabuse: A descriptive study. Pediatrics **86:** 428–439.
2. Adams, J. A., *et al.* 1994. Examination findings in legally confirmed child sexual abuse: It's normal to be normal. Pediatrics **94**(3): 310–317.

SUGGESTED READING

1. Bays, J. & D. Chadwick. 1993. Medical Diagnosis of the sexually abused child. Child Abuse Neglect **17:** 91–110.
2. Emans, S. J., E. R. Woods, N. T. Flagg & A. Freeman. 1987. Genital findings in sexually abused, symptomatic and asymptomatic girls. Pediatrics **79:** 778–785.
3. Kerns, D. & M. Ritter. 1992. Concave hymenal variations in suspected child sexual abuse. Pediatrics **2:** 265–272.
4. Muram, D. 1989. Child sexual abuse: Relationship between sexual acts and genital findings. Child Abuse Neglect **13:** 211–216.

Oral Contraceptive Compliance during Adolescence

D. SERFATY

Saint-Louis Hospital
9 rue de Villersexel
75007 Paris, France

According to Paula Adams Hillard, compliance is "the extent to which a patient's behavior coincides with the clinical prescription."[1] Compliance, therefore, means the correct, consistent, and continued use of any medical treatment including contraception.[2] Although a large number of effective contraceptive methods are available, we must note that failures of these methods occur, resulting in undesired pregnancies and abortions. Poor compliance with oral contraception is currently a major problem for adolescents as well as for family-planning providers.

ORAL CONTRACEPTIVE NONCOMPLIANCE: THE PROBLEMS

> In clinical trials OCs' [oral contraceptives] efficacy rates of 0.12 to 0.34 pregnancies per 100 woman/years were reported. Clinical trials show that, when used correctly, the new low-dose combined estrogen–progestin OCs have an estimated annual method failure rate of 0.1%. Failure rates in clinical practice, however, are higher than those reported in clinical trials. A 3% annual failure rate from clinical trials of married women increases to 6% when single women are included. In addition, marital status, age, race, and demographics affect method success. For diverse populations in both developed and developing countries, rates may go as high as 12% to 20%. While biological factors, such as individual variations in levels of steroids hormones, may play a role, several recent studies suggest that the gap between expected (or theoretical) and actual efficacy may be related to compliance. (Paula Adams Hillard, "Oral Contraceptive Noncompliance: The Extent of the Problem"[1])

According to John Guillebaud,[3] OC failure rates tend to be higher with younger than with older women, presumably because of their relative inexperience with contraceptive practice, but also because of a higher frequency of intercourse, higher intrinsic fertility, and more frequent stopping and switching of contraceptive methods.

Oral noncompliance is a common although often unrecognized problem in clinical practice.[4]

Following are the conclusions of a recent survey on the attitudes and knowledge of 10,317 young European women regarding the use of oral contraceptives and the incidence of poor compliance among OC users.[5]

Incidence of OC Use by Age Group

The incidence of OC use is the following: 19% in women aged 16 to 19 (1270/6676); 38% in women aged 20 to 24 (2556/6676); 40% in women aged 25 to 30.

Unplanned Pregnancy

Ten percent of all women (aged 16–30) have experienced at least one unplanned pregnancy; 18% of those were OC users at time of the unplanned pregnancy. Only 32% of women who stop taking the pill and experience an unplanned pregnancy have consulted their doctor before stopping the pill. FIGURE 1 lists the reasons for becoming pregnant while on the pill. Among these reasons the most prominent is having forgotten to take the pill. About 10% of voluntary abortions carried out in my service at the Saint-Louis Hospital seem to be due to OC noncompliance.[6] In 1995, more than 25% of women consulting a doctor for iterative induced abortion in the same hospital seem to be OC noncompliant, and 28.5% of repeated abortions are accomplished in women under 25. FIGURE 2 lists the reasons for stopping the pill before unplanned pregnancy in the Wycon Survey. Among these reasons, the most prominent are nuisance side effects and poor cycle control.

Discontinuation and Poor Compliance

In the Wycon Survey, 38% of OC users never discontinued; 32% have been on more than one formulation of pill; and 30% tried one pill formulation only, discontin-

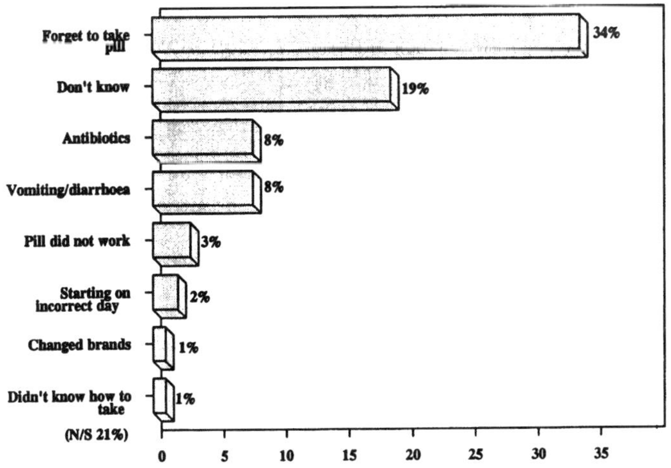

FIGURE 1. Unplanned pregnancies: Reasons for becoming pregnant while on the pill. Base: all respondents using OC at time of unplanned pregnancy. From Wycon Survey[5]; used with permission.

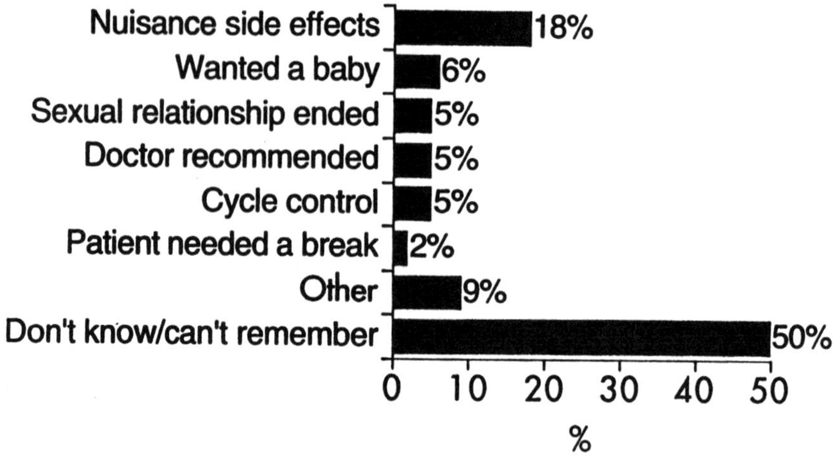

FIGURE 2. Reasons for stopping the pill before unplanned pregnancy. From Wycon Survey[5]; used with permission.

ued, and did not restart. Only 31% of the total number of women who discontinue OCs consult their doctor before stopping. In the Wycon Survey, nuisance side effects constitute 25% of the total reasons for discontinuation, and cycle control problems constitute 6% of the total reasons for discontinuation. In brief, oral contraceptive compliance seems adversely affected by three medical factors: side effects (whether they are really experienced by the patient or whether they are only fears and misinformation about OC side effects), poor cycle control, and patient's fears of serious diseases.[7] In the Wycon Survey, one in five young European women on the pill forgot to take their pill at least once in a cycle. In the survey conducted by Wyeth-Ayerst[5] only 39% of OC users/ex-users use back-up contraception if they miss two pills in a row.

Attitudes and Knowledge Regarding OC Use

FIGURE 3 lists the reasons patients give for not using the pill. Among these reasons, the most prominent is fear of side effects; 24% of all women believe there are no benefits from oral contraceptive use apart from contraception.

In the Wycon Survey, awareness of noncontraceptive health benefits is different in each age group. In European adolescents aged 16 to 19, this awareness includes the following benefits: regulating periods, 47%; improving acne, 24%; improving dysmenorrhea, 25%; long-term health benefits, only 2%. This awareness must influence OC compliance.

Which single feature would young women most want a pill to have? FIGURE 4 lists the young European women's wishes according to the Wycon Survey. The first one is contraceptive protection without weight gain.

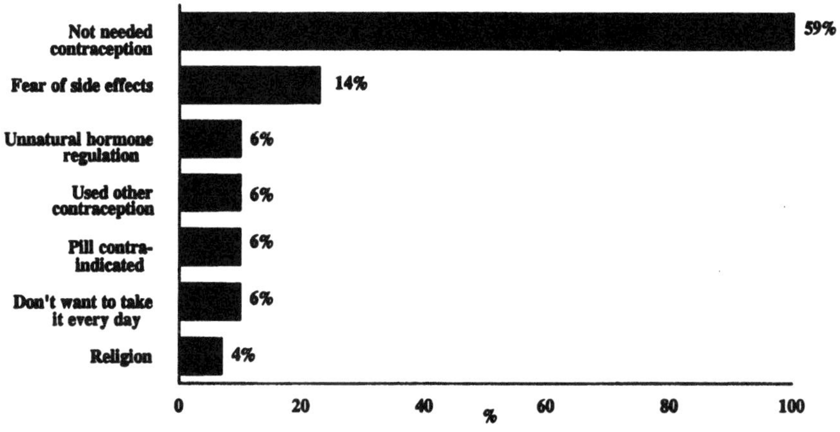

FIGURE 3. Attitudes: Reasons for not using the pill. Base: nonusers (No. 3,526). From Wycon Survey[5]; used with permission.

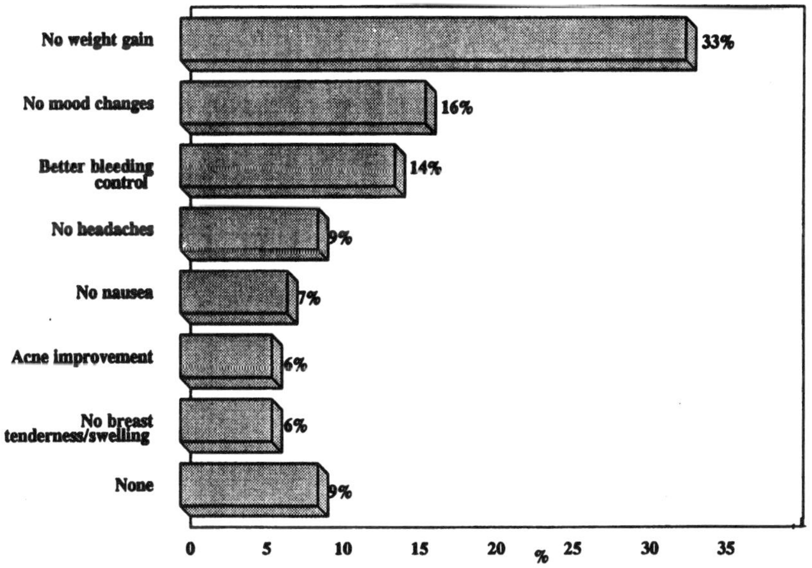

FIGURE 4. Side effects: Which single feature would women most want a pill to have. Base: all users and former users (No. 6,676). From Wycon Survey[5]; used with permission.

ORAL CONTRACEPTIVE NONCOMPLIANCE: PROPOSALS FOR SOLUTIONS

According to the International Health Foundation,[2] correct, consistent, and continued use of OCs means that several important requirements are met:

- No pills in the pack are missed;
- The pill-free interval is strictly respected;
- The pills are taken in the right order (e.g., bi and triphasics) or at the same time each day (e.g., progestogen-only pills);
- Another back-up method is used when certain medications are taken (e.g., certain antiepileptics or antibiotics) or in case of diarrhea or vomiting;
- Use is continued without interruption as long as contraception is necessary.

Missing a Pill

Services and counseling adapted to the individual patient should fight against this very frequent form of noncompliance. The basic approach should incorporate the following elements:

- Simple and short advice (how to take the pill? what to do in case of missing 1 or 2 pills?), avoiding the pitfall of swamping the adolescent with too much advice based on too many hypotheses;
- Avoid bi- or triphasic OCs if they are not specifically indicated and packaged as Sunday Starters (which, by the way, are minimally introduced in Europe) which make counseling too complex in the case of forgetfulness, particularly for many adolescents;
- Lessen the anxiety of patients (cause of missing pills) by informing them in a few words about the favorable balance of the benefits–risks ratio of oral contraception;
- Take action to improve the accessibility of supplies and advice including weekends and when one is abroad;
- Be available;
- Create an atmosphere of confidence.

Personally, I mistrust recent but *repeated* forgetfulness of pills in a patient, mainly young patients, who until then had been perfectly compliant. I interpret this as a sign of refusal or lassitude vis à vis the OC and would then be inclined to explore other contraceptive solutions with the patient.

Pill-Free Interval

Key concepts to impress upon the patient include the following:

- Insist on the importance of not starting a new pack late or missing a few pills at the start of a pack, which are the most hazardous times in the cycle to miss a pill;

- Give preference perhaps to 28-day pills (which surprisingly have little success in Europe in contrast with their success in the United States and Canada) when they are available.

Right Order

The key concepts to convey in counseling are to avoid bi- or triphasic OCs when they are not specifically indicated because for some adolescents they are more difficult to take than the monophasics.

Same Time Each Day

This is indicated solely for progestogen-only pills. These pills should be avoided when they are not indispensable (that is to say, they should be reserved for cardiovascular and metabolic contraindications for combined OCs, which are very rare during adolescence) even more so, as their gynecological tolerance is not always perfect.

Drug Interactions with Oral Contraceptives

The possibility of drug interactions with oral contraceptives should be brought up with *all* patients. In the case of adolescents with epilepsy, it is preferable, as far as possible, to use drugs without interactions (such as Valproic acid or Vigabatrin, antiepileptic by second intention). Other solutions when one fears drug interference could be the high-dose pills (which should remain on the market, as the FDA Advisory Group recommends), the decreased pill-free interval, and the back-up methods. Here, particularly, the role, complementary to that of pharmacists, of package inserts and the media is fundamental.

Vomiting and Diarrhea

According to Brook *et al.* (1991), who are quoted in Reference 2, in a UK study, 48% of pill users ignore the fact that vomiting and diarrhea interfere with the efficacy of the pill. Such episodes are not usually brought to the attention of physicians.[2] Counseling on this issue should consist of bringing the problem to the attention of all adolescents.

Pill Discontinuation

Prevention of pill discontinuation consists of the following measures:

- Informing users of the possibility of side effects;
- Choosing, *a priori,* pills having the least possible side effects and respecting the cycle control as much as possible;

- Informing users of the benefits–risks balance of the pill, which weighs in more and more heavily on the side of benefits;
- Mention in no uncertain terms the necessity of another form of contraception in case of stopping the pill as well as the existence of postcoital contraception if necessary.
- If one considers the hypothesis that the duration of the prescription, too long or too short, is a factor in discontinuation, one must adapt the prescription duration to each individual client and take action so that the prescription of pills by nondoctors is possible (as in case of midwives in Sweden) if one is convinced that this approach is well founded. Another possibility would be to permit pharmacists to extend prescriptions.
- One possibility to consider would be for OCs to be bought over the counter. According to M. Poots[8] "on risk/benefit grounds, OCs should be obtainable from vending machines, whereas cigarettes should be on prescription only." But "an initiative to make pills available over the counter in Sweden, more than a decade ago, ended in failure. The initiative did not work primarily because women stopped taking their pills after experiencing nuisance side effects, and there was no source the women could turn to for information. It was difficult to regain the ground that was lost once they stopped taking the pill."[9]
- Does the price of contraception influence its rate of use? According to a survey carried out by the International Health Foundation in eight Western industrialized countries, it appears that for oral contraception the price that must be paid by the users does not seem to play a part in a woman's decision for or against pill use.[2] It would be interesting to confirm this idea among adolescents and to study this problem in developing countries.

The efforts of physicians to prevent pill discontinuation should naturally be supported by pharmacists, the media, and other health care professionals.

ORAL CONTRACEPTION AND NONCOMPLIANCE: GENERAL RECOMMENDATIONS

Role of Physicians

As the persons charged with the task of medical screening and counseling, physicians naturally have a big responsibility in their patients' degree of compliance with contraception. Physicians should first of all recognize that certain adolescents have a high risk of noncompliance. Who are these adolescents? Adolescents who are chronically "pill forgetful," "abortion recidivists," drug addicts, whose socioeconomic and cultural status is disadvantageous, and whose physicians are not well suited to the adolescent patient (see definition below) have a high risk of noncompliance. These adolescents need particularly attentive and appropriate counseling, favoring, *a priori,* high-dose oral contraceptives and methods that one would define as "passive":

- IUDs (keeping in mind that IUDs are not recommended for adolescents in numerous European countries),

- Implants (hoping that they will not be accompanied by irregular bleeding),
- Injectables (hoping that they will be clinically well tolerated).

Physicians should then endeavor not to be contributing factors to noncompliance. Physicians who are not available, who give too much or too little information, who are unable to adapt easily to the personality and needs of the patient requesting contraception, who are not very well versed in contraception, or who are blasé will be at a high risk of patient noncompliance.

In practicing counseling, physicians can usefully follow the recent conclusions of a study of the International Planned Parenthood Federation.[10] This study was carried out in Guatemala, Hong Kong, Jordan, Kenya, Nepal, Trinidad, and Tobago from 1984 to 1986, on 11,532 women, all consulting with physicians for the first time about contraception. The study of existing relationships between counseling and use-continuation of contraceptive methods was the principal aim of the study.

The conclusions of this study were the following:

1. Neither the amount of medical screening nor the expressed satisfaction of the client appeared to exert an influence on use-continuation for any method in any of the six countries.
2. High-level counseling (which refers to the number of items included in the counseling given to clients), tends to be associated with higher risk of discontinuation.
3. Women who do not obtain the method that they had in mind are more likely to discontinue use.
4. The most consistent predictor of continued use is the adolescent's motivation.
5. It is also important that the adolescent knows that her partner, if any, will agree with the use of the method.

These conclusions enabled the IPPF to make four recommendations, which I fully support, in counseling patients about contraceptives:

1. Counseling on contraception should be focused mainly on the *essential* information and discussions needed by the adolescent to make an adequate contraceptive choice and for using the method properly and consistently.
2. Counseling should be restricted to the number of issues that can be *properly* discussed within the available time.
3. The amount of information provided during a counseling session should be in accordance with what the client can understand and retain in her memory.
4. The counseling should be tailored to the characteristics and needs of the individual clients.

One can conclude that the *quality* of counseling appears more important than the *quantity* of information given to users.

Role of the Media

The media certainly plays an important role in the field of oral contraceptive compliance. It is desirable that they become less alarmist concerning health risks, until such side effects have been proven, and that they report with maximum objectivity on the real side effects of methods of contraception. Reports should cover any timely announcements of the progress and good news concerning contraceptive methods as well as their many beneficial effects. Finally, the task of the media is to complete the counseling given by the physicians and above all to inform the users of the over-the-counter methods. In return, the duty of the physicians and the pharmaceutical industry is to inform the media more closely about their scientific work relating to birth control.

Role of Pharmaceutical Firms

The role of the pharmaceutical industry in matters of compliance is also very important. Pharmaceutical firms should continue their activities of fundamental and clinical research on contraception in order to put safe and efficient methods at the disposal of users. Moreover, these methods must be associated with good cycle control, have fewer side effects, be as easy to use as possible, and hinder the sexual life of users to the least extent possible.

On the other hand, pharmaceutical firms can facilitate compliance in contraception by paying special attention to package inserts, which are first of all intended to recall the directions for the use of contraceptives (which should be clear, simple, short, and, if necessary, printed in several languages); one can but deplore those unattractive package inserts that require a magnifying glass to be deciphered and many minutes to read. The firms can also practice a policy of providing services that are systematically associated with contraceptives (for example, by including in pill boxes a condom, a booklet about STDs, and/or an audio cassette of information on the use of the contraceptive), and by facilitating users' access to contraceptives by establishing a policy of reasonable prices.

Role of Pharmacists

The pharmacist, the obligatory intermediary between the physician and the adolescents, plays a primordial role, which is, in my opinion, insufficiently explored and exploited, in the field of compliance with contraception. The pharmacist should, in fact, complete the counseling begun by the physicians and explain to adolescents the use of their prescriptions whenever necessary and, because he or she is easily accessible, reply to their first questions about birth control methods (OCs supplies, drug interference, missed pills, emergency contraception, etc.).

CONCLUSION

Adolescent oral contraceptive noncompliance is a multifactorial problem that demands a multifactorial solution. Thanks to the combined efforts of the physicians, the media, the pharmaceutical firms, the pharmacists, to which one must add other non-doctors (such as midwives, nurses, conjugal counselors) when, by luck, they exist in the doctor's environment, it is possible to hope for *reasonable* improvement in compliance for oral contraception, particularly in adolescents.

I have no illusions, however, because there will always be a certain degree of noncompliance. The users of contraception are, after all, human beings and therefore fallible. There will, thus, always be a need to resort to postcoital contraception (which could be better named emergency contraception) of which all adolescents should know the possibilities and the limits. Postcoital pills could, in fact, cut unplanned pregnancies by half.[11]

There will also always be a certain number of unwanted pregnancies among adolescents due to noncompliance, and one must endeavor to help the patient profit from the process of receiving abortion care by promoting good-quality contraception with the maximum likelihood of good compliance.

REFERENCES

1. Adams Hillard, P. J. 1992. Oral contraceptive noncompliance: The extent of the problem. ADV Contrac. **8**(Suppl. 1): 13–20.
2. International Health Foundation (Brussels). 1993. Compliance Part I: Oral contraceptives. Newsletter **1:** 10–12.
3. Guillebaud, J. 1994. Oral contraceptive compliance: What you and your patients need to know. Churchill Livingstone. London. 118 pp.
4. International Working Group on Enhancing Patient Compliance and Oral Contraceptive Efficacy. 1993. A consensus statement enhancing patient compliance and oral contraceptive efficacy. Br. J. Fam. Plann. **18:** 126–129.
5. Wyeth Ayerst. 1993. Wyeth Ayerst Contraception Survey in Europe (Wycon). Isis Research Ltd. London.
6. Serfaty, D. 1994. Contraceptive noncompliance: Problems and solutions. Proceedings of the 3rd Congress of the European Society of Contraception. Dublin, Ireland, June 15–18, 1994. G. Creatsas, D. Serfaty & S. Skouby, Eds.: 55–68. Entopia. Athens.
7. Serfaty, D. 1992. Medical aspects of oral contraceptive discontinuation. ADV Contrac. **8**(Suppl. 1): 21–33.
8. 1993. Editorial. OCs o-t-c? Lancet **342**(8871): 565–566.
9. 1993. Poor compliance plagues over the counter experience. Contracep. Technol. Update **8:** 125–126.
10. Huezo, C. & U. Malhotra. 1993. Choice and use continuation of methods of contraception. A multicenter study. International Planned Parenthood Federation. London.
11. 1994. When it comes to prescribing emergency contraception, "Just do it." Contracept. Technol. Update **15**(5): 57–61.

Long-Acting Hormonal Contraception

DAVID R. BROMHAM

Department of Obstetrics and Gynaecology
St. James's University Hospital
Beckett Street
Leeds, LS9 7TF, United Kingdom

INTRODUCTION

There is not now and almost certainly never will be, an "ideal" contraceptive (TABLE 1) that will suit all users at all times in their lives. Similarly, there is no such thing as a contraceptor who will find all methods of contraception equally acceptable. It is for this reason that it is important to have a wide selection of different contraceptives to allow users to choose methods meeting, as nearly as possible, their priorities.

It must be remembered that there are important differences among adolescents throughout the world. In developing countries there is usually a tendency to earlier marriage and pregnancy with contraceptive use reserved mainly for pregnancy spacing and after family completion. In developed countries the young often become sexually active before marriage and, in most cases, before there is any intention to conceive and establish parenthood. This is well illustrated by a recent comparison of Norplant® users in Indonesia and England (TABLE 2).

For more than 30 years (nearly three generations) the combined oral contraceptive pill has been seen as the most appropriate contraceptive for young women. This perception finds expression in the fact that most young women requesting contraceptive advice will inform their chosen family-planning adviser that they "want to go on the pill." The reflexive prescription of this method, without discussion of alternatives that might actually be more appropriate to their needs, serves only to perpetuate this perception. However, the potential range of contraceptive options open to the adolescent are as great as to women of other ages.[3]

In this article the characteristics and utilization by adolescents of long-acting hormonal contraceptive methods will be considered. Although the range of injectables and implants is currently increasing, we will concentrate on those methods for which there is a reasonable volume of relevant experience in the literature: namely, depot medroxyprogesterone acetate (Depo-Provera®) and levonorgestrel subdermal implants (Norplant®). The system for the intrauterine release of levonorgestrel (Levonova® or Mirena®) will also be discussed here because some of its features are of particular relevance to adolescents. These three long-acting progestogen-only hormonal methods share a number of characteristics in common, the most important of which is their high efficacy and virtually zero possibility of "user-failure" (FIG. 1). This gives them all one obvious advantage over the combined pill which, particularly among adolescents,[4] has considerably greater potential for poor compliance and consequent failure, resulting in pregnancy. In one study from the United States, depot

TABLE 1. The Hypothetical "Ideal" Contraceptive[a]

- 100% reliable (no method or user failure pregnancies occur)
- 100% reversible (fertility returns to normal immediately after use is discontinued)
- 100% safe (no increase in mortality or morbidity in any user)
- Non-medicalized (does not require medical supervision of use)
- Not coitally related (does not interfere with sexual spontaneity)
- Discrete (use not obvious to another person)
- Cheap (low cost to user or health care system)
- Wide public acceptance (use not opposed on religious or similar grounds)
- Beneficial effects (e.g., protection against infection, malignancy, or menstrual disturbance)

[a]Table was adapted from Bromham (1995).[1]

medroxyprogesterone acetate (dMPA) and Norplant® were significantly more likely to be chosen by adolescents who had previously experienced pregnancy than was the combination pill.[5]

DEPO-PROVERA®

Even before the licensing of dMPA for contraception by the U.S. Food & Drug Administration (FDA), it was apparent that physicians familiar with the contraceptive problems of adolescents were prepared to prescribe this drug.[6] This seemed to be significantly more likely for female physicians, and there was a greater proportion of pediatricians than gynecologists who took this attitude. Mental retardation was seen as a particularly strong potential indication for use in this group. Although there are considerable variations between nations with regard to views on the ethics of using long-acting reversible or irreversible contraception or sterilization for those incompetent to give consent, the potential advantages of this method seem to have been appreciated by the physicians questioned in this study. In addition to a high order of efficacy, probably better than with any other contraceptive method, dMPA has the advantages, compared to the combined pill, of ease of compliance and use and absence of estrogenic side effects and, compared to intrauterine and implantable contraceptives, ease of initiation and discontinuation of the method. In addition, the method, although requiring medical contact at 12-weekly intervals, is otherwise discrete,

TABLE 2. Characteristics of English and Indonesian Norplant Acceptors[a]

	English Clinic (n = 70)	Indonesian Clinic (n = 44)
Age <21 years	10%	0%
Unmarried	19%	0%
No children	19%	0%

[a]Data adapted from Wilson and Marley (1995).[2]

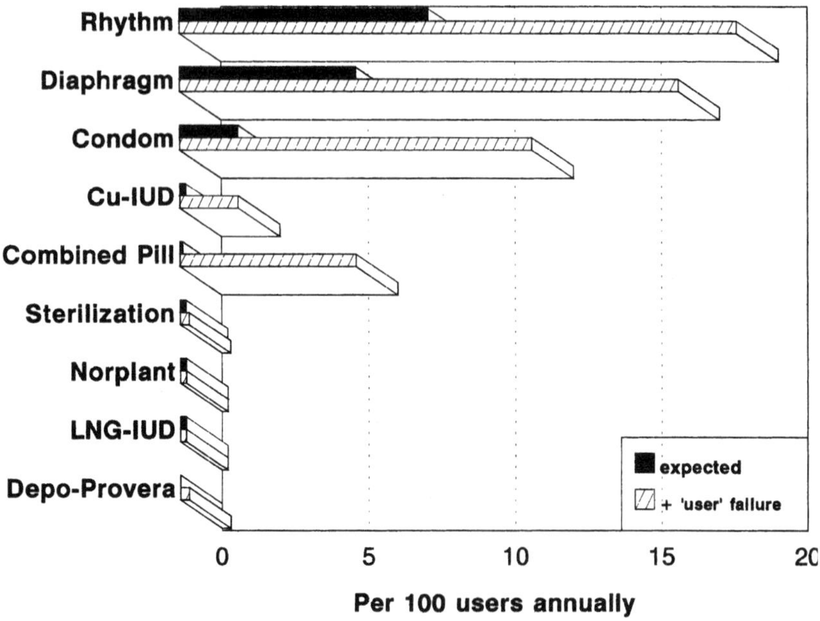

FIGURE 1. Contraceptive failure rates. (Data adapted from various sources.) Abbreviations: Cu-IUD = copper-medicated intrauteine device; LNG-IUD = levonorgestrel releasing intrauterine device. User failure = unintended conception because of misuse of the method by the contraceptor and/or poor advice or management by the provider.

there being no overt evidence of its use. The most significant side effects of this method relate to the derangement of menstrual pattern: frequent bleeding and spotting in the early months of use, oligo- and amenorrhea with longer continuation. These features relating to a greater suppression of endogenous estrogen output are more marked with dMPA than with the other methods under discussion. As with all hormonal methods, a relatively small proportion (5–10%) of users will experience effects such as weight and mood change and headaches. One Scandinavian study[7] showed that the frequency and severity of headaches and of adverse moods actually improved rather than worsened overall and that in those gaining weight (by no means all) half the increase was attributable to age change. The possibility that long-term use of this method, associated with high frequencies of amenorrhea, may contribute to bone mineral loss has been raised. This might be of particular importance in a younger woman seeking long-term deferment of an initial pregnancy, but as yet the evidence is inconclusive.

One U.S. Study[8] showed that over 80% of adolescents using this method were happy overall with it. Effectiveness, duration of effect, ease of compliance, and its discrete nature were each cited by about one-third of users as being import advantages. It was nonmenstrual side effects that seemed to be associated with most dissatisfaction. Continuation rates were 72% after one year and 6% after five years.

NORPLANT®

As discussed above the uptake of levonorgestrel subdermal contraceptive implants (Norplant®) by adolescent contraceptors is a feature of developed countries. Early reports from the U.S. indicated that a very high proportion of those demanding Norplant were adolescents,[9,10] that is, 43% with 14% aged 16 years or under.[10] Conversely, in one year half of those attending a Teen Pregnancy Program chose Norplant.[11] This effect has not been so dramatic in the United Kingdom (U.K.), but some centers have found up to 12.4% of acceptors being under 20 years old.[12] Features of the method that appeal to users,[13] specifically, ease of compliance, long duration, and efficacy, are similar to those discussed above for dMPA. There is very little evidence that continuation rates are lower among adolescents than older women.[9,14] This is similar to the experience in our own clinic (FIG. 2). Reasons for discontinuation in adolescents and older women seem to relate mainly to menstrual and nonmenstrual side effects. Although the potential for visibility of the implants is sometimes perceived as a potential disadvantage,[12] representing loss of discretion as well as cosmetic problems, it is not a frequent main indication for removal. The need for experienced, adequately trained personnel for the insertion and removal of this method may

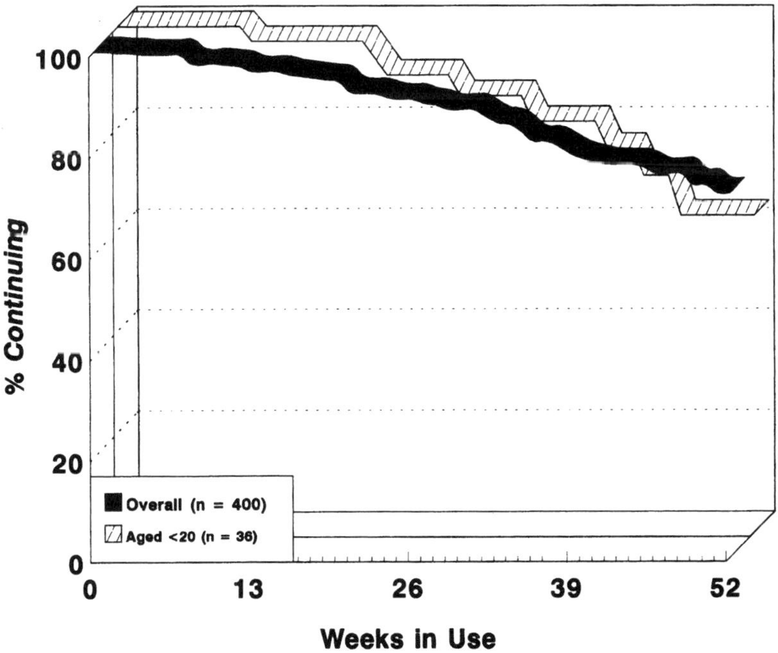

FIGURE 2. Continuation rates calculated weekly to 52 weeks by life-table method for patients attending St. James's University Hospital, Leeds. These rates are lower than for most other UK clinics but are not significantly different in young attenders.

be seen as potential disadvantages. However, between these events the Norplant user is largely "demedicalized." The ease of use of this contraceptive method is reflected in the poor attendance for follow-up visits among both adults and adolescents.[14]

LEVONOVA® OR MIRENA®

This levonorgestrel-releasing intrauterine contraceptive system (LNG-IUD) combines some of the characteristics of long-acting hormonal methods with those of intrauterine contraception. The use of intrauterine contraception has traditionally been avoided among young, nulliparous women for two reasons.

First are the anatomical considerations associated with fitting devices through a nulliparous cervix. This is not usually an important consideration with modern medicated devices. With the exception of the copper T 380A (Paragard®), most can be introduced through the nulliparous cervix, including the Multiload® series.[15] The latter device has an insertion diameter little different from that of the LNG-IUD, and the use of this in nulliparous adolescents is a possibility. Attention has been drawn to the potential benefit of using cervical local anesthetic techniques for the insertion of this and other devices.[16]

A more important consideration with regard to the use of IUDs by young women is the risk of pelvic inflammatory disease (PID). This is related to the frequency of intercourse and change of sexual partner in this age group and not purely to age itself.[17] It is known the hormonal methods may convey some protection from PID, however, presumably at the cervical mucus level, against the ascent of infecting organisms to the upper genital tract. In comparison to inert or copper-medicated IUDs, such protection might be anticipated with the LNG-IUD. Such a protective effect has indeed been shown in some studies.[18,19] The effect is most marked when considering women aged 25 years or under.[19] Although this observation may represent a particular advantage for adolescents considering intrauterine contraception, it must be acknowledged that relative protection against PID, when the LNG-IUD is compared to copper-medicated devices, is not a universal finding.[20,21] Furthermore, it is important that all contraceptors, particularly adolescents, are aware that any protection against PID does not equate to protection against acquiring or transmitting sexual infection.

LONG-ACTING HORMONAL CONTRACEPTION AND PROTECTION AGAINST SEXUALLY TRANSMITTED DISEASES

For some time, concerns have been expressed regarding confusion in young people over the dual role of the male condom in providing both contraception and protection from infection, notably with HIV.[22] Response to encouragement of condom use for the latter purpose may be jeopardized in the aftermath of unplanned pregnancy in those relying on condoms as a sole contraceptive agent.[23] Counseling for those likely to accept a long-acting hormonal contraceptive method should always emphasise the need to use condoms as protection against infection. This is emphasized by the experience in one U.S. study of 762 Norplant users (45% under 21 years of age).[24] Of these, 43% used condoms regularly before Norplant fitting, but only 20% indicated that they planned regular, continuous use. Although there was a greater proportion among younger women, it still seemed that many at risk of sexual infection would abandon condoms once provided with highly effective prevention of pregnancy.

CONCLUSION

The range of contraceptive methods available to adolescents includes, as it does for older women, long-acting hormonal contraceptives, and the uptake of these methods is remarkably high when they are offered to younger women. They provide high efficacy, greater than that often achieved with the combined oral contraceptive pill in this age group. This advantage relates to ease of compliance and continued contraceptive cover until positive steps to interrupt the method are taken. In addition, an element of greater discretion and privacy over the method may be attractive to some users. No contraceptive is without some drawbacks, and the side effects and risks of these methods should always be discussed with a potential user before commencement. This includes the fact that any protection offered against sexual infection relates only to a relative reduction in the incidence of PID. Fuller protection requires the continued use of condoms. This advice is of particular importance in adolescents, who statistically may be at greater risk.

SUMMARY

For 30 years, the combined oral contraceptive pill has been an almost automatic choice for effective contraception in sexually active adolescent women. Nevertheless, consideration of the criteria of a hypothetical "ideal" contraceptive suggests that long-acting progestogen-only methods may have considerable advantages for some adolescents. These would include greater efficacy, easier compliance, avoidance of estrogenic side effects, and potentially greater privacy. The disadvantages of menstrual irregularity, progestogenic side effects including weight gain, and the initial greater medicalization of the method, particularly implants, must be weighed against the wishes and preferences of the adolescent. A number of studies of the uptake and utilization of these methods in adolescence have arisen, particularly from the United States. These are reviewed together with experience from programs in the United Kingdom.

REFERENCES

1. Bromham, D. R. 1995. Overview of contraception in general practice. *In* Contraception. Update Postgraduate Centre Series. D. Bromham, Ed.: 7–10. Reed Healthcare Communications. Sutton, Surrey, UK.
2. Wilson, S. & C. Marley. 1995. A comparative study of users of Norplant in England and Indonesia. Br. J. Fam. Plann. **21**(3): 98–101.

3. WENT, D. 1995. Teenage contraception. *In* Contraception. Update Postgraduate Centre Series. D. Bromham, Ed.: 46–49. Reed Healthcare Communications. Sutton, Surrey, UK.
4. SERFATY, D. 1997. Oral contraceptive compliance during adolescence. Ann. N.Y. Acad. Sci. This volume.
5. CROMER, B. A., R. D. SMITH, J. MCA. BLAIR, J. DWYER & R. T. BROWN. 1994. A prospective study of adolescents who choose among levonorgestrel implant (Norplant), medroxyprogesterone acetate (Depo-Provera), or the combined oral contraceptive pill as contraception. Pediatrics **94**(5): 687–694.
6. ISART, F., F. T. WEBER, C. L. MERRICK & S. ROWE. 1992. Use of injectable progestin (medroxyprogesterone acetate) in adolescent health care. Contraception **46:** 41–48.
7. SOLHEIM, F. 1992. An assessment of quality of life in women treated with Depo-Provera in Sweden. *In* Depo-Provera® (Medroxyprogesterone Acetate) for Contraception. A Current Perspective of Scientific, Clinical & Social Issues. D. Zambrano, Ed.: 61–72. Oxford Clinical Communications. Oxford, UK.
8. SMITH, R. D., B. A. CROMER, J. R. HAYES & R. T. BROWN. 1995. Medroxyprogesterone acetate (Depo-Provera) use in adolescents: Uterine bleeding and blood pressure patterns, patient satisfaction, and continuation rates. Adolesc. Pediatr. Gynecol. **8:** 24–28.
9. CROSBY, U. D., B. E. SCHWARZ, K. L. GLUCK & S. F. HEARTWELL. 1993. A preliminary report of Norplant implant insertions in a large family planning program. Contraception **48**(4): 359–366.
10. FRANK, M. L., A. N. POINDEXTER, M. L. JOHNSON & L. BATEMAN. 1992. Characteristics and attitudes of early contraceptive implant acceptors in Texas. Fam. Plann. Perspect. **24**(5): 208–213.
11. MASHBURN, M. Levonorgestrel implant amongst adolescents. 1994. J. Pediatr. Health Care. **8**(6): 255–260.
12. BLAIN, S., J. LOVELADY, E. OLOTO, V. RANE & D. BROMHAM. 1995. Reasons for commencing and discontinuing contraception with Norplant—a review of local experience. Br. J. Fam. Plann. **21**(Suppl. 1): 17–21.
13. BROMHAM, D. 1995. Initial UK experience with Norplant: A first report from the UK Multicentre Study. Br. J. Fam. Plann. **21**(Suppl. 1): 5–8.
14. CULLINS, V. E., R. E. REMSBURG, P. D. BLUMENTHAL & G. R. HUGGINS. 1994. Comparison of adolescent and adult experiences with Norplant levonorgestrel contraceptive implants. Obstet. Gynecol. **83**(6): 1026–1032.
15. PETERSEN, K. R., L. BROOKS, B. JACOBSEN & S. O. SKOUBY. 1991. Intrauterine devices in nulliparous women. Adv. Contracept. **7:** 333–338.
16. HOLLINGWORTH, B. 1995. Pain control during insertion of an intrauterine device. Br. J. Fam. Plann. **21**(3): 102–103.
17. STRUTHERS, B. J. 1991. Copper IUDs, PID and fertility in nulliparous women. Adv. Contracept. **7:** 211–230.
18. TOIVONEN, J., T. LUUKAINEN & H. ALLONEN. 1991. Protective effective of intrauterine release of levonorgestrel on pelvic infection: Three years comparative experience of levonorgestrel- and copper-releasing intrauterine devices. Obstet. Gynecol. **77:** 261–264.
19. ANDERSSON, K., V. ODLIND & G. RYBO. 1994. Levonorgestrel-releasing and copper-releasing (Nova T) IUDs during five years of use: A randomized comparative trial. Contraception **49:** 56–72.
20. SIVIN, I., S. EL MAHGOUB & T. MCCARTHY. 1990. Long-term contraception with the levonorgestrel 20mcg/day (Lng 20) and the Copper T 380 Ag intrauterine devices: A five-year randomized study. Contraception **42:** 361–378.
21. SIVIN, I. & J. STERN. 1994. Health during prolonged use of levonorgestrel 20 μg/d and the Copper T Cu 380Ag intrauterine contraceptive devices: A multicenter study. Fertil. Steril. **61**(1): 70–77.

22. PERSSON, E. 1991. Family planning and prevention strategies for sexually transmitted diseases. Adv. Contracept. **7**(2/3): 181–186.
23. PIHOS, I. A., R.S. CARTMILL & D. R. BROMHAM. 1993. Impact of unplanned pregnancy & termination on intended future contraception in young women. Recent Developments on Pediatric-Adolescent Gynecology and Endocrinology. Program Abstracts.: 74. Entopia Editorial Productions. Athens, Greece.
24. FRANK, M. L., L. BATEMAN & A. N. POINDEXTER. 1993. Planned condom use by women with Norplant implants. Adv. Contracept. **9**(3): 227–232.

Intrauterine Contraception in Adolescent Women

The Gynefix Intrauterine Implant

DIRK WILDEMEERSCH,[a] HENRI VAN KETS, MARC VRIJENS, WILLY DELBARGE, YVES VAN TRAPPEN, MARLEEN TEMMERMAN, HERMAN DEPYPERE, AND MICHEL THIERY

International Study Group on Intrauterine Drug Delivery
Department of Obstetrics and Gynaecology
University of Ghent
De Pintelaan 185, 9000 Ghent, Belgium

INTRODUCTION

Of the more than 500 million young women between 15 and 19 years of age in the world today, up to 10%, depending on the country, become accidentally pregnant each year notwithstanding the numerous efforts to avoid this problem, such as providing sex education programs and contraceptive services, and despite the widespread availability and use of contraceptives.[1] Nonuse of a birth control method, discontinuation of use, contraceptive noncompliance, and method failure are the main reasons for the occurrence of an unintended pregnancy.[2]

A high proportion of these teenage pregnancies frequently end in abortion, and many of the abortions are obtained under unsafe conditions, mainly in countries where abortion is illegal. The estimated yearly number of induced abortions is at least 5 million, and the numbers are increasing rapidly, especially in the densely populated urban regions of the world such as in many Asian countries.[1,3]

It is doubtful that the problem of adolescent pregnancy will be solved or reduced by stimulating the use of birth control methods that depend on user compliance because of the very high rate of discontinuation and noncompliance in this group of young women. Although implantation methods, such as Norplant, also have weak points, it has been shown that they could play a very important part in the prevention of pregnancy in adolescents.[4]

Since 1985, the International Study Group on Intrauterine Drug Delivery has used the frameless, copper-releasing intrauterine implant (IUI) in young nulligravid women from the age of 14 and has published several studies demonstrating its high performance and its high acceptability.[5–7] This paper discusses the use of the implant system in nulligravid women based on long-term clinical experience in this age group and reconsiders the positioning of this new contraceptive as a strategy to be recommended to help reduce the number of teenage pregnancies. The clinical data reported in this paper have been discussed at length elsewhere.[7]

[a]Address for correspondence: Dr. D. Wildemeersch, Coordinator of Clinical Trials, Piers de Raveschootlaan 125, 8300 Knokke-Heist, Belgium.

MATERIALS AND METHODS

The GyneFix® Implant System

The GyneFix implant and insertion system has been described previously.[5] A short description of the implant is, however, appropriate. It consists of a non-biodegradable suture thread made of surgical 00 monofilament polypropylene on which six copper tubes (each 5 mm in length and 2.2 mm in diameter) are threaded, providing a total surface area of 330 mm^2. The upper and lower tubes are crimped onto the thread to keep the tubes in place. The upper extremity of the thread is provided with a knot that serves as an anchor. The knot is implanted into the fundal myometrium with a specially designed insertion instrument, allowing reliable anchoring, thereby permanently securing the device in the uterine cavity (FIG. 1).

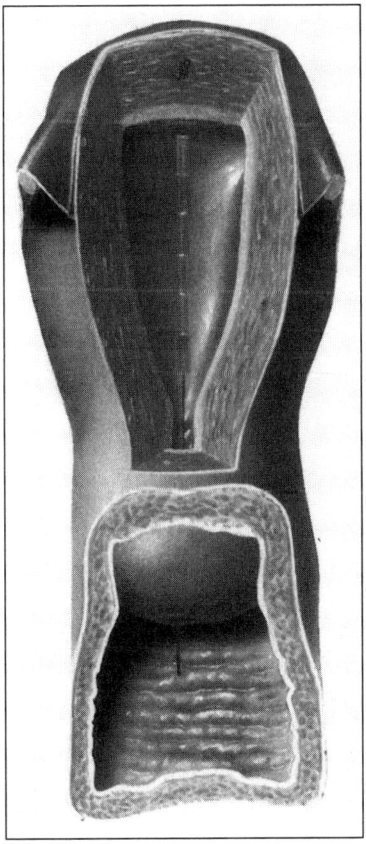

FIGURE 2. GyneFix® at insertion.

Candidates

The subjects who participated in this multicenter study were women between 14 and 48 years of age requesting contraception. The women were selected according to a list of inclusion and exclusion criteria, which includes a monogamous sexual relationship and absence of infection. Written or oral consent was obtained, and the trial was approved by the Ethical Committee of the University Hospital of Gent, Belgium and other institutions. 1039 GyneFix devices were inserted at various times during the menstrual cycle; 278 devices were inserted in nulligravid women of which 43 were young women below the age of 20. Insertions in nulligravid women were only done in Belgium.

Paracervical block or intracervical anesthesia, using a dental syringe with a fine needle, was performed, particularly in anxious patients, using the method described by Thiery.[8] Following insertion, women were advised neither to use tampons nor to have intercourse for the first 7 days. Follow-up examinations were scheduled at 1 month after insertion and every 6 months thereafter, and pertinent data were recorded on specially designed forms.

Investigators

The majority of the investigators in this international multicenter study were not actually trained in the insertion technique. They were instructed using a model and drawings of the insertion procedure.

STATISTICS

Life-table rates were calculated as suggested by Tietze and Lewit.[9] Statistical significance of rate differences was assessed by comparison between two proportions. Age and parity distribution of the acceptors is given in TABLE 1. TABLE 2 shows the overall results, and in TABLE 3 the groups are separated according to gravidity.

RESULTS

Pregnancy

Only two intrauterine pregnancies were recorded during the study (total group), yielding a gross cumulative pregnancy rate of 0.5 at 36 months. One pregnancy was located in the device-free cavity of a didelphic uterus. No ectopic pregnancies were registered.

Expulsion

Only six devices were expelled during the whole study, amounting to 0.7 at 36 months. Five devices were expelled during the first three month after insertion in

TABLE 1. GyneFix: Distribution of Acceptors According to Age and Gravidity

Age (years)	Number	Percent	Gravidity	Number	Percent
< 20	43	4.1	0	278	26.7
21–25	133	13.3	1+	716	73.3
26–30	274	26.3			
31–35	228	22.0			
> 35	356	34.3			
Total	1039	100.0			

TABLE 2. GyneFix (n = 1039): Number of Women, Woman-Months of Experience, and Gross Cumulative Event Rates per 100 Users at 12, 24, and 36 Months, Total Group[a]

	Months		
	12	24	36
No. of women completing 36 months	706	317	211
Woman-months of use	10051	16075.5	19029
Events			
Pregnancy	0.1	0.1	0.5
Expulsion	0.5 (0.2–1.2)	0.7 (0.2–1.4)	0.7 (0.2–1.4)
Removal for:			
Bleeding/pain	1.9 (1.0–2.9)	2.7 (1.6–3.9)	3.8 (2.3–5.3)
Other medical reasons	0.1 (0.0–0.7)	0.5 (0.1–1.5)	0.5 (0.1–1.5)
Planned pregnancy	2.0 (1.0–2.9)	7.4 (5.2–9.5)	12.8 (9.7–15.9)
Other personal reasons	0.3 (0.0–0.9)	1.2 (0.4–2.5)	1.6 (0.6–3.3)
Continuation rate	95.2	87.9	81.2
Lost to follow-up	6.8 (5.3–8.4)	7.8 (6.0–9.5)	8.7 (6.8–10.6)

[a]Values in parentheses give upper and lower confidence limits at 95% level.

four different centers, shortly after the centers started collaborating in the study, indicating improper insertion of the anchor due to unfamiliarity with the new insertion technique. Gravidity was not found to influence expulsion of the GyneFix (TABLE 3).

Removal for Medical Reasons

Removal rates for medical reasons amounted to 4.3 at 36 months in the total group. The most common side effect was bleeding, but the rate for removal for bleeding and pain was low (3.8 at 36 months). In the nulligravid group, this rate was only 1.2 at 36 months (TABLE 3).

TABLE 3. GyneFix (n = 1039): Number of Women, Woman-Months of Experience, and Gross Cumulative Event Rates per 100 Users at 36 months, According to Gravidity[a]

	Nulligravid	Nulliparous and Parous
No. of women completing 36 months	78	133
Woman-months of use	5629	13400
Events		
Pregnancy	1.4 (0.2–5.0)	0.0 (0.0–0.0)
Expulsion	0.9 (0.1–3.3)	0.6 (0.2–1.4)
Removal for:		
Bleeding/pain	1.2 (0.1–4.4)	4.9 (2.8–6.9)
Other medical reasons	1.2 (0.1–4.3)	0.2 (0.0–1.2)
Planned pregnancy	25.2 (18.2–32.1)	5.8 (3.3–8.3)
Other personal reasons	1.8 (0.4–5.2)	1.5 (0.4–4.0)
Continuation rate	70.1	87.6
Lost to follow-up	7.2 (3.8–10.5)	9.4 (7.1–11.7)

[a]Values in parentheses give upper and lower confidence limits at 95% level.

Adverse Events

No serious complications, for example, pelvic inflammatory disease (PID) or uterine perforations, were observed.

Continuation

The continuation rate amounted to 81.2% at 36 months in the total group of women and was 70.1% at 36 months in the nulligravid group, mostly because of a high number of removals for planned pregnancy (12.8% and 25.2%, respectively).

DISCUSSION

Pelvic Inflammatory Disease

The controversy over providing an IUD for nulligravid/nulliparous women lies in the possible effect that IUDs may have on future fertility of the young woman who selects the IUD as a method of contraception. Studies published in the 70s and early 80s showed that pelvic inflammatory disease is more frequent in nulliparous IUD users than in women using other methods of contraception.[10] Nevertheless, recent studies conclude that the PID risk is minimal in women who are at low risk for sexually transmitted diseases (STDs), in other words, among couples in mutually monogamous relationships.[11,12] Moreover, it was found that the risk of PID was higher in the first three weeks following insertion. According to the World Health Organization, many studies conducted in the past overdiagnosed PID in IUD users. There were also a number of methodologic problems in these studies such as using the wrong or inappropriate comparison groups (pill users).[12]

The present study confirms the low risk of PID, since no PID cases were diagnosed. We can conclude, therefore, that the nonprescription of IUDs to young nulligravid/nulliparous women because of the fear of PID is no longer justified. It is neither age nor the nulliparity, but sexual activity that increases the risk of infection. In some areas with a high prevalence of STDs in young women, screening for *Neisseria gonorrhoeae* and *Chlamydia trachomatis* may be important before the fitting of an IUD. Frequently, this is neither feasible nor practical. However, if the wet smear shows signs of infection, insertion of an IUD should be deferred until the cause is established and the infection is cured.

Why no proven PID cases have been recorded in all clinical trials with the GyneFix so far, in contrast with the T-shaped device, is hypothetical. The absence of transverse arms seems the most obvious reason for the absence of these infectious complications. Research has shown that pointed IUD projections commonly become embedded in the uterine wall or the uterine ostia of the fallopian tubes and can cause tissue proliferation and damage to the endometrial areas in which the IUD projections have penetrated.[13–15] It is probable that these changes predispose the user to infectious complications, including PID.

Performance and Tolerance

When selecting an IUD for nulligravid/nulliparous women, the consequences of disharmony between the IUD and the uterine cavity, accidental pregnancy due to displacement and expulsion, and a high removal rate due to side effects should be taken into consideration. The low tolerance rate and significantly lower performance rates of "framed" IUDs in nulliparous women compared to parous women have contributed to the low acceptance of IUDs in general and the bad reputation attributed to IUDs in the media.[29] With regard to effectiveness, literature data show that the 3-year cumulative pregnancy rates in nulliparous women using traditional IUDs are usually greater than four.[16–20] The younger the women, the higher the rate. It is evident that the frameless IUD should be recommended as the first choice intrauterine contraceptive in nulligravid/nulliparous women because of its very high effectiveness and optimal tolerance.

Furthermore, a "total" expulsion rate of over 10% at 3 years is usual in nulliparous women wearing a traditional IUD. This is caused by incompatibility between the IUD frame and the reduced dimensions of the uterine cavity.[29] Total expulsion puts the woman at risk of an unintended pregnancy. However, undetected and uncorrected partial expulsion is probably also a very important contributor to IUD failure, as Kaivola indicated.[21]

Pain and/or bleeding are major reasons for discontinuing use of the IUD and were an important motive for the development of the frameless IUI. As a consequence of disharmony, a young nulliparous woman is more likely to require removal of her IUD because of bleeding and pain. Cumulative removal rates at 3 years for pain/bleeding vary between 12 and 26% in large multicenter studies are usual for framed IUDs, as was also found by the study group.[20,29]

Implants versus the Birth Control Pill

It is becoming unlikely that birth control pills will ever be able to reduce the number of accidental adolescent pregnancies. The reports are clear: Poor compliance and discontinuation result in oral contraceptive (OC) failure rates in the general population that range from 3% to as high as 20%.[22] First-year discontinuation rates as high as 50 to 60% have been reported, mainly due to physical problems such as nuisance side effects and menstrual irregularities.[23] In a comparative study in 100 "postpartum" adolescents of whom 50 selected oral contraceptives and 48 Norplant, one subject in the Norplant group and 19 in the oral contraceptive group became pregnant during the first postpartum year! This is a further indication that OCs perform poorly in this group of women. On the other hand, the selection of Norplant is associated with high rates of continued use (95% for Norplant vs. 33% for OCs) and lower "new" pregnancy rates.[4]

Although Norplant is an effective contraceptive method offering distinct advantages over OCs in terms of prevention of teenage pregnancy, there are several disadvantages: the presence of systemic side effects such as weight gain, hair loss, acne, prolonged or irregular bleeding, and the hypo-estrogenic effect common to all systemic progestogen-only contraceptives which may affect bone mass and density. Pain at the site of insertion, the visibility of the implants and the high price are other disadvantages (TABLE 4). The implants can usually, but not always, be removed without undue delay and with little discomfort.[24]

Emergency Insertion and Insertion Immediately after Pregnancy Termination

For women exposed to unprotected sexual intercourse, emergency insertion of the IUI can be used to avoid an unwanted pregnancy. The IUI is particularly useful when the woman considers its use for long-term contraception and when more than 48 to 72 hours have elapsed, excluding the use of OCs (Yuzpe method) for emergency con-

TABLE 4. Use-Related Factors: Comparison between Different Methods Used by Adolescent Women

	Pill	Norplant	GyneFix
Failure after one year (%)	3 (up to 20)	< 1	< 1
Noncompliance	+++	—	—
Side effect/complications (range 0–3)	3	1–2	0–1
Insertion/removal problems	—	Frequent	Rare
Price	Moderate	High	Low

traception.[25] However, women at increased risk of STDs should be adequately counseled.

Preliminary clinical studies have shown that the GyneFix implant can be successfully inserted immediately following spontaneous or induced abortion.[26] Immediate post-abortal IUD insertion is a very convenient and opportune moment to provide contraception: The motivation for contraception is usually high, it is convenient for the woman as well as the provider, the cervix is dilated, and one has the assurance that the woman is protected before leaving the clinic. Additionally, the reduced cost may also be important. The most important advantage of immediate post-abortal IUD insertion is the prevention of repeat abortion. In most studies, however, the expulsion rates of traditional IUDs are higher than when the IUD is inserted post-menstrually. It should be remembered that the contribution of IUD expulsion to unintended pregnancies and abortions, worldwide, is tremendous.[27] The IUI can be helpful not only to reduce this number but also to reduce the number of abortions.

Aspects Related to Insertion in Young Nulligravid/Nulliparous Women

Certain insertion-related techniques should be considered when inserting IUDs, especially in young, nulliparous women. To make the insertion procedure more acceptable, especially when the young woman is anxious, the use of intracervical anesthetics is recommended. One of the authors (DW) uses intracervical block anesthesia routinely in nulligravid and nulliparous women. The use of a dental syringe with an extra fine needle is particularly convenient.[8] Apart from the reduction of pain during and after insertion, fewer vasovagal attacks and fewer removals for pain and bleeding have been reported in the first year. If a vasovagal syncope should occur, atropine sulfate 0.2 mg i.v. and 0.2 mg s.c. results in prompt recovery.

Counseling

Counseling is an essential part of every family-planning provider's role. There are several important elements to family-planning counseling:

1. To obtain information about contraceptive method needs and a brief medical history.
2. To inform the woman about birth control methods and help her choose a method. The provider should list the available birth control methods and clearly describe those that interest the client—how they work, advantages and disadvantages, and possible side effects. The effectiveness of various methods should be discussed in the light of the risks and problems of an unintended pregnancy. The final decision to use a frameless IUD—or any other method—must be an informed choice by the client. When counseling nulligravid or nulliparous women, a number of young women believe that they cannot use the IUD until they have been pregnant. It is important to explain them that there is no link between intrauterine contraception and PID for women with low exposure to STDs and that additional protection, such as a condom, is needed be-

fore starting a new sexual relationship. Counseling should also include an explanation about the mechanism of action. The generally accepted mechanism of action is that the copper creates an environment which induces foreign body cells that are hostile to sperm. When the foreign body cells die, they liberate an endotoxin that is toxic to sperm. There is therefore little doubt that the IUD acts as a true contraceptive and not as an abortifacient agent.

3. To inform the young women about the frameless IUD (why the GyneFix was developed, the importance of harmony, clinical effectiveness of GyneFix) and counsel her about the insertion. Once the decision has been taken to use the frameless IUD, the provider should explain how the insertion is done to remove anxiety about the insertion procedure and that, in case of anxiety, local or loco-regional anesthesia can be provided.

CONCLUSION

The frameless intrauterine implant system was selected in 1988 by the National Academy of Sciences of the United States.[28] The IUI is approved for marketing in the European Union and was recently introduced in a number of European countries.

The harmonious design characteristics of the implant system providing optimal tolerance, its high effectiveness, its strictly local action, and the absence of systemic side effects in contrast with oral or injectable hormonal methods are powerful arguments not to refuse or withhold this unique contraceptive method for use by young nulligravid/nulliparous women at low risk for sexually transmitted diseases.

The frameless intrauterine implant system should be recommended as an important new contraceptive option for interval, emergency, and immediately postabortal contraception in order to reduce the high number of unintended/unwanted pregnancies, and induced abortions, in adolescent women.

SUMMARY

Pregnancy rates among adolescents have not decreased over the last 10 years, despite numerous efforts. To solve this important health problem, the major strategy recommended is to encourage contraceptive use among sexually active teenagers. An important means of obtaining this is by promoting methods that are not dependent on daily administration in order to avoid noncompliance. One such method (Norplant) has already shown to be much more effective than the combination pill in preventing pregnancy in adolescent women.

The frameless intrauterine implant system (fixed, frameless, and completely flexible) has been studied since 1985 in women between 14 and 50 years of age. The results in young nulligravid women confirm its very high effectiveness (cumulative pregnancy rate at 36 months: 1.4%), its low expulsion rate (cumulative rate at 36 months: 0.9%) and its optimal tolerance (cumulative removal rate for medical reasons at 36 months: 2.4%), resulting in a high acceptance of the implant and a high continued use.

The system (GyneFix®) offers long-term protection (5 years), and its insertion, with or without anesthetic, is easily accomplished in the office. The GyneFix should therefore be recommended as an excellent alternative for birth control pills for young women with low risk for STDs, especially when compliance is a problem, without an increased risk for complications and without systemic side effects. Removal of the device is accomplished by traction on the tail. It can also be used for emergency contraception and for insertion immediately after termination of pregnancy.

ACKNOWLEDGMENTS

Data were analyzed by Eureca, Belgium. We thank Mrs G. Allaerts for secretarial assistance.

The International Study Group on Intrauterine Drug Delivery was created by a group of gynecologists at the University of Gent, Belgium, with experience in intrauterine contraception, in order to study innovative technologies for the sustained target delivery of drugs the uterine cavity. The main objective of the multidisciplinary group is to find more acceptable approaches to the prevention and treatment of gynecological conditions and to birth control with the aim to facilitate access and to improve safety, acceptability, user compliance, and quality of life for women. The International Study Group conducts clinical research in collaboration with leading centers and organizations worldwide.

REFERENCES

1. 1994. Youth at risk: Meeting the Sexual Health Needs of Adolescents—Questions and Answers, Population Policy Information Kit, No. 9, April. Available from Population Action International, 1120, 19th Street, N.W., Suite 550, Washington, DC 20036.
2. GUILLEBAUD, J. 1995. Oral Contraceptive Compliance. What You and Your Patients Need to Know. Churchill Livingstone. London.
3. 1988. U.S. teen pregnancy. F.H.I. Network, Volume 10, No. 1, Fall
4. POLANECZKY, M., G. SLAP, C. FORKE, A. RAPPAPORT & S. SONDHEIMER. 1994. The use of levonorgestrel implants (Norplant) for contraception in adolescent mothers. N. Engl. J. Med. **331**(18): 1201–1230.
5. WILDEMEERSCH, D., H. VAN KETS, H. VAN DER PAS, M. VRIJENS, Y. VAN TRAPPEN, J. J. AMY, I. BATAR, P. BARRI, F. MARTINEZ, L. IGLESIAS-CORTIT & M. THIERY. 1994. IUD tolerance in nulligravid and parous women: Optimal acceptance with the frameless CuFix implant system. Br. J. Fam. Plann. **20:** 2–5.
6. VAN KETS, H., D. WILDEMEERSCH, H. VAN DER PAS, M. VRIJENS, Y. VAN TRAPPEN, J. J. AMY, I. BATAR, P. BARRI, F. MARTINEZ, L. IGLESIAS-CORTIT, WU SHANGCHUN, CAO XIAOMING, FENG ZUAN-CHONG & M. THIERY. 1995. IUD expulsion solved with implant technology. Contraception **51:** 87–92.
7. H. VAN KETS, M. VRIJENS, Y. VAN TRAPPEN, W. DELBARGE, H. VAN DER PAS, M. TEMMERMAN, I. BATAR, P. BARRI, F. MARTINEZ, L. IGLESIAS-CORTIT, D. WILDEMEERSCH, E. PIZARRO, A. ANDRADE, M. THIERY, J. WU, X. CAO, Z. C. FENG & M. H. WU. 1995. Gyne-Fix® intrauterine copper releasing implant system: A major improvement in efficacy, expulsion and tolerance. Adv. Contracept. **11:** 131–142.
8. THIERY, M. 1985. Pain relief at insertion and removal of an IUD: A simplified technique for paracervical block. Adv. Contracept. **1:** 167–170.
9. TIETZE, C. & S. LEWIT. 1973. Recommended procedures for the statistical evaluation of intrauterine contraception. Stud. Fam. Plann. **4:** 35–46.

10. WESTROM, L. 1980. Incidence, prevalence, and trends of acute PID and its consequence to industrialized countries. Am. J. Obstet. Gynecol. **138:** 880–892.
11. STRUTHERS, B.J. 1991. Copper IUDs, PID, and fertility in nulliparous women. *Adv. Contracept.* **7:** 211–230.
12. FARLEY, T. M., M. J. ROSENBERG, P. J. ROWE, *et al.* 1992. Intrauterine devices and pelvic inflammatory disease: An international perspective. Lancet **239:** 785–788.
13. ATRASH, H. K., A. FRYE & C. J. R. HOGUE. 1994. Incidence of morbidity and mortality with IUD in situ in the 1980s and 1990s. A New Look at IUDs—Advancing Contraceptive Choices. IUD Conference, New York, March 1992. Butherworth-Heinemann. Boston. pp. 76–87.
14. SHEPPARD, B. L. 1987. Endometrial morphological changes in IUD users: A review. Contraception **36:** 1–10.
15. PIZARRO, E. G. SCHÖENSTEDT, G. MEHECH, M. HIDALGO, C. ROMERO & G. MUÑOS. 1989. Uterine cavity and the location of IUDs following administration of meclofenamic acid to menorrhagic women. Contraception **40:** 413–423.
16. JAIN, A. K. 1975. Safety and effectiveness of intrauterine devices. Contraception **19:** 243–248.
17. WEINER, R. *et al.* 1978. Copper intrauterine contraception in adolescent nullipara. Br. J. Obstet. Gynaecol. **85:** 204–206.
18. HIRVONEN, E. & S. KAIVOLA. 1983. A new copper IUD (Fincoid) in adolescent and young nulliparous women. Contracept. Deliv. Syst. **4:** 149–152.
19. SAURE, A., E. HIRVONEN, A. KIVIJÄRVI & H. TIMONEN. 1984. Comparative performance of Fincoid, Nova-T, and Multiload 375 IUDs. *In* Intrauterine Contraception: Advances and Future Prospects. G. I. Zatuchni, A. Goldsmith, J. J. Sciarra, Eds.: 104–108. Harper & Rowe. Philadelphia.
20. VAN KETS, H. 1990. Clinical Performance of Intrauterine Devices. Ph.D. dissertation, State University Gent, Faculty of Medicine, Gent, Belgium.
21. KAIVOLA, S. 1990. Postremoval assessment of the intrauterine position of the IUDs: An analysis of 1012 removals with special reference to pregnancy risk and dislocation. Presentation at the Annual Meeting of the Society for the Advancement of Contraception, November 4–11, Singapore.
22. Wyeth-Ayerst Contraceptive Survey in Europe (WYCON). 1993. ISIS Research Ltd. London.
23. POTTER, L. S. 1991. Oral contraceptive compliance and its role in the effectiveness of the method. *In* Patient Compliance in Medical Practice and Clinical Trials. J. A. Cramer & B. Spilker, Eds.: 195–207. Raven Press. New York.
24. FRANK, M. L., A. N. POINDEXTER III, L. M. CORNIN, C. A. COX & L. BATEMAN. 1993. One-year experience with subdermal contraceptive implants in the United States. Contraception **48:** 229–243.
25. KUBBA, A. 1995. Emergency Contraception—Guidelines for Doctors. Faculty of the Family Planning and Reproductive Health Care of the Royal College of Obstetricians and Gynaecologists. London.
26. BATAR, I., D. WILDEMEERSCH, M. VRIJENS, W. DELBARGE. 1997. Immediate post-abortal insertion of the frameless intrauterine implant (IUI): International Study Group on Intrasuterine Drug Delivery. Data on file. Address: Department of Obstetrics, University Hospital Gent, De Pintelaan 185, 9000 Ghent, Belgium.
27. UNFPA Project Report. Study of Stainless Steel Ring And Copper T IUD. Efficacy, Use, Cost/Benefit and Conversion in China. UNFPA Project CPR/91/P43: 1–53, May 21, 1992.
28. 1988. More contraceptive choices likely by the end of the century. Outlook **6:** 2–8.
29. PETERSEN, K. R., L. BROOKS, B. JACOBSEN & S. O. SKOUBY. 1991. Intrauterine devices in nulliparous women. Adv. Contracept. **7:** 333–338.

Anti-STD Vaginal Contraceptive Sponges

E. HASSAN,[a,b] G. CREATSAS,[c] A. GRAVANIS,[d]
V. GEORGOULIAS,[d] AND A. PSYCHOYOS[e]

[b]*Department of Obstetrics and Gynecology*
University of Crete
Heraklion, Greece

[c]*First Department of Obstetrics and Gynecology*
University of Athens
"Alexandra" Hospital
Athens, Greece

[d]*Department of Pharmacology*
School of Medicine
University of Crete
Heraklion, Greece

[e]*Hôpital Bicêtre (INSERM)*
Kremlin-Bicêtre, France

Women face two main health risks from the decision to be sexually active: unintended pregnancy and sexually transmitted diseases (STDs). Actions taken to prevent a pregnancy may also influence either the occurrence of STDs or the consequences of infection. The introduction during the last three decades of oral contraceptives and intrauterine devices has considerably reduced the use of vaginal contraception.[1] This is in spite of several advantages and specific indications for the latter among adolescents[2] and premenopausal women.[3] Contraceptive methods that also prevent STDs are urgently needed at the present. This crucial need emerges from the acquired immunodeficiency syndrome pandemic, but also from the recent recrudescence of other STDs. Special educational programs and other approaches to control this epidemic are needed. To date, the only effective methods for the prevention of STDs, including acquired immunodeficiency syndrome, is the male condom. However, the condom is unacceptable to many men and women. It is used once, put in place just before coitus, and women have little control over its use.

Means for women to protect themselves from STDs and human immunodeficiency virus are few.[4] Most preventive strategies are designed around having fewer partners and the use of latex condoms, but women cannot always reduce the number of partners and male partners might not cooperate in the use of condoms. Methods of disease prevention that women can control are needed, and vaginal application of chemicals that are bactericidal and virucidal may be one way to achieve this goal.[5] There is an intuitive feeling that barrier contraceptive methods should reduce the likelihood of acquiring most STDs. Evidence of the protective effect of barrier meth-

[a]Address for correspondence: Elsheikh Hassan, Pindarou 1A, 145 65 Ekali, Greece.

ods of contraception on the risk of STDs has been published, but there has been no quantitative assessment of the protection.[6] Spermicide-impregnated sponges combine the actions of a physical barrier that blocks the cervix with a material that absorbs the ejaculate and a spermicide.[7] Spermicides are not a single class of chemicals. For instance, nonoxynol-9 is classified as a surfactant,[8] benzalkonium chloride is a disinfectant, and sodium cholate is a strong spermicidal and antiviral agent.[9]

The active ingredient of most commercially available spermicides is nonoxynol-9, a highly polar molecule that immobilizes sperm by disrupting the cell membrane. Laboratory investigations indicate that nonoxynol-9 inhibits a variety of sexually transmissible organisms, including those responsible for gonorrhea, chlamydial infection, candidiasis, genital herpes, syphilis, trichomoniasis and the acquired immunodeficiency syndrome.[10–12] Nonoxynol-9 at concentrations of 0 to 5% or more inactivated HTLV-111 and HIV-1 *in vitro*, whereas 1% or more reduced the live counts of the target lymphocytes.[11,13] Commercially available spermicides contain 1 to 5% nonoxynol-9 and are often included in contraceptive jellies and foams used by women in combination with another barrier method. In April 1983, the United States Food and Drug Administration approved the Today contraceptive sponge (VLI Corporation, Irvine, California) for over-the-counter sales. It was the first new mode of contraception to be approved in the United States in two decades. It was also the first barrier method of contraception to undergo the clinical testing for safety and efficacy that is required for prescription drugs and devices. Since then it has been approved for use and is being sold in a number of other countries including Korea, Sweden, Switzerland, and the United Kingdom. The Today sponge is made of proprietary polyurethane and contains 1 gm of the spermicide nonoxynol-9, as well as small amounts of preservatives (citric, sorbic, and benzoic acids) that help maintain its pH at about 4 to 5.[14]

Cholic acid (sodium cholate) was found to exhibit a strong spermicidal and antiviral (anti-human immunodeficiency virus [HIV]-1) activity. The same effects are observed for F-5 gel. Both cholic acid and F-5 gel exert a dose-dependent, *in vitro* inhibitory effect on the activity of HIV-1–associated reverse transcriptase in an acellular system and on the potential of HIV-1 to efficiently infect human lymphocytes.[9] It was found that both cholic acid and F-5 gel at doses >2.5 mM and 10^{-4} vol/vol, respectively, may inhibit the proliferation of normal human lymphocytes and CEM leukemia cells.[9] In addition, recently reported data demonstrate that bile salts may destroy HIV-1–infected T cells *in vitro*.[15,16] Consequently, these agents may be useful in the selective destruction of HIV-infected cells as well as in the inhibition of HIV-1 itself. This possibility becomes more apparent in cases where the HIV is presented in cavities, such as the vagina. *In vitro* benzolkonium choride has a direct inhibitory effect on HIV-1,[17] and nonoxynol-9 inhibits the growth of several infective agents, such as *Treponema pallidum*,[18] *Neisseria gonorrhoeae*,[18] *Chlamydia trachomatis*,[19–21] HSV,[19] and CMV,[22] but not bovine papilloma virus (BPV-1) and BK virus (BKV).[22] Because BPV-1 is closely related to HPV, it is reasonable to assume that nonoxynol-9 does not inactivate the latter either. Of course, certain pharmacological problems may be introduced by the local application of these compounds, such as a local cytotoxic-irritational effect on the vaginal mucosa, as well as systemic effects after absorption and transfer into the circulation. Such criticisms have been expressed in particular for nonoxynol-9 as used in certain barrier contraceptives at high concentrations.[23] Spermicides can alter the vaginal flora. A nonoxynol-9 user has a significantly higher risk of vaginal colonization with *Escherichia coli*, *Candida*, enterococci, and staphylococci than nonusers.[24] Nonoxynol-9 was also associated with a significantly higher frequency of ulcerative genital diseases, vulvitis, and a non-significant reduction of genital warts infection.[25]

Chlamydia trachomatis is one of the most prevalent sexually transmitted pathogens responsible for a large number of infections in men and women. It is the most common sexually transmitted organism in the United States[26] and causes cervicitis, pelvic inflammatory disease, and infertility in women; nongonococcal urethritis and epididymitis in men; and pneumonia and conjunctivitis in newborns. It is of particular concern because its clinically indolent course allows many infected persons to go untreated, with extensive medical and economic consequences. Indications have been found that the effect of nonoxynol-9 on *Chlamydia trachomatis* is to inhibit the organisms,[10,20,21] whereas others have found that it does not affect the elementary bodies that initiate and spread infection.[27]

A survey among female prostitutes in the United States found a reduced risk of hepatitis B virus infection among black and Hispanic women who used spermicide and/or diaphragm, but no such protection among white prostitutes. Among non-Hispanic prostitutes, the use of a sponge during the past five years was associated with a lower risk of infection.[28] Considering risk factors for hepatitis C virus (HCV) seropositivity, the odds ratio for women whose partners used condoms was 1–5 (95% Cl = 0.6–4.2).[29] However, another study indicates that the risk of sexual transmission of HCV is nil or very low when condoms are used.[30]

It has been suggested that the use of nonoxynol-9 may disrupt the vaginal epithelium,[31] making it easier for an infection to become established.[32] Chlorhexidine is now under study as a spermicide: it is less irritating to mucosal cells than nonoxynol-9. Work has been carried out for several years at Manchester University on this antiseptic.[33] This agent has spermicidal properties but is not a surfactant and is positively charged. It is compatible with cervical mucus, and thickens midcycle mucus, a property that would tend to prevent the entrance of sperm into the uterus.[34] Clearance of chlorohexidine from the vagina is delayed, unlike spermicides containing nonoxynol-9, which tend to trickle out, and it does not seem to disrupt the vaginal epithelium. Apart from its potential as a spermicide *in vivo*, it is also active *in vitro* against HIV in low concentrations.[35] Further work may show that chlorhexidine used vaginally can form an important part of the barrier vaccine strategy.

Epidemiological studies and clinical trials should provide quantitative estimates of the level of protection provided by barrier methods of contraception and should indicate which factors affect the level of protection. The studies should also indicate the method that combines the highest level of protection, ease of use, and acceptability, in order to promote their use in preventive campaigns. To evaluate the efficacy of the F-5 gel-impregnated contraceptive sponge in affecting the incidence of endocervical and vaginal infections caused by different pathogens, we conducted a randomized comparative study using two forms of the new contraceptive vaginal sponge Protectaid®. The Protectaid contraceptive sponge consists of a modern contraceptive protective sponge with soft polyurethane and interconnecting "open" cells specially designed for medical use. It provides contraception, bacterial, and antiviral protection. It can be easily inserted and retrieved and offers many features of a modern spermicidal protective device. Impregnated with F-5 gel, it provides protection from common pathogens (aerobic-anaerobic). The spermicidal action is effective within 30 seconds. The F-5 gel ruptures the spermatozoid's flagellum, thus impeding any movement or migration. It also destroys the spermatozoid head's acrosome. This second feature prevents accidental fertilization by a mutilated spermatozoon. The sponge, when compressed during intercourse, releases additional gel and/or absorbs seminal and vaginal fluids. Its design (two opposite cut loops) makes it simple to use.

The efficacy, irritability, and acceptability of two regimens of Protectaid contraceptive sponge (Axcan, Ltd. Mont St. Hilaire, Canada) were studied. Both types were impregnated with F-5 gel but each carried a different dose of nonoxynol 9. The first regimen consisted of 1.0% benzalkonium chloride, 0.5% nonoxynol 9, 0.5% sodium cholate, dimethylpolysiloxane (dispersing agent), and methylcellulose (carrier). The dose of nonoxynol-9 in the second regimen was 0.125%.

The sponge was given to 35 women 20 to 35 years of age who were randomly allocated into two groups. For the first group, consisting of 20 women, the regimen with 0.5% nonoxynol-9 was given. The second group, consisting of 15 women, received the regimen with 0.125% nonoxynol 9. Pretreatement examination showed normal ovulation and intact internal genitalia. All women had a single sexual partner with normal sperm examination. Written consent was obtained from each woman before enrollment in the study. Pregnant women and those with positive cervical cultures were excluded from the study, as well as men with positive urethral cultures. All women were instructed on how to insert the sponge, that is, to insert it within the 30 minutes preceding the first act of sexual intercourse regardless of the day of the cycle, and to remove it 4 to 6 hours after the last intercourse. In no case were they to leave the sponge in place for more than 24 hours following insertion. Endocervical and vaginal cultures for isolation and identification of aerobic-anaerobic pathogens, chlamydia, mycoplasma, and fungi species were performed before treatment and at 3-, 6-, 9-, and 12-month intervals. Colposcopic examination was performed before treatment and 24 hours after the first insertion to evaluate any irritation.

During a twelve-month use, the Protectaid contraceptive sponge efficacy was 100% in both groups. Cervical cultures at the 6-month interval showed the presence of *Mycoplasma hominis* and *Candida albicans* in one and two cases, respectively, in the first group. In the second group cervical cultures at the 3-month interval showed *Gardnerella vaginalis* and β hemolitic streptococcus in 1 and 2 cases, respectively. Those patients were properly treated and had minor clinical symptoms. Colposcopy examination showed no cervical or vaginal lesion in either group. In the first group one case of irritation and one case of hyperemia in the vagina were found. In the second group no change was noted. The acceptability of the sponge was ideal: No women complained of inconvenience or discomfort.

Protectaid contraceptive sponge with F-5 gel is a modern contraceptive method that allows easy insertion and retrieval and variable fit. It is undetectable by either partner during sexual intercourse. Our results do not indicate that the contraceptive sponge should be the only prophylaxis against STDs, since it does not protect all possible sites of infection. A low concentration of nonoxynol-9 decreases the possibility of vaginal irritation but does not affect contraceptive efficacy.

REFERENCES

1. COHEN, J. 1991. Le point sur la contraceptive locale dans le monde. Gynecol. Observ. **247:** 5.
2. CREATSAS, G. 1991. Adolescent contraception and pregnancy. Newslett. Eur. Soc. Contracept. **3:** 1–2.
3. ERNY, R. & H. PORTE. 1991. Efficacite des spermicides. Contracept. Fertil. Sexual. **19:** 289–291.
4. STEIN, Z. A. 1990. HIV prevention: The need for methods women can use. Am. J. Publ. Health **80:** 460–462.
5. NIRUTHISARD, S., R. RODDY & S. CHUTIVONGSE. 1992. Use of nonoxynol-9 and reduction in rate of gonococcal and chlamydial cervical infections. Lancet **339:** 1371–1375.
6. D'ORO, L. C., F. PARAZZINI, L. NALDI & C. L., VECCHIA. 1994. Barrier methods of contraception, spermicides and sexually transmitted diseases: A review. Genitourin Med. **70:** 410–417.
7. ROSENBERG, M. J. & E. L., GOLLUB. 1992. Commentary: Methods women can use that may prevent sexually transmitted disease, including HIV. Am. J. Pub. Health **82:** 1473–1478.
8. MARTINDALE. 1989. The Extra Pharmacopoeia. 29th edit. The Pharmaceutical Press. London.
9. PSYCHOYOS, A., G. CREATSAS, E. HASSAN, V. GEORGOULIAS & A. GRAVANIS. 1993. Spermicidal and antiviral properties of cholic acid: Contraceptive efficacy of a new vaginal sponge (Protectaid®) containing sodium cholate. Hum. Reprod. **8**(6): 866–869.
10. ALLICOTTI, G. M., R. H. JENSEN *et al.* 1985. Prophylactic properties of the Today contraceptive sponge. Read before the annual meeting of the association of Planned Parenthood Professionals, Seattle, WA.
11. HICKS, D. R., L. S., MARTIN, *et al.* 1985. Inactivation of HTLV-111/LAV-infected cultures of normal human lymphocytes by nonoxynol-9 in vitro. Lancet **2:** 1422–1423.
12. JICK, H., M. T. HANNAN, *et al.* 1982. Vaginal spermicides and gonorrhea. JAMA **248:** 1619–1621.
13. POLSKY, B., P. BARON, *et al.* 1988. In vitro inactivation of HIV-1 by contraceptive sponge containing nonoxynol-9. Lancet **2:** 1456.
14. EDELMAN, D. & B. NORTH. 1987. Updated pregnancy rates for the Today contraceptive sponge. Am. J. Obstet. Gynecol. **157:** 1164–1165.
15. LLOYD, G., T. ATKINSON & P. M. SUTTON. 1988. Effect of bile salts and of fusidic acid on HIV-1 infection of cultured cells. Lancet **2:** 1418–1421.
16. BABA, M., D. SCHOLS, *et al.* 1989. Selective activity of several cholic acid derivatives against human immunodeficiency virus replication in vitro. J. AIDS **2:** 264–271.
17. WAINBERG, M. A., B. SPIRA, *et al.* 1990. Inactivation of human immunodeficiency virus Type 1 in tissue culture fluid and in genital secretions by the spermicide benzalkonium chloride. J Clin Microbiol 28, 156–158.
18. SINGH, B., J. C. CUTLER & H. M. D. UTIDJIAN. 1972. Studies on the development of a vaginal preparation providing both prophylaxis against venereal disease and other genital infections and contraception: Effect in vitro of vaginal contraceptive and non-contraceptive preparations on Treponema pallidum and Neisseria gonorrhoeae. Br. J. Venereal Dis. **48:** 57–64.
19. JUDSON, F. N., J. M. EHRET, *et al.* 1989. In vitro evaluations of condoms with and without nonoxynol-9 as physical and chemical barriers against *Chlamydia trachomatis*, herpes simplex virus type 2 and human immunodeficiency virus. Sex. Transm. Dis. **16:** 51–56.
20. BENES, S. & W. M., MCCORMACK. 1985. Inhibition of growth of Chlamydia trachomatis by nonoxynol-9 in vitro. Antimicrob. Agents Chemother. **27:** 724–726.

21. KELLY, J. P., R. B. REYNOLDS, *et al.* 1985. In vitro activity of the spermicide nonoxynol-9 against *Chlamydia trachomatis*. Antimicrob. Agents Chemother. **27:** 760–762.
22. HERMONAT, P. L., R. W. DANIEL & K. V. SHAH. 1992. The spermicide does not inactivate papillomavirus. Sex. Transm. Dis. **19:** 203–205.
23. NIRUTHISARD, S., R. RODDY & S. CHUTIVONGSE. 1991. The effects of frequent nonoxynol-9 use on the vaginal and cervical mucosa. Sex. Transm. Dis. **18:** 176–179.
24. HOOTON, T. M., S. HILIER, *et al.* 1991. *Escherichia coli* bacteriuria and contraceptive methods. JAMA **265:** 64–69.
25. KREISS, J., E. NGYGI, K. HOLMES, *et al.* 1992. Efficacy of nonoxynol-9 contraceptive sponge use in preventing heterosexual acquisition of HIV in Nairobi prostitutes. JAMA **268:** 477–482.
26. ROSENBERG, M., W. ROJANAPITHAYAKORN, *et al.* 1987. Effect of the contraceptive sponge on clamydial infection, gonorrhea and candidiasis. JAMA **257:** 2308–2312.
27. KAPPUS, E. W. & T. C., QUINN. 1986. The spermicide nonoxynol-9 does not inhibit *Chlamydia trachomatis* in vitro. Sex. Transm. Dis. **13:** 134–137.
28. ROSENBLUM, L., W. DARROW, J. WITTE, *et al.* 1992. Sexual practices in the transmission of hepatitis B virus and prevalence of hepatitis delta virus infection in female prostitutes in the United States. JAMA **267:** 2477–2481.
29. OSMOND, D. H., N. S. BADIAN, *et al.* 1993. Risk factors for hepatitis C virus seropositivity in heterosexual couples. JAMA **269:** 361–365.
30. BRESTERS, D., E. P. MANSER-BUNSCHOTEN, *et al.* 1993. Sexual transmission of hepatitis C virus. Lancet **342:** 210–211.
31. O'FARREL, N. & D. BARLOW. 1992. Use of nonoxynol-9. Lancet **340:** 179.
32. KLEBANOFF, S. J. 1992. Effects of the spermicidal agent nonoxynol-9 on vaginal microbial flora. J. Infect. Dis. **165:** 19–25.
33. CHANTLER, E. 1992. Vaginal spermicides: some current concerns. Br. J. Fam. Plann. **17:** 118–119.
34. CHANTLER, E. 1990. New and existing spermicides with virusidal properties. *In* Heterosexual Transmission of AIDS: Proceedings of the Second Contraceptive Research and Development Program International Workshop 1989. N. J. Alexander, H. L. Gabelnick & J. M. Spieler, Eds.: 303–310. Wiley-Liss. New York.
35. ANONYMOUS. 1992. Multipurpose spermicides. Lancet **340:** 211–213.

Minimizing the Problem of Poor Compliance in Adolescents

Clinical Experience with a Modern Low-Dose Gestodene-Containing Oral Contraceptive

KLAUS BRILL

German Operation Gynecology
Schering A.G.
Berlin, Germany

INTRODUCTION

The problem of compliance with oral contraceptive use is an issue of major importance, where any improvement can have the potential to significantly reduce the large number of abortions and unplanned pregnancies that occur every year. It has been estimated that if compliance could be improved and the failure rate of oral contraceptives reduced by just 1% worldwide, approximately 63,000 fewer women would have unwanted pregnancies each year. Compliance is, however, a complex problem, and improving compliance requires a multifactorial approach. Compliance is usually divided into two categories: first, incorrect or inconsistent pill use and, second, pill discontinuation. Both forms of poor compliance appear to have common origins, rooted in a lack of knowledge about oral contraception and real or perceived problems with adverse events. Although problems with compliance can affect all groups of women, one group, namely adolescents, represent a particular problem.

It has been reported that 84% of pregnancies in women under the age of 20 are unplanned,[1] and in the United States approximately one-third of all abortions are performed on women less than 20 years old. Pregnancy in adolescents is also a major reason for dropping out of school. The problem of contraception in adolescents is of major importance, because a high proportion of young people are sexually active. Again, in the United States, 70% of all unmarried 19-year-old women and half of all teenagers are reported to be sexually active.[2,3]

It is now generally accepted that oral contraceptives are the most effective method of contraception for healthy adolescents. Unfortunately, this group is more likely to stop taking the pill because of undesired adverse events, including weight gain, fluid retention, and intermenstrual bleeding, than their older counterparts.[4] Also, adolescents are known to have their own particular problems. They often have an ambivalent attitude towards becoming pregnant, and cost factors and parental objections to the pill can all contribute to noncompliant behavior. Also, young women may stop pill use at the end of each relationship, and use no back-up method of contraception while they are between long-term relationships. These factors not only increase the incidence of inconsistent pill use, but also increase the likelihood of pill discontinuation.[5]

A number of common reasons may be given by all groups of women when asked why they have discontinued use of an oral contraceptive. A problem with cycle control is one common reason, but there are others regularly cited. A recent survey into compliance[6] investigated a wide range of aspects of oral contraceptive use among women in Europe. This survey found that when asked about why they discontinued pill-use, cycle control, problems with adverse events, and weight gain were the most frequently cited reasons. This is probably a fairly representative result that could be extrapolated to most groups of women; however, the question of weight gain is one that is of particular concern to adolescents, who are at a stage in their life when appearance is of paramount importance.

Although adolescents represent a particular problem with respect to oral contraceptive compliance, it is nevertheless clear that much can be done to overcome this problem. Providing a clear understanding of both the benefits and possible adverse events associated with oral contraceptive use is an important factor. Often it is a misunderstanding, coupled with misinformation from unreliable sources such as friends and parents, that leads to poor compliance and discontinuation of oral contraceptive use. Time must be taken to explain in detail about the pill and its use. With adolescents, it may be necessary to spend more time than usual ensuring that the patient fully understands what is said. It is important to ensure that the patient understands what adverse events she may experience and that if she does have cycle control problems or headaches that these will most likely disappear after 2 or 3 cycles. Wherever possible, the patient should be seen regularly, thus giving an opportunity for any further questions to be answered.

Compliance can also be improved by ensuring that an oral contraceptive is chosen that minimizes the problems that are known to be related to pill discontinuation. No one oral contraceptive formulation can suit every woman, and therefore it may be necessary to change from one oral contraceptive to another until the best result is obtained. For adolescents, it is important to select an oral contraceptive that is easy to use, has a low incidence of intermenstrual bleeding, a low incidence of adverse events, and is not associated with weight gain.

Oral contraceptives differ with respect to estrogen and progestogen dose, and comparative clinical studies have clearly shown that preparations containing gestodene are associated with superior cycle control when compared with those containing either desogestrel or norgestimate.[7] Furthermore, there is clinical evidence that a monophasic preparation containing 30 μg ethinylestradiol and 75 μg gestodene is well tolerated by adolescents. Data has been analyzed from 5,602 subjects under the age of 18 years, who were recruited within a multicenter clinical trial of gestogene[8] that involved over 100,000 women.

CLINICAL EXPERIENCE WITH GESTODENE IN ADOLESCENTS

Study Design

The six-cycle study, which was designed to assess contraceptive reliability, cycle control, and tolerability of 30 μg ethinylestradiol/75 μg gestodene, involved 5,602 adolescents under the age of 18 years. The age range was 12 to 17, with an average age of 16.4 years; however, only 12 patients (0.2%) were under the age of 14. Of the adolescents in the study, 87.1% were receiving oral contraceptive therapy for the first time, and 12.9% were switching from another oral contraceptive preparation. Of those subjects switching from another preparation, 45.0% changed because of intolerance to their previous oral contraceptive.

Compliance

The clinical status of all subjects on admission to the study is given in TABLE 1. Throughout the investigation, the general health of the study population remained unchanged. Overall clinical status at the end of the study period (cycle 6) is summarized in TABLE 2.

Out of the 5,602 women who entered the trial, 4,746 (84.7%) completed the six cycles. Of the 15.3% who withdrew from the study prematurely, only 4.4% gave treatment-related adverse events as the cause. Of the remainder, 0.3% withdrew to start a family, 0.1% withdrew because of pregnancy, and 10.6% failed to complete the six cycles of the study (TABLE 2). Where adverse events (not related to the menstrual cycle) were given as the cause for withdrawal from the study, weight gain (0.7%), nausea (0.5%), and headache (0.5%) were the reasons most frequently cited.

Compliance throughout the study was generally good, with 89.7% of subjects taking all pills according to the clinicians' instructions. Dosing errors were reported in 10.3% of the study population. Of these, 8.2% failed to take all pills, 1.2% did not observe the pill-free period, and 0.9% both missed pills and took pills during the pill-free period. The relative incidence of intake errors was greatest in those subjects taking oral contraceptives for the first time. Overall, the incidence of intake errors decreased during the course of the study.

Contraceptive Efficacy

During the course of the study, there were five pregnancies, all of which occurred in the group taking an oral contraceptive for the first time. Of these pregnancies,

TABLE 1. Clinical Status at Baseline

	All Subjects	Pill Starters	Switchers
Mean age (years)	16.4 ± 0.8	16.3 ± 0.8	16.6 ± 0.6
Mean body weight (kg)	57.0 ± 7.6	56.7 ± 7.5	58.6 ± 8.0
Cycle length < 28 days	14.3%	14.7%	11.6%
28 days	52.9%	49.2%	79.0%
> 28 days	32.7%	36.1%	9.4%
Withdrawal bleeding			
Duration 4 days	28.9%	27.7%	36.8%
5 days	71.1%	72.3%	63.2%
Amount: Normal	75.6%	75.0%	79.2%
Scanty	8.1%	7.7%	10.4%
Heavy	16.4%	17.2%	10.4%

TABLE 2. Withdrawals from the Study

Reason	Number of Subjects (%)
Adverse reactions	244 (4.4)
Cycle control related	74 (1.3)
Adverse events (e.g., weight gain, nausea, etc.)	170 (3.0)
Wish for pregnancy	16 (0.3)
Pregnancy	5 (0.1)
Lost to follow-up	593 (10.6)

three were associated with errors in dosing, while two were attributed to method failure. This resulted in Pearl indices of 0.08 for method failure and 0.13 for user failure.

Cycle Control

At baseline, 52.9% of the study population had a cycle length of 28 days, 32.7% had a cycle length of greater than 28 days, and 14.3% had a cycle length less than 28 days. During the course of the study, the number of subjects with a 28-day cycle increased, reaching 78.9% by cycle 3 and 81.3% by cycle 6 (TABLE 3). The stabilizing effect of monophasic gestodene on initially prolonged cycles was observed mainly in those subjects taking an oral contraceptive for the first time.

Monophasic gestodene had a beneficial effect on the intensity of menstrual bleeding. The number of subjects with heavy bleeding decreased from 17.0% at baseline to 2.5% at cycle 3 and 1.3% at cycle 6. The corresponding incidence of those subjects with light bleeding rose from 8.6% at cycle 0 to 28.6% at cycle 6. This trend was observed in both subjects receiving an oral contraceptive for the first time and those switching from another preparation.

Cycle control with monophasic gestodene was remarkable, with the incidence of

TABLE 3. Clinical Status after Six Cycles of Monophasic Gestodene

		All Subjects	Pill Starters	Switchers
Mean body weight (kg)		57.3 ± 7.6	57.1 ± 7.5	58.8 ± 8.1
Cycle length	< 28 days	15.9%	16.4%	12.6%
	28 days	81.3%	80.9%	83.8%
	> 28 days	2.8%	2.7%	3.6%
Withdrawal bleeding				
Duration	4 days	61.7%	62.2%	58.7%
	5 days	38.3%	37.8%	41.3%
Amount:	Normal	70.1%	69.3%	75.8%
	Scanty	28.6%	29.6%	21.0%
	Heavy	1.3%	1.1%	3.2%

both spotting and breakthrough bleeding declining throughout the six cycles of the study. For breakthrough bleeding, the incidence was significantly lower than the pretreatment value, even in cycle 1 (FIG. 1). The overall incidence of intermenstrual bleeding (spotting and breakthrough bleeding combined) decreased from 18.7% of subjects at baseline to 2.0% at cycle 6.

Cycle control was observed to be significantly affected by user compliance. The incidence of both spotting and breakthrough bleeding were found to be considerably lower in those women who did not miss any pills (3.7% and 1.8%, respectively) compared with those who did miss pills (30.0% and 15.7%).

Absence of withdrawal bleeding occurred relatively infrequently in the study and was clearly dependent on whether or not the subject had a predisposition towards amenorrhea. For subjects with no history of amenorrhea, the overall incidence was 0.4% of all cycles, with no significant difference between those women receiving an oral contraceptive for the first time and those switching from another preparation. For women with a frequent history of amenorrhea, the incidence was much higher at 4.4%, and for this group the incidence was significantly higher in the women receiving an oral contraceptive for the first time. In all groups, including those with and without a history of amenorrhea, the incidence declined over the course of the study.

Dysmenorrhea was also affected by prior medical history, and the incidence was markedly higher in those women presenting with a history of the condition. Whereas dysmenorrhea in women with no prior medical history fell from 2.2% at cycle 1 to 0.8% at cycle 6, the corresponding figures for those women with a prior history were 36.4% and 20.3%.

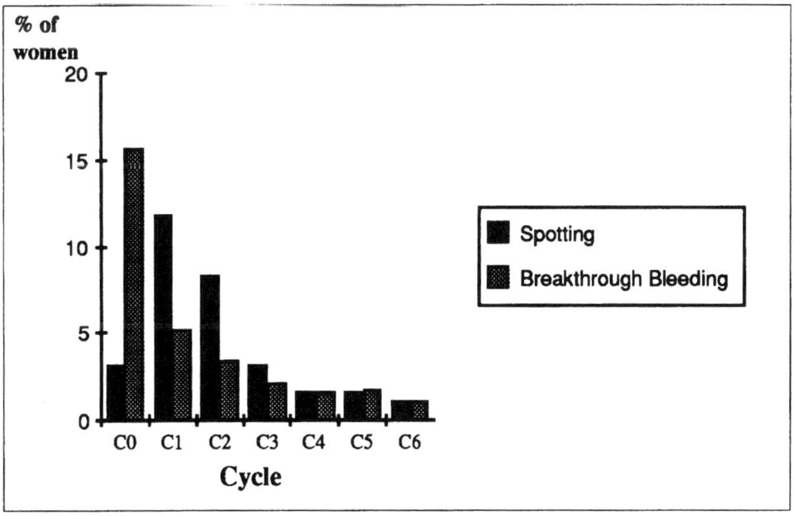

FIGURE 1. The incidence of intermenstrual bleeding.

Tolerability

Monophasic gestodene was well tolerated by both groups of women, those taking an oral contraceptive for the first time and those switching from another preparation. Only two adverse events were reported by more than 1% of the women in the study, these being headache (2.1%) and nausea (1.8%). Where adverse events were reported, investigators considered approximately 16.3% not to be treatment related, 44.5% to be "possible" treatment related, and the remaining 39.2% to be "probably" treatment related. The incidence of all of the most frequently reported adverse events declined throughout the course of the study (FIG. 2). There was one case of superficial thrombophlebitis, but this did not lead to withdrawal from the study.

Throughout the study, body weight remained relatively unchanged. When weight at cycle 6 was compared with pretreatment weight, 91.2% of women had either lost weight or their weight had remained unchanged. Weight change in 87.8% of women did not exceed the physiological range of ± 2 kg. Increases and decreases of greater than 5 kg were observed in only 1.4% and 0.6% of women, respectively. FIGURE 3 shows the distribution of weight change at cycle 6, compared to pretreatment values.

At the end of the study, a standard assessment form was used to evaluate the acceptance of monophasic gestodene: 85.0% of women in the study rated the preparation as good and 9.6% as satisfactory. There was no difference in acceptance between the group taking an oral contraceptive for the first time and those switching from another preparation.

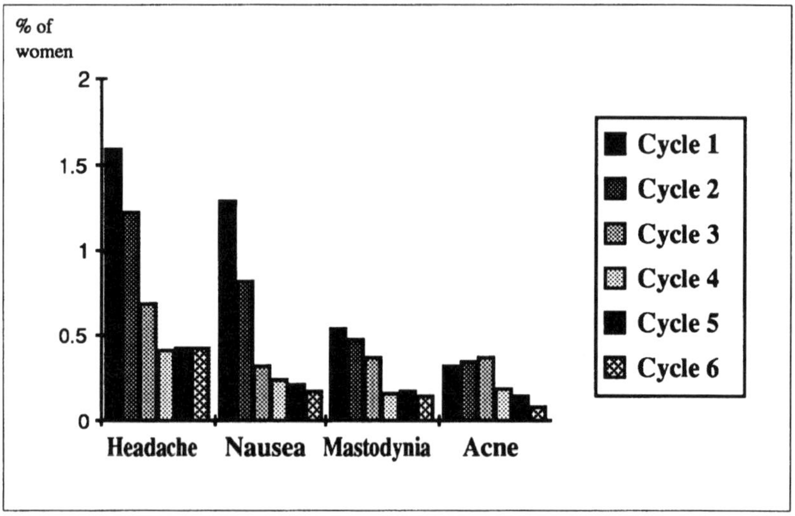

FIGURE 2. The incidence of adverse events.

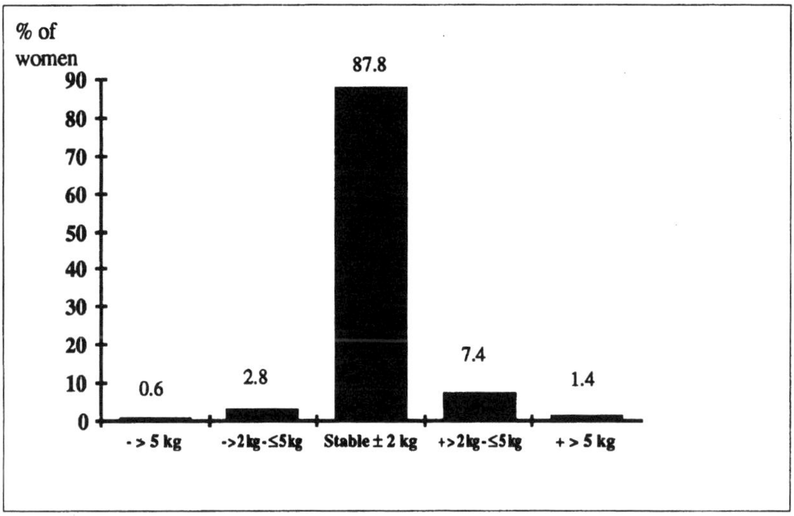

FIGURE 3. The effect of monophasic gestodene on body weight.

DISCUSSION

Analysis of the results from this large-scale clinical trial in adolescents under the age of 18 years demonstrates that 30 μg ethinylestradiol combined with 75 μg gestodene is an appropriate oral contraceptive for use in this age group. It was shown to have good contraceptive efficacy, to provide good cycle control, and to be well tolerated. Compliance in the study was high, and 89.7% of women did not miss any pills. Of those who admitted to intake errors, the incidence was greatest in those using an oral contraceptive for the first time. As might be expected, the incidence of intake errors fell throughout the six cycles of the study.

Because adolescents are a high-risk group for poor compliance and discontinuation, cycle control and tolerability is of particular importance. It is well known that a high rate of intermenstrual bleeding may limit the acceptability of low-dose oral contraceptives and that it is one of the most common reasons given by teenagers for discontinuing the use of oral contraceptives.[9] In this study, cycle control was found to be excellent. Both spotting and breakthrough bleeding declined over the course of the study, both reaching an incidence of 1.0% by cycle 6. Breakthrough bleeding in particular was low in this study, falling significantly below pretreatment values even in cycle 1. The intensity of menstrual bleeding also declined during the study and by cycle 6, only 1.3% of women reported heavy bleeding compared with 17.0% at baseline.

Tolerability with monophasic gestodene was also good, and the overall incidence of adverse events reported was low. Only two adverse events, nausea and headache, were reported by more than 1% of the study population. All frequently reported events declined throughout the course of the study, and only 4.4% of women who entered the trial withdrew because of adverse events. Of particular interest in this study was the minimal effect on body weight. As with cycle control, this is an aspect of oral contraceptive therapy that can be a major reason for withdrawal. Adolescents, more than most other groups, are concerned about their appearance, and any increase in body weight can be seen as unacceptable. In this study, 91.2% of women experienced no significant increase in weight, and only 1.4% gained more than 5 kg.

If a woman discontinues oral contraceptive use, or if she does not begin to use an oral contraceptive in the first place, she is not only missing one of the most reliable forms of contraception available today, but she is also missing the additional associated health benefits, including protection from ovarian and endometrial cancer. For the adolescent, improvement in dysmenorrhea can also be a particularly important benefit, since this is a condition that is most common and problematic in younger women. Use of an oral contraceptive usually brings a significant improvement in symptoms within two to three cycles, and it is benefits such as this, as well as the longer term benefits, that should be stressed when initially prescribing an oral contraceptive to an adolescent patient.

Solving the problem of compliance in adolescents can be seen to require a number of mutually supporting actions. Providing good information is perhaps the most important way forward, since if a young woman knows what to expect in terms of possible adverse events and what to do if they forget to take a pill, then she will be far less likely to discontinue unnecessarily. Choosing the right pill is possibly the next most important factor, and if you can find a pill that suits the patient in question, provides good cycle control, and does not appear to cause weight gain, this should also help to improve compliance.

SUMMARY

Adolescents represent a particularly difficult group with respect to compliance. Not only is incorrect pill intake a common problem, but unnecessary discontinuation also occurs regularly. Reasons for poor compliance are varied, but inadequate information and problems with cycle control and weight gain are particularly important. Choosing a well-tolerated oral contraceptive can help to improve compliance, and clinical experience from a large, multicenter trial suggests that monophasic gestodene (75 μg gestodene/30 μg ethinylestradiol) is a suitable preparation for this group of women. An investigation of 5,602 adolescents with an average age of 16.4 years found good contraceptive reliability and excellent cycle control. The incidence of spotting and breakthrough bleeding was low and declined during the course of the study. The preparation was tolerated well, and the incidence of adverse events was low, with only 4.4% of women withdrawing from the study due to adverse events. An increase in body weight was uncommon. At the end of the study, 85.0% of adolescents rated monophasic gestodene as good and 9.6% as satisfactory.

REFERENCES

1. Jones, E. F., J. Forrest, N. Goldman, S. Henshaw, R. Lincoln, J. Rossof, C. Westoff & D. Wulf. 1985. Teenage pregnancy in developed countries: Determinants and policy implications. Fam. Plann. Perspect. **17:** 53–63.

2. McAnarney, E. R. & W. R. Hendee. 1989. The prevention of adolescent pregnancy. J. Am. Med. Assoc. **262:** 78–82.
3. Hofferth, S. L., J. R. Kahn & W. Baldwin. 1987. Premarital sexual activity among US teenage women over the past three decades. Fam. Plann. Perspect. **19:** 46–54.
4. Oddens, B. J., H. M. Vemer, A. Visser & E. Ketting. 1993. Contraception in Germany. Adv. Contracept. **9:** 105–116.
5. Steinberg, W. M. 1995. Oral contraceptive user compliance: How to improve it. Gynecol. Endocrinol. **9**(Suppl. 1): 1–4.
6. Rosenberg, M. J., M. S. Waugh & T. E. Meehan. 1995. Use and misues of oral contraceptives: Risk indicators for poor pill taking and discontinuation. Contraception **51:** 283–288.
7. Wilde, M. I. & J. A. Balfour. 1995. Gestodene—A review of its pharmacology, efficacy, and tolerability in combined contraceptive preparations. Drugs **50:** 364–395.
8. Brill, K., T. Norpoth, J. Schnitker & M. Albring. 1991. Clinical experience with a modern low-dose oral contraceptive in almost 100,000 users. Contraception **43:** 101–110.
9. Bossemeyer, R. P., L. F. Aquiar, R. P. Andrade, *et al.* 1993. Multicenter open study of monophasic gestogene and athinylestradiol in teenagers. Gynecol. Endocrinol. **7**(Suppl.): 13–18.

Female Adolescent Sexuality

The Risks and Management

KATERINA HAKA-IKSE[a]

Department of Paediatrics
The University of Toronto Medical School and
The Hospital for Sick Children
Toronto, Ontario

Several concerns exist about adverse psychosocial outcomes arising from poor resolution of female adolescent sexuality issues. Consequently, physicians are faced with the challenge of providing anticipatory guidance and support to their pediatric female patients in order to assist healthy unfolding of sexuality development.

For those physicians who are treating female adolescents, there are two important premises to consider in regard to sexuality:

First, sexuality should be seen as a developmental process from birth on, going through various stages before reaching full maturity in meaning and expression.

Second, sexuality does not consist only of its obvious physical components: Cognitive and psychosocial processes are basic aspects of it. Such aspects include the capacity to communicate, develop mutual respect, experience intimacy, and assume responsibility. A parallel can be drawn between sexuality and menarche. In the latter the onset of menarche does not indicate full reproductive maturity. As an example, it has been suggested that the blood supply to the cervix and the uterus is not fully developed to support adequate fetal nutrition and that the still-growing adolescent body (at least between the ages of 13 and 17 years) competes with the fetus for nutrients. In the same way, coital capacity and sexual activity in adolescence is usually not matched by the capacity to understand the implications or even the mechanics of such activity, to exercise control over the sexual behavior, or master the full range of the social-emotional issues associated with it.

Consequently, adolescent sexuality, despite its vigor, intensity, and unique thrill, is a period that is full of risks. Although the entire adolescent population shares these risks when involved in and experimenting with various sexual behaviors, there are certain adolescent groups that are particularly vulnerable to dysfunctional use and outcomes related to sexuality.

As we follow the developmental perspective, it becomes evident that many of the risk factors that operate in the adolescent period have their antecedents in earlier life.[1] Moreover, dysfunctionalities related to sexuality in adolescence may continue to exist in one form or another well past the adolescent period.

Pediatricians and adolescent medicine specialists are particularly interested in early identification of these vulnerable adolescents and use preventative intervention to

[a]Address for correspondence: K. Haka-Ikse, M.D., Suite 908, 123 Edward Street, Toronto, Ontario M5G 1E2, Canada.

alleviate risks.[2] With this preventative perspective in mind, it is imperative to consider closely the early signs that may predict sexuality-related risks in the adolescent. In many situations these signs can be detected in early life, including not only the school-aged period but even the preschool years.

The factors that are related to sexuality risks in adolescence can be classified as *biological* and *psychosocial*.

Biological risk factors: These may involve areas that are not immediately associated with sexual functioning, yet they may have important implications for it. Such factors may be chronic illnesses in young people, physical or intellectual challenges, and exceptionalities that include learning disabilities and attention deficit disorders with or without hyperactivity. In all these situations, the female adolescent is prone to experience poor self-esteem, exclusion from the same-age mainstream, and feelings of being isolated and rejected. Premature sexual activity in such circumstances may be used as a compensatory mechanism to ensure acceptance, inclusion, and status within the peer group and give an identity and vicarious sense of self-worth to the affected adolescent. It is well known that, together with premature sexual activity, other, co-morbid situations arise: promiscuity, adolescent pregnancy, higher high school drop-out rate, substance abuse, suicidal behavior, delinquency and possible criminality, other risk-taking behaviors, and sexually transmitted disease.[3] Many of these co-morbid situations may have a life-long impact on physical health as well as in social outcomes such as limited education; few or no work skills; and entry into the cycle of poverty, dependency, and welfare.

A group of female adolescents considered to be at biological risk are the early maturers.[4] Although there is no clear relationship between levels of pubertal hormones and behavior, the timing of the puberty greatly affects the experiences of adolescence, particularly within a certain social context.[5] Early maturers have been found to have lower self-esteem and be socially more restricted by their families.[6] Generally, adolescent girls are purported to have decreased self-esteem but considerably more so when pubertal onset is early. Breast development and adiposity may contribute to this negative self-image,[6] and this has been found true regardless of the timing of the puberty. Early maturers present a higher prevalence of early depressive symptoms[7] and panic disorder.[8] They have been found to present more sexual-coital activity and delinquent behaviors. Earlier maturers have more contact with delinquent teens.[9] A Finnish study in a group of 14-to 16-year-old girls indicates a higher prevalence of psychosomatic symptoms.[10] Although in the past decade there has been a small decline in the prevalence of pregnancy in the adolescent group as a whole, in the United States the prevalence of pregnancy in earlier maturers shows a slight increase. A possible explanation may be the lack of cognitive understanding of the consequences of coital activity or knowledge of contraceptive measures.[11]

Psychosocial (intrapsychic and sociocultural) risk factors: These risks arise from lack of a consistent, supportive environment, family or parenting dysfunctionality, physical and sexual abuse, neglect, and other forms of sociocultural deprivation. These risk factors usually pre-exist the adolescent period, but the symptoms and signs of the problems in the female adolescent become apparent mainly during the teen years. An example of this is the observation that preschool and early school-aged girls may not manifest important psychopathology at the time of parental separation and divorce, but these same girls tend to present a higher prevalence of sexual activity and acting out behaviors upon reaching adolescence.

A *consistent* environment is considered to be a protective factor for sexuality-related risks in female adolescents. The structure and parental control appear to be the important protective variables. Girls who live in a two-parent household are also more protected than those who grow up in a single-parent family.[10]

On the contrary, *parental dysfunctionality* in various forms affects the psychosocial and sexuality development of girls much before the teen years.[1] Parents who are ambivalent tend to form an insecure attachment and to be in conflict with the child. Needy parents who were themselves deprived or who face major crises cannot fulfill their child's needs for closeness and security or the development of a clear sense of identity and self-worth. These parents may be neglectful of the child's physical needs as well. Permissive, indulging parents limit the child's drive for independence and achievement motivation. Attitudes and practices in certain families, although not actually abusive, create an overtly sexualized climate at a time that young children have no cognitive skills to grasp what is happening and have no control over regulation of their emotions. Practices such as co-sleeping, co-bathing, exposure to adult nudity and intimacies, discussion of sexual matters, inappropriate reading material, and exposure to media do have a deep effect on the child's own feelings about and attitudes toward sexuality. Often such attitudes and practices result from the parents' own needs for acceptance, closeness, and vicarious fulfillment of intimacy. Certain lifestyles confront children with tenuous family relationships such as casual change of sexual partners or sexual expression that is aggressive, violent, and used to control others. These family scripts show an intergenerational transmission pattern and perpetuate the sexual dysfunction.

Sexually abusive actions ranging from inappropriate comments addressed to the child to a variety of sexual acts often of an aggressive nature perpetrated by a parent, family member, or others are deeply traumatic events with life-long consequences.

Verbally and physically abusive families affect the girl's development as she cannot experience trust, becomes submissive-hostile, or may develop aggressive, abusive tendencies.

Membership in a minority, usually an economically and socially deprived group, is also a major risk factor. It does lead to the tendency to achieve a sense of identity and worth through early sexual activity and motherhood, which provides the adolescent with social assistance and affiliation with a peer group sharing the same lifestyle.

The dynamics leading to psychopathology in adolescence are diverse and so may be the expression of psychopathology. Such expression depends on the type of the insult, the time and duration of it, the temperament of the particular adolescent, and possible protective factors. The usual results are vulnerability to exploitation; premature, indiscriminate sexual activity; and related co-morbidity due to the adolescent girl's low self-esteem, need to establish herself as a sexual object to compensate for her feelings of being unloved, and/or intent to experience some control over others through the sexual activity. At times the adolescent uses the sexual activity to counteract depression. Adolescent pregnancy may be wanted and repeated in the vain hope that the infant will fulfill the adolescent mother's unmet dependency needs. The traumas that underlie such adolescent behaviors usually affect several levels of psychosocial functioning and extend through the whole life cycle, possibly intergenerationally.

One particular area of psychosocial and sexual dysfunction that becomes more worrisome in adolescent years is gender identity disorder.[12] Although present in the preschool and latency period, this disorder may be dismissed in the early years. It does involve preoccupation and the wish to identify with and behave as though belonging to the opposite sex. The gender identity disorders are considered to be the outcome of particular family dysfunctionality that leads to devaluation of, and a threat generated by acknowledging and adhering to, one's own gender. Association of gender identity disorders with homosexuality is postulated, although not so far documented. Such an association may expose the adolescent girl with this disorder to depression and suicidality to which adolescents with homosexual strivings are particularly prone.

MEDICAL PREVENTATIVE AND THERAPEUTIC INTERVENTION

Physicians who deal with youth and particularly pediatricians should keep in mind that the foundation for healthy sexuality development is laid in early childhood. Therefore, it must be considered and supported early.

Such support should be provided through education of parents and children. Despite scientific evidence and availability of information about childhood sexuality, both the community and individual members of it continue largely to ignore and repress the issue. Physicians can serve as an important source of education and attitude change at different levels in the community.

Information about good caregiving that promotes healthy development and sexuality can be provided during health care visits; in the form of reading material; through talks to parents and caregivers' groups; and consultation to day-care centers, schools, and the community at large. School board policies and programs can be influenced positively through the physicians' advocacy.

Anticipatory guidance: An important part of physicians' ongoing contact with families is to support parent–child relationships based on trust, flexibility, open communication, and understanding of the child's needs. This is essential for children to develop good self esteem, feelings of competence, a sense of responsibility, and a healthy attitude toward sexuality. Also, the physician should be available to invite questions related to psychosocial concerns and sexuality with children of all ages, in a way that makes them comfortable and respond to queries with age-appropriate information and reassurance. Information and guidance about use of contraceptives and protection from sexually transmitted diseases is essential.

Special attention should be given to children who are biologically or psychosocially at risk. Expert interviewing is needed to create an atmosphere of trust that will elicit discussion about factual information, concerns about feelings, anxieties, sexual identity, sexual functioning, and activity. In all instances but suicidal behavior, the child should be assured of full confidentiality.

Management of problems: The information obtained from the parents, the child, and from the physical examination of the child is meant to be used for therapeutic intervention. Such may be in the form of supportive counseling, realistic reassurance, and assisting the parents and the adolescent in conflict resolution. Referral of the adolescent to a pediatric psychiatrist is at times necessary, especially when depression and suicidal behavior are issues of concern.

Family problems can be alleviated if the physician is acquainted with community resources, social services, and referral processes that can be mobilized on the adolescent's and the family's behalf.

The physician's ability to interview, enter into a therapeutic alliance with the adolescent and her family, and become an advocate for both are skills that should increasingly become an important part of medical education.

SUMMARY

Human sexuality goes through many stages from birth onward before reaching adult meaning and expression. Apart from the physical aspects, sexuality involves complex cognitive and social-emotional developmental processes including capacity for intimacy, affiliation, communication, mutual respect and responsibility. A variety of risks may affect sexuality development at any stage and facet of it. To support healthy sexuality functioning in the female adolescent, physicians need to identify early risk markers, some of which are biological and others intrapsychic or sociocultural. Identification should lead to preventative action in support of the adolescent.

REFERENCES

1. HAKA-IKSE, K. & M. MIAN. 1993. Pediatr. Rev. **14:** 401–497.
2. LITT, I. F. 1995. Pediatr. Rev. **16:** 243–247.
3. ORR, D. P., M. BEITER & G. INGERSOLL. 1991. Premature sexual activity as an indication of psychosocial risk. Pediatrics **87:** 141–147.
4. DORM, L. D., L. I. CRICKETT & A. C. PETERSEN. 1988. The relations of pubertal status to intrapersonal changes in young adolescents. J. Early Adolesc. **8:** 405–419.
5. LERNER, R. M. 1985. Adolescent maturational changes and psychosocial development: A dynamic interactional perspective. J. Youth Adolesc. **14:** 355–372.
6. ANDERSON, E. R., E. M. HETHERINGTON & W. G. CLINGEMPEEL. 1989. Transformations in family at puberty: Effects of family context. J. Early Adolesc. **9:** 310–324.
7. ANGOLD, A. & M. RUTTER. 1992. Effects of age and pubertal states on depression in a large clinical sample. Dev. Psychopathol. **4:** 5–28.
8. HAYWORD, C., J. D. KILLEN & L. D. HAMMER. 1992. Pubertal stage and panic attack history in sixth- and seventh-grade girls. Am. J. Psychiat. **149:** 1239–1243.
9. SILBERSTEIN, R. K., A. C. PETERSEN & H. L. ALBRECHT. 1989. Maturational timing and the development of problem behaviour: Longitudinal studies in adolescence. J. Early Adolesc. **9:** 247–268.
10. ARO, H. & V. TAIPALE. 1987. The impact of timing of puberty on psychosomatic symptoms among fourteen- to sixteen-year-old Finnish girls. Child Dev. **58:** 261–268.
11. JASKIEWITZ, J. A. & E. R. MCANARNEY. 1994. Pregnancy during adolescence. Pediat. Rev. **15:** 32–38.
12. Diagnostic and Statistical Manual of Mental Disorders. (DSM-IV). 1994. 4th Edit. American Psychiatric Association. Washington, DC.

Index of Contributors